Steroids: Chemistry and Applications in Drug Design and Delivery

Steroids: Chemistry and Applications in Drug Design and Delivery

Editor: Lura Faucit

AMERICAN
MEDICAL PUBLISHERS
www.americanmedicalpublishers.com

AMERICAN
MEDICAL PUBLISHERS
www.americanmedicalpublishers.com

Cataloging-in-Publication Data

Steroids : chemistry and applications in drug design and delivery / edited by Lura Faucit.
p. cm.
Includes bibliographical references and index.
ISBN 979-8-88740-476-9
1. Steroid drugs. 2. Steroids. 3. Steroid drugs--Design. 4. Drug delivery systems.
5. Pharmaceutical chemistry. 6. Pharmacology. I. Faucit, Lura.
RM297.S74 S744 2023
615.36--dc23

American Medical Publishers,
41 Flatbush Avenue,
1st Floor, New York,
NY 11217, USA

ISBN 979-8-88740-476-9 (Hardback)

Contents

Preface

A steroid is an organic molecule having four rings organized in a specific molecular configuration that is biologically active. Steroids serve two principal biological functions. First, they are important components of cell membranes that affect membrane fluidity. Second, they act as signaling molecules. Animals, plants, and fungi all contain hundreds of steroids. Steroid hormones influence metabolism and the biological processes. These hormones affect endocrine functions such as sexual differentiation and reproductive life. The pharmaceutical industry has used steroids for making anticancer, anti-inflammatories, anticonvulsants, contraceptives, and fertility drugs. Steroid dimers are a class of chemicals that are produced by a variety of marine creatures and can also be manufactured in laboratories. This class of compounds has a wide range of pharmacological and biological properties, and can be utilized to make molecular umbrellas for drug delivery. This book explores all the important aspects of steroids in the present-day scenario. It is a valuable compilation of topics, encompassing their chemistry as well as applications in drug design and delivery. This book is a vital tool for all researching or studying steroids.

Significant researches are present in this book. Intensive efforts have been employed by authors to make this book an outstanding discourse. This book contains the enlightening chapters which have been written on the basis of significant researches done by the experts.

Finally, I would also like to thank all the members involved in this book for being a team and meeting all the deadlines for the submission of their respective works. I would also like to thank my friends and family for being supportive in my efforts.

Editor

1

The Importance of Steroid Uptake and Intracrine Action in Endometrial and Ovarian Cancers

Tea Lanišnik Rižner[1], Theresia Thalhammer[2*†] and Csilla Özvegy-Laczka[3†]*

[1] Institute of Biochemistry, Faculty of Medicine, University of Ljubljana, Ljubljana, Slovenia, [2] Department of Pathophysiology and Allergy Research, Centre for Pathophysiology, Infectiology and Immunology, Medical University of Vienna, Vienna, Austria, [3] Momentum Membrane Protein Research Group, Research Centre for Natural Sciences, Institute of Enzymology, Hungarian Academy of Sciences, Budapest, Hungary

***Correspondence:**
Tea Lanišnik Rižner
tea.lanisnik-rizner@mf.uni-lj.si
Theresia Thalhammer
theresia.thalhammer@meduniwien.ac.at

† These authors have contributed equally to this work.

Endometrial and ovarian cancers predominately affect women after menopause, and are more frequently observed in developed countries. These are considered to be hormone-dependent cancers, as steroid hormones, and estrogens in particular, have roles in their onset and progression. After the production of estrogens in the ovary has ceased, estrogen synthesis occurs in peripheral tissues. This depends on the cellular uptake of estrone-sulfate and dehydroepiandrosterone-sulfate, as the most important steroid precursors in the plasma of postmenopausal women. The uptake through transporter proteins, such as those of the organic anion-transporting polypeptide (OATP) and organic anion-transporter (OAT) families, is followed by the synthesis and action of estradiol E2. Here, we provide an overview of the current understanding of this intracrine action of steroid hormones, which depends on the availability of the steroid precursors and transmembrane transporters for precursor uptake, along with the enzymes for the synthesis of E2. The data is also provided relating to the selected transmembrane transporters from the OATP, OAT, SLC51, and ABC-transporter families, and the enzymes involved in the E2-generating pathways in cancers of the endometrium and ovary. Finally, we discuss these transporters and enzymes as potential drug targets.

Keywords: sulfatase, aromatase, 17beta-hydroxysteroid dehydrogenase, transporters, OATP, ABC-transporter

HORMONE-DEPENDENT CANCERS

Steroid hormones have important roles in human physiology, and the disruption of androgen, estrogen, and progesterone actions are implicated in the development of hormone-dependent cancers and benign hormone-dependent diseases. Hormone-dependent cancers include prostate, breast, endometrial, and ovarian cancers, which comprise more than 20% of all cancers in humans, and more than 35% of cancers in women (Ferlay et al., 2013). Indeed, in women, breast cancer is the most frequent cancer in the developed world. In 2012, 1,671,149 new cases of breast cancer were estimated worldwide, with 521,907 associated deaths. In the developed world, endometrial cancer is the most common among gynecological cancers. Worldwide, there were 319,605 new cases and 76,160 deaths from endometrial cancer in 2012 alone (Ferlay et al., 2013). The most deadly of the hormone-dependent cancers is ovarian cancer. Worldwide, there were 238,719 new cases and 151,905 deaths from ovarian cancer in 2012 (Ferlay et al., 2013).

Cancers of the endometrium and ovary predominately affect women after menopause, and they are more frequently observed in developed countries. These enormous numbers of patients and deaths attributed to these hormone-dependent diseases demonstrate the uttermost importance of detailed understanding of their pathophysiology, including the roles of the steroid hormones.

Endometrial Cancer and Steroid Hormones

Endometrial cancer is the fourth most prevalent among all cancers, and the eighth most deadly cancer in North American and European women (Ferlay et al., 2013). The incidence of endometrial cancer is also increasing, with more patients from the premenopausal and peri-menopausal population (Sanderson et al., 2017). Based on its histopathology, clinical manifestation, and epidemiology, endometrial cancer cases can be classified into two groups. Estrogen-dependent type I endometrial cancer with endometrioid or mucinous histology includes 70–80% of all cases. Type II endometrial cancer is characterized by serous papillary or clear-cell histology, originates from atrophic endometrium, and develops from intraepithelial carcinoma (Amant et al., 2005; Ryan et al., 2005). Type II endometrial cancer includes 20% of all cases, and it is usually considered as estrogen independent.

Endometrial cancers also differ in their genetic alterations. Type I tumors are commonly associated with microsatellite instability and mutations in the *PTEN, PIK3CA, K-RAS, CTNNB1*, and *FGFR* genes (Yeramian et al., 2013). Type II endometrial cancers are associated with inactivation of the *TP53* and *TP16* genes, and with amplification of the *ERBB, CCND1*, and *CCNE1* genes (Yeramian et al., 2013; Murali et al., 2014). Based on the recent integrated genomic characterization of endometrial cancer, its classification into four categories has been suggested: (i) cancers with mutations in DNA polymerase ε; (ii) hypermutated cancers with microsatellite instability; (iii) cancers with low frequency of DNA amplifications; and (iv) cancers with high frequency of DNA amplifications (Kandoth et al., 2013). The first three groups comprise endometrioid endometrial cancers, and the last group includes serous and endometriod types of endometrial cancers (Kandoth et al., 2013). The endometrioid types have usually been considered as type I endometrial cancers, while the poorly differentiated endometrioid endometrial cancer (grade 3) was recently classified as type II endometrial cancer (Murali et al., 2014).

Epidemiological studies have identified several risk factors for the development of endometrial cancer, which include obesity (Jenabi and Poorolajal, 2015), estrogen-only therapy, early menarche, late menopause, and nulliparity, among others. Recent studies have shown that both type I and type II endometrial cancers share several risk factors (Setiawan et al., 2013), and patients with these cancers show no difference in E2 and progesterone blood levels, which suggest similar pathogenesis (Wan et al., 2016). Obesity is an important risk factor for the development of endometrial cancer. It is associated with higher levels of circulating estrogens in postmenopausal women, as adipose tissue can serve as a source of estrogens that are formed from inactive precursors of adrenal or ovarian origin (Blouin et al., 2009). Additionally, the high-risk population includes patients treated with tamoxifen. This is the standard therapy for the majority of the 1.6 million breast cancer patients identified yearly worldwide (Ferlay et al., 2013), and also for patients with Lynch syndrome, with over one million cases in Europe alone (Hampel and de la Chapelle, 2011).

Most of the risk factors for the development of endometrial cancer can be explained by the unopposed estrogen hypothesis. According to this hypothesis, the exposure to endogenous or exogenous estrogens in the absence of progesterone or synthetic progestins increases the proliferation of endometrial cells and the concurrent DNA replication errors. This can result in somatic mutations and malignant transformations (Henderson and Feigelson, 2000; Akhmedkhanov et al., 2001). In endometrial cancer, estrogens drive proliferation *via* estrogen receptor α (ERα), which belongs to the superfamily of nuclear receptors and is encoded by *ESR1*. The presence of ERα is related to early-stage cancer, while a shift in the ratio between ERα and estrogen receptor β (ERβ) or loss of ERα are associated with shorter disease-free survival (Saegusa and Okayasu, 2000; Sakaguchi et al., 2002; Hu et al., 2005; Mylonas, 2010; Zannoni et al., 2013). Progesterone opposes the action of estrogens and stimulates differentiation, as supported by association of the genetic variations in genes that encode the PRA and PRB progesterone receptors with increased risk of endometrial cancer (Lee et al., 2010).

Epidemiological evidence suggests that also elevated blood levels of androgens, including testosterone, androstenedione, and dehydroepiandrosterone-sulfate (DHEA-S), are associated with greater risk of endometrial cancer (Lukanova et al., 2004). Significantly increased serum concentrations of DHEA, androstenedione, and testosterone were seen in patients with type I endometrial cancer when compared to healthy women (Audet-Walsh et al., 2011). Interestingly, an epidemiological study in premenopausal women revealed no associations between androgens and endometrial cancer (Clendenen et al., 2016). The importance of androgens as etiological factors has been supported also by the expression of the androgen receptor and the presence of androgen-metabolizing enzymes in well and moderately differentiated endometrial cancer (Gibson et al., 2014). However, in contrast to epidemiological studies, these *in-vitro* reports have suggested protective effects of androgens. Currently, the role of androgens in endometrial cancer is thus not well-defined, although higher blood concentrations of androgens seen in patients with type I endometrial cancer, together with the presence of the androgen receptor and androgen-metabolizing enzymes in tissue samples, have suggested that androgens do not serve only as precursors of estrogens, but probably have discrete roles in the pathophysiology of this gynecological cancer.

Ovarian Cancer and Steroid Hormones

Ovarian cancer is a heterogeneous disease that encompasses five major types of tumors that show different etiologies, risk factors, origins, molecular features, and clinical behaviors. These tumors are mainly derived from non-ovarian tissues that have colonized the ovaries. As much as 90% of all ovarian cancers are epithelial ovarian cancers. With a frequency of 70%, the most common ovarian cancer is high-grade serous carcinoma (which originates from serous tubal intraepithelial carcinomas in the Fallopian tubes). This is followed by endometrioid carcinoma and clear-cell carcinoma (both of which originate from endometrial cells), at 10% frequency each, and then low-grade serous carcinoma (which originates from benign lesion in the ovary) and mucinous carcinoma (which originates from gastrointestinal tissue), at 5% of all epithelial cancers (Binder et al., 2015; Prat, 2015; Ramalingam, 2016). High-grade serous ovarian carcinoma carries *TP53* mutations, while low-grade serous ovarian carcinoma has wild-type *TP53*, but mutations in *K-RAS*, *B-RAF*, and other oncogenes (Rojas et al., 2016). Most patients with ovarian cancer are diagnosed with advanced stage disease and consequently have poor prognosis. Only 46% of these patients survive for 5 years, and compared to other cancers, the overall survival has not increased significantly in the last 40 years (Bast, 2011).

Data from epidemiological studies suggest that ovarian cancer depend on estrogens, although the precise roles of estrogens have not yet been defined (Chura et al., 2009a). Epidemiological studies (Women's Health Initiative and Million Women Study) (Anderson et al., 2003; Beral et al., 2007, 2015) have indicated that both estrogen only and combined estrogen–progestin hormone replacement therapies increase the risk of serous and endometrioid ovarian cancer, but not of other types. Also, genetic susceptibility studies have supported estrogens in the etiology of ovarian cancer, as a single nucleotide polymorphism (SNP) in the *ESR2* gene, which codes for ERβ, and which is considered a tumor suppressor, is associated with significantly increased risk of ovarian cancer (Lurie et al., 2011). Moreover, in clinical samples of ovarian cancer, ERα is widely expressed, while the levels of ERβ expression are progressively lost during ovarian cancer progression toward metastatic tumors (Rutherford et al., 2000). Estrogens have also been reported to stimulate ovarian cancer proliferation and to increase metastatic potential (Bai et al., 2000; Park et al., 2008).

The observed beneficial effects of pregnancy and increased incidence of ovarian carcinoma among women with progesterone deficiency (Diep et al., 2015) imply that progesterone and progestins might prevent the development of ovarian cancer (Modan et al., 1998; Ho, 2003; Modugno et al., 2012; Jeon et al., 2016). Protective effects of progesterone have also been supported by the reduced PRA levels in ovarian carcinoma compared to benign ovarian tissue (Ho, 2003). On the other hand, a SNP in the *PGR* gene that influences the levels of the encoded PRA and PRB does not affect the risk of ovarian cancer (Pearce et al., 2008; Modugno et al., 2012). Some epidemiological studies have indicated that circulating androgens might also have roles in ovarian cancer, while other studies have not supported androgens as an etiological factor (for review, see Modugno et al., 2012).

The epidemiological data on the involvement of steroid hormones in the etiology of ovarian cancer are thus currently inconclusive, and in some cases contradictory. As ovarian cancer predominately affects women after menopause, it might be explained by a greater importance of steroid biosynthesis from adrenergic precursors and their actions in tumor tissue compared to the circulating hormone levels (Modugno et al., 2012). This is supported by the presence and activity of androgen and estrogen biosynthetic enzymes in epithelial ovarian cancer (Chura et al., 2009b).

INTRACRINE ACTIONS OF STEROID HORMONES

In higher primates and humans, steroid hormones act in endocrine, paracrine, autocrine, and intracrine manners. In these species, steroid hormones are formed in the endocrine glands and also in peripheral tissues, from inactive precursors of adrenal origin or *de-novo* from cholesterol. The biosynthesis and actions of steroid hormones in humans thus differ importantly from the situation in animal models, where steroid hormones are formed exclusively in the endocrine glands and act in the target tissues (Luu-The and Labrie, 2010). In humans, steroid hormones thus act in the same (i.e., intracrine, autocrine) or the neighboring (i.e., paracrine) cell(s) where they are formed. Steroid hormones that are formed in a particular cell can activate the corresponding intracellular receptors of the nuclear receptor superfamily, which act as transcription factors. The activated receptor dimer then binds to the hormone-responsive elements of DNA, which is followed by binding of co-activators/co-repressors and other indispensable components of the transcription machinery. In this manner, steroid hormones regulate the expression of the target genes over a time period of hours or days (for review, see Hewitt et al., 2016). As genes that encode steroid hormone receptors have several transcripts and splice variants, this brings additional complexity to their mechanisms of action (for review, see Prossnitz and Barton, 2011; Thomas and Gustafsson, 2011; Hattori et al., 2016).

Steroid hormones can also activate membrane-bound receptors, in terms of the covalently modified, palmitoylated classical receptors of the nuclear receptor superfamily (Levin, 2011), or G-protein-coupled receptors (Prossnitz et al., 2008), or newly identified membrane receptors (Romero-Sánchez et al., 2008). In this manner, they activate intracellular signaling pathways, and can thus have rapid effects that occur in the time frame of minutes or hours.

It has been known for more than 30 years that steroid hormones can be formed from inactive steroid precursors in target peripheral tissues. The terms intracrine action and intracrinology were coined by Labrie to describe the mechanism of action where steroids are formed in the same cell in which they exert their action (Labrie, 1991). Active androgens and estrogens can be formed from inactive or less active precursor steroid hormones, mainly DHEA, DHEA-S, androstenedione, and estrone-sulfate (E1-S). The local formation of steroid hormones thus has major roles in both normal tissues, such as breast, muscle, skin, and bone (Suzuki et al., 2005), and also in hormone-dependent tumor tissues, which comprise up to 20% of all cancers (Ferlay et al., 2013).

DHEA-S as a Precursor for Androgen and Estrogen Formation

Humans and other primates are unique in that their adrenal glands (*zona reticularis*) produce large quantities of the inactive steroid precursors DHEA, DHEA-S, and androstenedione, which can be metabolized in peripheral tissues into active androgens and estrogens. These reactions depend on the presence of androgen and estrogen forming and inactivating enzymes (Labrie et al., 1998, 2015). In this manner peripheral target tissues can control and adjust the formation and inactivation of steroid hormones according to local requirements.

Labrie et al. (1998) estimated that 30–50% of androgens in men in their 50 and 60 s are formed in peripheral tissues from inactive precursors from the adrenal gland, mainly as DHEA and DHEA-S. In women after menopause, intracrine formation is even more important, with up to 100% of estrogens formed from the adrenal precursors DHEA and DHEA-S, and *de-novo* synthesis of the androgen androstenedione from cholesterol in the ovaries (Labrie et al., 1998; Fogle et al., 2007).

Serum concentrations of DHEA change through life, with production of DHEA and DHEA-S increasing during adrenarche, after the age of 6–8 years. These increased circulating levels of DHEA and DHEA-S are then maintained for two decades, before they start to decline after the third decade of life (Labrie et al., 1997). The levels of DHEA thus regress with advanced age, where the rate of this regression differs among races; e.g., lower decreases in circulating DHEA-S levels have been reported in Japanese women compared to Caucasians (Crawford et al., 2009). In spite of this decline, the plasma concentrations of DHEA and DHEA-S in adult men and women are still 200–3,000-fold higher than those of testosterone, 2,000–20,000-fold higher than those of 5α-dihydrotestosterone (5αDHT), and 30,000–800,0000-fold higher than those of estradiol (E2) (Labrie et al., 1998; Audet-Walsh et al., 2011; Giton et al., 2011) (**Table 1**), with large inter-individual variability seen. Interestingly, increased concentrations of DHEA-S have been reported for menopausal transition, which might be related to the rise of luteinizing hormone (Yasui et al., 2012).

In postmenopausal women, the daily production of DHEA is 6–8 mg, with about 50% of this originating from the adrenal gland, 20% from the ovarian theca cells, and the remaining 30% from the circulating DHEA-S, through the action of sulfatase (Yasui et al., 2012). In these women, plasma concentrations of DHEA and DHEA-S are relatively high; at approximately 6.6 nM and 1.6 μM, respectively (**Table 1**). In contrast, plasma concentrations of E1 and E2 are much lower, at 60 and 12–15 pM, respectively. DHEA and DHEA-S can serve as sources for the local formation of androgens and estrogens. In peripheral tissues, E2 can be synthesized from adrenal DHEA and DHEA-S, and also from adrenal or ovarian androstenedione (**Figure 1**). Androstenedione formed from DHEA or DHEA-S can be further activated to testosterone, by the action of 17-ketosteroid reductase type 5, which is better known as aldo-keto reductase 1C3 (AKR1C3). Testosterone can also be further activated to the most potent androgen 5α-DHT, by 5α-reductases type 1 and 2 (**Figure 1**). In patients with endometrial cancer, plasma DHEA, and androstenedione concentrations are increased (Audet-Walsh et al., 2011) and are related to increased risk of endometrial cancer (Potischman et al., 1996; Lukanova et al., 2004). Also, a strong association between DHEA-S and breast cancer risk has been reported (Key et al., 2002), while no association with DHEA or androstenedione was seen for ovarian cancer (Modugno et al., 2012).

Estrone Sulfate as a Precursor for Estrogen Formation

Estrone-sulfate (E1-S) represents the most abundant estrogen in the peripheral blood and an important steroid precursor for estrogen formation after activation by sulfatase (STS) and 17-ketosteroid reductases (HSD17B1, HSD17B7, or HSD17B12) (**Figure 1**), with relatively high concentrations in postmenopausal women (0.5–0.6 nM). E1-S levels are associated with high body mass index (Jasonni et al., 1984), which implies that E1-S originates mainly from adipose tissue. Indeed, high concentrations of E1-S have been reported for visceral adipose tissue as compared to blood, where local concentrations are up to 60-fold higher compared to serum (Labrie, 2003).

About 3-fold higher E1-S plasma concentrations were reported for postmenopausal patients with endometrial cancer type I, compared to control healthy women, while no significant difference was seen between endometrial cancer type II and healthy women (Audet-Walsh et al., 2011). This suggests that in type I endometrial cancer, E1-S might represent a source for local E2 formation, or might reflect increased metabolism of estrogens in cancer tissue. The levels of E1-S are significantly decreased in patients with endometrial cancer with less-differentiated tumors and in patients with myometrial invasion and lympho-vascular space invasion. On the other hand, the circulating levels of E1-S are 2-fold higher in recurrent cases compared to non-recurrent cases (Audet-Walsh et al., 2011). Also, in ovarian cancer, E1-S may serve as a precursor for biosynthesis of E2. Chura et al. (2009a) reported that the great majority of epithelial ovarian cancer samples show E1 sulfatase activity and 17-ketosteroid reductase activity, which promote the activation of E1-S to the most potent estrogen E2. Additionally, ovarian cancer cell lines have capacity for metabolism of E1-S to E1 and E2 (Ren et al., 2015).

DHEA-S and E1-S can serve as precursors for active steroid hormones. Although the levels of DHEA-S and E1-S decrease after menopause, serum concentrations of these precursors in postmenopausal women are sufficient for the local formation and actions of steroid hormones. To reach the sites of intracrine or paracrine action, DHEA-S and E1-S have to cross several biological membranes. First, they have to be extruded from their site of synthesis, and when they reach the peripheral tissue, they have to be taken up by individual cells.

Transporters for DHEA-S and E1-S

The key determinants of the efflux and uptake of DHEA-S and E1-S are the membrane proteins known as ATP-binding-cassette (ABC)-transporters (Ween et al., 2015),

TABLE 1 | Serum steroid hormone levels in healthy premenopausal and postmenopausal women.

Steroid hormone Mw (g/mol)	Pre-menopausal women			Post-menopausal women		
	Age (years)/BMI (kg/m^2)	Concentration (number of women)	Reference	Age (years)/BMI (kg/m^2)	Concentration (number of women)	Reference
DHEA-S (368.6)	30–35/–	1.27 ± 0.62 µg/ml **3.44 ± 1.68 µM** (47) (mean ± *SD*)	Labrie et al., 2006	55–65/–	0.59 ± 0.36 µg/ml **1.60 ± 0.98 µM** (377) (mean ± *SD*)	Labrie et al., 2006
	30 (19–40)/ 27.8 (21.1–33.3) (2.5, 97.5th percentile)	1.94 µg/ml (0.36–3.78) **5.26 µM** (0.97–10.26) (42, folicular phase) (2.5, 97.5th percentile)	Keefe et al., 2014	58.3 ± 5.6/27.0 ± 5.4 (mean ± *SD*)	0.60 (0.23–1.29) µg/ml **1.63 (0.62–3.50) µM** (110) (10–90th percentile)	Audet-Walsh et al., 2011
DHEA (288.4)	30–35/–	4.47 ± 2.19 ng/ml **15.50 ± 7.59 nM** (47) (mean ± *SD*)	Labrie et al., 2006	55–65/–	1.95 ± 1.18 ng/ml **6.76 ± 4.09 nM** (377) (mean ± *SD*)	Labrie et al., 2006
	30 (19–40)/27.8 (21.1–33.3) (2.5, 97.5th percentile)	3.89 ng/ml (0.67–10.94) **13.49 (2.32–37.93) nM** (42, folicular phase) (2.5, 97.5th percentile)	Keefe et al., 2014	58.3 ± 5.6/27.0 ± 5.4 (mean ± *SD*)	1.91 (0.84–4.34) ng/ml **6.62 (2.91–15.05) nM** (110) (10–90th percentile)	Audet-Walsh et al., 2011
A-dione (286.4)	30–35/–	0.96 ± 0.35 ng/ml **3.35 ± 1.22 nM** (47) (mean ± *SD*)	Labrie et al., 2006	55–65/–	0.40 ± 0.18 ng/ml **1.39 ± 0.63 nM** (377) (mean ± *SD*)	Labrie et al., 2006
	30 (19–40)/27.8 (21.1–33.3) (2.5, 97.5th percentile)	1.06 ng/ml (0.69–2.23) **3.70 (2.41–7.79) nM** (42, folicular phase) (2.5, 97.5th percentile)	Keefe et al., 2014	58.3 ± 5.6/27.0 ± 5.4 (mean ± *SD*)	0.44 (0.24–0.80) ng/ml **1.54 (0.84–2.79) nM** (110) (10–90th percentile)	Audet-Walsh et al., 2011
Testosterone (288.4)	30–35/–	0.18 ± 0.07 ng/ml **0.62 ± 0.24 nM** (47) (mean ± *SD*)	Labrie et al., 2006	55–65/–	0.14 ± 0.07 ng/ml **0.49 ± 0.24 nM** (377) (mean ± *SD*)	Labrie et al., 2006
	30 (19–40)/27.8 (21.1–33.3)	0.242 ng/ml	Keefe et al., 2014	58.3 ± 5.6/27.0 ± 5.4	0.14 (0.06–0.24) ng/ml	Audet-Walsh et al., 2011

(Continued)

TABLE 1 | Continued

Steroid hormone Mw (g/mol)	Pre-menopausal women			Post-menopausal women		
	Age (years)/BMI (kg/m^2)	Concentration (number of women)	Reference	Age (years)/BMI (kg/m^2)	Concentration (number of women)	Reference
	(2.5, 97.5th percentile)	(0.10–0.588) **0.76 (0.35–2.04) nM** (42, folicular phase) (2.5, 97.5th percentile)		(mean ± *SD*)	**0.49 (0.21–0.83) nM** (110) (10–90th percentile)	
DHT (290.4)	30–35/–	70 ± 30 pg/ml **241.05 ± 103.31 pM** (47) (mean ± *SD*)	Labrie et al., 2006	55–65/–	40 ± 30 pg/ml **137.74 ± 103.31 pM** (377) (mean ± *SD*)	Labrie et al., 2006
		82.12 ± 25.10 pg/ml **282.78 ± 86.43 pM** (10) (mean ± *SD*)	Caron et al., 2009	58.3 ± 5.6/27.0 ± 5.4 (mean ± *SD*)	30.00 (10.00–70.00) pg/ml **103.31 (34.44–241.05) pM** (110) (10–90th percentile)	Audet-Walsh et al., 2011
Estrone (270.4)	30–35/–	53.96 ± 23.28 pg/ml **199.56 ± 86.09 pM** (47) (mean ± *SD*)	Labrie et al., 2009	58.3 ± 5.6/27.0 ± 5.4 (mean ± *SD*)	18.36 (10.01–35.45) pg/ml **67.90 (37.02–131.10) pM** (110) (10–90th percentile)	Audet-Walsh et al., 2011
	32.1 ± 7.9/– (mean ± *SD*)	38.50 ± 11.86 pg/ml **142.38 ± 43.86 pM** (19, follicular) 75.84 ± 31.62 pg/ml **280.47 ± 116.94 pM** (19, luteal) (mean ± *SD*)	Caron et al., 2009	55–74/–	14.59 (13.67–16.07) pg/ml **53.95 (50.54–59.43) pM** (423) (median, 10–90th percentile)	Fuhrman et al., 2012
Estradiol (272.4)	30–35/–	82.05 ± 42.19 pg/ml **301.21 ± 154.88 pM** (47) (mean ± *SD*)	Labrie et al., 2009	58.3 ± 5.6/27.0 ± 5.4 (mean ± *SD*)	3.35 (1.00–9.67) pg/ml **12.30 (3.67–35.50) pM** (110) (10–90th percentile)	Audet-Walsh et al., 2011
	32.1 ± 7.9/– (mean ± *SD*)	38.40 ± 20.40 pg/ml **140.97 ± 74.89 pM** (19, follicular) 103.66 ± 73.27 pg/ml **380.54 ± 268.98 pM** (19, luteal) (mean ± *SD*)	Caron et al., 2009	55–74/–	4.21 (3.96–4.57) pg/ml **15.45 (14.54–16.77) pM** (423) (median, 10–90th percentile)	Fuhrman et al., 2012

(Continued)

TABLE 1 | Continued

Steroid hormone Mw (g/mol)	Pre-menopausal women			Post-menopausal women		
	Age (years)/BMI (kg/m^2)	**Concentration (number of women)**	**Reference**	**Age (years)/BMI (kg/m^2)**	**Concentration (number of women)**	**Reference**
Estrone-S (350.4)	32.1 ± 7.9/– (mean ± *SD*)	0.64 ± 0.37 ng/ml **1.83 ± 1.06 nM** (19, follicular) 1.92 ± 1.09 ng/ml **5.48 ± 3.11 nM** (19, luteal) (mean ± *SD*)	Caron et al., 2009	55–65/–	0.22 ± 0.01 ng/ml **0.63 ± 0.03 nM** (377)	Labrie et al., 2009
				58.3 ± 5.6/27.0 ± 5.4 (mean ± *SD*)	0.17 (0.04–0.52) ng/ml **0.49 (0.11–1.48) nM** (110)	Audet-Walsh et al., 2011

All steroid hormone concentrations included in this table were measured by GC-MS or LC-MS/MS. Molar concentrations are in bold.

organic anion-transporting polypeptides (OATPs) (Obaidat et al., 2012; Roth et al., 2012), organic anion transporters (OAT) (Burckhardt and Burckhardt, 2011), and transporters encoded by the members of solute carrier family 51 (*SLC51*) (Ballatori et al., 2013) (**Table 2**). In peripheral tissues, these uptake transporters have crucial roles in providing the steroid precursors for local androgen and estrogen formation.

Organic Anion-Transporting Polypeptides

The OATPs are encoded by genes of the solute carrier for organic anions *(SLCO)* family, where this OATP/*SLCO* family comprises 11 members in humans. OATPs have been detected in various cells and tissues of the human body (Roth et al., 2012). Some OATPs, like OATP1A2, OATP2B1, and OATP4A1, are ubiquitous, while OATP1B1 and OATP1B3 are restricted to hepatocytes (Hagenbuch and Stieger, 2013). However, under pathological conditions, such as in cancers, the OATP expression pattern is changed (Obaidat et al., 2012). OATPs are anion exchangers that mediate the cellular uptake of large (>300 Da) organic, mostly negatively charged, molecules in a Na^+- and ATP-independent manner (Roth et al., 2012). Their physiological substrates are bilirubin, bile acids, prostaglandins, thyroid hormones, and conjugated steroid hormones, such as DHEA-S and E1-S. OATP1A2, OATP1B1, OATP1B3, and OATP2B1 mediate the uptake of DHEA-S, while OATP1A2, OATP1B1, OATP1B3, OATP2B1, OATP4A1, and OATP4C1 catalyze the uptake of E1-S (**Table 2**). At least four members of the family (i.e., OATP1A2, OATP1B1, OATP1B3, OATP2B1) transport various clinically applied drugs, in addition to endobiotics. Therefore, these proteins are also key determinants of drug absorption, distribution, and excretion (Kovacsics et al., 2016).

Organic Anion Transporters

The OATs are anion exchangers that are encoded by members of the *SLC22* gene family. Most OATs are polyspecific, as they can transport structurally diverse, relatively hydrophilic, low molecular mass (<500 Da) compounds. Several members of the *SLC22* gene family, including OAT1 and OAT3, are well-established determinants of renal clearance, intestinal absorption, and hepatic elimination of drugs (Burckhardt and Burckhardt, 2011; Koepsell, 2013). On the other hand, OATs are also important in neurotransmitter homeostasis in the brain, and at least four members of this family (i.e., OAT2, OAT3, OAT4, OAT7) transport E1-S, while OAT3, OAT4, and OAT7 transport DHEA-S (Koepsell, 2013) (**Table 2**). OAT2 is expressed in the liver and kidney (Koepsell, 2013), and in adipose tissue (Human Protein Atlas). OAT3 is expressed in the kidney, and also in the blood-brain barrier (Burckhardt and Burckhardt, 2011), while OAT4 localizes to the kidney, and is also present in the placenta, where it mediates the uptake of DHEA-S that is crucial for placental estrogen synthesis (Ugele et al., 2003).

Transporters Encoded by Solute Carrier (*SLC) 51* Gene Family (OSTα, OSTβ)

The human *SLC51* gene family has only two members, *SLC51A* and *SLC51B*, which are also known as organic solute transporter (OST)α and OSTβ (Ballatori et al., 2013). OSTα and OSTβ are

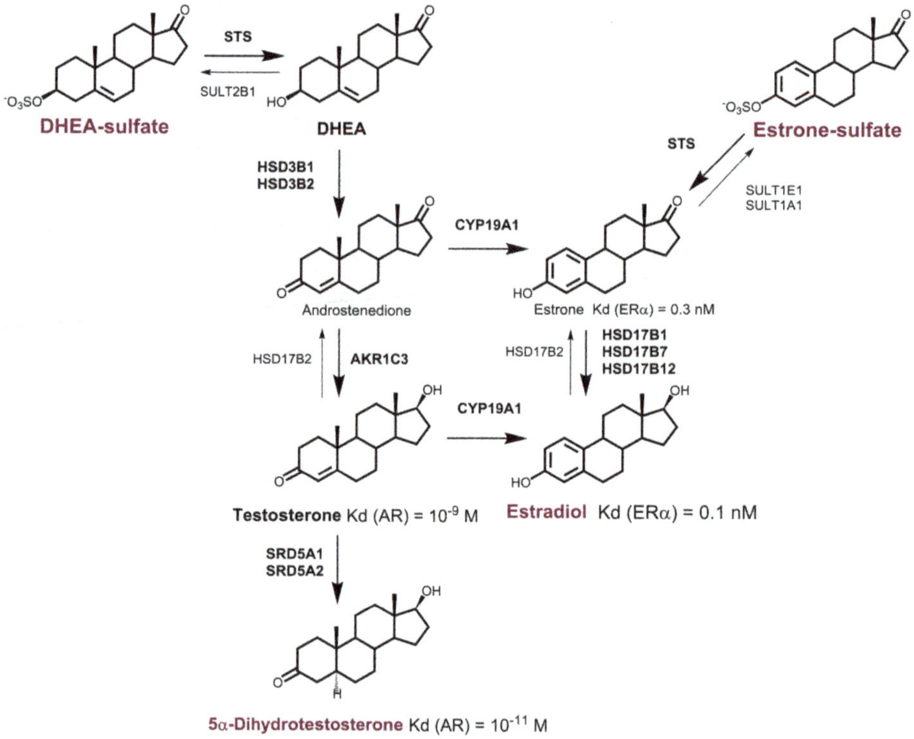

FIGURE 1 | Formation of active steroid hormones from DHEA-S and E1-S. In peripheral tissues, dehydroepiandrosterone sulfate (DHEA-S), and estrone-sulfate (E1-S) serve as precursors for formation of active steroid hormones. DHEA-S can be activated to estradiol (E2) via androstenedione by the actions of sulfatase (STS), 3β-hydroxysteroid dehydrogenases type 1 and 2 (HSD3B1, HSD3B2), aromatase (CYP19A1), and the reductive 17β-hydroxysteroid dehydrogenases (HSD17B1, HSD17B7, 17HSD12) or aldo-keto reductase (AKR1C3). E2 can also be formed from estrone sulfate (E1-S) by the action of sulfatase (STS) and reductive HSD17B. DHEA-S can be activated to active androgens. The most potent androgen 5α-dihydrotestosterone can be formed from DHEA-S by the actions of STS and HSD3B1, or HSD3B2 and AKR1C3, and 5α-reductases types 1 and 2 (SRD5A1, SRD5A2).

TABLE 2 | Characteristics of the most relevant E1-S and DHEA-S transporters.

Family	Protein	Gene	K_m for E1-S (μM)	Reference	K_m for DHEAS (μM)	Reference
OATPs	1A2	SLCO1A2	16–59	Lee W. et al., 2005	7	Kullak-Ublick et al., 1998
	1B1	SLCO1B1	0.3–45	Tamai et al., 2001; Roth et al., 2012	22	Kullak-Ublick et al., 2001; Roth et al., 2012
	1B3	SLCO1B3	58	Gui et al., 2008	>30	Cui et al., 2001
	2B1	SLCO2B1	21	Tamai et al., 2001; Pizzagalli et al., 2003	9	Pizzagalli et al., 2003
	4A1	SLCO4A1	n.d.	Tamai et al., 2000	–	–
	4C1	SLCO4C1	26.6	Yamaguchi et al., 2010	–	–
OATs	OAT2	SLC22A7	n.d.	Kobayashi et al., 2005	–	–
	OAT3	SLC22A8	2.2 and 21.2	Burckhardt and Burckhardt, 2011	13	Nozaki et al., 2007
	OAT4	SLC22A11	1.01 and 21.7	Burckhardt and Burckhardt, 2011	0.63 and 29.2	Burckhardt and Burckhardt, 2011
	OAT7	SLC22A9	8.7	Burckhardt and Burckhardt, 2011	2.2	Burckhardt and Burckhardt, 2011
ABC	ABCC1/MRP1		0.9	Conrad et al., 2002	5	Zelcer et al., 2003
	ABCC4/MRP4		–		2	Zelcer et al., 2003
	ABCC11/MRP8		–	Arlanov et al., 2016	21	Bortfeld et al., 2006
	ABCG2/BCRP		6.8	Imai et al., 2003	–	Lee Y. J. et al., 2005
SLC51	OSTα/β	SLC51A/B	n.d.	Ballatori et al., 2005	n.d.	Ballatori et al., 2005

n.d.: not measured

obligate heterodimers that transport bile acids and conjugated steroids; i.e., E1-S and DHEA-S. OSTα and OSTβ act down the concentration gradient of their substrates, and therefore they may be involved in both efflux and uptake processes (Ballatori et al., 2013, 2008). In humans, the *SLC51A* and *SLC51B* mRNAs have been reported for many tissues, including intestine, kidney, liver, testes, ovary, uterus, prostate, adrenal, and mammary gland (Seward et al., 2003).

ATP-Binding-Cassette Transporters

There are 48 distinct ABC-transporters in humans, which have been grouped into seven subfamilies, from ABC-A to ABC-G (Ween et al., 2015). The ABC-transporters mediate the active transport of various compounds across extracellular and intracellular membranes, with the energy derived from hydrolysis of ATP. Many ABC-transporters work as efflux pumps, to extrude their substrates from cells. ABC-transporters recognize a large variety of endogenous substances, and also chemically distinct molecules, including clinically applied drugs (Sarkadi et al., 2006). Overexpression of polyspecific ABC-transporters in tumors results in increased extrusion of drugs and can lead to resistance against multiple anti-cancer agents, termed as multi-drug resistance (MDR) (Schinkel and Jonker, 2003). The three major ABC-transporters implicated in MDR are ABCB1 (Pgp, P-glycoprotein) (Sharom, 2014), ABCC1, which is better known as MDR-associated protein 1 (MRP1) (Cole, 2014), and ABCG2, which is also known as breast cancer resistance protein (BCRP) or mitoxantrone resistance protein (MXR) (Ishikawa and Nakagawa, 2009). The multispecific MDR transporters are proven determinants of drug absorption, distribution, and excretion (Szakacs et al., 2008).

Members of ABC-transporter family C (i.e., ABCC1, ABCC4, ABCC11, ABCG2) transport large, negatively charged molecules. ABCC1 (MRP1) is ubiquitous in the body, and its main physiological substrates are leukotriene C4, and various glutathione-conjugated, glucuronidated, or sulfated compounds, including E1-S (Bodo et al., 2003; Cole, 2014). ABCC4 (MRP4) is found throughout the human body and transports molecules that are involved in cellular signaling, such as cyclic nucleotides, eicosanoids, and conjugated steroids (Slot et al., 2011). ABCC11 (MRP8) is found in brain, breasts, lungs, liver, kidney, placenta, prostate, testes, and apocrine glands, as well as in cancerous tissues (Kruh et al., 2007). Its substrates are lipophilic anions, as well as cyclic nucleotides and anticancer drugs (Bortfeld et al., 2006; Matsumoto et al., 2014). ABCC1, ABCC11, and ABCG2 transport E1-S, while ABCC1, ABCC4, ABCC11, and ABCG2 mediate excretion of DHEA-S (**Table 2**).

Concerted (and possibly co-regulated) actions of OATPs, OATs, transporters encoded by the *SLC51* gene family, ABC-efflux pumps, and biotransformation enzymes are needed for the handling of potentially toxic endogenous (e.g., bile acids) and exogenous (e.g., drugs) compounds (Sarkadi et al., 2006). Similarly, united actions of these transporters and the intracellular enzymes are required for maintenance of normal steroid hormone homeostasis.

DISTURBED TRANSPORT AND ESTROGEN ACTIONS IN GYNECOLOGICAL CANCERS

Changes in Uptake and Excretion of Steroid Conjugates

Altered expression of OATPs (usually as up-regulation) has been documented in different types of cancers. As these transporters serve as mediators of the uptake of nutrients for tumor growth and survival, and as they also bring anticancer agents into cancer cells, they may have significant impact on cancer therapies (Li and Shu, 2014). High levels of the steroid transporting OATPs (i.e., OATP1A2, OATP2B1, OATP1B3, OATP4A1, OATP4C1) have been suggested for breast cancer cells, as compared to normal tissue (Pizzagalli et al., 2003; Al Sarakbi et al., 2006; Meyer zu Schwabedissen et al., 2008; Wlcek et al., 2008). OATP1B3 has also been observed in endometrial carcinoma, where high levels significantly correlated with type I tumors and longer disease-free survival (Ogane et al., 2013) (**Table 3**). High levels of OATP1B3 and lower levels of OATP1B1 have also been reported in ovarian cancer samples (Arakawa et al., 2012; Furihata et al., 2015; Thakkar et al., 2015) and cancer cell lines (Cho et al., 2009; Chay et al., 2010; Svoboda et al., 2011; Lancaster et al., 2013) (**Table 3**). In addition to OATP1B3 and OATP1B1, also OATP2B1, OATP3A1, and OATP4A1 have been detected at the mRNA level in ovarian cancer samples (Tamai et al., 2000).

Among the transporters encoded by the *SLC22* genes, OAT2 has been detected in colorectal cancer (Tashiro et al., 2014), while to date there are no studies on the expression of the *SLC22* genes that encode the OAT2, OAT3, OAT4, and OAT7 proteins, nor on the transporters from the OST/SLC51 family in endometrial and ovarian cancers.

ABC-transporters are commonly up-regulated in chemoresistant cancers, and increased expression and activity of these drug efflux pumps results in reduced cellular accumulation of drugs (Ween et al., 2015). In endometrial cancer, chemoresistance is the major problem in advanced and recurrent cases (Chaudhry and Asselin, 2009). However, the data on expression of *ABC-transporters* in endometrial cancer are very limited. Among the steroid-transporting ABC-transporters, ABCG2 has been observed at the mRNA and protein levels in CD133^{+} Ishikawa endometrial cancer cells, which have characteristics of cancer stem cells (Nakamura et al., 2010, 2014), (Ween et al., 2015). Expression of *ABCC4* was detected in the HEC-1A endometrial cancer cell line, where the mRNA levels were suppressed by down-regulation of transcription factor *KLF9*. Decreased expression of *KLF9* has previously been observed in endometrial cancers of stages II to IV (Simmen et al., 2008).

In ovarian cancer, chemoresistance is typically observed after initial sensitivity to platin-based and taxol-based therapies. The great majority of patients with advanced ovarian cancer develop MDR due to the overexpression of the ABC-transporters (Auner et al., 2010). In ovarian cancer, expression of *ABCC1* has been observed at the mRNA and protein levels in serous, mucinous, clear-cell, endometrioid, and undifferentiated ovarian cancer tissues (for recent review, see Ween et al., 2015). Across multiple studies, positive immunohistochemical staining for

TABLE 3 | DHEA-S and E1-S transporters and estrogen biosynthetic enzymes in endometrial cancer.

Gene	Level	Cell line		Tumor tissue	
		Regulation	**Reference**	**Regulation**	**Reference**
OATP1B3	Protein			Cancer/adjacent tissue ↑	Ogane et al., 2013
ABCC4	mRNA	β HEC-1A after down-regulation of KLF9	Simmen et al., 2008		
ABCG2	mRNA	CD+133 Ishikawa cells, Expressed	Nakamura et al., 2014		
	Protein	CD+133 Ishikawa cells, Expressed	Nakamura et al., 2014		
HSD3B1	mRNA	HHUA, Expressed	Sugawara et al., 2004	Cancer/adjacent tissue ≈	Sinreih et al., 2013
		HIEEC, Ishikawa, HEC-1A Expressed ↑ HEC-1A/HIEEC	Hevir-Kene and Rižner, 2015		
HSD3B2	mRNA	HOUA, Expressed	Sugawara et al., 2004	Cancer/adjacent tissue ≈	Sinreih et al., 2013
		HIEEC, Ishikawa, HEC-1A Expressed ↑ HEC-1A/HIEEC	Hevir-Kene and Rižner, 2015		
CYP19A1	mRNA	HHUA, HOUA, No expression	Sugawara et al., 2004	Cancer/adjacent tissue, Low expression, ≈	Pathirage et al., 2006; Smuc and Rizner, 2009; Lépine et al., 2010; Cornel et al., 2012
		HIEEC, Ishikawa, HEC-1A Low expression ↑ HEC-1A/Ishikawa	Hevir-Kene and Rižner, 2015		
	Protein			Cancer/pre-/post-menopausal endometrium, No staining	Human Protein Atlas
	Activity	HEC-1, HEC-1B, RL-95, Ishikawa; No activity	Fournier and Poirier, 2009		
		HIEEC, Ishikawa, HEC-1A, No activity	Hevir-Kene and Rižner, 2015		
HSD17B1	mRNA	HIEEC, Ishikawa, HEC-1A Expressed, ↑ HEC-1A/HIEEC	Hevir-Kene and Rižner, 2015	Cancer/adjacent tissue, Low levels	Smuc et al., 2006; Lépine et al., 2010; Cornel et al., 2012
				Decreased	Smuc and Rizner, 2009; Lépine et al., 2010
				Increased in G1, ERα	Cornel et al., 2012
	Protein			Cancer/pre-/postmenopausal endometrium: 9% Cancer, weak/negative/negative	Human Protein Atlas
HSD17B7	mRNA	HIEEC, Ishikawa, HEC-1A Expressed, ↑ HEC-1A/HIEEC	Hevir-Kene and Rižner, 2015	Cancer/adjacent tissue Decreased	Smuc and Rizner, 2009; Lépine et al., 2010
				Unchanged	Lépine et al., 2010; Cornel et al., 2012
	Protein			Cancer/pre-/postmenopausal endometrium: 45% Cancer, weak/weak/weak	Human Protein Atlas
HSD17B12	mRNA	HIEEC, Ishikawa, HEC-1A Expressed, ↑ HEC-1A/HIEEC	Hevir-Kene and Rižner, 2015	Cancer/adjacent tissue, Unchanged	Smuc and Rizner, 2009
				No significant difference	Cornel et al., 2012
				EC type 2; Increased	Lépine et al., 2010
	Protein			Cancer/pre-/postmenopausal endometrium: 45% Cancer, weak/weak/weak	Human Protein Atlas

(Continued)

TABLE 3 | Continued

Gene	Level	Cell line		Tumor tissue	
		Regulation	Reference	Regulation	Reference
HSD17B2	mRNA	HIEEC, Ishikawa, HEC-1A Expressed ≈	Hevir-Kene and Rižner, 2015	Cancer/adjacent tissue, EC type 2; Increased	Lépine et al., 2010
				EC type 1; ≈ Increased in G2	Cornel et al., 2012
				EC type 1 postmenopausal; Increased	Lépine et al., 2010; Sinreih et al., 2013
	Protein			Cancer/pre-/postmenopausal endometrium; Moderate/ moderate/moderate	Human Protein Atlas
AKR1C3	mRNA	HIEEC, Ishikawa, HEC-1A Expressed, ↑ Ishikawa, HEC-1A/HIEEC	Hevir-Kene and Rižner, 2015	Cancer/adjacent tissue; Increased in individual patients	Rizner et al., 2006
				No sign. difference	Smuc and Rizner, 2009
				Cancer/adjacent tissue; Increased trend in G2/G3 EC	Cornel et al., 2012
	Protein			Cancer/pre-/post-menopausal endometrium: 45% Cancer moderate/strong/strong	Human Protein Atlas
STS	mRNA	HIEEC, Ishikawa, HEC-1A Expressed	Hevir-Kene and Rižner, 2015	Cancer/adjacent tissue; ≈	Smuc and Rizner, 2009
				Increased	Lépine et al., 2010
	Protein			Cancer/pre-/postmenopausal endometrium: 82% Cancer weak-moderate/weak/weak	Human Protein Atlas
	Activity E1-S	HEC-1A, HEC-1B, RL-95, Ishikawa; Low activity in whole cells, higher activity in homogenates	Fournier and Poirier, 2009		
		AC-258	Milewich and Porter, 1987		
SULT1E1	mRNA	Control HIEEC, Ishikawa, HEC-1A Expressed ≈	Hevir-Kene and Rižner, 2015	Cancer/adjacent tissue type 1 and 2; Borderline increase	Lépine et al., 2010
				Cancer/adjacent tissue type 1 ≈	Hevir et al., 2011
	Protein			Cancer/pre-/postmenopausal endometrium: Not detected, Negative/moderate/negative, Not detected	Human Protein Atlas
SULT2B1	mRNA	HIEEC, Ishikawa, HEC-1A Expressed, ↑ Ishikawa and HEC-1A/HIEEC	Hevir-Kene and Rižner 2015	Cancer/adjacent tissue; Increased	Hevir et al., 2011
	Protein			Cancer/pre-/postmenopausal endometrium: Moderate/ moderate/moderate	Human Protein Atlas

Endometrial cancer cell lines: HHUA, Ishikawa, well differentiated cell lines; RL-95, moderately differentiated cell line; HOUHA, HEC-1A, HEC-1B poorly differentiated cell line; HIEEC: control cell line of normal endometrium (pre-menopausal).

ABCC1 (MRP1) has been seen in 22–68% of paraffin sections from ovarian cancers (for review. see Ween et al., 2015), with association with higher tumor grade reported (Bagnoli et al., 2013). Also *ABCC4* is expressed in ovarian cancers. In a study that included 127 patients with ovarian cancer, ABCC4 (MRP4) was associated with shorter progression-free survival (Bagnoli et al., 2013; Ween et al., 2015). Finally, ABCC11 and ABCG2 have also been detected in ovarian cancers; the ABCG2 as a marker of side-populations of ovarian cancer cells that show stem-cell characteristics (Ween et al., 2015). In the *ABCG2* gene, several SNPs with functional consequences have been described, although controversial data have been reported considering their association with the outcome of ovarian cancers (for review, see Ween et al., 2015). *ABCG2* was induced in patients after their chemotherapy, and also by estrogens in the PA-1 ovarian cancer cell line after stable transfection with the gene encoding ERα (for

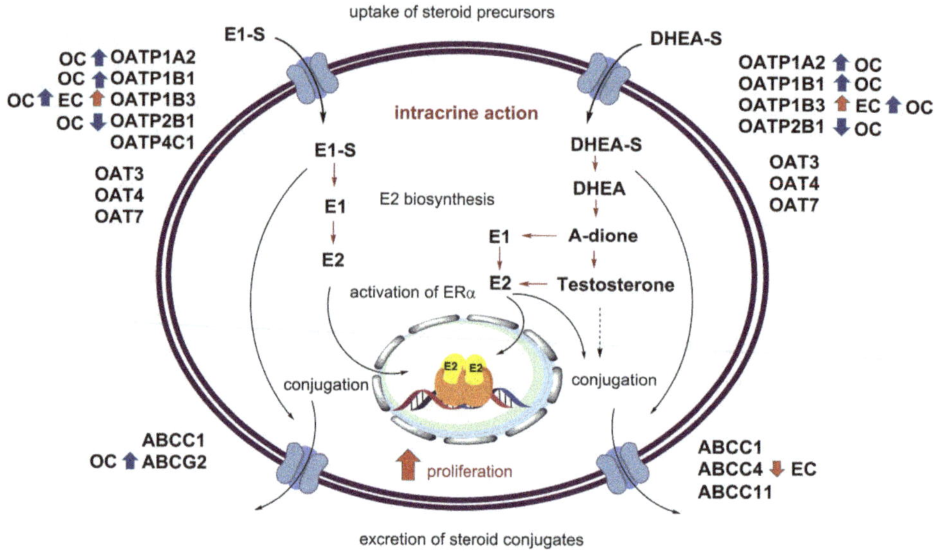

FIGURE 2 | Uptake, intracrine action, and excretion of steroid hormones. The major players in intracrine estrogen action are depicted, with the additional data on the levels of OATP, OAT, and ABC-transporters in endometrial (red arrows) and ovarian cancers (blue arrows).

review, see Ween et al., 2015). Recent systematic genomic analysis and biological properties of ovarian cancer cell lines showed that many commonly used "ovarian cancer" cell lines are unlikely to originate from high-grade serous ovarian cancer (Domcke et al., 2013; Haley et al., 2016). Therefore, novel cancer cells lines recently established will provide better models (Kreuzinger et al., 2015).

Analysis of The Cancer Genome Atlas data for the *SLCO* and *SLC22* genes in endometrial and ovarian cancers (cbioportal; http://www.cbioportal.org) (Cerami et al., 2012; Gao et al., 2013) has provided further information. The *SLCO1A2, SLCO1B1, SLCO1B3, SLCO1C1, SLCO2B1*, and *SLCO4A1* genes were amplified in <1% of patients, but showed mutations (as mainly missense mutations), in 3.1–5.6% of 240 patients with endometrial cancer. A similar trend was seen for the *SLC22* genes. Mutations were detected in all four *SLC22A* genes (i.e., *SLC22A7, SLC22A8, SLC22A11, SLC22A9*), in 2.6–5.1% of all patients. Among the *ABC* genes, there were mutations in all four genes involved in the efflux of steroid conjugates (i.e., *ABCC1, ABCC4, ABCC11, ABCG2*), in 5.7–8.3% of patients with endometrial cancer. In contrast, the *SLCO1A2, SLCO1B1, SLCO1B3, SLCO1C1, SLCO2B1*, and *SLCO4A1* genes were amplified in 4.7–7.4% of a total of 316 patients with serous ovarian cancer, with concurrent amplification of *SLCO1A2/1B1/1B3/1C1* and *SLCO1B1/1B3/1C1*, and also *SLCO1B3/1C1*. Among the *SLC22* and *ABC* genes, *SLC22A7* and *ABCC1* were amplified in 3.5 and 2.5% of patients, respectively, with serous ovarian cancers.

Although, the current knowledge on transporters in endometrial cancer are scarce, the currently available data suggest that E1-S and DHEA-S might enter cancerous cells via OATP1B3, which is present mainly in type I tumors (Ogane et al., 2013) (**Table 3**, **Figure 2**). This uptake might be affected by the missense mutations seen in 5.1% of patients (cbioportal; http://www.cbioportal.org). On the other hand, excretion of steroid conjugates can be catalyzed by ABCC4, a high affinity DHEA-S transporter that shows down-regulated expression in advanced stages of cancer (III-IV) (Simmen et al., 2008) (**Table 4**, **Figure 2**). Similarly, increased levels of ABCG2 were observed in CD133+ Ishikawa cells (Nakamura et al., 2014). Again, further regulation is achieved by mutations of *ABCC4* and *ABCG2*, in 6.2 and 5.7% of patients, respectively (cbioportal; http://www.cbioportal.org).

The published data reveal that in ovarian cancer, E1-S and DHEA-S can enter cancer cells via higher levels of OATP1B3, and also other OATPs might contribute, such as OATP1B1 (**Table 2**). Uptake of these steroids might be further regulated by *SLCO* gene amplification (cbioportal; http://www.cbioportal.org). This uptake is opposed by the excretion that is catalyzed by ABCC1, ABCC4, and ABCG2, where ABCC1 and ABCG2 have the highest affinities for E1-S and DHEA-S, respectively. Amplification of genes such as *ABCC1* and *ABCG2* further modulate the excretion (cbioportal; http://www.cbioportal.org).

Altered Formation of Androgens and Estrogens

In endometrial and ovarian cancers, several genes that encode the enzymes for local androgen and estrogen formation from precursor steroid conjugates are expressed, and some are differentially regulated (**Tables 3, 4**).

Expression of the individual estrogen and androgen biosynthetic genes in endometrial cancer has been studied by several groups (for review, see Rižner, 2013). Expression of *STS*, which is required for the hydrolysis of E1-S and DHEA-S, was seen to be high and unchanged (Smuc and Rizner, 2009) or increased (Lépine et al., 2010) in cancer tissues compared

TABLE 4 | DHEA-S and E1-S transporters and estrogen biosynthetic enzymes in ovarian cancer.

Gene	Level	Cell line		Tumor tissue	
		Regulation	Reference	Regulation	Reference
OATP1B1	mRNA			↑ Serous epithelial adenocarcinoma/control tissue	Svoboda et al., 2011
OATP1B3	mRNA	IGROV1, OVCAR-3, OVCAR-4, OVCAR5, OVCAR-8, SK-OV-3, Expressed	Lancaster et al., 2013	Cancer/control tissue ↑	Lancaster et al., 2013
		OVCAR-3, SK-OV-3, Expressed, ↑ OVCAR-3/SK-OV-3	Svoboda et al., 2011	↑ Serous epithelial adenocarcinoma/control tissue	Svoboda et al., 2011
OATP2B1	mRNA			↑ Serous epithelial adenocarcinoma/control tissue	Svoboda et al., 2011
OATP4A1	mRNA	↑YDOV-151 (mucinous adenocarcinoma), SK-OV-3/HOSE	Cho et al., 2009	≈ Serous epithelial adenocarcinoma/control tissue	Svoboda et al., 2011
		↑YDOV-139 (serous carcinoma)	Chay et al., 2010		
OATP4C1	mRNA			≈ Serous epithelial adenocarcinoma/control tissue	Svoboda et al., 2011
ABCC1	mRNA			Expressed in serous, mucinous, clear cell, endometrioid, undifferentiated cancer	Reviewed by (Ween et al., 2015)
	Protein			Positive IHC in 22–68% of ovarian cancers	Reviewed by (Ween et al., 2015)
ABCC4	Protein			127 OC patients; association with shorter progress free survival	Bagnoli et al., 2013
ABCG2	Protein	Induced in PA-1 OC cell line transfected with ESR1	Ee et al., 2004	Expressed in OC, a marker of of OC stem cells	Zhang et al., 2008
				↑ resistant OC (carboplatin + paclitaxel)	Ween et al., 2015
STS	mRNA			≈ EOC (9–10)/OSE (17)	Ren et al., 2015
	Protein			70% clear cell (32/45); 33% serous (6/18); and 50% mucinous adenocarcinoma (4/8)	Okuda et al., 2001
				Expressed EOC and OSE	Ren et al., 2015
				17% Cancer low/moderate, Normal ovary low (stromal cells)	Human Protein Atlas
	Activity E1-S	↑ SKOV-3, PEO-1 vs. OSE	Ren et al., 2015	↑ STS ↓ progression-free survival, epithelial OC (48), serous OC (34)	Chura et al., 2009a,b
		OC-117	Milewich and Porter, 1987		
SULT1E1	mRNA			↓ EOC (9–10)/OSE (17)	Ren et al., 2015
	Protein	Expressed EOC and OSE	Ren et al., 2015	17% Cancer moderate/normal ND	Human Protein Atlas
				Expressed	Ren et al., 2015
	Activity E1	↑ SKOV-3, PEO-1 vs. OSE	Ren et al., 2015		
HSD17B1	Activity E1→E2	↑ SKOV-3, PEO-1 vs. OSE	Ren et al., 2015		
HSD17B2	mRNA			↓ EOC (9–10)/OSE (17)	Ren et al., 2015
	Protein			Expressed	Ren et al., 2015
	Activity E2			Epithelial OC (48), serous OC (34)	Chura et al., 2009b

(Continued)

TABLE 4 | Continued

Gene	Level	Cell line		Tumor tissue	
		Regulation	Reference	Regulation	Reference
AKR1C3	mRNA			↓ EOC (9–10)/OSE (17)	Ren et al., 2015
	Protein			Expressed	Ren et al., 2015
	Activity T			Epithelial OC (48), serous OC (34)	Chura et al., 2009b
HSD3B1/2	Activity DHEA			Epithelial OC (48), serous OC (34)	Chura et al., 2009b

EOC, epithelial ovarian carcinoma; OSE, ovarian surface epithelia; OCCA, ovarian clear-cell adenocarcinoma, IGROV1, OVCAR-3, OVCAR-4, OVCAR5, OVCAR-8, SK-OV-3, AC-258, OC-117, PEO-1; ovarian cancer cell lines.

to control endometrial tissue. SULT1E1 opposes the action of STS. However, the expression data for *SULT1E1* mRNA are controversial, with low and increased (Lépine et al., 2010) or unchanged (Hevir et al., 2011) expression reported for cancer tissue, as compared to control endometrium. In model cell lines for well (Ishikawa cells), moderately (RL-95 cells), and poorly (HEC-1A, HEC-1B cells) differentiated endometrial cancer (see Supplementary Table 1) sulfatase activity was detected in whole cells and in cell homogenates (Fournier and Poirier, 2009). There was no difference in the expression of *SULT1E1* between the HIEEC control endometrial cell line and the HEC-1A endometrial cancer cell line (Supplementary Table 1) (Hevir-Kene and Rižner, 2015). Among the enzymes that catalyze the activation of E1 to E2 (**Figure 1**), the mRNA levels of *HSD17B1* were low (Smuc et al., 2006; Lépine et al., 2010; Cornel et al., 2012), decreased (Smuc and Rizner, 2009; Lépine et al., 2010), or increased in ERα-positive G1 cancers (Cornel et al., 2012). The expression of *HSD17B7* was unchanged (Lépine et al., 2010; Cornel et al., 2012) or decreased (Smuc and Rizner, 2009), and the expression of *HSD17B12* was unchanged (Smuc and Rizner, 2009; Cornel et al., 2012) or increased (Lépine et al., 2010), in endometrial cancer. In model cell lines, the *HSD17B1*, *HSD17B7*, and *HSD17B12* genes were up-regulated in HEC-1A vs. HIEEC cells (Hevir-Kene and Rižner, 2015).

HSD17B2 catalyzes the oxidation of E2 back to the less potent E1, and expression of the corresponding gene *HSD17B2* was increased in endometrial cancer (Lépine et al., 2010; Cornel et al., 2012; Sinreih et al., 2013), while there was no difference in expression of *HSD17B2* among control and cancer cell lines (Hevir-Kene and Rižner, 2015). The *CYP19A1* gene encodes aromatase and is responsible for the biosynthesis of E2 *via* androstenedione or testosterone; this was weakly expressed in cancer tissue, with no significant differences seen between cancer and control endometrium (Pathirage et al., 2006; Smuc and Rizner, 2009; Lépine et al., 2010; Cornel et al., 2012). In the HHUA and HOUA model cell lines, *CYP19A1* was not expressed (Supplementary Table 1) (Sugawara et al., 2004), and there was low expression in HIEEC, Ishikawa, and HEC-1A cells (Hevir-Kene and Rižner, 2015). In tissue samples, several reports showed immunohistochemical staining for CYP19A1 in paraffin sections of endometrial cancer, where both stromal and epithelial cells were stained, and several reports have shown a lack of specific staining (for review, see Rižner, 2013). Together with our current experimental data (Sinreih et al., in review to Frontiers in Pharmacology Research Topic), it appears that in endometrial cancer the sulfatase pathway has a more important role in E2 formation.

Among enzymes that catalyze local androgen formation from DHEA-S, in addition to STS, genes encoding *HSD3B1*, and *HSD3B2* showed no differences in expression between endometrial cancer and control tissue (Sinreih et al., 2013) (**Figure 1**). Also in the HHUA, HOUA, Ishikawa, HEC-1A, and HIEEC model cell lines (Supplementary Table 1), these two genes *HSD3B1* and *HSD3B2* were expressed, with higher mRNA levels in the HEC-1A cells as compared to the control HIEEC cells (Sugawara et al., 2004; Hevir-Kene and Rižner, 2015). Additionally, the gene that encodes AKR1C3, which catalyzes the activation of androstenedione to testosterone, was expressed in cancer tissue, but with no significant difference seen between cancer and adjacent control tissue, although with particularly increased levels in individual patients (Rizner et al., 2006). There was also a trend for increased expression of *AKR1C3* in G2/G3 cancers compared to G1 cancers (Cornel et al., 2012), but there were also decreased levels of AKR1C3 reported in cancer compared to control endometrium (Zakharov et al., 2010). Interestingly, *AKR1C3* was up-regulated in Ishikawa and HEC-1A cells vs. the control HIEEC cells (Hevir-Kene and Rižner, 2015). These data thus supports the capacity of cancerous endometrium for formation of androgens from DHEA and DHEA-S.

In ovarian cancer, *STS* is expressed at the mRNA and protein levels in primary cell cultures, tissue samples, and model cell lines (see Supplementary Table 2) (Ren et al., 2015; Okuda et al., 2001), with no significant differences seen between ovarian carcinoma and ovarian surface epithelial cells. Using immunohistochemistry, STS was detected in 70% of clear cells, and in 33% of serous and 50% of mucinous tumors (Okuda et al., 2001). High STS activity was detected in epithelial ovarian cancer tissue (Chura et al., 2009a), and also in the SKOV-3 and PEO-1 ovarian cancer cell lines (Supplementary Table 2). STS activity was higher in the model cell lines than in control ovarian surface epithelia cells (Ren et al., 2015). Significantly decreased expression of *SULT1E1* was seen at the mRNA level in epithelial ovarian cancer cells compared to ovarian surface epithelial cells (Ren et al., 2015).

In addition to STS activity, other enzymatic activities that are also necessary for local formation of androgens and estrogen have been observed in tissue samples of ovarian cancer, including conversion of DHEA to androstenedione, and conversions between E2, E1, testosterone, and androstenedione (Chura et al., 2009b). The enzymes that catalyze these reactions (i.e., HSD17B2, AKR1C3, SULT1E1) were detected by immunohistochemistry in ovarian cancer tissue samples (Ren et al., 2015). The importance of the local formation of E2 *via* the sulfatase pathway is supported by high levels of STS and significantly down-regulated *SULT1E1* together with metabolism of E1-S to E1 (Milewich and Porter, 1987; Chura et al., 2009a) and E2 (Ren et al., 2015) in tissue samples and model cell lines of ovarian cancer. In ovarian cancer samples, androstenedione can be formed from DHEA (Chura et al., 2009a), although Ren et al. (Ren et al., 2015) found no evidence for further formation of estrogens via the aromatase pathway or activation of androstenedione to testosterone and 5α-dihydrotestosterone, as also supported by down-regulation of *AKR1C3*. However, in other studies, CYP19A1 was expressed in stroma cells of ovarian cancers (Manna et al., 2016), and has been considered a target for an endocrine therapy (Langdon et al., 2017).

PHARMACOLOGICAL INTERVENTIONS THAT TARGET INTRACRINE ACTIONS

Endometrial and ovarian cancers are considered to be hormone-dependent cancers. As they develop mainly in postmenopausal women, they depend on local formation of active estrogens, while the roles of androgens are currently not fully understood. After menopause, the intracrine production of estrogens from the steroid precursors E1-S and DHEA-S in cancer cells can theoretically be blocked in a number of ways, including: (i) prevention of transporter-mediated uptake of E1-S and DHEA-S from the circulation; (ii) inhibition of enzymes in the intracrine pathway for the formation of active estrogens by the so-called selective intracrine modulators; (iii) prevention of estrogen actions via ERα; and (iv) induction of estrogen inactivation and excretion from cancer cells via the ABC-efflux pumps, which will decrease their intracellular concentrations. Strategies for targeting transporters, receptors and enzymes in intracrine pathways in endometrial and ovarian cancers are discussed in more detail in the following sections, with comparisons also from several studies in breast cancer.

Sulfatase and 17-Ketosteroid Reductase Type 1 as Novel Drug Targets

Previous studies have suggested that in the endometrium and ovary of postmenopausal women, hydrolysis of sulfated precursors is the major pathway for the generation of active estrogens. Indeed, STS inhibitors have been successfully tested in preclinical and animal models of hormone-dependent cancers (for an extensive review on E1 sulfatase inhibitors and their efficacy in animal and human tumor models, see Thomas and Potter, 2015; Rižner, 2016). Irosustat (STX64) is a potent tricylic coumarin-based sulfamate that irreversibly blocks STS activity, and it has been examined in phase II clinical trials for the treatment of patients with advanced hormone-dependent breast and endometrial cancers (Stanway et al., 2007). Although the breast cancer data have not yet been published (ClinicalTrials.gov Identifier: NCT01662726) https://clinicaltrials.gov/ct2/show/NCT01662726), the effects in endometrial cancer were not as good as the effects of medroxyprogesterone acetate, which is in clinical use for cases of advanced/ recurrent cancer (Pautier et al., 2012).

Estrone formed by the sulfatase pathway has to be activated by reductive HSD17B enzymes, where HSD17B1 has the highest catalytic efficiency (Rižner, 2013). The inhibitors of reductive HSD17B1 enzymes can block the conversion of E1 to E2, and have potential for application to hormone-sensitive cancer therapy. Although the mRNA and protein levels of HSD17B1 are very low, this approach might be interesting for treatment of endometrial cancer, as recent reports have shown correlations between increased *HSD17B1* mRNA levels and poor prognosis (Cornel et al., 2017). This approach might also be useful in ovarian cancer, as increased reduction of E1 to E2 has been seen in ovarian cancer cells (Ren et al., 2015). Indeed, compounds have been developed that show promising inhibition of E2 formation from E1 *in vitro* (Brozic et al., 2008; Mazumdar et al., 2009), although none of these have been studied in clinical trials to date. Most likely they will not be highly effective as mono-therapeutic agents, because they prevent the conversion of a weak estrogenic E1 to the most potent estrogen E2 only, but they might be useful in combination with other inhibitors, such as inhibitors of STS.

Even if the production of E2 via the sulfatase pathway exceeds that of the aromatase pathway, blocking one enzyme might up-regulate the others. Such a mechanism was recently reported for ERα-positive breast cancer cell lines, where resistance to aromatase inhibitors was associated with up-regulation of *STS* and E1-S transporting *OATPs* (Higuchi et al., 2016). Therefore, as a consequence of inhibition of STS, the low expression levels of *CYP19A1* in endometrial and ovarian cancers (Manna et al., 2016) might be up-regulated as well. In this case, a combination of inhibitors for STS and CYP19A1 might be useful. After the introduction in around 1980 of aminoglutethimide as the first aromatase inhibitor with documented anti-cancer efficacy (Samojlik et al., 1980), the third-generation aromatase inhibitors letrozole and anastrozole, and exemestane, are currently used for treatment of postmenopausal breast cancer (Smith and Dowsett, 2003). However, in endometrial cancer, aromatase inhibitors have shown only weak effects (Bogliolo et al., 2016). For recurrent ovarian cancer their application has been suggested as well and remarkably positive effects were reported for a patient with endometrioid ovarian cancer (Pan and Kao, 2010). Dual CYP19A1-STS inhibitors have also already been designed, where the sulfatase inhibitory pharmacophore was integrated into an established aromatase inhibitor (sulfamate derivatives of letrozole and anastrozole), or *vice versa* (Woo et al., 2010; Harrelson and Lee, 2016). In a similar manner, dual HSD17B1/ STS inhibitors also represent a plausible approach in future drug discovery.

For further drug development, compounds from natural sources with dual aromatase and sulfatase inhibitory activities might also be of interest, such as a traditional Chinese herbal formula (Shu-Gan-Liang-Xue decoction) that is used for treatment of patients with breast cancer in traditional Chinese medicine (Zhou et al., 2014).

Estrogen Receptor α as a Drug Target

The activation of ERα by estrogens can be prevented by antagonists or selective estrogen receptor modulators (SERMs). There is an important difference between these compounds, as antagonists block estrogen action in all tissues, while SERMs can act as agonists in certain tissues, and as antagonists in other tissues, where their actions depend on the availability of co-activators and co-repressors (Traboulsi et al., 2017). The best studied SERM is tamoxifen, which has been successfully applied in the treatment of hormone-receptor-positive breast cancer for more than 40 years (see Scharl and Salterberg, 2016). In endometrium, tamoxifen has estrogenic effects and stimulates cell proliferation, which leads to hyperplasia, and eventually, to endometrial cancer (Ellis et al., 2015). Only recently has concern arisen that tamoxifen might also increase the risk of ovarian cancer, as it promotes lesions in the fallopian tubes and ovaries (Chene et al., 2014). Novel SERMs have been developed to combat estrogen-dependent cancers, including toremifene and raloxifene, together with the selective ER down-regulators, such as selective receptor downregulator fulvestrant (for reviews, see Bogliolo et al., 2017; Traboulsi et al., 2017). Further clinical studies on patients with endometrial and ovarian cancer are currently awaited.

OAT, OATP, and ABC-Transporters as Novel Drug Targets?

The E1-S– and DHEA-S–transporting OATPs are up-regulated in endometrial and ovarian cancers. To prevent OATP-mediated uptake of steroid hormone precursors into tumor cells, blocking OATP transport would be required. Inhibition of OATP-mediated uptake has been studied extensively using synthetic and natural inhibitors of OATP1B3 and OATP1B1 to block the uptake of statins and other substrates of these OATPs, both *in vitro* and in animal studies. However, blocking the function of these two liver-specific OATPs can change the hepatic clearance of drugs, which can result in their altered pharmacokinetics (i.e., elevated plasma levels of drugs are usually expected). This may cause serious adverse reactions, such as statin-induced myotoxicity, as has been demonstrated by co-administration of cyclosporine-A and gemfibrozil with statins (for review, see Kalliokoski and Niemi, 2009; Maeda, 2015).

Moreover, studies in breast cancer have revealed that prevention of the expression of a single *OATP* is not sufficient to inhibit steroid hormone uptake (Higuchi et al., 2016). Therefore, simultaneous blocking of various OATPs would be required. However, this would also influence the physiological functions of OATPs, and would disturb the metabolic homeostasis and protection against toxins. Therefore, the clinical application of such a simultaneous block is questionable (Stieger and Hagenbuch, 2014). Furthermore, in general, this block would only work with the particular isoforms of the transporters that are restricted to the cancerous tissues (Thakkar et al., 2015). To date, only one cancer-specific isoform (cancer-type OATP1B3) has been identified, although only in colon and pancreatic cancers (Furihata et al., 2015). As the *SLCO* and *SLC* genes are amplified in a subset of patients with ovarian cancer, their targeted inhibition might be considered. Also mutations in *SLCO* and *SLC* in endometrial cancer patients might allow the development of mutation-specific inhibitors.

However, the evaluation of OATP and OAT transporters as drug targets is currently precluded by the lack of complete information about their biological functions, substrate specificities, and mechanisms of action, and the importance of the corresponding *SLCO* and *SLC* gene amplifications and mutations in patients with endometrial and ovarian cancers.

Another option would theoretically be to limit the concentrations of steroid precursors in tumor cells by increasing steroid hormone efflux via ABC-transporters. Many ABC-proteins are expressed at physiological barriers where they protect cells and tissues against toxic compounds, which include anticancer drugs (Chen et al., 2016). Some of these ABC proteins are associated with drug resistance in ovarian and endometrial cancers. For example, overexpression of ABCC1 and ABCG2 in serous ovarian cancer reduces the cellular accumulation of anticancer drugs, and this leads to the development of MDR and poor prognosis (Kunicka and Soucek, 2014; Elsnerova et al., 2016). Furthermore, ABCC1 is associated with higher tumor grade, and ABCC4 with reduced progression-free survival of patients with ovarian cancer (Ween et al., 2015). Moreover, in endometrial cancer, *ABCG2* is expressed in the Ishikawa model cell line, which is enriched in CD133 and has cancer stem cell characteristics (Nakamura et al., 2010). Inhibitors of ABC-transporters have thus been included in several clinical studies that have targeted mainly ABCB1, and also ABCC1 and ABCG2 (for extensive review, see Ween et al., 2015). However, these have not shown sufficient efficacy to block ovarian cancer progression. Higher expression of these *ABC*s should also lead to increased extrusion of steroid hormone conjugates from the cancer cells. However, in terms of the usually negative correlation between the expression levels of these ABC-transporters and patient prognosis (see above), the benefit of targeting these ABC-transporters with concurrent decreased hormone levels will not counterweigh the MDR induced.

Current Status and Future Prospects

In patients with advanced endometrial and ovarian cancers, targeting ERα or enzymes for estrogen activation has not proven to be successful to date (Secky et al., 2013; Mueller et al., 2015). As a small subgroup of patients (~20%) still responds to estrogen-deprivation therapy, better stratification of patients for menopausal status, hormone receptor status, and presence of estrogen biosynthetic enzymes, among other factors, could select a subpopulation that would most likely benefit from estrogen-deprivation therapy. The development of resistance to estrogen-deprivation therapy may be of major concern, and therefore a combination of drugs instead of monotherapy with one agent may extend the period of sensitivity to these therapeutics. In this respect, dual STS/CYP191 inhibitors might be important, as drugs also targeting ERα (ERα antagonists) might be given together with STS and/or HSD17B1 inhibitors. Very promising data have been reported for breast cancer, where a combination of aromatase inhibitors and novel agents that target overexpressed kinases has led to enhanced therapeutic responses (Zhao and Ramaswamy, 2014; Daldorff et al., 2017). Elucidation of such novel approaches for endometrial and ovarian cancer-specific pathways in combination with the use of selective intracrine modulators or selective estrogen-receptor modulators may lead to the development of novel therapeutic approaches to improve the success of cancer chemotherapy.

AUTHOR CONTRIBUTIONS

TLR contributed to conception and design of the review, TLR, TT, and CÖL contributed to the final version of the manuscript, and all authors read and approved the final manuscript.

ACKNOWLEDGMENTS

The preparation of this manuscript was supported by grant J3-5510 to TLR from the Slovenian Research Agency, an OTKA K 109423 grant from the National Research, Development and Innovation Office (CÖL), and by the MedInProt Programme (CÖL). CÖL is a recipient of the Bolyai János Fellowship of the Hungarian Academy of Sciences. The authors thank Dr. Chris Berrie for critical reading of the manuscript.

REFERENCES

Akhmedkhanov, A., Zeleniuch-Jacquotte, A., and Toniolo, P. (2001). Role of exogenous and endogenous hormones in endometrial cancer: review of the evidence and research perspectives. *Ann. N. Y. Acad. Sci.* 943, 296–315. doi: 10.1111/j.1749-6632.2001.tb03811.x

Al Sarakbi, W., Mokbel, R., Salhab, M., Jiang, W. G., Reed, M. J., and Mokbel, K. (2006). The role of STS and OATP-B mRNA expression in predicting the clinical outcome in human breast cancer. *Anticancer Res.* 26, 4985–4990.

Amant, F., Moerman, P., Neven, P., Timmerman, D., Van Limbergen, E., and Vergote, I. (2005). Endometrial cancer. *Lancet* 366, 491–505. doi: 10.1016/S0140-6736(05)67063-8

Anderson, G. L., Judd, H. L., Kaunitz, A. M., Barad, D. H., Beresford, S. A., Pettinger, M., et al. (2003). Effects of estrogen plus progestin on gynecologic cancers and associated diagnostic procedures: the Women's Health Initiative randomized trial. *JAMA* 290, 1739–1748. doi: 10.1001/jama.290.13.1739

Arakawa, H., Nakanishi, T., Yanagihara, C., Nishimoto, T., Wakayama, T., Mizokami, A., et al. (2012). Enhanced expression of organic anion transporting polypeptides (OATPs) in androgen receptor-positive prostate cancer cells: possible role of OATP1A2 in adaptive cell growth under androgen-depleted conditions. *Biochem. Pharmacol.* 84, 1070–1077. doi: 10.1016/j.bcp.2012.07.026

Arlanov, R., Lang, T., Jedlitschky, G., Schaeffeler, E., Ishikawa, T., Schwab, M., et al. (2016). Functional characterization of common protein variants in the efflux transporter ABCC11 and identification of T546M as functionally damaging variant. *Pharmacogenomics J.* 16, 193–201. doi: 10.1038/tpj.2015.27

Audet-Walsh, E., Lépine, J., Grégoire, J., Plante, M., Caron, P., Têtu, B., et al. (2011). Profiling of endogenous estrogens, their precursors, and metabolites in endometrial cancer patients: association with risk and relationship to clinical characteristics. *J. Clin. Endocrinol. Metab.* 96, E330–E339. doi: 10.1210/jc.2010-2050

Auner, V., Sehouli, J., Oskay-Oezcelik, G., Horvat, R., Speiser, P., and Zeillinger, R. (2010). ABC transporter gene expression in benign and malignant ovarian tissue. *Gynecol. Oncol.* 117, 198–201. doi: 10.1016/j.ygyno.2009.10.077

Bagnoli, M., Beretta, G. L., Gatti, L., Pilotti, S., Alberti, P., Tarantino, E., et al. (2013). Clinicopathological impact of ABCC1/MRP1 and ABCC4/MRP4 in epithelial ovarian carcinoma. *Biomed. Res. Int.* 2013:143202. doi: 10.1155/2013/143202

Bai, W., Oliveros-Saunders, B., Wang, Q., Acevedo-Duncan, M. E., and Nicosia, S. V. (2000). Estrogen stimulation of ovarian surface epithelial cell proliferation. *In Vitro Cell. Dev. Biol. Anim.* 36, 657–666. doi: 10.1290/1071-2690(2000)036<0657:ESOOSE>2.0.CO;2

Ballatori, N., Christian, W. V., Lee, J. Y., Dawson, P. A., Soroka, C. J., Boyer, J. L., et al. (2005). OSTalpha-OSTbeta: a major basolateral bile acid and steroid transporter in human intestinal, renal, and biliary epithelia. *Hepatology* 42, 1270–1279. doi: 10.1002/hep.20961

Ballatori, N., Christian, W. V., Wheeler, S. G., and Hammond, C. L. (2013). The heteromeric organic solute transporter, OSTalpha-OSTbeta/SLC51: a transporter for steroid-derived molecules. *Mol. Aspects Med.* 34, 683–692. doi: 10.1016/j.mam.2012.11.005

Ballatori, N., Fang, F., Christian, W. V., Li, N., and Hammond, C. L. (2008). Ostalpha-Ostbeta is required for bile acid and conjugated steroid disposition in the intestine, kidney, and liver. *Am. J. Physiol. Gastrointest Liver Physiol.* 295, G179–G186. doi: 10.1152/ajpgi.90319.2008

Bast, R. C. (2011). Molecular approaches to personalizing management of ovarian cancer. *Ann. Oncol.* 22(Suppl. 8), viii5–viii15. doi: 10.1093/annonc/mdr516

Beral, V., Bull, D., Green, J., Reeves, G., and Collaborators, M. W. S. (2007). Ovarian cancer and hormone replacement therapy in the Million Women Study. *Lancet* 369, 1703–1710. doi: 10.1016/S0140-6736(07)60534-0

Beral, V., Gaitskell, K., Hermon, C., Moser, K., Reeves, G., and Peto, R. (2015). Menopausal hormone use and ovarian cancer risk: individual participant meta-analysis of 52 epidemiological studies. *Lancet* 385, 1835–1842. doi: 10.1016/S0140-6736(14)61687-1

Binder, P. S., Prat, J., and Mutch, D. G. (2015). Molecular staging of gynecological cancer: what is the future? *Best Pract. Res. Clin. Obstet. Gynaecol.* 29, 776–789. doi: 10.1016/j.bpobgyn.2015.01.008

Blouin, K., Veilleux, A., Luu-The, V., and Tchernof, A. (2009). Androgen metabolism in adipose tissue: recent advances. *Mol. Cell. Endocrinol.* 301, 97–103. doi: 10.1016/j.mce.2008.10.035

Bodo, A., Bakos, E., Szeri, F., Varadi, A., and Sarkadi, B. (2003). The role of multidrug transporters in drug availability, metabolism and toxicity. *Toxicol. Lett.* 140–141, 133–143. doi: 10.1016/S0378-4274(02)00497-6

Bogliolo, S., Cassani, C., Dominoni, M., Orlandini, A., Ferrero, S., Iacobone, A. D., et al. (2017). The role of fulvestrant in endometrial cancer. *Expert Opin. Drug Metab. Toxicol.* 13, 537–544. doi: 10.1080/17425255.2016.1244264

Bogliolo, S., Gardella, B., Dominoni, M., Musacchi, V., Cassani, C., Zanellini, F., et al. (2016). Effectiveness of aromatase inhibitors in the treatment of advanced endometrial adenocarcinoma. *Arch. Gynecol. Obstet.* 293, 701–708. doi: 10.1007/s00404-015-3974-9

Bortfeld, M., Rius, M., Konig, J., Herold-Mende, C., Nies, A. T., and Keppler, D. (2006). Human multidrug resistance protein 8 (MRP8/ABCC11), an apical efflux pump for steroid sulfates, is an axonal protein of the CNS and peripheral nervous system. *Neuroscience* 137, 1247–1257. doi: 10.1016/j.neuroscience.2005.10.025

Brozic, P., Lanisnik Risner, T., and Gobec, S. (2008). Inhibitors of 17beta-hydroxysteroid dehydrogenase type 1. *Curr. Med. Chem.* 15, 137–150. doi: 10.2174/092986708783330629

Burckhardt, G., and Burckhardt, B. C. (2011). *In vitro* and *in vivo* evidence of the importance of organic anion transporters (OATs) in drug therapy. *Handb. Exp. Pharmacol.* 201, 29–104. doi: 10.1007/978-3-642-14541-4_2

Caron, P., Audet-Walsh, E., Lépine, J., Bélanger, A., and Guillemette, C. (2009). Profiling endogenous serum estrogen and estrogen-glucuronides by liquid chromatography-tandem mass spectrometry. *Anal. Chem.* 81, 10143–10148. doi: 10.1021/ac9019126

Cerami, E., Gao, J., Dogrusoz, U., Gross, B. E., Sumer, S. O., Aksoy, B. A., et al. (2012). The cBio cancer genomics portal: an open platform for exploring multidimensional cancer genomics data. *Cancer Discov.* 2, 401–404. doi: 10.1158/2159-8290.CD-12-0095

Chaudhry, P., and Asselin, E. (2009). Resistance to chemotherapy and hormone therapy in endometrial cancer. *Endocr. Relat. Cancer* 16, 363–380. doi: 10.1677/ERC-08-0266

Chay, D., Cho, H., Lim, B. J., Kang, E. S., Oh, Y. J., Choi, S. M., et al. (2010). ER-60 (PDIA3) is highly expressed in a newly established serous ovarian cancer cell line, YDOV-139. *Int. J. Oncol.* 37, 399–412. doi: 10.3892/ijo_00000688

Chen, Z., Shi, T., Zhang, L., Zhu, P., Deng, M., Huang, C., et al. (2016). Mammalian drug efflux transporters of the ATP binding cassette (ABC) family in multidrug resistance: a review of the past decade. *Cancer Lett.* 370, 153–164. doi: 10.1016/j.canlet.2015.10.010

Chene, G., Radosevic-Robin, N., Tardieu, A. S., Cayre, A., Raoelfils, I., Dechelotte, P., et al. (2014). Morphological and immunohistochemical study of ovarian and tubal dysplasia associated with tamoxifen. *Eur. J. Histochem.* 58:2251. doi: 10.4081/ejh.2014.2251

Cho, H., Lim, B. J., Kang, E. S., Choi, J. S., and Kim, J.-H. (2009). Molecular characterization of a new ovarian cancer cell line, YDOV-151, established from mucinous cystadenocarcinoma. *Tohoku J. Exp. Med.* 218, 129–139. doi: 10.1620/tjem.218.129

Chura, J. C., Blomquist, C. H., Ryu, H. S., and Argenta, P. A. (2009a). Estrone sulfatase activity in patients with advanced ovarian cancer. *Gynecol. Oncol.* 112, 205–209. doi: 10.1016/j.ygyno.2008.08.037

Chura, J. C., Ryu, H. S., Simard, M., Poirier, D., Tremblay, Y., Brooker, D. C., et al. (2009b). Steroid-converting enzymes in human ovarian carcinomas. *Mol. Cell. Endocrinol.* 301, 51–58. doi: 10.1016/j.mce.2008.07.015

Clendenen, T. V., Hertzmark, K., Koenig, K. L., Lundin, E., Rinaldi, S., Johnson, T., et al. (2016). Premenopausal circulating androgens and risk of endometrial cancer: results of a prospective study. *Horm. Cancer* 7, 178–187. doi: 10.1007/s12672-016-0258-1

Cole, S. P. (2014). Multidrug resistance protein 1 (MRP1, ABCC1), a "multitasking" ATP-binding cassette (ABC) transporter. *J. Biol. Chem.* 289, 30880–30888. doi: 10.1074/jbc.R114.609248

Conrad, S., Kauffmann, H. M., Ito, K., Leslie, E. M., Deeley, R. G., Schrenk, D., et al. (2002). A naturally occurring mutation in MRP1 results in a selective decrease in organic anion transport and in increased doxorubicin resistance. *Pharmacogenetics* 12, 321–330. doi: 10.1097/00008571-200206000-00008

Cornel, K. M., Krakstad, C., Delvoux, B., Xanthoulea, S., Jori, B., Bongers, M. Y., et al. (2017). High mRNA levels of 17beta-hydroxysteroid dehydrogenase type 1 correlate with poor prognosis in endometrial cancer. *Mol. Cell. Endocrinol.* 442, 51–57. doi: 10.1016/j.mce.2016.11.030

Cornel, K. M., Kruitwagen, R. F., Delvoux, B., Visconti, L., Van de Vijver, K. K., Day, J. M., et al. (2012). Overexpression of 17β-hydroxysteroid dehydrogenase type 1 increases the exposure of endometrial cancer to 17β-estradiol. *J. Clin. Endocrinol. Metab.* 97, E591–E601. doi: 10.1210/jc.2011-2994

Crawford, S., Santoro, N., Laughlin, G. A., Sowers, M. F., McConnell, D., Sutton-Tyrrell, K., et al. (2009). Circulating dehydroepiandrosterone sulfate concentrations during the menopausal transition. *J. Clin. Endocrinol. Metab.* 94, 2945–2951. doi: 10.1210/jc.2009-0386

Cui, Y., Konig, J., Leier, I., Buchholz, U., and Keppler, D. (2001). Hepatic uptake of bilirubin and its conjugates by the human organic anion transporter SLC21A6. *J. Biol. Chem.* 276, 9626–9630. doi: 10.1074/jbc.M004968200

Daldorff, S., Mathiesen, R. M., Yri, O. E., Odegard, H. P., and Geisler, J. (2017). Cotargeting of CYP-19 (aromatase) and emerging, pivotal signalling pathways in metastatic breast cancer. *Br. J. Cancer* 116, 10–20. doi: 10.1038/bjc.2016.405

Diep, C. H., Daniel, A. R., Mauro, L. J., Knutson, T. P., and Lange, C. A. (2015). Progesterone action in breast, uterine, and ovarian cancers. *J. Mol. Endocrinol.* 54, R31–R53. doi: 10.1530/JME-14-0252

Domcke, S., Sinha, R., Levine, D. A., Sander, C., and Schultz, N. (2013). Evaluating cell lines as tumour models by comparison of genomic profiles. *Nat. Commun.* 4:2126. doi: 10.1038/ncomms3126

Ee, P. L., Kamalakaran, S., Tonetti, D., He, X., Ross, D. D., and Beck, W. T. (2004). Identification of a novel estrogen response element in the breast cancer resistance protein (ABCG2) gene. *Cancer Res.* 64, 1247–1251. doi: 10.1158/0008-5472.CAN-03-3583

Ellis, A. J., Hendrick, V. M., Williams, R., and Komm, B. S. (2015). Selective estrogen receptor modulators in clinical practice: a safety overview. *Expert Opin. Drug Saf.* 14, 921–934. doi: 10.1517/14740338.2015.1014799

Elsnerova, K., Mohelnikova-Duchonova, B., Cerovska, E., Ehrlichova, M., Gut, I., Rob, L., et al. (2016). Gene expression of membrane transporters: importance for prognosis and progression of ovarian carcinoma. *Oncol. Rep.* 35, 2159–2170. doi: 10.3892/or.2016.4599

Ferlay, J., Soerjomatraram, I., Ervik, M., Dikshit, R., Eser, S., Mathers, C., et al. (2013). *GLOBOCAN 2012 v1.0, Cancer Incidence and Mortality Worldwide: IARC CancerBase No.11 (Internet).*

Fogle, R. H., Stanczyk, F. Z., Zhang, X., and Paulson, R. J. (2007). Ovarian androgen production in postmenopausal women. *J. Clin. Endocrinol. Metab.* 92, 3040–3043. doi: 10.1210/jc.2007-0581

Fournier, M.-A., and Poirier, D. (2009). Estrogen formation in endometrial and cervix cancer cell lines: involvement of aromatase, steroid sulfatase and 17β-hydroxysteroid dehydrogenases (types 1, 5, 7 and 12). *Mol. Cell. Endocrinol.* 301, 142–145. doi: 10.1016/j.mce.2008.08.027

Fuhrman, B. J., Schairer, C., Gail, M. H., Boyd-Morin, J., Xu, X., Sue, L. Y., et al. (2012). Estrogen metabolism and risk of breast cancer in postmenopausal women. *J. Natl. Cancer Inst.* 104, 326–339. doi: 10.1093/jnci/djr531

Furihata, T., Sun, Y., and Chiba, K. (2015). Cancer-type organic anion transporting polypeptide 1B3: current knowledge of the gene structure, expression profile, functional implications and future perspectives. *Curr. Drug Metab.* 16, 474–485. doi: 10.2174/1389200216666150812142715

Gao, J., Aksoy, B. A., Dogrusoz, U., Dresdner, G., Gross, B., Sumer, S. O., et al. (2013). Integrative analysis of complex cancer genomics and clinical profiles using the cBioPortal. *Sci. Signal.* 6:pl1. doi: 10.1126/scisignal.2004088

Gibson, D. A., Simitsidellis, I., Collins, F., and Saunders, P. T. (2014). Evidence of androgen action in endometrial and ovarian cancers. *Endocr. Relat. Cancer* 21, T203–T218. doi: 10.1530/ERC-13-0551

Giton, F., Fiet, J., Cornu, J. N., Cussenot, O., Bélanger, A., Urien, S., et al. (2011). Serum sex steroids measured in middle-aged European and African-Caribbean men by gas chromatography-mass spectrometry. *Eur. J. Endocrinol.* 165, 917–924. doi: 10.1530/EJE-11-0551

Gui, C., Miao, Y., Thompson, L., Wahlgren, B., Mock, M., Stieger, B., et al. (2008). Effect of pregnane X receptor ligands on transport mediated by human OATP1B1 and OATP1B3. *Eur. J. Pharmacol.* 584, 57–65. doi: 10.1016/j.ejphar.2008.01.042

Hagenbuch, B., and Stieger, B. (2013). The SLCO (former SLC21) superfamily of transporters. *Mol. Aspects Med.* 34, 396–412. doi: 10.1016/j.mam.2012.10.009

Haley, J., Tomar, S., Pulliam, N., Xiong, S., Perkins, S. M., Karpf, A. R., et al. (2016). Functional characterization of a panel of high-grade serous ovarian cancer cell lines as representative experimental models of the disease. *Oncotarget* 7, 32810–32820. doi: 10.18632/oncotarget.9053

Hampel, H., and de la Chapelle, A. (2011). The search for unaffected individuals with Lynch syndrome: do the ends justify the means?. *Cancer Prev. Res.* 4, 1–5. doi: 10.1158/1940-6207.CAPR-10-0345

Harrelson, J. P., and Lee, M. W. (2016). Expanding the view of breast cancer metabolism: promising molecular targets and therapeutic opportunities. *Pharmacol. Ther.* 167, 60–73. doi: 10.1016/j.pharmthera.2016.07.014

Hattori, Y., Ishii, H., Munetomo, A., Watanabe, H., Morita, A., Sakuma, Y., et al. (2016). Human C-terminally truncated ERα variants resulting from the use of alternative exons in the ligand-binding domain. *Mol. Cell. Endocrinol.* 425, 111–122. doi: 10.1016/j.mce.2016.01.026

Henderson, B. E., and Feigelson, H. S. (2000). Hormonal carcinogenesis. *Carcinogenesis* 21, 427–433. doi: 10.1093/carcin/21.3.427

Hevir, N., Sinkovec, J., and Rižner, T. L. (2011). Disturbed expression of phase I and phase II estrogen-metabolizing enzymes in endometrial cancer: lower levels of CYP1B1 and increased expression of S-COMT. *Mol. Cell. Endocrinol.* 331, 158–167. doi: 10.1016/j.mce.2010.09.011

Hevir-Kene, N., and Rižner, T. L. (2015). The endometrial cancer cell lines Ishikawa and HEC-1A, and the control cell line HIEEC, differ in expression of estrogen biosynthetic and metabolic genes, and in androstenedione and estrone-sulfate metabolism. *Chem. Biol. Interact.* 234, 309–319. doi: 10.1016/j.cbi.2014.11.015

Hewitt, S. C., Winuthayanon, W., and Korach, K. S. (2016). What's new in estrogen receptor action in the female reproductive tract. *J. Mol. Endocrinol.* 56, R55–R71. doi: 10.1530/jme-15-0254

Higuchi, T., Endo, M., Hanamura, T., Gohno, T., Niwa, T., Yamaguchi, Y., et al. (2016). Contribution of estrone sulfate to cell proliferation in aromatase inhibitor (AI) -resistant, hormone receptor-positive breast cancer. *PLoS ONE* 11:e0155844. doi: 10.1371/journal.pone.0155844

Ho, S. M. (2003). Estrogen, progesterone and epithelial ovarian cancer. *Reprod. Biol. Endocrinol.* 1:73. doi: 10.1186/1477-7827-1-73

Hu, K., Zhong, G., and He, F. (2005). Expression of estrogen receptors ERalpha and ERbeta in endometrial hyperplasia and adenocarcinoma. *Int. J. Gynecol. Cancer* 15, 537–541. doi: 10.1111/j.1525-1438.2005.15321.x

Imai, Y., Asada, S., Tsukahara, S., Ishikawa, E., Tsuruo, T., and Sugimoto, Y. (2003). Breast cancer resistance protein exports sulfated estrogens but not free estrogens. *Mol. Pharmacol.* 64, 610–618. doi: 10.1124/mol.64.3.610

Ishikawa, T., and Nakagawa, H. (2009). Human ABC transporter ABCG2 in cancer chemotherapy and pharmacogenomics. *J. Exp. Ther. Oncol.* 8, 5–24.

Jasonni, V. M., Bulletti, C., Franceschetti, F., Bonavia, M., Bolelli, G., Ciotti, P., et al. (1984). Estrone sulphate plasma levels in postmenopausal women with and without endometrial cancer. *Cancer* 53(12), 2698–2700. doi: 10.1002/1097-0142(19840615)53:12<2698::AID-CNCR2820531223>3.0.CO;2-O

Jenabi, E., and Poorolajal, J. (2015). The effect of body mass index on endometrial cancer: a meta-analysis. *Public Health* 129, 872–880. doi: 10.1016/j.puhe.2015.04.017

Jeon, S. Y., Hwang, K. A., and Choi, K. C. (2016). Effect of steroid hormones, estrogen and progesterone, on epithelial mesenchymal transition in ovarian cancer development. *J. Steroid Biochem. Mol. Biol.* 158, 1–8. doi: 10.1016/j.jsbmb.2016.02.005

Kalliokoski, A., and Niemi, M. (2009). Impact of OATP transporters on pharmacokinetics. *Br. J. Pharmacol.* 158, 693–705. doi: 10.1111/j.1476-5381.2009.00430.x

Kandoth, C., Schultz, N., Cherniack, A. D., Akbani, R., Liu, Y., Shen, H., et al. (2013). Integrated genomic characterization of endometrial carcinoma. *Nature* 497, 67–73. doi: 10.1038/nature12113

Keefe, C. C., Goldman, M. M., Zhang, K., Clarke, N., Reitz, R. E., and Welt, C. K. (2014). Simultaneous measurement of thirteen steroid hormones in women with polycystic ovary syndrome and control women using liquid chromatography-tandem mass spectrometry. *PLoS ONE* 9:e93805. doi: 10.1371/journal.pone.0093805

Key, T., Appleby, P., Barnes, I., Reeves, G., and Group, E. H. A. B. C. C. (2002). Endogenous sex hormones and breast cancer in postmenopausal women: reanalysis of nine prospective studies. *J. Natl. Cancer Inst.* 94, 606–616. doi: 10.1093/jnci/94.8.606

Kobayashi, Y., Ohshiro, N., Sakai, R., Ohbayashi, M., Kohyama, N., and Yamamoto, T. (2005). Transport mechanism and substrate specificity of human organic anion transporter 2 (hOat2 [SLC22A7]). *J. Pharm. Pharmacol.* 57, 573–578. doi: 10.1211/0022357055966

Koepsell, H. (2013). The SLC22 family with transporters of organic cations, anions and zwitterions. *Mol. Aspects Med.* 34, 413–435. doi: 10.1016/j.mam.2012.10.010

Kovacsics, D., Patik, I., and Ozvegy-Laczka, C. (2016). The role of organic anion transporting polypeptides in drug absorption, distribution, excretion and drug-drug interactions. *Expert Opin. Drug Metab. Toxicol.* 13, 409–424. doi: 10.1080/17425255.2017.1253679

Kreuzinger, C., Gamperl, M., Wolf, A., Heinze, G., Geroldinger, A., Lambrechts, D., et al. (2015). Molecular characterization of 7 new established cell lines from high grade serous ovarian cancer. *Cancer Lett.* 362, 218–228. doi: 10.1016/j.canlet.2015.03.040

Kruh, G. D., Guo, Y., Hopper-Borge, E., Belinsky, M. G., and Chen, Z. S. (2007). ABCC10, ABCC11, and ABCC12. *Pflugers Arch.* 453, 675–684. doi: 10.1007/s00424-006-0114-1

Kullak-Ublick, G. A., Fisch, T., Oswald, M., Hagenbuch, B., Meier, P. J., Beuers, U., et al. (1998). Dehydroepiandrosterone sulfate (DHEAS): identification of a carrier protein in human liver and brain. *FEBS Lett.* 424, 173–176. doi: 10.1016/S0014-5793(98)00168-9

Kullak-Ublick, G. A., Ismair, M. G., Stieger, B., Landmann, L., Huber, R., Pizzagalli, F., et al. (2001). Organic anion-transporting polypeptide B (OATP-B) and its functional comparison with three other OATPs of human liver. *Gastroenterology* 120, 525–533. doi: 10.1053/gast.2001.21176

Kunicka, T., and Soucek, P. (2014). Importance of ABCC1 for cancer therapy and prognosis. *Drug Metab. Rev.* 46, 325–342. doi: 10.3109/03602532.2014.901348

Labrie, F. (1991). Intracrinology. *Mol. Cell. Endocrinol.* 78, C113–C118. doi: 10.1016/0303-7207(91)90116-A

Labrie, F. (2003). Extragonadal synthesis of sex steroids: intracrinology. *Ann. Endocrinol.* 64, 95–107.

Labrie, F., Bélanger, A., Bélanger, P., Bérubé, R., Martel, C., Cusan, L., et al. (2006). Androgen glucuronides, instead of testosterone, as the new markers of androgenic activity in women. *J. Steroid Biochem. Mol. Biol.* 99, 182–188. doi: 10.1016/j.jsbmb.2006.02.004

Labrie, F., Bélanger, A., Luu-The, V., Labrie, C., Simard, J., Cusan, L., et al. (1998). DHEA and the intracrine formation of androgens and estrogens in peripheral target tissues: its role during aging. *Steroids* 63, 322–328. doi: 10.1016/S0039-128X(98)00007-5

Labrie, F., Cusan, L., Gomez, J. L., Martel, C., Bérubé, R., Bélanger, P., et al. (2009). Comparable amounts of sex steroids are made outside the gonads in men and women: strong lesson for hormone therapy of prostate and breast cancer. *J. Steroid Biochem. Mol. Biol.* 113, 52–56. doi: 10.1016/j.jsbmb.2008.11.004

Labrie, F., Diamond, P., Cusan, L., Gomez, J. L., Bélanger, A., and Candas, B. (1997). Effect of 12-month dehydroepiandrosterone replacement therapy on bone, vagina, and endometrium in postmenopausal women. *J. Clin. Endocrinol. Metab.* 82, 3498–3505. doi: 10.1210/jcem.82.10.4306

Labrie, F., Ke, Y., Gonthier, R., and Bélanger, A. (2015). Letter to the editor: superior mass spectrometry-based estrogen assays should replace immunoassays. *J. Clin. Endocrinol. Metab.* 100, L86–L87. doi: 10.1210/jc.2015-2930

Lancaster, C. S., Sprowl, J. A., Walker, A. L., Hu, S., Gibson, A. A., and Sparreboom, A. (2013). Modulation of OATP1B-type transporter function alters cellular uptake and disposition of platinum chemotherapeutics. *Mol. Cancer Ther.* 12, 1537–1544. doi: 10.1158/1535-7163.MCT-12-0926

Langdon, S. P., Gourley, C., Gabra, H., and Stanley, B. (2017). Endocrine therapy in epithelial ovarian cancer. *Expert Rev. Anticancer Ther.* 17, 109–117. doi: 10.1080/14737140.2017.1272414

Lee, E., Hsu, C., Haiman, C. A., Razavi, P., Horn-Ross, P. L., Van Den Berg, D., et al. (2010). Genetic variation in the progesterone receptor gene and risk of endometrial cancer: a haplotype-based approach. *Carcinogenesis* 31, 1392–1399. doi: 10.1093/carcin/bgq113

Lee, W., Glaeser, H., Smith, L. H., Roberts, R. L., Moeckel, G. W., Gervasini, G., et al. (2005). Polymorphisms in human organic anion-transporting polypeptide 1A2 (OATP1A2): implications for altered drug disposition and central nervous system drug entry. *J. Biol. Chem.* 280, 9610–9617. doi: 10.1074/jbc.M411092200

Lee, Y. J., Kusuhara, H., Jonker, J. W., Schinkel, A. H., and Sugiyama, Y. (2005). Investigation of efflux transport of dehydroepiandrosterone sulfate and mitoxantrone at the mouse blood-brain barrier: a minor role of breast cancer resistance protein. *J. Pharmacol. Exp. Ther.* 312, 44–52. doi: 10.1124/jpet.104.073320

Lépine, J., Audet-Walsh, E., Grégoire, J., Têtu, B., Plante, M., Ménard, V., et al. (2010). Circulating estrogens in endometrial cancer cases and their relationship with tissular expression of key estrogen biosynthesis and metabolic pathways. *J. Clin. Endocrinol. Metab.* 95, 2689–2698. doi: 10.1210/jc.2010-2648

Levin, E. R. (2011). Minireview: extranuclear steroid receptors: roles in modulation of cell functions. *Mol. Endocrinol.* 25, 377–384. doi: 10.1210/me.2010-0284

Li, Q., and Shu, Y. (2014). Role of solute carriers in response to anticancer drugs. *Mol. Cell. Ther.* 2:15. doi: 10.1186/2052-8426-2-15

Lukanova, A., Lundin, E., Micheli, A., Arslan, A., Ferrari, P., Rinaldi, S., et al. (2004). Circulating levels of sex steroid hormones and risk of endometrial cancer in postmenopausal women. *Int. J. Cancer* 108, 425–432. doi: 10.1002/ijc.11529

Lurie, G., Wilkens, L. R., Thompson, P. J., Shvetsov, Y. B., Matsuno, R. K., Carney, M. E., et al. (2011). Estrogen receptor beta rs1271572 polymorphism and invasive ovarian carcinoma risk: pooled analysis within the Ovarian Cancer Association Consortium. *PLoS ONE* 6:e20703. doi: 10.1371/journal.pone.0020703

Luu-The, V., and Labrie, F. (2010). The intracrine sex steroid biosynthesis pathways. *Prog. Brain Res.* 181, 177–192. doi: 10.1016/S0079-6123(08)81010-2

Maeda, K. (2015). Organic anion transporting polypeptide (OATP)1B1 and OATP1B3 as important regulators of the pharmacokinetics of substrate drugs. *Biol. Pharm. Bull.* 38, 155–168. doi: 10.1248/bpb.b14-00767

Manna, P. R., Molehin, D., and Ahmed, A. U. (2016). Dysregulation of Aromatase in breast, endometrial, and ovarian cancers: an overview of therapeutic strategies. *Prog. Mol. Biol. Transl. Sci.* 144, 487–537. doi: 10.1016/bs.pmbts.2016.10.002

Matsumoto, H., Tsuchiya, T., Yoshiura, K., Hayashi, T., Hidaka, S., Nanashima, A., et al. (2014). ABCC11/MRP8 expression in the gastrointestinal tract and a novel role for pepsinogen secretion. *Acta Histochem. Cytochem.* 47, 85–94. doi: 10.1267/ahc.13040

Mazumdar, M., Fournier, D., Zhu, D. W., Cadot, C., Poirier, D., and Lin, S. X. (2009). Binary and ternary crystal structure analyses of a novel inhibitor with 17beta-HSD type 1: a lead compound for breast cancer therapy. *Biochem. J.* 424, 357–366. doi: 10.1042/BJ20091020

Meyer zu Schwabedissen, H. E., Tirona, R. G., Yip, C. S., Ho, R. H., and Kim, R. B. (2008). Interplay between the nuclear receptor pregnane X receptor and the uptake transporter organic anion transporter polypeptide 1A2 selectively enhances estrogen effects in breast cancer. *Cancer Res.* 68, 9338–9347. doi: 10.1158/0008-5472.CAN-08-0265

Milewich, L., and Porter, J. C. (1987). *In situ* steroid sulfatase activity in human epithelial carcinoma cells of vaginal, ovarian, and endometrial origin. *J. Clin. Endocrinol. Metab.* 65, 164–169. doi: 10.1210/jcem-65-1-164

Modan, B., Ron, E., Lerner-Geva, L., Blumstein, T., Menczer, J., Rabinovici, J., et al. (1998). Cancer incidence in a cohort of infertile women. *Am. J. Epidemiol.* 147, 1038–1042. doi: 10.1093/oxfordjournals.aje.a009397

Modugno, F., Laskey, R., Smith, A. L., Andersen, C. L., Haluska, P., and Oesterreich, S. (2012). Hormone response in ovarian cancer: time to reconsider as a clinical target? *Endocr. Relat. Cancer* 19, R255–R279. doi: 10.1530/ERC-12-0175

Mueller, J. W., Gilligan, L. C., Idkowiak, J., Arlt, W., and Foster, P. A. (2015). The regulation of steroid action by sulfation and desulfation. *Endocr. Rev.* 36, 526–563. doi: 10.1210/er.2015-1036

Murali, R., Soslow, R. A., and Weigelt, B. (2014). Classification of endometrial carcinoma: more than two types. *Lancet Oncol.* 15, e268–e278. doi: 10.1016/S1470-2045(13)70591-6

Mylonas, I. (2010). Prognostic significance and clinical importance of estrogen receptor alpha and beta in human endometrioid adenocarcinomas. *Oncol. Rep.* 24, 385–393. doi: 10.3892/or_00000871

Nakamura, M., Kyo, S., Zhang, B., Zhang, X., Mizumoto, Y., Takakura, M., et al. (2010). Prognostic impact of CD133 expression as a tumor-initiating cell marker in endometrial cancer *Hum. Pathol.* 41, 1516–1529. doi: 10.1016/j.humpath.2010.05.006

Nakamura, M., Zhang, X., Mizumoto, Y., Maida, Y., Bono, Y., Takakura, M., et al. (2014). Molecular characterization of CD133+ cancer stem-like cells in endometrial cancer. *Int. J. Oncol.* 44, 669–677. doi: 10.3892/ijo.2013.2230

Nozaki, Y., Kusuhara, H., Kondo, T., Hasegawa, M., Shiroyanagi, Y., Nakazawa, H., et al. (2007). Characterization of the uptake of organic anion transporter (OAT) 1 and OAT3 substrates by human kidney slices. *J. Pharmacol. Exp. Ther.* 321, 362–369. doi: 10.1124/jpet.106.113076

Obaidat, A., Roth, M., and Hagenbuch, B. (2012). The expression and function of organic anion transporting polypeptides in normal tissues and in cancer. *Annu. Rev. Pharmacol. Toxicol.* 52, 135–151. doi: 10.1146/annurev-pharmtox-010510-100556

Ogane, N., Yasuda, M., Kameda, Y., Yokose, T., Kato, H., Itoh, A., et al. (2013). Prognostic value of organic anion transporting polypeptide 1B3 and copper transporter 1 expression in endometrial cancer patients treated with paclitaxel and carboplatin. *Biomed. Res.* 34, 143–151. doi: 10.2220/biomedres.34.143

Okuda, T., Saito, H., Sekizawa, A., Shimizu, Y., Akamatsu, T., Kushima, M., et al. (2001). Steroid sulfatase expression in ovarian clear cell adenocarcinoma: immunohistochemical study. *Gynecol. Oncol.* 82, 427–434. doi: 10.1006/gyno.2001.6322

Pan, Y., and Kao, M. S. (2010). Endometrioid ovarian carcinoma benefits from aromatase inhibitors: case report and literature review. *Curr. Oncol.* 17, 82–85. doi: 10.3747/co.v17i6.676

Park, S. H., Cheung, L. W., Wong, A. S., and Leung, P. C. (2008). Estrogen regulates Snail and Slug in the down-regulation of E-cadherin and induces metastatic potential of ovarian cancer cells through estrogen receptor alpha. *Mol. Endocrinol.* 22, 2085–2098. doi: 10.1210/me.2007-0512

Pathirage, N., Di Nezza, L. A., Salmonsen, L. A., Jobling, T., Simpson, E. R., and Clyne, C. D. (2006). Expression of aromatase, estrogen receptors, and their coactivators in patients with endometrial cancer. *Fertil. Steril.* 86, 469–472. doi: 10.1016/j.fertnstert.2005.12.057

Pautier, P., Lobbedez, F., Melchar, B., Kutarska, E., Hall, G., and Reed, N. (2012). A phase II multicentre randomized open-label study of oral steroid sulphatase (STS) inhibitor irosustat (BN83495) versus megestrol acetate (MA) in women with advanced/recurrent endometrial cancer. *AnnalsOncol.* 23(Suppl. 9), 329.

Pearce, C. L., Wu, A. H., Gayther, S. A., Bale, A. E., Beck, P. A., Beesley, J., et al. (2008). Progesterone receptor variation and risk of ovarian cancer is limited to the invasive endometrioid subtype: results from the Ovarian Cancer Association Consortium pooled analysis. *Br. J. Cancer* 98, 282–288. doi: 10.1038/sj.bjc.6604170

Pizzagalli, F., Varga, Z., Huber, R. D., Folkers, G., Meier, P. J., and St-Pierre, M. V. (2003). Identification of steroid sulfate transport processes in the human mammary gland. *J. Clin. Endocrinol. Metab.* 88, 3902–3912. doi: 10.1210/jc.2003-030174

Potischman, N., Hoover, R. N., Brinton, L. A., Siiteri, P., Dorgan, J. F., Swanson, C. A., et al. (1996). Case-control study of endogenous steroid hormones and endometrial cancer. *J. Natl. Cancer Inst.* 88, 1127–1135. doi: 10.1093/jnci/88.16.1127

Prat, J. (2015). Staging classification for cancer of the ovary, fallopian tube, and peritoneum: abridged republication of guidelines from the international Federation of Gynecology and Obstetrics (FIGO). *Obstet. Gynecol.* 126, 171–174. doi: 10.1097/AOG.0000000000000917

Prossnitz, E. R., and Barton, M. (2011). The G-protein-coupled estrogen receptor GPER in health and disease. *Nat. Rev. Endocrinol.* 7, 715–726. doi: 10.1038/nrendo.2011.122

Prossnitz, E. R., Arterburn, J. B., Smith, H. O., Oprea, T. I., Sklar, L. A., and Hathaway, H. J. (2008). Estrogen signaling through the transmembrane G protein-coupled receptor GPR30. *Annu. Rev. Physiol.* 70, 165–190. doi: 10.1146/annurev.physiol.70.113006.100518

Ramalingam, P. (2016). Morphologic, immunophenotypic, and molecular features of epithelial ovarian cancer. *Oncology* 30, 166–176.

Ren, X., Wu, X., Hillier, S. G., Fegan, K. S., Critchley, H. O., Mason, J. I., et al. (2015). Local estrogen metabolism in epithelial ovarian cancer suggests novel targets for therapy. *J. Steroid Biochem. Mol. Biol.* 150, 54–63. doi: 10.1016/j.jsbmb.2015.03.010

Rižner, T. L. (2013). Estrogen biosynthesis, phase I and phase II metabolism, and action in endometrial cancer. *Mol. Cell. Endocrinol.* 381, 124–139. doi: 10.1016/j.mce.2013.07.026

Rižner, T. L. (2016). The important roles of steroid sulfatase and sulfotransferases in gynecological diseases. *Front. Pharmacol.* 7:30. doi: 10.3389/fphar.2016.00030

Rizner, T. L., Smuc, T., Rupreht, R., Sinkovec, J., and Penning, T. M. (2006). AKR1C1 and AKR1C3 may determine progesterone and estrogen ratios in endometrial cancer. *Mol. Cell. Endocrinol.* 248, 126–135. doi: 10.1016/j.mce.2005.10.009

Rojas, V., Hirshfield, K. M., Ganesan, S., and Rodriguez-Rodriguez, L. (2016). Molecular characterization of epithelial ovarian cancer: implications for diagnosis and treatment. *Int. J. Mol. Sci.* 17:2113. doi: 10.3390/ijms171 22113

Romero-Sánchez, M., Peiper, S. C., Evans, B., Wang, Z., Catasús, L., Ribe, A., et al. (2008). Expression profile of heptahelical putative membrane progesterone receptors in epithelial ovarian tumors. *Hum. Pathol.* 39, 1026–1033. doi: 10.1016/j.humpath.2007.11.007

Roth, M., Obaidat, A., and Hagenbuch, B. (2012). OATPs, OATs and OCTs: the organic anion and cation transporters of the SLCO and SLC22A gene superfamilies. *Br. J. Pharmacol.* 165, 1260–1287. doi: 10.1111/j.1476-5381.2011.01724.x

Rutherford, T., Brown, W. D., Sapi, E., Aschkenazi, S., Muñoz, A., and Mor, G. (2000). Absence of estrogen receptor-β expression in metastatic ovarian cancer. *Obstet. Gynecol.* 96, 417–421. doi: 10.1016/S0029-7844(00)00917-0

Ryan, A. J., Susil, B., Jobling, T. W., and Oehler, M. K. (2005). Endometrial cancer. *Cell Tissue Res.* 322, 53–61. doi: 10.1007/s00441-005-1109-5

Saegusa, M., and Okayasu, I. (2000). Changes in expression of estrogen receptors alpha and beta in relation to progesterone receptor and pS2 status in normal and malignant endometrium. *Jpn. J. Cancer Res.* 91, 510–518. doi: 10.1111/j.1349-7006.2000.tb00975.x

Sakaguchi, H., Fujimoto, J., Aoki, I., Toyoki, H., Khatun, S., and Tamaya, T. (2002). Expression of oestrogen receptor alpha and beta in uterine endometrial and ovarian cancers. *Eur. J. Cancer* 38(Suppl. 6), S74–S75. doi: 10.1016/S0959-8049(02)00296-4

Samojlik, E., Veldhuis, J. D., Wells, S. A., and Santen, R. J. (1980). Preservation of androgen secretion during estrogen suppression with aminoglutethimide in the treatment of metastatic breast carcinoma. *J. Clin. Invest.* 65, 602–612. doi: 10.1172/JCI109705

Sanderson, P. A., Critchley, H. O., Williams, A. R., Arends, M. J., and Saunders, P. T. (2017). New concepts for an old problem: the diagnosis of endometrial hyperplasia. *Hum. Reprod. Update* 23, 232–254. doi: 10.1093/humupd/dmw042

Sarkadi, B., Homolya, L., Szakacs, G., and Varadi, A. (2006). Human multidrug resistance ABCB and ABCG transporters: participation in a chemoimmunity defense system. *Physiol. Rev.* 86, 1179–1236. doi: 10.1152/physrev.00037.2005

Scharl, A., and Salterberg, A. (2016). Significance of ovarian function suppression in endocrine therapy for breast cancer in pre-menopausal women. *Geburtshilfe Frauenheilkd* 76, 516–524. doi: 10.1055/s-0042-106389

Schinkel, A. H., and Jonker, J. W. (2003). Mammalian drug efflux transporters of the ATP binding cassette (ABC) family: an overview. *Adv. Drug Deliv. Rev.* 55, 3–29. doi: 10.1016/S0169-409X(02)00169-2

Secky, L., Svoboda, M., Klameth, L., Bajna, E., Hamilton, G., Zeillinger, R., et al. (2013). The sulfatase pathway for estrogen formation: targets for the treatment and diagnosis of hormone-associated tumors. *J. Drug Deliv.* 2013:957605. doi: 10.1155/2013/957605

Setiawan, V. W., Yang, H. P., Pike, M. C., McCann, S. E., Yu, H., Xiang, Y. B., et al. (2013). Type I and II endometrial cancers: have they different risk factors?. *J. Clin. Oncol.* 31, 2607–2618. doi: 10.1200/JCO.2012.48.2596

Seward, D. J., Koh, A. S., Boyer, J. L., and Ballatori, N. (2003). Functional complementation between a novel mammalian polygenic transport complex and an evolutionarily ancient organic solute transporter, OSTalpha-OSTbeta. *J. Biol. Chem.* 278, 27473–27482. doi: 10.1074/jbc.M301106200

Sharom, F. J. (2014). Complex interplay between the p-glycoprotein multidrug efflux pump and the membrane: its role in modulating protein function. *Front. Oncol.* 4:41. doi: 10.3389/fonc.2014.00041

Simmen, F. A., Su, Y., Xiao, R., Zeng, Z., and Simmen, R. C. (2008). The Krüppel-like factor 9 (KLF9) network in HEC-1-A endometrial carcinoma cells suggests the carcinogenic potential of dys-regulated KLF9 expression. *Reprod. Biol. Endocrinol.* 6:41. doi: 10.1186/1477-7827-6-41

Sinreih, M., Hevir, N., and Rižner, T. L. (2013). Altered expression of genes involved in progesterone biosynthesis, metabolism and action in endometrial cancer. *Chem. Biol. Interact.* 202, 210–217. doi: 10.1016/j.cbi.2012.11.012

Slot, A. J., Molinski, S. V., and Cole, S. P. (2011). Mammalian multidrug-resistance proteins (MRPs). *Essays Biochem.* 50, 179–207. doi: 10.1042/bse0500179

Smith, I. E., and Dowsett, M. (2003). Aromatase inhibitors in breast cancer. *N. Engl. J. Med.* 348, 2431–2442. doi: 10.1056/NEJMra023246

Smuc, T., and Rizner, T. L. (2009). Aberrant pre-receptor regulation of estrogen and progesterone action in endometrial cancer. *Mol. Cell. Endocrinol.* 301, 74–82. doi: 10.1016/j.mce.2008.09.019

Smuc, T., Rupreht, R., Sinkovec, J., Adamski, J., and Rizner, T. L. (2006). Expression analysis of estrogen-metabolizing enzymes in human endometrial cancer. *Mol. Cell. Endocrinol.* 248, 114–117. doi: 10.1016/j.mce.2005.10.013

Stanway, S. J., Delavault, P., Purohit, A., Woo, L. W., Thurieau, C., Potter, B. V., et al. (2007). Steroid sulfatase: a new target for the endocrine therapy of breast cancer. *Oncologist* 12, 370–374. doi: 10.1634/theoncologist.12-4-370

Stieger, B., and Hagenbuch, B. (2014). Organic anion-transporting polypeptides. *Curr. Top. Membr.* 73, 205–232. doi: 10.1016/B978-0-12-800223-0.00005-0

Sugawara, T., Nomura, E., and Fujimoto, S. (2004). Expression of enzyme associated with steroid hormone synthesis and local production of steroid hormone in endometrial carcinoma cells. *J. Endocrinol.* 180, 135–144. doi: 10.1677/joe.0.1800135

Suzuki, T., Miki, Y., Nakamura, Y., Moriya, T., Ito, K., Ohuchi, N., et al. (2005). Sex steroid-producing enzymes in human breast cancer. *Endocr. Relat. Cancer* 12, 701–720. doi: 10.1677/erc.1.00834

Svoboda, M., Wlcek, K., Taferner, B., Hering, S., Stieger, B., Tong, D., et al. (2011). Expression of organic anion-transporting polypeptides 1B1 and 1B3 in ovarian cancer cells: relevance for paclitaxel transport. *Biomed. Pharmacother.* 65, 417–426. doi: 10.1016/j.biopha.2011.04.031

Szakacs, G., Varadi, A., Ozvegy-Laczka, C., and Sarkadi, B. (2008). The role of ABC transporters in drug absorption, distribution, metabolism, excretion and toxicity (ADME-Tox). *Drug Discov. Today* 13, 379–393. doi: 10.1016/j.drudis.2007.12.010

Tamai, I., Nezu, J., Uchino, H., Sai, Y., Oku, A., Shimane, M., et al. (2000). Molecular identification and characterization of novel members of the human organic anion transporter (OATP) family. *Biochem. Biophys. Res. Commun.* 273, 251–260. doi: 10.1006/bbrc.2000.2922

Tamai, I., Nozawa, T., Koshida, M., Nezu, J., Sai, Y., and Tsuji, A. (2001). Functional characterization of human organic anion transporting polypeptide B (OATP-B) in comparison with liver-specific OATP-C. *Pharm. Res.* 18, 1262–1269. doi: 10.1023/A:1013077609227

Tashiro, A., Tatsumi, S., Takeda, R., Naka, A., Matsuoka, H., Hashimoto, Y., et al. (2014). High expression of organic anion transporter 2 and organic cation transporter 2 is an independent predictor of good outcomes in patients with metastatic colorectal cancer treated with FOLFOX-based chemotherapy. *Am. J. Cancer Res.* 4, 528–536.

Thakkar, N., Lockhart, A. C., and Lee, W. (2015). Role of organic anion-transporting polypeptides (OATPs) in cancer therapy. *AAPS J.* 17, 535–545. doi: 10.1208/s12248-015-9740-x

Thomas, C., and Gustafsson, J.-Å. (2011). The different roles of ER subtypes in cancer biology and therapy. *Nat. Rev. Cancer* 11, 597–608. doi: 10.1038/nrc3093

Thomas, M. P., and Potter, B. V. (2015). Estrogen O-sulfamates and their analogues: clinical steroid sulfatase inhibitors with broad potential. *J. Steroid Biochem. Mol. Biol.* 153, 160–169. doi: 10.1016/j.jsbmb.2015.03.012

Traboulsi, T., El Ezzy, M., Gleason, J. L., and Mader, S. (2017). Antiestrogens: structure-activity relationships and use in breast cancer treatment. *J. Mol. Endocrinol.* 58, R15–R31. doi: 10.1530/JME-16-0024

Ugele, B., St-Pierre, M. V., Pihusch, M., Bahn, A., and Hantschmann, P. (2003). Characterization and identification of steroid sulfate transporters of human placenta. *Am. J. Physiol. Endocrinol. Metab.* 284, E390–E398. doi: 10.1152/ajpendo.00257.2002

Wan, J., Gao, Y., Zeng, K., Yin, Y., Zhao, M., Wei, J., et al. (2016). The levels of the sex hormones are not different between type 1 and type 2 endometrial cancer. *Sci. Rep.* 6:39744. doi: 10.1038/srep39744

Ween, M. P., Armstrong, M. A., Oehler, M. K., and Ricciardelli, C. (2015). The role of ABC transporters in ovarian cancer progression and chemoresistance. *Crit. Rev. Oncol. Hematol.* 96, 220–256. doi: 10.1016/j.critrevonc.2015.05.012

Wlcek, K., Svoboda, M., Thalhammer, T., Sellner, F., Krupitza, G., and Jaeger, W. (2008). Altered expression of organic anion transporter polypeptide (OATP) genes in human breast carcinoma. *Cancer Biol. Ther.* 7, 1450–1455. doi: 10.4161/cbt.7.9.6282

Woo, L. W., Jackson, T., Putey, A., Cozier, G., Leonard, P., Acharya, K. R., et al. (2010). Highly potent first examples of dual aromatase-steroid sulfatase inhibitors based on a biphenyl template. *J. Med. Chem.* 53, 2155–2170. doi: 10.1021/jm901705h

Yamaguchi, H., Sugie, M., Okada, M., Mikkaichi, T., Toyohara, T., Abe, T., et al. (2010). Transport of estrone 3-sulfate mediated by organic anion transporter OATP4C1: estrone 3-sulfate binds to the different recognition site for digoxin in OATP4C1. *Drug Metab. Pharmacokinet.* 25, 314–317. doi: 10.2133/dmpk.25.314

Yasui, T., Matsui, S., Tani, A., Kunimi, K., Yamamoto, S., and Irahara, M. (2012). Androgen in postmenopausal women. *J. Med. Invest.* 59, 12–27. doi: 10.2152/jmi.59.12

Yeramian, A., Moreno-Bueno, G., Dolcet, X., Catasus, L., Abal, M., Colas, E., et al. (2013). Endometrial carcinoma: molecular alterations involved in tumor development and progression. *Oncogene* 32, 403–413. doi: 10.1038/onc.2012.76

Zakharov, V., Lin, H. K., Azzarello, J., McMeekin, S., Moore, K. N., Penning, T. M., et al. (2010). Suppressed expression of type 2 3alpha/type 5 17beta-hydroxysteroid dehydrogenase (AKR1C3) in endometrial hyperplasia and carcinoma. *Int. J. Clin. Exp. Pathol.* 3, 608–617.

Zannoni, G. F., Monterossi, G., De Stefano, I., Gargini, A., Salerno, M. G., Farulla, I., et al. (2013). The expression ratios of estrogen receptor alpha (ERalpha) to estrogen receptor beta1 (ERbeta1) and ERalpha to ERbeta2 identify poor clinical outcome in endometrioid endometrial cancer. *Hum. Pathol.* 44, 1047–1054. doi: 10.1016/j.humpath.2012.09.007

Zelcer, N., Reid, G., Wielinga, P., Kuil, A., van der Heijden, I., Schuetz, J. D., et al. (2003). Steroid and bile acid conjugates are substrates of human multidrug-resistance protein (MRP) 4 (ATP-binding cassette C4). *Biochem. J.* 371(Pt 2), 361–367. doi: 10.1042/bj20021886

Zhang, S., Balch, C., Chan, M. W., Lai, H. C., Matei, D., Schilder, J. M., et al. (2008). Identification and characterization of ovarian cancer-initiating cells from primary human tumors. *Cancer Res.* 68, 4311–4320. doi: 10.1158/0008-5472.CAN-08-0364

Zhao, M., and Ramaswamy, B. (2014). Mechanisms and therapeutic advances in the management of endocrine-resistant breast cancer. *World J. Clin. Oncol.* 5, 248–262. doi: 10.5306/wjco.v5.i3.248

Zhou, N., Han, S. Y., Zhou, F., and Li, P. P. (2014). Anti-tumor effect of Shu-Gan-Liang-Xue decoction in breast cancer is related to the inhibition of aromatase and steroid sulfatase expression. *J. Ethnopharmacol.* 154, 687–695. doi: 10.1016/j.jep.2014.04.045

2

Steroidal Pyrimidines and Dihydrotriazines as Novel Classes of Anticancer Agents against Hormone-Dependent Breast Cancer Cells

Alexander M. Scherbakov[1], Alexander V. Komkov[2], Anna S. Komendantova[2], Margarita A. Yastrebova[1], Olga E. Andreeva[1], Valerii Z. Shirinian[2], Alakananda Hajra[3], Igor V. Zavarzin[2] and Yulia A. Volkova[2*]*

[1] Department of Experimental Tumor Biology, N.N. Blokhin National Medical Research Center of Oncology, Moscow, Russia, [2] N.D. Zelinsky Institute of Organic Chemistry, Russian Academy of Sciences, Moscow, Russia, [3] Department of Chemistry, Visva-Bharati University, Santiniketan, India

Correspondence:
Alexander M. Scherbakov
alex.scherbakov@gmail.com
Yulia A. Volkova
yavolkova@gmail.com

Most breast and prostate tumors are hormone-dependent, making it possible to use hormone therapy in patients with these tumors. The design of effective endocrine drugs that block the growth of tumors and have no severe side effects is a challenge. Thereupon, synthetic steroids are promising therapeutic drugs for the treatment of diseases such as hormone-dependent breast and prostate cancers. Here, we describe novel series of steroidal pyrimidines and dihydrotriazines with anticancer activities. A flexible approach to unknown pyrimidine and dihydrotriazine derivatives of steroids with selective control of the heterocyclization pattern is disclosed. A number of 18-nor-5α-androsta-2,13-diene[3,2-d]pyrimidine, androsta-2-ene[3,2-d]pyrimidine, $\Delta^{1,3,5(10)}$-estratrieno[16,17-d]pyrimidine, and 17-chloro-16-dihydrotriazine steroids were synthesized by condensations of amidines with β-chlorovinyl aldehydes derived from natural hormones. The synthesized compounds were screened for cytotoxicity against breast cancer cells and showed IC_{50} values of 7.4 μM and higher. Compounds were tested against prostate cancer cells and exhibited antiproliferative activity with IC_{50} values of 9.4 μM and higher comparable to that of cisplatin. Lead compound **4a** displayed selectivity in ERα-positive breast cancer cells. At 10 μM concentration, this heterosteroid inhibited 50% of the E2-mediated ERα activity and led to partial ERα down-regulation. The ERα reporter assay and immunoblotting were supported by the docking study, which showed the probable binding mode of compound **4a** to the estrogen receptor pocket. Thus, heterosteroid **4a** proved to be a selective ERα modulator with the highest antiproliferative activity against hormone-dependent breast cancer and can be considered as a candidate for further anticancer drug development. In total, the synthesized heterosteroids may be considered as new promising classes of active anticancer agents.

Keywords: heterosteroids, steroidal pyrimidines, steroidal dihydrotriazines, breast cancer, prostate cancer, estrogen receptor α, anticancer drugs

INTRODUCTION

Breast cancer is the most common cancer in women worldwide, with more than 1.5 million new cases recorded every year; it is also the fifth highest cause of cancer death (Nathan and Schmid, 2017). Estrogens are steroid hormones that play a critical role in the regulation of growth, differentiation, and metabolism of mammary cells, including malignant cells. Due to the ability of estrogens to significantly stimulate the growth of mammary cells, these hormones are involved in the progression of breast cancer. For more than 40 years, the antiestrogen tamoxifen (ICI 46474) is considered as the absolute leader in the endocrine therapy of hormone-dependent breast cancers (Jameera Begam et al., 2017). Tamoxifen belongs to selective estrogen receptor modulators (SERMs) (Cosman and Lindsay, 1999; Jameera Begam et al., 2017), which, in certain circumstances, perform the role of estrogen agonists or antagonists and modulate the effect of hormones in the target cells; otherwise, SERMs are also called estrogen agonists/antagonists. Due to convenient dosage forms for oral use, high efficiency, and low cost of the prolonged course of therapy, tamoxifen is considered as the "gold standard" for the treatment of patients with ERα-positive breast cancer. On the other hand, the effectiveness of tamoxifen may be limited by the development of resistance, an increased risk of endometrial cancer, and individual drug intolerance (Scherbakov et al., 2006; Ali et al., 2016; Traboulsi et al., 2017). This is why the development of novel classes of agents that effectively inhibit the growth of ERα-positive tumors and have no severe side effects is a challenge (Tryfonidis et al., 2016).

Synthetic steroids encompass a wide range of compounds with various specific anticancer activities, e.g., aromatase inhibitors such as formestane and exemestane (Carlini et al., 2001), antiproliferative agents such as 2-methoxyestradiol (Lakhani et al., 2003), androgen signaling inhibitors such as galeterone and abiraterone (Bryce and Ryan, 2012), the SERM compound PSK3471, the steroid sulfatase inhibitor EMATE (Purohit and Foster, 2012), and the selective estrogen receptor degrader (SERD) fulvestrant (Nathan and Schmid, 2017; **Figure 1**).

Aromatase and steroid sulfatase inhibitors, SERDs, and SERMs synthetically derived from natural hormones are of great interest for the development of new breast cancer treatment regimens, especially for metastatic forms of the disease (Singer et al., 2006; Scherbakov et al., 2013; Secky et al., 2013; Boer, 2017; Kaklamani and Gradishar, 2017). Fulvestrant is an estrogen receptor degrader that binds with high selectivity to target cells, causes their degradation, resulting in the complete inhibition of the estrogen-mediated growth of breast cancer cells (Nathan and Schmid, 2017). First approved in the US in 2002, fulvestrant is not associated with tamoxifen-like agonist side effects, is not cross-resistant to tamoxifen or exemestane, and produces very high response rates in breast cancer patients. A combination of fulvestrant with other drugs seems to be very promising. In this regards, the combination of anastrozole and fulvestrant is superior to anastrozole alone or sequential anastrozole and fulvestrant for the treatment of ERα-positive metastatic breast cancer (Mehta et al., 2012).

In fulvestrant, the alkylsulfinyl moiety is attached to the endogenous estrogen receptor ligand, 17β-estradiol, at the 7-position, providing a structure similar to that of natural hormones but showing reverse biological activity. Recently, we have demonstrated that the modification of 17β-estradiol with imidazo[1,2-a]pyridine pendant at the 17α-position has the same effect (Rassokhina et al., 2016). 17α-Imidazopyridine-17β-methoxyestradiol showed remarkable effects as a selective ERα receptor modulator. In this study, we turned to an investigation of the structure—ERα-modulator activity relationship for two novel classes of heterosteroids possessing an *N*-heterocycle attached at the 16-position and fused to the A/D ring of the steroid core. We report the unique derivatives of the androstene and estrane series containing A/D-ring annulated pyrimidine or linked dihydrotriazine moieties. The antiproliferative potential of all synthesized compounds was evaluated in the MCF-7 and MDA-MB-231 breast cancer cell lines. The compounds were also tested toward two prostate cancer cell lines PC3 and 22Rv1. Taking into account activities of the compounds against hormone-dependent breast cancer ERα was analyzed as possible target for this series. Four compounds proved to be active as ERα antagonists. Steroidal dihydrotriazine **4a** was selected as the lead compound and analyzed by the ERα-reporter assay, immunoblotting, and docking simulation. Finally, the binding of compound **4a** to the estrogen receptor pocket was discussed using different docking models.

MATERIALS AND METHODS

Chemistry

General Information

NMR spectra were acquired on Bruker Avance 600 and 300 spectrometers at 293, 303, and 333 K; the chemical shifts δ were measured in ppm relative to the solvent (^{1}H: DMSO-d_6, δ 2.50 ppm; ^{13}C: DMSO-d_6, δ 39.50 ppm). Splitting patterns are designated as s, singlet; d, doublet; t, triplet; q, quartet; m, multiplet; dd, double doublet; ddd, double double doublet; dt, doublet triplet. The coupling constants (*J*) are in Hertz. The structures of compounds were established using 1D NMR (^{1}H, ^{13}C) and 2D NMR (^{1}H-^{1}H COSY, ^{13}C-^{1}H HMBC, ^{13}C-^{1}H HSQC) spectroscopy. Infrared spectra were measured on a FT-IR spectrometer in KBr pellets. High-resolution mass spectra (HRMS) were measured using electrospray ionization (ESI) in positive ion mode (interface capillary voltage 4,500 V); the mass range was from m/z 50 to 3,000 Da; external/internal calibration was performed using an electrospray calibrant solution. A syringe injection was used for solutions in CH_3CN (flow rate 3 ml/min). Nitrogen was applied as a dry gas and the interface temperature was set at 180°C. Melting points were measured on a Boetius capillary melting point apparatus and are uncorrected. Analytical thin-layer chromatography (TLC) was carried out on silica gel plates (silica gel 60 F254 aluminum supported plates); the visualization was accomplished with

Abbreviations: SERM, Selective estrogen receptor modulator; SERD, selective estrogen receptor degrader; ER, estrogen receptor; MTT, methylthiazolyldiphenyl-tetrazolium bromide; ERE, estrogen response element; DCC serum, dextran-coated charcoal-treated serum; AR, androgen receptor; E2, 17β-estradiol.

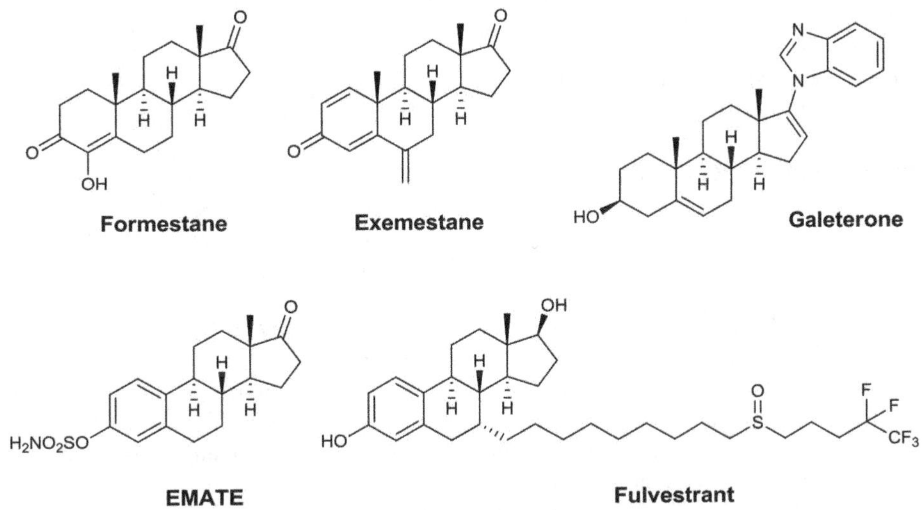

FIGURE 1 | Steroidal anticancer agents.

an UV lamp (254/365 nm) and using chemical staining with $[Ce(SO_4)_2/H_2SO_4]$. Column chromatography was performed on silica gel 60 (230–400 mesh, Merck). Androst-5-en-3β-ol-17-one-3β-acetate, 17β-hydroxy-5α-androstan-3-one, estrone, phosphorus oxychloride, guanidine salts, and acetimidamide hydrochloride were commercially available and were used as purchased. The spectroscopic data for steroidal chlorovinyl aldehydes **2a–c** are consistent with those reported previously (Komkov et al., 2015; Volkova et al., 2016). All reactions were carried out in freshly distilled and dry solvents.

3-Hydroxy-2′-methyl-$\Delta^{1,3,5(10)}$-estratrieno[17,16-d]pyrimidine (3a)

Chloro-16-formyl-$\Delta^{1,3,5(10)}$-estratetraen-3-ol **2a** (113 mg, 0.36 mmol) was added to a suspension of acetamidine hydrochloride (51 mg, 0.54 mmol) and potassium carbonate (120 mg, 0.89 mmol) in DMF (4 mL). The mixture was stirred at 80°C for 9 h until the complete conversion of the intermediates (TLC monitoring). The resulting mixture was cooled to room temperature and diluted with water (30 mL). The precipitate that formed was filtered, dried, and washed with water (3 × 5 mL). The product was isolated by column chromatography using petroleum ether/ethyl acetate, 1:1, to obtain colorless solid (34 mg, 30% yield). R_f 0.27 (petroleum ether:EtOAc, 1:2; visualized by UV light at 254 nm); m.p. 264–266°C. ^1H NMR (600 MHz, DMSO-d_6), δ: 0.92 (s, 3H, 18-CH_3), 1.35–1.41 (m, 1H, 7-CH_2), 1.50–1.56 (m, 1H, 11-CH_2), 1.61–1.69 (m, 2H, 8-CH_2, 12-CH_2), 1.70–1.76 (m, 1H, 14-CH), 1.90–1.95 (m, 1H, 7-CH), 2.14–2.18 (m, 1H, 12-CH_2), 2.21–2.27 (m, 1H, 9-CH), 2.37–2.42 (m, 1H, 11-CH_2), 2.48–2.54 (m, 1H, 15-CH_2), 2.56 (s, 3H, 2′-CH_3), 2.73–2.85 (m, 3H, 6-CH_2, 15-CH_2), 6.47 (s, 1H, 4-CH), 6.53 (dd, J = 2.4, 8.4 Hz, 1H, 2-CH), 7.07 (d, 1H, J = 8.4 Hz, 1-CH), 8.46 (s, 1H, 4-CH), 9.00 (br.s, 1H, OH). ^{13}C NMR (125 MHz, DMSO-d_6), δ: 17.1 (18-CH_3), 25.5 (2′-CH_3), 25.8 (11-CH_2), 26.9 (7-CH_2), 27.0 (15-CH_2), 28.9 (6-CH_2), 32.7 (12-CH_2), 37.2 (8-CH), 43.7 (9-CH), 45.8 (13-C), 54.3 (14-CH), 112.8 (2-CH), 115.0 (4-CH), 125.8 (1-CH), 130.1 (10-C), 130.5 (16-C), 137.0 (5-C), 151.8 (4′-CH), 155.0 (3-C), 165.1 (2′-C), 181.0 (17-C). IR (KBr), cm^{-1}: 3179 (OH), 2986, 2929, 2859 (CH), 1607, 1585, 1555, 1501 (C=C, C=N). HRMS (ESI) for $C_{21}H_{25}N_2O$ ($[M+H]^+$): calcd 321.1961, found 321.1951.

2′-Amino-3-hydroxy-$\Delta^{1,3,5}$(10)-estratrieno[17,16-d]pyrimidine (3b)

17-Chloro-16-formyl-$\Delta^{1,3,5(10)}$-estratetraen-3-ol **2a** (142 mg, 0.45 mmol) was added to a suspension of guanidine acetate (80 mg, 0.67 mmol) and potassium carbonate (180 mg, 1.34 mmol) in methanol (10 mL). The mixture was refluxed for 6 h until the complete conversion of the intermediates (TLC monitoring). The resulting mixture was cooled to room temperature and the solvent was removed under reduced pressure. The solid reside was washed with water (10 mL) and dried. The workup afforded the analytically pure product as colorless solid (129 mg, 89% yield). R_f 0.31 ($CHCl_3$:MeOH, 5:0.2; visualized by UV light at 254 nm). The spectral data are consistent with those reported by Forgo and Vincze (2002); m.p. 285–287°C [m.p.$_{lit}$ (Forgo and Vincze, 2002) = 284–286°C]. ^1H NMR (600 MHz, DMSO-d_6), δ: 0.89 (s, 3H, 18-CH_3), 1.32–1.36 (m, 1H, 7-CH_2), 1.45–1.50 (m, 1H, 11-CH_2), 1.54–1.64 (m, 2H, 8-CH_2, 12-CH_2), 1.65–1.68 (m, 1H, 14-CH), 1.86–1.90 (m, 1H, 7-CH_2), 2.03–2.08 (m, 1H, 12-CH_2), 2.20–2.25 (m, 1H, 9-CH), 2.31–2.38 (m, 2H, 11-CH_2, 15-CH_2), 2.62 (dd, J = 6.6, 14.4 Hz, 1H, 15-CH_2), 2.69 (dt, J = 5.4, 16.2 Hz, 1H, 6-CH_2), 2.77 (dt, J = 11.4, 16.2 Hz, 1H, 6-CH_2), 6.36 (br.s, 2H, NH_2), 6.40 (s, 1H, 4-CH), 6.45 (dd, J = 1.8, 8.4 Hz, 1H, 2-CH), 6.98 (d, 1H, J = 8.4 Hz, 1-CH), 8.00 (d, J = 1.8 Hz, 1H, 4-CH) (the signal of OH group was not observed in the ^1H NMR spectrum). ^{13}C NMR (125 MHz, DMSO-d_6), δ: 17.1 (CH_3), 26.0 (11-CH_2), 26.6 (15-CH_2), 27.1 (7-CH_2), 29.1 (6-CH_2), 32.9 (12-CH_2), 37.4 (8-CH), 43.9 (9-CH), 45.8 (13-C), 54.4 (14-CH), 113.5

(2-CH), 115.6 (4-CH), 121.0 (16-C), 125.6 (1-CH), 128.2 (10-C), 136.7 (5-C), 152.6 (4′-CH), 157.5 (3-C), 162.9 (2′-C), 182.0 (17-C). IR (KBr), cm^{-1}: 3361, 3181 (OH), 2930, 2858 (CH), 1637 (NH_2), 1608, 1560 (C=C, C=N). HRMS (ESI) for $C_{20}H_{24}N_3O$ ($[M+H]^+$): calcd 322.1914, found 322.1903.

3β-Acetoxy-3′-methyl-5-androsteno[17,16-d]pyrimidine (3c)

3β-Acetoxy-17-chloro-16-formylandrosta-5,16-diene **2b** (130 mg, 0.34 mmol) was added to a suspension of acetamidine hydrochloride (65 mg, 0.69 mmol) and potassium carbonate (190 mg, 1.36 mmol) in DMF (5 mL). The mixture was stirred at 80°C for 6.5 h until the complete conversion of the intermediates (TLC monitoring). The resulting mixture was cooled to room temperature and the solvent was removed under reduced pressure. The crude product was isolated by column chromatography using petroleum ether/ethyl acetate, 1:2, to obtain colorless solid (52 mg, 40% yield). R_f 0.47 (petroleum ether:EtOAc, 1:2; visualized by UV light at 254 nm). The spectral data are consistent with those reported by Gogoi et al. (2013). m.p. 169–171°C [m.p.$_{lit}$ (Gogoi et al., 2013) = 165–167°C]. ^1H NMR (600 MHz, DMSO-$d_{6\,at\,303K}$), δ: 0.91 (s, 3H, 18-CH_3), 1.05 (s, 3H, 19-CH_3), 1.07–1.13 (m, 2H, 1-CH_2, 9-CH), 1.49 (dt, J = 4.2, 12.6 Hz, 1H, 12-CH_2), 1.53–1.65 (m, 4H, 2-CH_2, 11-CH_2, 12-CH_2, 14-CH), 1.67–1.73 (m, 2H, 7-CH_2, 11-CH_2), 1.74–1.82 (m, 2H, 2-CH_2, 8-CH), 1.86 (dt, J = 3.6, 13.2 Hz, 1H, 1-CH_2), 1.99 (s, 3H, CH_3CO), 2.05–2.12 (m, 1H, 7-CH_2), 2.28–2.32 (m, 2H, 4-CH_2), 2.47 (dd, J = 15.0 Hz, 1H, 15-CH_2), 2.54 (s, 3H, 2′-CH_3), 2.72 (dd, J = 6.6,15.0 Hz, 1H, 15-CH_2), 4.43–4.48 (m, 1H, 3-CH), 5.39–5.40 (m, 1H, 6-CH), 8.43 (s, 1H, H-4′). ^{13}C NMR (125 MHz, DMSO-$d_{6\,at\,303K}$), δ: 16.7 (18-CH_3), 18.9 (19-CH_3), 20.0 (11-CH_2), 21.0 (CH_3), 25.4 (2′-CH_3), 27.3 (2-CH_2), 27.3 (15-CH_2), 30.1 (8-CH), 30.6 (7-CH_2), 32.4 (12-CH_2), 36.3 (10-C), 36.3 (1-CH_2), 37.7 (4-CH_2), 45.4 (13-C), 49.8 (9-CH), 55.0 (14-CH), 73.1 (3-CH), 121.6 (6-CH), 130.5 (16-C), 139.8 (5-C), 151.8 (4′-CH), 165.1 (2′-C), 169.7 (CO), 180.8 (17-C). IR (KBr), cm^{-1}: 2941, 2903, 2858 (CH), 1732 (CO), 1589, 1556 (C=C, C=N). HRMS (ESI) for $C_{24}H_{33}N_2O_2$ ($[M+H]^+$): calcd 381.2537, found 381.2535.

3β-Hydroxy-3′-methyl-5-androsteno[17,16-d]pyrimidine (3d)

A mixture of steroidal pyrimidine **3c** (50 mg, 0.13 mmol) and potassium carbonate (200 mg, 1.44 mmol) in MeOH (8 mL) was refluxed for 3 h until the complete conversion of the starting material (TLC monitoring). The resulting mixture was cooled to room temperature and the solvent was removed under reduced pressure. The crude product was washed with water (6 mL) and dried to get colorless solid (42 mg, 95% yield). R_f 0.28 ($CHCl_3$:MeOH, 5:0.1; visualized by UV light at 254 nm); m.p. 182–183°C. ^1H NMR (600 MHz, DMSO-d_6 + CCl_4), δ: 0.92 (s, 3H, 18-CH_3), 1.03 (s, 3H, 19-CH_3), 0.99–1.09 (m, 2H, 1-CH_2, 9-CH), 1.32–1.38 (m, 1H, 2-CH_2), 1.48 (dt, J = 4.2, 12.6 Hz, 1H, 12-CH_2), 1.50–1.55 (m, 1H, 14-CH), 1.58–1.73 (m, 4H, 2-CH_2, 7-CH_2, 11-CH_2), 1.74–1.82 (m, 2H, 1-CH_2, 8-CH), 2.04–2.19 (m, 4H, 4-CH_2, 7-CH_2, 12-CH_2), 2.46 (dd, J = 14.4 Hz, 1H, 15-CH_2), 2.55 (s, 3H, 2′-CH_3), 2.72 (dd, J = 14.4 Hz, 1H, 15-CH_2), 3.22–3.32 (m, 1H, 3-CH), 5.28–5.30 (m, 1H, 6-CH), 8.39 (s, 1H, H-4′) (the signal of OH group was not observed in the ^1H NMR spectrum). ^{13}C NMR (125 MHz, DMSO-d_6 + CCl_4), δ: 16.7 (18-CH_3), 19.1 (19-CH_3), 20.0 (11-CH_2), 25.3 (2′-CH_3), 27.4 (15-CH_2), 30.2 (8-CH), 30.7 (7-CH_2), 31.3 (2-CH_2), 32.5 (12-CH_2), 36.3 (10-C), 36.8 (1-CH_2), 42.2 (4-CH_2), 45.4 (13-C), 50.1 (9-CH), 55.2 (14-CH), 69.9 (3-CH), 119.8 (6-CH), 130.4 (16-C), 141.6 (5-C), 151.5 (4′-CH), 164.9 (2′-C), 180.7 (17-C). IR (KBr), cm^{-1}: 3378 (OH), 2965, 2938, 2858, 2818 (CH), 1599, 1554 (C=C, C=N). HRMS (ESI) for $C_{22}H_{31}N_2O$ ($[M+H]^+$): calcd 339.2431, found 339.2431.

2′-Amino-3β-hydroxy-5-androsteno[17,16-d]pyrimidine (3e)

3β-Acetoxy-17-chloro-16-formylandrosta-5,16-diene **2b** (122 mg, 0.32 mmol) was added to a suspension of guanidine acetate (58 mg, 0.48 mmol) and potassium carbonate (134 mg, 0.97 mmol) in methanol (10 mL). The resulting mixture was refluxed for 6 h until the complete conversion of the intermediates (TLC monitoring). The resulting mixture was cooled to room temperature. The precipitate that formed was filtered, washed with H_2O (5 mL), and dried. The workup afforded the analytically pure product as colorless solid (92 mg, 84% yield). R_f 0.56 ($CHCl_3$:MeOH, 5:0.2; visualized by UV light at 254 nm). The spectral data are consistent with those reported by Matsumoto et al. (2003). m.p. 342–344°C [m.p.$_{lit}$ (Matsumoto et al., 2003) = 308–312°C]. ^1H NMR (600 MHz, DMSO-$d_{6\,at\,333K}$), δ: 0.90 (s, 3H, 18-CH_3), 1.03 (s, 3H, 19-CH_3), 0.98–1.10 (m, 2H, 1-CH_2, 9-CH), 1.34–1.42 (m, 1H, 2-CH_2), 1.42–1.50 (m, 1H, 12-CH_2), 1.44–1.52 (m, 1H, 14-CH), 1.55–1.83 (m, 6H, 1-CH_2, 2-CH_2, 7-CH_2, 8-CH, 11-CH_2), 1.99–2.09 (m, 2H, 7-CH_2, 12-CH_2), 2.09–2.22 (m, 2H, 4-CH_2), 2.29 (dd, J = 6.0, 13.8 Hz, 1H, 15-CH_2), 2.55 (dd, J = 6.0, 13.8 Hz, 1H, 15-CH_2), 3.24–3.32 (m, 1H, 3-CH), 4.41 (br.s, 1H, OH), 5.30–5.32 (m, 1H, 6-CH), 6.11 (br.s, 2H, NH_2), 7.98 (s, 1H, H-4′). ^{13}C NMR (125 MHz, DMSO-$d_{6\,at\,333K}$), δ: 16.4 (18-CH_3), 18.8 (19-CH_3), 19.9 (11-CH_2), 26.6 (15-CH_2), 30.1 (7-CH_2), 30.5 (8-CH), 31.2 (2-CH_2), 32.5 (12-CH_2), 36.1 (10-C), 36.6 (1-CH_2), 42.0 (4-CH_2), 45.0 (13-C), 50.0 (9-CH), 55.1 (14-CH), 69.7 (3-CH), 119.6 (6-CH), 121.0 (16-C), 141.5 (5-C), 152.2 (4′-CH), 162.6 (2′-C), 181.5 (17-C). IR (KBr), cm^{-1}: 3535 (OH), 3368, 3314, 3159 (NH_2), 2935, 2893, 2844 (CH), 1647 (NH_2), 1608, 1559 (C=C, C=N). HRMS (ESI) for $C_{21}H_{30}N_3O$ ($[M+H]^+$): calcd 340.2383, found 340.2382. Anal. calcd for $C_{21}H_{29}N_3O$:C, 74.30; H, 8.6; N, 12.38. Found: C, 73.83; H, 8.65; N, 12.15.

2′-Amino-17β-hydroxy-5α-androstano[2,3-d]pyrimidine (3f)

3-Chloro-2-formyl-17β-formyloxy-5α-androstane **2c** (108 mg, 0.30 mmol) was added to a suspension of guanidine acetate (53 mg, 0.45 mmol) and potassium carbonate (124 mg, 0.90 mmol) in methanol (10 mL). The mixture was refluxed for 4 h until the complete conversion of the intermediates (TLC monitoring). The resulting mixture was cooled to room temperature. The precipitate that formed was filtered, washed with water (5 mL), and dried. The workup afforded analytically pure product as colorless solid (91 mg, 89% yield). R_f 0.67 ($CHCl_3$:MeOH, 5:0.2; visualized by UV light at 254 nm). The spectral data are consistent with those reported by

De Ruggieri et al. (1962). m.p. > 350°C (m.p.$_{lit}$ > 300°C). ^{1}H NMR (600 MHz, DMSO-d$_6$), δ: 0.68 (s, 3H, 18-CH$_3$), 0.69 (s, 3H, 19-CH$_3$), 0.78–0.84 (m, 1H, 9-CH), 0.86–0.95 (m, 2H, 7-CH$_2$, 14-CH), 0.98–1.06 (m, 1H, 12-CH$_2$), 1.14–1.29 (m, 2H, 6-CH$_2$, 15-CH$_2$), 1.32–1.42 (m, 3H, 8-CH, 11-CH$_2$, 16-CH$_2$), 1.49–1.56 (m, 3H, 5-CH, 6-CH$_2$, 15-CH$_2$), 1.58–1.64 (m, 1H, 11-CH$_2$), 1.64–1.70 (m, 1H, 7-CH$_2$), 1.77–1.82 (m, 1H, 12-CH$_2$), 1.83–1.89 (m, 1H, 16-CH$_2$), 2.16 (d, J = 15.6 Hz, 1H, 1-CH$_2$), 2.24 (dd, J = 12.6, 18.0 Hz, 1H, 4-CH$_2$), 2.43–2.56 (m, 2H, 4-CH$_2$, 1-CH$_2$), 3.47 (t, J = 8.4 Hz, 1H, 17-CH), 4.18 (br.s, 1H, OH), 5.90 (br.s, 2H, NH$_2$), 7.91 (s, 1H, H-4′). ^{13}C NMR (125 MHz, DMSO-d$_6$), δ: 10.8 (18-CH$_3$), 10.9 (19-CH$_3$), 20.2 (11-CH$_2$), 22.7 (15-CH$_2$), 27.8 (6-CH$_2$), 29.6 (16-CH$_2$), 30.5 (7-CH$_2$), 34.5 (10-C), 35.0 (8-CH), 35.2 (4-CH$_2$), 36.3 (12-CH$_2$), 38.4 (1-CH$_2$), 40.8 (5-CH), 42.1 (13-C), 50.4 (14-CH), 53.0 (9-CH), 79.8 (17-CH), 116.7 (2-C), 157.9 (4′-CH), 161.6 (2′-C), 164.2 (3-C). IR (KBr), cm^{-1}: 3322, 3169 (NH$_2$), 2969, 2923, 2905, 2849 (CH), 1659 (NH$_2$), 1596, 1561 (C=C, C=N). HRMS (ESI) for $C_{21}H_{32}N_3O$ ([M+H]$^+$): calcd 342.2540, found 342.2538.

16-(4,6-Dimethyl-1,2-dihydro-1,3,5-triazin-2-yl)-17-chloro-Δ$^{1,3,5(10),16}$-estratetraen-3-ol (4a)

17-Chloro-16-formyl-Δ$^{1,3,5(10)}$-estratetraen-3-ol **2a** (100 mg, 0.32 mmol) was added to a suspension of acetamidine hydrochloride (150 mg, 1.3 mmol) and potassium carbonate (260 mg, 1.92 mmol) in DMF (4 mL). The mixture was stirred at 80°C for 8 h until the complete conversion of the intermediates (TLC monitoring). The resulting mixture was cooled to room temperature and diluted with water (30 mL). The precipitate that formed was filtered and washed with water (5 mL) and hot benzene (5 mL). The workup afforded the analytically pure product as colorless solid (40 mg, 32% yield). R$_f$ 0.37 (petroleum ether:EtOAc, 1:2; visualized by UV light at 254 nm); m.p. 209–210°C. ^{1}H NMR (600 MHz, DMSO-d$_6$), δ: 0.84 (s, 3H, 18-CH$_3$), 1.30–1.36 (m, 1H, 7-CH$_2$), 1.37–1.50 (m, 3H, 8-CH, 11-CH$_2$, 12-CH$_2$), 1.58–1.62 (m, 1H, 14-CH), 1.75–1.83 (m, 2H, 7-CH$_2$, 12-CH$_2$), 1.80 (s, 3H, 4′-CH$_3$), 1.82 (s, 3H, 6′-CH$_3$), 1.95 (dd, J = 12.0, 14.4 Hz, 1H, 15-CH$_2$), 2.14 (dd, J = 6.6, 14.4 Hz, 1H, 15-CH$_2$), 2.18–2.22 (m, 1H, 9-CH), 2.31–2.36 (m, 1H, 11-CH$_2$), 2.68–2.78 (m, 2H, 6-CH$_2$), 5.35 (s, 1H, 2′-CH), 6.44 (d, J = 2.4 Hz, 1H, 4-CH), 6.51 (dd, 1H, J = 2.4, 9.0 Hz, 2-CH), 7.02 (d, 1H, J = 9.0 Hz, 1-CH), 9.03 (br.s, 1H), 9.37 (br.s, 1H). ^{13}C NMR (150 MHz, DMSO-d$_6$), δ: 15.0 (18-CH$_3$), 20.2 (4′-CH$_3$, 6′-CH$_3$), 25.8 (11-CH$_2$), 26.7 (7-CH$_2$), 28.9 (15-CH$_2$, 6-CH$_2$), 33.6 (12-CH$_2$), 36.9 (8-CH), 43.7 (9-CH), 47.9 (13-C), 53.1 (14-CH), 67.8 (2′-CH), 112.7 (2-CH), 115.0 (4-CH), 125.6 (1-CH), 130.2 (10-C), 135.4 (17-C), 137.0 (5-C), 138.6 (16-C), 151.6 (4′-C, 6′-C), 155.0 (3-C). IR (KBr), cm^{-1}: 3198 (NH), 2929, 2857 (CH), 1703, 1611 (C=C, C=N), 1499, 1456, 1435, 1378, 1287, 1248. HRMS (ESI) for $C_{23}H_{29}ClN_3O$ ([M+H]$^+$): calcd 398.1994, found 398.1995.

3β-Acetoxy-16-(4,6-dimethyl-1,2-dihydro-1,3,5-triazin-2-yl)-17-chloroandrosta-5,16-diene (4b)

3β-Acetoxy-17-chloro-16-formylandrosta-5,16-diene **2b** (100 mg, 0.26 mmol) was added to a suspension of acetamidine hydrochloride (125 mg, 1.3 mmol) and potassium carbonate (220 mg, 1.6 mmol) in DMF (4 mL). The mixture was stirred at 80°C for 8 h until the complete conversion of the intermediates (TLC monitoring). The resulting mixture was cooled to room temperature and diluted with water (30 mL). The precipitate that formed was filtered, washed with water (5 mL), and dried. The crude product was purified by column chromatography using chloroform/MeOH, 10:1, to obtain colorless solid (45 mg, 30% yield). R$_f$ 0.45 (petroleum ether:EtOAc, 1:2; visualized by UV light at 254 nm); m.p. 158–160°C. ^{1}H NMR (600 MHz, DMSO-d$_6$), δ: 0.84 (s, 3H, 18-CH$_3$), 1.01 (s, 3H, 19-CH$_3$), 1.02–1.11 (m, 2H, 1-CH$_2$, 9-CH), 1.32 (dt, J = 4.2, 12.6 Hz, 1H, 12-CH$_2$), 1.36–1.41 (m, 1H, 14-CH), 1.43–1.49 (m, 1H, 11-CH$_2$), 1.51–1.65 (m, 4H, 2-CH$_2$, 7-CH$_2$, 8-CH, 11-CH$_2$), 1.69–1.73 (m, 1H, 12-CH$_2$), 1.76–1.84 (m, 2H, 1-CH$_2$, 2-CH$_2$), 1.79 (s, 3H, 4′-CH$_3$), 1.81 (s, 3H, 6′-CH$_3$), 1.88 (dd, J = 14.4, 15.0 Hz, 1H, 15-CH$_2$), 1.92–1.97 (m, 1H, 7-CH$_2$), 1.98 (s, 3H, CH$_3$CO), 2.07 (dd, 1H, J = 6.6, 15.0 Hz, 15-CH$_2$), 2.26–2.31 (m, 2H, 4-CH$_2$), 4.42–4.48 (m, 1H, 3-CH), 5.32 (s, 1H, 2′-CH), 5.34–5.36 (m,1H, 6-CH), 9.40 (br.s, 1H, NH). ^{13}C NMR (125 MHz, DMSO-d$_6$), δ: 14.8 (18-CH$_3$), 18.8 (19-CH$_3$), 19.9 (11-CH$_2$), 20.3 (4′-CH$_3$, 6′-CH$_3$), 20.9 (CH$_3$COO), 27.3 (2-CH$_2$), 29.2 (15-CH$_2$), 29.9 (8-CH), 30.3 (7-CH$_2$), 33.4 (12-CH$_2$), 36.3 (1-CH$_2$), 36.3 (10-C), 37.6 (4-CH$_2$), 47.5 (13-C), 49.8 (9-CH), 53.6 (14-CH), 67.4 (2′-CH), 73.1 (3-CH), 121.8 (6-CH), 135.4 (17-C), 138.5 (16-C), 139.8 (5-C), 152.0 (4′-C, 6′-C), 169.7 (CO). IR (KBr), cm^{-1}: 3183 (NH), 2945, 2857 (CH), 1735 (COO),1704, 1629 (C=C, C=N). HRMS (ESI) for $C_{26}H_{37}ClN_3O_3$ ([M+H]$^+$): calcd 458.2569, found 458.2558.

17β-Hydroxy-2-(4,6-dimethyl-1,2-dihydro-1,3,5-triazin-2-yl)-3-chloro-5α-androstane (4c)

3-Chloro-2-formyl-17β-formyloxy-5α-androstane **2c** (120 mg, 0.34 mmol) was added to a suspension of acetamidine hydrochloride (160 mg, 1.69 mmol) and potassium carbonate (280 mg, 2.0 mmol) in DMF (5 mL). The mixture was stirred at 60–65°C for 6 h until the complete conversion of the intermediates (TLC monitoring). The resulting mixture was cooled to room temperature and the solvent was removed under reduced pressure. The product was purified by column chromatography using chloroform/MeOH, 6:1, to obtain colorless solid (41 mg, 29% yield). R$_f$ 0.30 (CHCl$_3$:MeOH, 5:0.3; visualized by UV light at 254 nm); m.p. 210–212°C. ^{1}H NMR (600 MHz, DMSO-d$_6$), δ: 0.62 (s, 3H, 18-CH$_3$), 0.68 (s, 3H, 19-CH$_3$), 0.65–0.71 (m, 1H, 9-CH), 0.78–0.88 (m, 2H, 7-CH$_2$, 14-CH), 0.90–0.96 (m, 1H, 12-CH$_2$), 1.11–1.18 (m, 2H, 6-CH$_2$, 15-CH$_2$), 1.22–1.39 (m, 5H, 8-CH, 11-CH$_2$, 16-CH$_2$), 1.40–1.50 (m, 3H, 5-CH, 6-CH$_2$, 15-CH$_2$), 1.60 (d, J = 12.0 Hz, 1H, 7-CH$_2$), 1.64 (d, J = 16.8 Hz, 1H, 1-CH$_2$), 1.71 (d, J = 12.6 Hz, 1H, 12-CH$_2$), 1.80 (s, 3H, 4′-CH$_3$), 1.82 (s, 3H, 6′-CH$_3$), 2.00–2.05 (m, 1H, 4-CH$_2$), 2.06 (d, J = 16.8 Hz, 1H, 1-CH$_2$), 2.14–2.19 (m, 1H, 4-CH$_2$), 3.39–3.43 (m, 1H, 17-CH), 4.40 (br.s, 1H), 5.48 (s, 1H, 2′-CH), 9.50 (br.s, 1H). ^{13}C NMR (150 MHz, DMSO-d$_6$), δ: 11.1 (18-CH$_3$), 11.6 (19-CH$_3$), 20.3 (4′-CH$_3$, 6′-CH$_3$), 20.4 (11-CH$_2$), 23.0 (15-CH$_2$), 27.2 (6-CH$_2$), 29.8 (16-CH$_2$), 30.6 (7-CH$_2$), 34.1 (10 C), 35.0 (8-CH), 36.4 (12-CH$_2$), 38.1 (4-CH$_2$), 39.1 (1-CH$_2$), 42.4 (13-C), 42.5 (5-CH), 50.4 (14-CH), 53.1 (9-CH), 70.7 (2′-CH), 80.0 (17-CH), 123.0 (3-C), 134.0 (2-C),

152.2 (4′-C, 6′-C). IR (KBr), cm^{-1}: 3205 (NH), 2926, 2872 (CH), 1708, 1665 (C=C, C=N), 1498, 1469, 1444, 1380, 1380, 1338, 1250. HRMS (ESI) for $C_{24}H_{37}ClN_3O$ ($[M+H]^+$): calcd 418.2620, found 418.2610.

Cell Cultures and Evaluation of Inhibitory Activity

The MCF-7 and MDA-MB231 human breast cancer cell lines and the PC3 and 22Rv1 prostate cancer cell lines were purchased from the ATCC collection. Cells were cultured in standard high glucose DMEM medium (Hyclone) supplemented with 10% fetal calf serum (FCS) (HyClone) and 0.1 mg/ml sodium pyruvate (Santa Cruz) at 37°C, 5% CO_2 and 80–85% humidity (NuAir CO_2 incubator). The cell growth was evaluated by the modified MTT (3-[4,5-dimethylthiazol-2-yl]-2,5-diphenyltetrazolium bromide) (Applichem) test (Iselt et al., 1989) as described in Volkova et al. (2016). Briefly, the cells were seeded at a density of 2.5 × 10^4 cells per well in 24-well plates (Corning) in 900 μL of the medium. The tested compounds were dissolved in DMSO (Applichem) to 10 mM before experiments and then were diluted in the medium to the required concentrations. Compounds with different concentrations in 100 μL of the medium were added 24 h after the seeding, and the cells were grown for 72 h. After incubation with the compounds, the medium was removed, and the MTT reagent dissolved in the medium was added to the final concentration of 0.2 mg/mL to each well and incubated for 3 h. Then the cell supernatants were removed and the MTT formazan purple crystals were dissolved in 100% DMSO (350 μL per well). Plates were gently shaken and the absorbance was measured at 571 nm with a MultiScan reader (ThermoFisher). The viability of the cells was assessed after subtraction of the blank value (the absorbance in the well w/o cells) from all wells. Dose-response curves were analyzed by regression analysis using sigmoidal curves (Log(concentration) vs. normalized absorbance). The half maximal inhibitory concentrations (IC_{50}) were determined with GraphPad Prism.

Transient Transfection and Measurement of Estrogen Receptor α Activity

To determine the transcriptional activity of the estrogen receptor α (ERα), MCF-7 cells were transfected with the plasmids containing luciferase reporter gene under the control of the promoter containing estrogen responsive elements. Assay was performed in steroid-free conditions (phenol red-free DMEM medium supplemented with 10% DCC serum). The reporter plasmid ERE-TK-LUC used in this work was kindly provided by Reid et al. (2003). The transfection was carried out for 24 h at 37°C using Metafectene (Biontex Laboratories). To control the efficiency and potential toxicity of the transfection, the cells were co-transfected with the β-galactosidase plasmid. The tested compounds were added to phenol red-free DMEM medium supplemented with 10% DCC serum. The luciferase activity was measured according to a standard protocol (Promega) using a Infinite M200 Pro luminometer (Tecan). The β-galactosidase activity was analyzed using a substrate, *p*-nitrophenyl β-D-galactopyranoside (ONPG). Briefly, cell lysates were mixed with 0.1 M phosphate buffer (pH 7.5) containing 1.0 mM $MgCl_2$, 3.3 mM ONPG and 53 mM β-mercaptoethanol. After incubation for 1 h at 37°C, the absorbances at 405 nm were measured on the MultiScan FC reader (ThermoFisher). The luciferase activity was calculated in arbitrary units evaluated as the ratio of the luciferase activity to the galactosidase activity.

Western Blot Analysis

The cells were removed from the dishes with 1.2 ml of phosphate buffer, twice washed, and incubated for 10 min on ice in the modified lysis buffer containing 50 mM Tris-HCl, pH 7.5, 0.5% Igepal CA-630, 150 mM NaCl, 1 mM EDTA, 1 mM DTT, 1 mM PMSF, 0.1 mM sodium orthovanadate and aprotinin, leupeptin, pepstatin (1 μg/mL each) as described earlier (Scherbakov et al., 2006). The protein content was determined by the Bradford method.

Cell lysates (40 μg protein) were separated in 10% SDS-PAGE under reducing conditions, transferred to a nitrocellulose membrane (SantaCruz), and processed according to the standard protocol. To prevent nonspecific absorption, the membranes were treated with 5% nonfat milk solution in TBS buffer (100 mM Tris, 150 mM NaCl, pH 7.5) with 0.1% Tween-20 and then incubated with primary antibodies overnight at 4°C.

Primary antibodies to ERα were purchased from Sigma-Aldrich (Merck); the antibodies against α-tubulin (Cell Signaling Technology) were added to standardize loading. Goat anti-rabbit IgGs (Jackson ImmunoResearch) conjugated to horseradish peroxidase were used as secondary antibodies. Signals were detected using the ECL reagent as described in Mruk and Cheng (2011) and an ImageQuant LAS4000 system (GE HealthCare). ImageJ software (NIH) was used for densitometry.

Statistical Analysis

Each biology experiment was repeated three times. Statistical analysis was performed using Microsoft Excel and GraphPad Prism. Results were expressed as mean ± S.D. (standard deviation value). Student's *t*-test was used to evaluate the significance of differences in comparisons. *P*-value of <0.05 was considered statistically significant.

Molecular Docking Analysis

In silico docking was performed using Autodock Vina (Trott and Olson, 2010) run through PyRx interface to manage the workflow and PyMol to visualize the results. Ligands were prepared by generating the energy-minimized 3D structures using ChemBioDraw3D followed by processing with Autodock Tools 1.5.4 to assign Gasteiger charges, merge nonpolar hydrogens, and set torsional bonds. Initial docking runs were performed within a 25–30 Å cubic search space surrounding the binding pocket, with solutions found using an exhaustiveness of 8, and output modes ranked according to binding affinity (BA). For a detailed comparison, multiple runs with a reduced search space were run with an increased exhaustiveness of 16 and 32. The Autodock Vina produced ligand poses with the best fit and strongest BA (global minima) using a stochastic algorithm to explore surfaces/pockets of the rigid macromolecule, through an iterative series of local optimizations evaluating both intermolecular (hydrophobic interactions, repulsions, hydrogen bonding, etc.) and intramolecular (torsion, rotational torque) factors. SAR insights are greatly aided by molecular docking analysis but must be taken as putative due to the rigid modeling of the protein target and the potential for conformational bias (Bissantz et al., 2010).

RESULTS

Chemistry

Our interest in the preparation of structurally diverse heterosteroids lead to a need for a facile flexible strategy, in which a common intermediate can be used in a conjunctive fashion to form an array of *N*-heterocycles attached or fused to the steroid core. Hence, we turned to β-chlorovinyl aldehydes, which are readily available by the Vilsmeier–Haack reaction (Tasneem, 2003) and proved to be highly reactive ambident electrophiles (Bera et al., 2008; Bezboruah et al., 2013; Brockmeyer et al., 2014; Kroger et al., 2015). Recently, we have reported the synthesis of steroidal pyridazines (Komkov et al., 2015; Volkova et al., 2016), thiadiazoles (Zavarzin et al., 2013), and 4,5-disubstituted pyrimidines (Komendantova et al., 2017) via condensation of β-chlorovinyl aldehydes with bis-nucleophiles such as oxamic acid thiohydrazides and amidines. Based on these results, we accomplished the efficient synthesis of heterosteroids possessing a six-membered *N*-heterocycle attached or fused to the A/D ring of the steroid core starting from readily available materials. Thus, the synthesis of derivatives of the androstene and estrane series containing A-/D-ring annulated pyrimidine (**Schemes 1, 3a–f**) or linked dihydrotriazine (**Schemes 1, 4a–c**) moieties was accomplished starting from natural hormones **1a–c** (estrone, dihydrotestosterone, and dehydroepiandrosterone) by the general two-step sequence involving: (1) the Vilsmeier–Haack reaction giving steroidal *β*-chlorovinyl aldehydes **2a–c**, (2) the condensation of the former with amidines (**Scheme 1**).

The heterocyclization pattern was directed to dihydrotriazines by increasing amidine excess up to 4–5 equivs. The dihydrotriazine ring was constructed from two acetimidamide molecules and one steroid molecule *via* the nucleophilic attack of two amidine molecules on the formyl group. The reaction of acetimidamide with potassium carbonate in DMF produced heterosteroids **4a–c** containing the dihydrotriazine substituent at the 16-C or 2-C position of the steroid core in 29–32% yields. The structural assignments for all compounds **3a–f** and **4a–c** were confirmed by 2D NMR (^{1}H-^{1}H COSY, ^{13}C-^{1}H HMBC, and ^{13}C-^{1}H HSQC, see Supplementary Material) techniques and HRMS.

Antitumor Evaluation

Cytotoxic Effects against Breast and Prostate Cancer Cells

The antiproliferative activity of all the synthesized compounds was evaluated against the human estrogen-responsive MCF-7 breast cancer cell line and ERα-negative MDA-MB231 cells using the MTT assay (Figures S1, S2). Cisplatin, a standard chemotherapy drug, was used as the reference compound. All compounds were also tested for cytotoxicity toward prostate cancer cells (Figures S3, S4). AR-negative PC3 cells and AR-positive 22Rv1 cells were used in this assay. The corresponding inhibitory concentrations IC_{50} (IC_{50} is the half maximal inhibitory concentration) are given in **Table 1.**

Most of the tested heterosteroids showed remarkable anticancer activity against ERα-positive MCF-7 cancer cells. Estranes **3a,b** containing the D-ring-fused pyrimidine moiety proved to be inactive, while their androstene analogs **3c–e** were active with the IC_{50} values in the range of 12.0–21.6 μM. It is remarkable that the IC_{50} value for compound **3d** containing the 3-OH group is higher than that for compound **3c** possessing the 3-OAc protected group. The solubility of steroidal A-ring annulated pyrimidine **3f** in DMSO is too low to perform the MTT assay.

Steroidal dihydrotriazines **4a–c** proved to be more active against MCF-7 cancer cells compared to steroidal fused pyrimidines. Androstene derivative **4c** bearing the dihydrotriazine moiety at C-2 had the IC_{50} value of 14.8 μM, while the IC_{50} value for compound **4b** modified at 16-C reached 11.2 μM. The 16-C dihydrotriazine-modified estrane **4a** was shown to be the most active derivative. Moreover, only steroidal dihydrotriazines **4a**, **4b**, and **4c** were active against ERα-negative MDA-MB231 cells; their IC_{50} values vary in the range of 12.2–19.1 μM.

All compounds were tested against 22Rv1 and PC3 prostate cancer cells. Among them, compounds **4a**, **4b**, and **4c** displayed antiproliferative activity. Estrane derivative **4a** inhibited the growth of PC3 and 22Rv1 prostate cancer cells with IC_{50} of 13.5 and 11.7 μM, respectively, while androstene derivative **4b** displayed cytotoxicity comparable to that of cisplatin in hormone-dependent 22Rv1 prostate cancer cells. Androstene derivative **4c** was less active against prostate cancer cells than compounds **4a** and **4b**, and revealed the IC_{50} value about 20 μM (**Table 1**).

ERα Activity and Immunoblotting

Considering indicated antiproliferative activity of compounds in ERα-positive MCF-7 breast cancer cells, ERα was analyzed as a possible target for these synthetic steroids. For this purpose the luciferase reporter assay was used to determine ERα activity in MCF-7 cells. The ERα-mediated reporter constructs were provided to express luciferase under the control of the promoter containing estrogen responsive elements (ERE-TK-LUC). Thus, ERα activity was correlated to luciferase activity measured in treated or control cells.

As can be seen in **Figure 2A**, estranes **3a,b** containing the D-ring-fused pyrimidine moiety did not inhibit ERα activity at 10 μM concentration. Moreover, these **3a** and **3b** stimulated ERα activity at low (10 nM) concentration acting as partial receptor agonists (Table S1). Androstene derivative **4b** proved to be inactive as ERα inhibitor. Compound **4c** showed weak inhibitory activity, while steroids **3c, 3d, 3e,** and **4a** highly inhibited E2-mediated ERα activity at 10 μM concentration. These compounds showed no ERα agonist activity in the luciferase reporter assay (Table S1).

Taking into consideration the two-fold gain in cytotoxicity of compound **4a** against ERα-positive breast cancer cells vs.

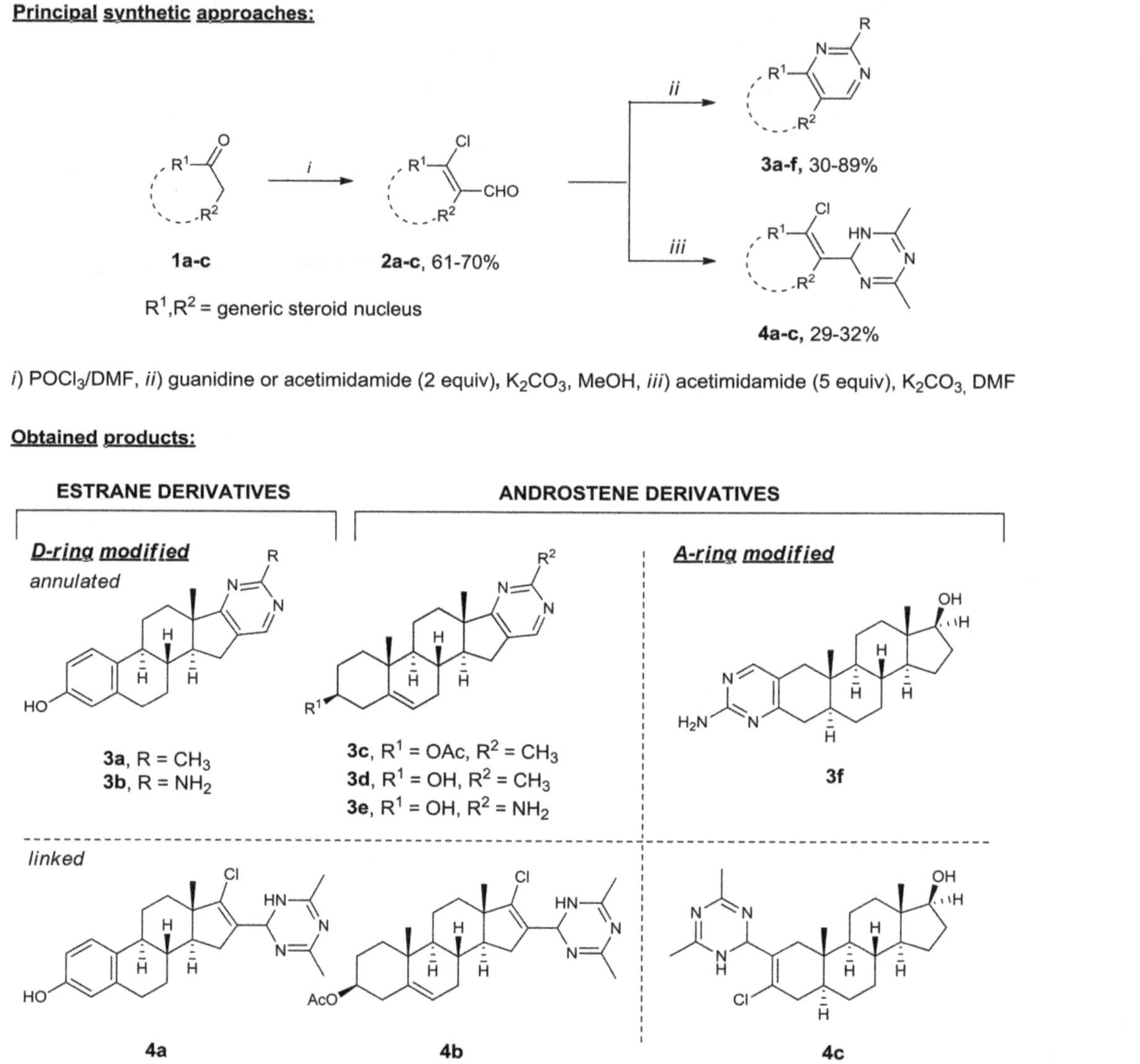

SCHEME 1 | Synthesis of A-/D-ring functionalized azasteroids of the androstene and estrane series. Steroidal β-chlorovinyl aldehydes **2** as ambident elecrophiles easily undergo cyclizations with bis-nucleophilic guanidine and acetimidamide under mild reaction conditions (2 equiv excess, under reflux in methanol with potassium carbonate) providing A-/D-fused steroidal pyrimidines **3a–f** in 30–89% yields. The reaction of acetimidamide with 2 equiv excess of potassium carbonate in DMF produced heterosteroids **4a–c** containing the dihydrotriazine substituent at the 16-C or 2-C position of the steroid core in 29–32% yields.

ERα-negative cells and its high activity as ERα inhibitor we performed immunoblotting of ERα in MCF-7 cells. The data obtained by immunoblotting confirmed that compound **4a** exerted ERα inhibitory activity. The incubation of MCF-7 cells with compound **4a** resulted in the partial suppression of ERα expression, as can be seen in **Figure 2B.** Tamoxifen was used as the standard reference drug and its application resulted in an increase in ERα expression, which may be attributed to tamoxifen-induced stabilization of inactive ERα in the cell cytoplasm as discussed in Wijayaratne and McDonnell (2001). As compared with tamoxifen, compound **4a** was found to be active as the partial ERα downregulator (**Figure 2B**).

Estrogen Receptor Docking Analysis

In order to gain insight into the structural basis of the observed ERα inhibitory effects of compound **4a**, we performed *in silico* docking analysis using Autodock Vina. Low-energy binding poses were generated by evaluating the combined energetic contributions of torsion, steric repulsion, hydrogen bonding, and hydrophobic interactions between the ligand and the protein binding pocket. Using the crystal structures of ERα in complexes with estradiol [PDB: 1GWR (Warnmark et al., 2002), **Figure 3A**] and the weak agonists 17α-modified estradiol analogs TFMPV-E2 [PDB: 2P15 (Nettles et al., 2007), **Figure 3B**] and EEu [PDB: 2YAT (Li et al., 2011), **Figure 3C**], we found that the steroidal moiety of compound **4a** in the docked poses differs

TABLE 1 | Antiproliferative activity of the synthesized heterosteroidal compounds.

Entry	IC_{50}, μM			
	Breast cancer		Prostate cancer	
	MCF-7	MDA-MB231	PC3	22Rv1
3a	NA	NA	NA	NA
3b	NA	NA	NA	NA
3c	21.6 ± 2.2	NA	NA	NA
3d	12.0 ± 1.4	NA	NA	NA
3e	14.9 ± 1.5	NA	NA	NA
4a	7.4 ± 0.9	14.7 ± 1.6	13.5 ± 1.5	11.7 ± 1.4
4b	11.2 ± 1.4	12.2 ± 1.4	12.9 ± 1.4	9.4 ± 1.0
4c	14.8 ± 1.6	19.1 ± 2.1	22.7 ± 2.4	18.1 ± 1.9
Cisplatin (reference drug)	6.5 ± 0.9	14.1 ± 1.7	4.9 ± 0.7	9.8 ± 1.1

NA indicates that the compound does not inhibit the growth by 50% at concentrations lower than 25 μM.

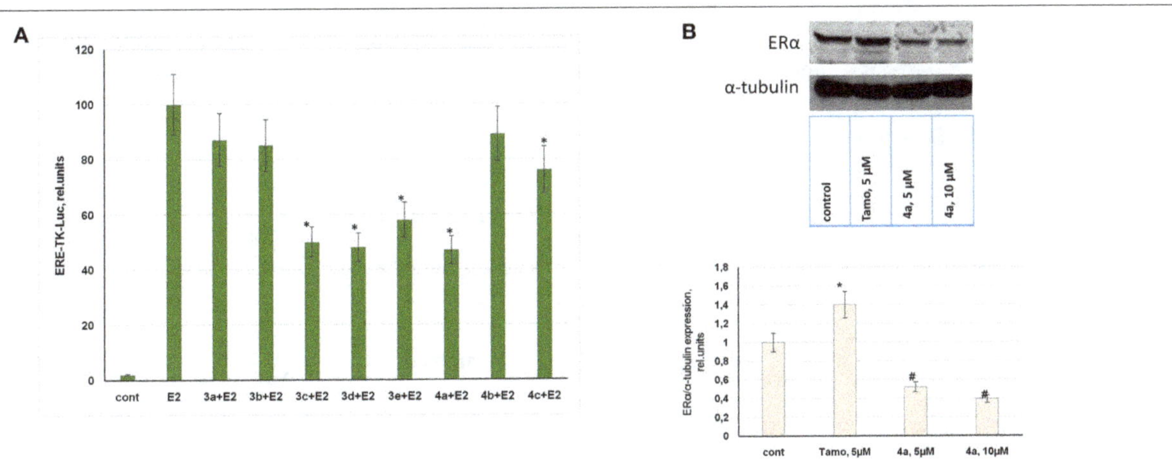

FIGURE 2 | Evaluation of ERα activity and expression. **(A)** MCF-7 human breast cancer cells were transfected with the ERE-TK-LUC plasmid containing the luciferase reporter gene under the estrogen responsive element (ERE) and co-transfected with β-galactosidase plasmid. The media was removed 24 h after transfection and 10 nM of 17β-estradiol was used to induce ERα activity. Synthesized compounds at 10 μM concentration or vehicle control (cont) was added to phenol-free DMEM supplemented with 10% steroid-free serum (Hyclone). The luciferase and β-galactosidase activities were determined in 24 h. The luciferase activity was calculated in relative units evaluated as the ratio of the luciferase activity to the galactosidase activity. *$P < 0.05$ vs. E2-treated cells. **(B)** MCF-7 cells were treated with or without tamoxifen or compound **4a**. The cell samples were subjected to Western blot analysis of ERα and α-tubulin as the loading control; Densitometry for ERα/α-tubulin ratio was carried out using ImageJ software with the densitometry protocol provided by The University of Queensland. *$P < 0.05$ vs. control cells, #$P < 0.05$ vs. tamoxifen-treated and control cells.

from the estradiol moieties of the original ligands (**Table 1, Figures 3A–C,E**).

Compound **4a** was found to be too big for the accommodation in the estradiol-binding pocket of ERa in the structure 1GWR. Meanwhile, the ligands TFMPV-E2 (PDB: 2P15) and EEu (PDB: 2YAT) are known to modulate the dynamics of the ERα helix 12 (shown in red, **Figures 3A–D**), resulting in an increase in the ligand-binding pocket surface of ER without changing the shape of the ligand-binding domain of ER due to the presence of bulky substituents at the 17α position of the estradiol core (Eignerova et al., 2010; Gryder et al., 2013). Compound **4a** bearing the bulky dihydrotriazine ring at the 16-position is docked against the ERα crystal structures 2P15 and 2YAT with reasonable binding affinity (−8.1 and −8.9 kcal/mol, respectively). However, the major binding modes of compound **4a** for 2P15 and 2YAT are as follows: the A-ring phenolic hydroxyl group points away the binding pocket of ER and the dihydrotriazine moiety points inward the binding pocket. The critical hydrogen-bonding interactions between the steroid estradiol, TFMPV-E2 and the A-ring phenolic hydroxyls of EEu with Arg-394/Glu-353 were not found for compound **4a** (**Figures 3A–C**), which can be attributed to steric hindrance caused by the bulky substituent at the 16-position and spatial aliasing of the estrane core due to the addition of the $C_{16}=C_{17}$ double bond.

Alternatively, compound **4a** docked against the crystal structure of ERα in complex with the ER antagonist 4-hydroxytamoxifen (PDB: 3ERT, **Figures 3D,E**) is able to fill the hydrophobic space and latch onto Arg-394/Glu-353.

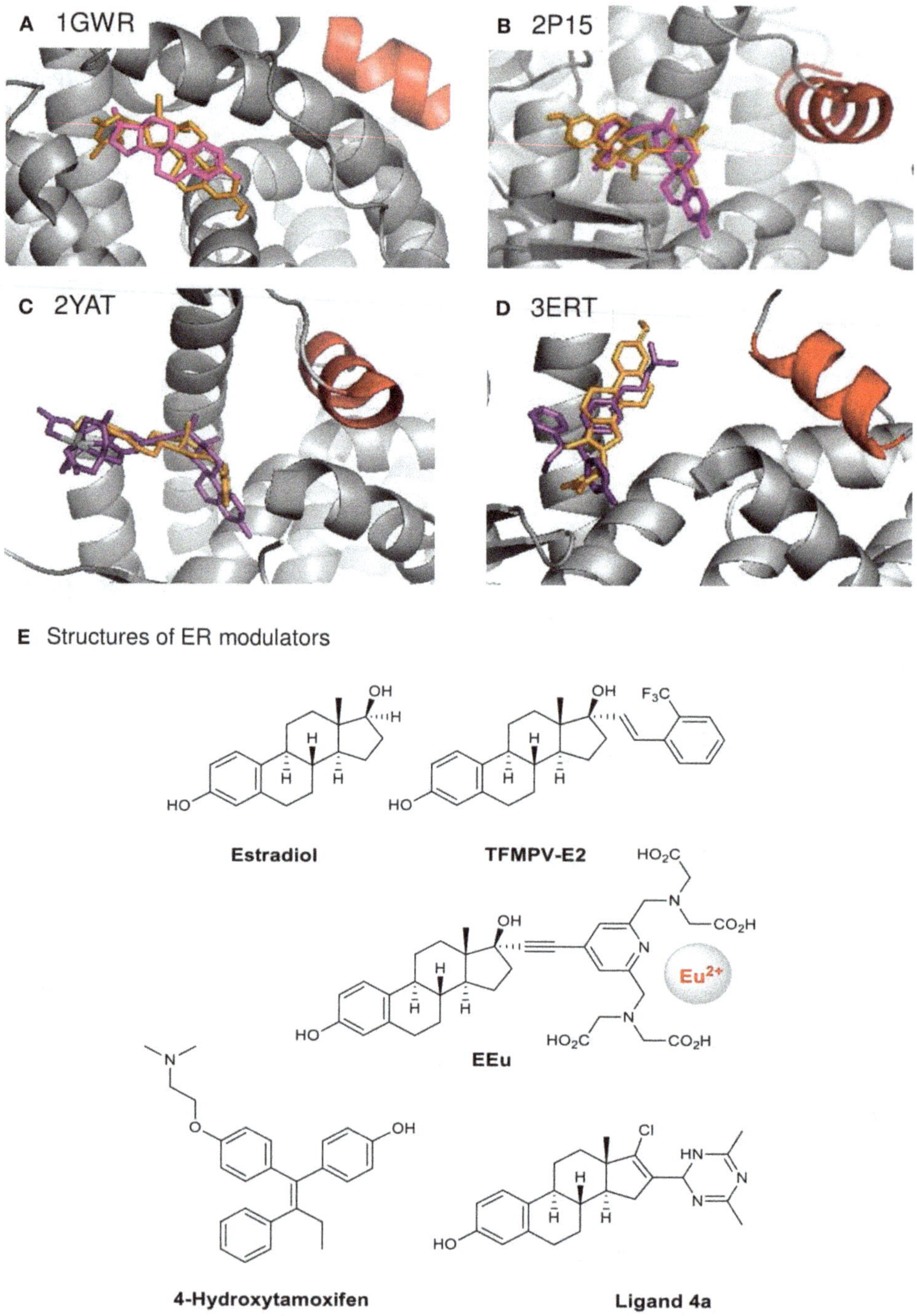

FIGURE 3 | Crystal structures of agonist-bound ERα 1GWR **(A)**, 2P15 **(B)**, 2YAT **(C)** and antagonist-bound 3ERT **(D)** used in the docking analysis of ER modulator **4a**. Their original ligands **(E)** are in purple, modulator **4a** in orange, and helix 12 in red. Only the highest ranked poses with the strongest BA were selected: **(A)** +0.1 kcal/mol, **(B)** −8.1 kcal/mol, **(C)** −8.9 kcal/mol, **(D)** −8.9 kcal/mol.

Tamoxifen prevents the helix 12 from closing properly upon the binding pocket of the ligand-binding domain, while compound **4a** can extend the steroidal moiety through the opening left by the displaced helix 12. The D ring of steroid **4a** modified at the 16-and 17-positions can go inside the pocket potentially stabilized by polar interactions with TRP-383, Phe-404, Leu-387, Met-388, and Leu-391. These docked structures may reflect the most probable mode of binding. Although the direct comparisons are speculative, our docking outputs are supported by our observation with compound **4a** in ER luciferase reporter assays. The antagonist effect of compound **4a** is interesting, because D-ring modifications of estradiol commonly result in weak ER agonists (Yang et al., 2000; Kreis et al., 2001).

DISCUSSION

The initial synthesis of annulated steroidal pyrimidines by the groups of Clinton (Ackerman et al., 1964) and Ruggieri (De Ruggieri and Gandolfi, 1965; De Ruggieri et al., 1965, 1966a,b) dates back to the mid-1960s. Their synthetic approach was based on condensation of guanidines with activated α,β-unsaturated ketones, primarily β-enol ethers, and have become widely applied in chemistry of steroids due to a great diversity of obtainable products (Romo et al., 1968; Bajwa and Sykes, 1978; Hajos and Snatzke, 1989; Mallamo et al., 1992; Hasan et al., 1995; Forgo and Vincze, 2002). Unfortunately, this method suffers from drawbacks, such as harsh reaction conditions, moderate yields and high labor content/cost of preparing starting materials. Therefore, over the years a considerable effort has been directed toward the development of alternative methods for steroidal pyrimidines synthesis. Improved solid phase protocol of β-enol ethers heterocyclization was elaborated toward synthesis of steroidal A-ring fused pyrimidines (Barthakur et al., 2009). Although there is an example of condensation using β-enamino ketones (Xu et al., 2012). Boruah group have developed a range of methods, among which are three-component condensation of steroidal ketones with aromatic aldehydes and amidine derivatives in presence of potassium tert-butoxide (Saikia et al., 2014), $Pd(OAc)_2$-catalyzed hetrocyclization of steroidal β-halo-α,β-unsaturated aldehydes with amidines (Gogoi et al., 2013) and $SmCl_3$-catalyzed condensation of β-formyl enamide with urea under microwave irradiation (Barthakur et al., 2007). Baran group reported synthesis of 4,5-disubstituted pyrimidines from steroidal ketones and formamidine acetate (Baran et al., 2006). Here we have achieved high-yielding syntheses of novel A- and D-rings annulated steroidal pyrimidines via developed by us metal-free condensations of β-chlorovinyl aldehydes with amidines (Komendantova et al., 2017). These reactions are efficiently occur under mild conditions, with the added advantage that heterocyclization pattern can be easily switch to steroidal dihydrotriazines, previously unexplored class of heterosteroids.

Steroidal pyrimidines may be considered as promising compounds for the design of novel antitumor drugs. This line of research has been extensively developed in recent years. In 2017, Ke et al. designed novel steroidal[17,16-d]pyrimidines derived from dehydroepiandrosterone and evaluated their *in vitro* inhibitory activity against liver and gastric cancer cells (Ke et al., 2017). Briefly, 16 steroidal[17,16-d]pyrimidines derived from dehydroepiandrosterone were designed and synthesized via a sequence transformation, and their activities were assessed by MTT. Ke et al. found that some of these heterocyclic steroidal[17,16-d]pyrimidines showed antiproliferative activities against HepG2, Huh-7, and SGC-7901 cell lines compared to the reference 5-fluorouracil. Eight novel compounds synthesized by Ke et al. exhibited excellent inhibitory activities against all three cell lines with 70–82% growth inhibition at the concentration of 40 μg/mL. Thus, steroidal[17,16-d]pyrimidines might be used as promising compounds for discovery of novel anticancer drugs for treatment of liver and gastric cancers.

Other promising steroidal pyrimidines were discussed by Ali et al. (2017). The antitumor activity of the B-ring fused steroidal pyrimidines was tested *in vitro* against the MDA-MB231, HeLa, and HepG2 cancer cell lines and the non-cancer normal cell line PBMCs (peripheral blood mononuclear cells) by the standard MTT assay. The compounds showed moderate to good activity and proved to be nontoxic to normal PBM cells. One of the synthesized compounds was found to be active against all three cancer cell lines but more specific against the MDA-MB231 cells with IC_{50} of about 9 μM, which is similar to our data on the activity of the compounds against breast cancer cells. Finally, the authors discussed the ability of steroidal compounds to interact with the protein HSA involved in drug delivery.

Metastatic bone tumors occur at particularly high rates in cancers of the breast, prostate, and lung, accounting more than 70% of all patients. Treatment of skeletal metastasis and development of new specific "blockers" of bone resorption are relevant. Pyrimidine-fused betulinic acid may be considered as promising compounds for the design of novel inhibitors of osteoclast differentiation and bone resorption. Jun Xu et coworkers synthesized over 20 heterocyclic ring-fused betulinic acid derivatives and evaluated their inhibition on RANKL-induced osteoclast formation in preosteoclast RAW264.7 cells (Xu et al., 2012). Some compounds exhibited potent inhibitory activity on RANKL-induced osteoclast formation by TRAP assay.

The elucidation of the mechanism of action of compounds in target cells and understanding of their common metabolism in human body are of interest. The structural optimization will be performed and the molecular mechanism of novel steroidal pyrimidines will be investigated in due course. On the other hand, the activity of steroidal dihydrotriazines against cancer cells is less well known described, and our study is very relevant.

CONCLUSION

Here, we describe novel series of steroidal anticancer agents. In summary, this study demonstrates that the cyclization of steroidal β-chlorovinyl aldehydes with bis-nucleophilic amidines provides an easy approach to various novel heterosteroids. Natural hormones **1a–c** (estrone, 3β-acetoxyandrostene, 3-keto-17β-hydroxyandrostane) were transformed into the corresponding A- and D-modified steroidal pyrimidines and dihydrotriazines in moderate to high yields (29–89%) using a two-step sequence involving the Vilsmeier–Haack reaction and condensation with amidines, such as guanidine and acetimidamide. The new compounds showed remarkable cytotoxic activity against breast and prostate cancer cells. Furthermore, lead compounds demonstrated selectivity toward ERα in MCF-7 breast cancer cells. Compound **4a** inhibits 50% of ERα activity at its cytotoxic concentration. Using immunoblotting, partial ERα downregulation was observed in compound **4a**-treated MCF-7 cells. Docking approaches confirmed the ability of compound **4a** to bind to ERα. Thus, compound **4a** may be considered as a candidate for future anticancer drug design, in particular, for ERα-positive breast cancers.

Despite a limited number of compounds in series, it provides significant novel insight into the structure–activity relationship of heterosteroids as anticancer agents. Biological studies show that annulation of androst-5-ene core with pyrimidine is efficient for development of novel selective compounds for treatment of hormone-dependent breast cancer. Moreover, installation of dihydrotriazine pendant at A- and D-rings of estrane and androst-5-ene cores results in strong antiproliferative activities against breast and prostate cancer cells comparable with cisplatine. The two-fold gain in cytotoxicity of 16-C dihydrotriazine-modified estrane against ERα-positive breast cancer cells vs. ERα-negative cells and its high activity as ERα inhibitor were shown while similar androstene derivative was less selective.

These results offer new knowledge about the binding site and receptor flexibility of ERα. The described heterosteroids will be useful lead agents for the development of more potent and selective SERMs.

AUTHOR CONTRIBUTIONS

AS carried out the immunoblotting, performed the statistical analysis and the transient transfection, drafted and prepared the manuscript for submission, worked with cell cultures; AVK synthesized steroidal compounds; ASK synthesized steroidal compounds, prepared the supporting information; MY worked with cell cultures; OA performed the reporter analysis, worked with plasmids; VS managed the project; IZ managed the project; AH managed the project; YV wrote the manuscript, conceived of the study, *in silico* analysis, and managed the project; All authors read and approved the final manuscript.

ACKNOWLEDGMENTS

The ERE-TK-LUC plasmid was kindly provided by Dr. George Reid. High resolution mass spectra were recorded at the Department of Structural Studies of the N.D. Zelinsky Institute of Organic Chemistry, Russian Academy of Sciences, Moscow. The densitometry protocol for immunoblotting was provided by The University of Queensland (https://di.uq.edu.au/community-and-alumni/sparq-ed/sparq-ed-services/using-imagej-quantify-blots).

REFERENCES

Ackerman, J. H., Potts, G. O., Beyler, A. L., and Clinton, R. O. (1964). Steroidal heterocycles. X. Steroidal(3,2-D)Pyrimidines and related compounds. *J. Med. Chem.* 7, 238–240. doi: 10.1021/jm00332a027

Ali, A., Asif, M., Alam, P., Jane Alam, M., Asif Sherwani, M., Hasan Khan, R., et al. (2017). DFT/B3LYP calculations, *in vitro* cytotoxicity and antioxidant activities of steroidal pyrimidines and their interaction with HSA using molecular docking and multispectroscopic techniques. *Bioorg. Chem.* 73, 83–99. doi: 10.1016/j.bioorg.2017.06.001

Ali, S., Rasool, M., Chaoudhry, H., Pushparaj, P. N., Jha, P., Hafiz, A., et al. (2016). Molecular mechanisms and mode of tamoxifen resistance in breast cancer. *Bioinformation* 12, 135–139. doi: 10.6026/97320630012135

Bajwa, J. S., and Sykes, P. J. (1978). Steroidal Heterocycles: 2-Thiocyanatoandrosteno-3,2-d. pyrimidines and -[I 7,16-d]pyrimidines. *J. Chem. Soc. Perkin Trans.* 1, 1618–1621. doi: 10.1039/P19780001618

Baran, P. S., Shenvi, R. A., and Nguyen, S. A. (2006). One-step syntesis of 4,5-disubstituted pyrimidines using commercially available and inexpensive reagents. *Heterocycles* 70, 581–588. doi: 10.3987/COM-06-S(W)27

Barthakur, M. G., Borthakur, M., Devi, P., Saikia, C. J., Saikia, A., Bora, U., et al. (2007). A novel and efficient lewis acid catalysed preparation of pyrimidines: microwave-promoted reaction of urea and b-formyl enamides microwave-promoted reaction of urea mad and b-aFormyl Ennamides. *Synlett* 2, 223–227. doi: 10.1055/s-2007-968018

Barthakur, M. G., Gogoi, S., Dutta, M., and Boruah, R. C. (2009). A facile three-component solid phase synthesis of steroidal A-ring fused pyrimidines under microwave irradiation. *Steroids* 74, 730–734. doi: 10.1016/j.steroids.2009.03.006

Bera, R., Dhananjaya, G., Singh, S. N., Ramu, B., Kiran, S. U., Kumar, P. R., et al. (2008). Revisiting the reaction of β-chloroacroleins with 2-aminophenol: a new observation. *Tetrahedron* 64, 582–589. doi: 10.1016/j.tet.2007.10.101

Bezboruah, P., Gogoi, P., Gogoi, J., and Boruah, R. C. (2013). KF/Al_2O_3/PEG-400: an efficient catalytic system for the fiesselmann-type synthesis of thiophene derivatives. *Synthesis* 45, 1341–1348. doi: 10.1055/s-0033-1338299

Bissantz, C., Kuhn, B., and Stahl, M. (2010). A medicinal chemist's guide to molecular interactions. *J. Med. Chem.* 53, 5061–5084. doi: 10.1021/jm100112j

Boer, K. (2017). Fulvestrant in advanced breast cancer: evidence to date and place in therapy. *Ther. Adv. Med. Oncol.* 9, 465–479. doi: 10.1177/1758834017711097

Brockmeyer, F., Schoemaker, R., Schmidtmann, M., and Martens, J. (2014). Multicomponent reaction for the first synthesis of 2,2-dialkyl- and 2-alkyl-2-aralkyl-5,6-diaryl-2H-1,3-thiazines as scaffolds for various 3,4-dihydro-2H-1,3-thiazine derivatives. *Org. Biomol. Chem.* 12, 5168–5181. doi: 10.1039/C4OB00866A

Bryce, A., and Ryan, C. J. (2012). Development and clinical utility of abiraterone acetate as an androgen synthesis inhibitor. *Clin. Pharmacol. Ther.* 91, 101–108. doi: 10.1038/clpt.2011.275

Carlini, P., Frassoldati, A., De Marco, S., Casali, A., Ruggeri, E. M., Nardi, M., et al. (2001). Formestane, a steroidal aromatase inhibitor after failure of non-steroidal aromatase inhibitors (anastrozole and letrozole): is a clinical benefit still achievable? *Ann. Oncol.* 12, 1539–1543. doi: 10.1023/A:1013180214359

Cosman, F., and Lindsay, R. (1999). Selective estrogen receptor modulators: clinical spectrum. *Endocr. Rev.* 20, 418–434. doi: 10.1210/er.20.3.418

De Ruggieri, P., and Gandolfi, C. (1965). Steroids. XIX. Steroid heterocyclics. [17,16-d]-Pyrimidines of androstane and [3,4-c]pyrazole, [17,16-d]pyrimidines of androstane and estrane. *Gazz. Chim. Ital.* 95, 338–350.

De Ruggieri, P., Gandolfi, C., and Chiaramonti, D. (1962). Steroidi nota xii. Eterociclici steroidali. Alcuni derivati eterociclici in positione 2,3 dell'androstano e relativi composti. *Gazz. Chim. Ital.* 92, 768–798.

De Ruggieri, P., Gandolfi, C., and Guzzi, U. (1965). Steroids. XX. Steroidal heterocyclics. [3,2-d] Pyrimidino [17,16-c] pyrazolo derivs. of androstanes and estranes. *Gazz. Chim. Ital.* 95, 455–464.

De Ruggieri, P., Gandolfi, C., and Guzzi, U. (1966a). Steroids. XXIII. Steroid heterocyclics. 6′-Amino, 2′,6′-diamino-, and 2′-hydroxy-6′-amino [3,2-d], [17,16-d]dipyrimidines of androstane and estrane. *Gazz. Chim. Ital.* 96, 152–178.

De Ruggieri, P., Gandolfi, C., and Guzzi, U. (1966b). Steroids. XXIV. Steroid heterocyclics. [3,2-c]-5′-aminoisoxazole intermediates in the synthesis of [3,2-d]-2′,6′-disubstituted pyrimidines. *Gazz. Chim. Ital.* 96, 179–185.

Eignerova, B., Sedlak, D., Dracinsky, M., Bartunek, P., and Kotora, M. (2010). Synthesis and biochemical characterization of a series of 17α-perfluoroalkylated estradiols as selective ligands for estrogen receptor α. *J. Med. Chem.* 53, 6947–6953. doi: 10.1021/jm100563h

Forgo, P., and Vincze, I. (2002). Syntheses and advanced NMR structure determination of androsteno-[17,16-d]-pyrimidine derivatives. *Steroids* 67, 749–756. doi: 10.1016/S0039-128X(02)00031-4

Gogoi, J., Gogoi, P., Bezbaruah, P., and Boruah, R. C. (2013). Microwave-assisted Pd-catalyzed synthesis of fused steroidal and non-steroidal pyrimidines from β-halo-α,β-unsaturated aldehydes. *Tetrahedron Lett.* 54, 7136–7140. doi: 10.1016/j.tetlet.2013.10.094

Gryder, B. E., Rood, M. K., Johnson, K. A., Patil, V., Raftery, E. D., Yao, L. P., et al. (2013). Histone deacetylase inhibitors equipped with estrogen receptor modulation activity. *J. Med. Chem.* 56, 5782–5796. doi: 10.1021/jm400467w

Hajos, G., and Snatzke, G. (1989). Synthesis and circular dichroism of cholestenopyrimidines. *Liebigs Ann. Chem.* 31–34. doi: 10.1002/jlac.198919890107

Hasan, M., Rashid, N., Khan, K. M., Snatzke, G., Duddeck, H., and Voelter, W. (1995). Syntheses and CD studies of 5α-cholesteno[3,2-d]-, -[2,3-d]- and -[3,4-d]pyrimidines. *Liebigs Annalen* 1995, 889–896. doi: 10.1002/jlac.1995199505130

Iselt, M., Holtei, W., and Hilgard, P. (1989). The tetrazolium dye assay for rapid *in vitro* assessment of cytotoxicity. *Arzneimittelforschung* 39, 747–749.

Jameera Begam, A., Jubie, S., and Nanjan, M. J. (2017). Estrogen receptor agonists/antagonists in breast cancer therapy: a critical review. *Bioorg. Chem.* 71, 257–274. doi: 10.1016/j.bioorg.2017.02.011

Kaklamani, V. G., and Gradishar, W. J. (2017). Endocrine therapy in the current management of postmenopausal estrogen receptor-positive metastatic breast cancer. *Oncologist* 22, 507–517. doi: 10.1634/theoncologist.2015-0464

Ke, S., Shi, L., Zhang, Z., and Yang, Z. (2017). Steroidal[17,16-d]pyrimidines derived from dehydroepiandrosterone: a convenient synthesis, antiproliferation activity, structure-activity relationships, and role of heterocyclic moiety. *Sci. Rep.* 7:44439. doi: 10.1038/srep44439

Komendantova, A. S., Komkov, A. V., Volkova, Y. A., and Zavarzin, I. V. (2017). Efficient synthesis of 4- and 5-Substituted 2-Aminopyrimidines by coupling of β-chlorovinyl aldehydes and guanidines. *Eur. J. Org. Chem.* 2017, 4260–4264. doi: 10.1002/ejoc.201700737

Komkov, A. V., Komendantova, A. S., Menchikov, L. G., Chernoburova, E. I., Volkova, Y. A., and Zavarzin, I. V. (2015). A straightforward approach toward multifunctionalized pyridazines via imination/electrocyclization. *Org. Lett.* 17, 3734–3737. doi: 10.1021/acs.orglett.5b01718

Kreis, W., Budman, D. R., and Calabro, A. (2001). A reexamination of PSC 833 (Valspodar) as a cytotoxic agent and in combination with anticancer agents. *Cancer Chemother. Pharmacol.* 47, 78–82. doi: 10.1007/s002800000191

Kroger, D., Brockmeyer, F., and Kahrs, C. (2015). A three-component reaction for rapid access to underexplored 1,3-thiazine-2-thiones. *Org. Biomol. Chem.* 13, 7223–7229. doi: 10.1039/C5OB00377F

Lakhani, N. J., Sarkar, M. A., Venitz, J., and Figg, W. D. (2003). 2-Methoxyestradiol, a promising anticancer agent. *Pharmacotherapy* 23, 165–172. doi: 10.1592/phco.23.2.165.32088

Li, M.-J., Greenblatt, H. M., Dym, O., Albeck, S., Pais, A., Gunanathan, C., et al. (2011). Structure of estradiol metal chelate and estrogen receptor complex: the basis for designing a new class of selective estrogen receptor modulators. *J. Med. Chem.* 54, 3575–3580. doi: 10.1021/jm200192y

Mallamo, J. P., Pilling, G. M., Wetzel, J. R., Kowalczyk, P. J., Bell, M. R., Kullnig, R. K., et al. (1992). Antiandrogenic steroidal sulfonyl heterocycles. Utility of electrostatic complementarity in defining bioisosteric sulfonyl heterocycles. *J. Med. Chem.* 35, 1663–1670. doi: 10.1021/jm00088a001

Matsumoto, T., Watanabe, M., Mataka, S., and Thiemann, T. (2003). Estrano[17,16-e]pyrimidine-peptide conjugates. *Steroids* 68, 751–757. doi: 10.1016/S0039-128X(03)00145-4

Mehta, R. S., Barlow, W. E., Albain, K. S., Vandenberg, T. A., Dakhil, S. R., Tirumali, N. R., et al. (2012). Combination anastrozole and fulvestrant in metastatic breast cancer. *N. Engl. J. Med.* 367, 435–444. doi: 10.1056/NEJMoa1201622

Mruk, D. D., and Cheng, C. Y. (2011). Enhanced chemiluminescence (ECL) for routine immunoblotting: an inexpensive alternative to commercially available kits. *Spermatogenesis* 1, 121–122. doi: 10.4161/spmg.1.2.16606

Nathan, M. R., and Schmid, P. (2017). A review of fulvestrant in breast cancer. *Oncol. Ther.* 5, 17–29. doi: 10.1007/s40487-017-0046-2

Nettles, K. W., Bruning, J. B., Gil, G., O'neill, E. E., Nowak, J., Guo, Y., et al. (2007). Structural plasticity in the oestrogen receptor ligand-binding domain. *EMBO Rep.* 8, 563–568. doi: 10.1038/sj.embor.7400963

Purohit, A., and Foster, P. A. (2012). Steroid sulfatase inhibitors for estrogen- and androgen-dependent cancers. *J. Endocrinol.* 212, 99–110. doi: 10.1530/JOE-11-0266

Rassokhina, I. V., Volkova, Y. A., Kozlov, A. S., Scherbakov, A. M., Andreeva, O. E., Shirinian, V. Z., et al. (2016). Synthesis and antiproliferative activity evaluation of steroidal imidazo[1,2-a]pyridines. *Steroids* 113, 29–37. doi: 10.1016/j.steroids.2016.06.001

Reid, G., Hubner, M. R., Metivier, R., Brand, H., Denger, S., Manu, D., et al. (2003). Cyclic, proteasome-mediated turnover of unliganded and liganded ERalpha on responsive promoters is an integral feature of estrogen signaling. *Mol. Cell* 11, 695–707. doi: 10.1016/S1097-2765(03)00090-X

Romo, J., Rodriguez-Hahnd, L., and Jimenez, M. (1968). Synthesis of steroidal pyrimidine N-oxides. *Can. J. Chem.* 46, 2807–2821. doi: 10.1139/v68-465

Saikia, P., Gogoi, S., Gogoi, S., and Boruah, R. C. (2014). An efficient route for annulation of pyrimidines to steroids and non-steroids via a base catalyzed one-pot three component reaction. *Steroids* 88, 1–6. doi: 10.1016/j.steroids.2014.06.015

Scherbakov, A. M., Krasil'nikov, M. A., and Kushlinskii, N. E. (2013). Molecular mechanisms of hormone resistance of breast cancer. *Bull. Exp. Biol. Med.* 155, 384–395. doi: 10.1007/s10517-013-2160-y

Scherbakov, A. M., Lobanova, Y. S., Shatskaya, V. A., Onopchenko, O. V., Gershtein, E. S., and Krasil'nikov, M. A. (2006). Activation of mitogenic pathways and sensitization to estrogen-induced apoptosis: two independent characteristics of tamoxifen-resistant breast cancer cells? *Breast Cancer Res. Treat.* 100, 1–11. doi: 10.1007/s10549-005-9075-x

Secky, L., Svoboda, M., Klameth, L., Bajna, E., Hamilton, G., Zeillinger, R., et al. (2013). The sulfatase pathway for estrogen formation: targets for the treatment and diagnosis of hormone-associated tumors. *J. Drug Deliv.* 2013:957605. doi: 10.1155/2013/957605

Singer, C. F., Fink-Retter, A., Gschwantler-Kaulich, D., Thalhammer, T., Hudelist, G., Mueller, R., et al. (2006). Selective spatial upregulation of intratumoral stromal aromatase in breast cancer patients: evidence for imbalance of local estrogen metabolism. *Endocr. Relat. Cancer* 13, 1101–1107. doi: 10.1677/erc.1.01230

Tasneem (2003). Vilsmeier-haack reagent (Halomethyleneiminium Salt). *Synlett* 2003, 138–139. doi: 10.1055/s-2003-36241

Traboulsi, T., El Ezzy, M., Gleason, J. L., and Mader, S. (2017). Antiestrogens: structure-activity relationships and use in breast cancer treatment. *J. Mol. Endocrinol.* 58, R15–R31. doi: 10.1530/JME-16-0024

Trott, O., and Olson, A. J. (2010). AutoDock Vina: improving the speed and accuracy of docking with a new scoring function, efficient optimization, and multithreading. *J. Comput. Chem.* 31, 455–461. doi: 10.1002/jcc.21334

Tryfonidis, K., Zardavas, D., Katzenellenbogen, B. S., and Piccart, M. (2016). Endocrine treatment in breast cancer: Cure, resistance and beyond. *Cancer Treat. Rev.* 50, 68–81. doi: 10.1016/j.ctrv.2016.08.008

Volkova, Y. A., Antonov, Y. S., Komkov, A. V., Scherbakov, A. M., Shashkov, A. S., Menchikov, L. G., et al. (2016). Access to steroidal pyridazines via modified thiohydrazides. *RSC Adv.* 6, 42863–42868. doi: 10.1039/C6RA06881B

Warnmark, A., Treuter, E., Gustafsson, J. A., Hubbard, R. E., Brzozowski, A. M., and Pike, A. C. (2002). Interaction of transcriptional intermediary factor 2 nuclear receptor box peptides with the coactivator binding site of estrogen receptor alpha. *J. Biol. Chem.* 277, 21862–21868. doi: 10.1074/jbc.M200764200

Wijayaratne, A. L., and McDonnell, D. P. (2001). The human estrogen receptor-α is a ubiquitinated protein whose stability is affected differentially by agonists, antagonists, and selective estrogen receptor modulators. *J. Biol. Chem.* 276, 35684–35692. doi: 10.1074/jbc.M101097200

Xu, J., Li, Z., Luo, J., Yang, F., Liu, T., Liu, M., et al. (2012). Synthesis and biological evaluation of heterocyclic ring-fused betulinic acid derivatives as novel inhibitors of osteoclast differentiation and bone resorption. *J. Med. Chem.* 55, 3122–3134. doi: 10.1021/jm201540h

Yang, X., Ferguson, A. T., Nass, S. J., Phillips, D. L., Butash, K. A., Wang, S. M., et al. (2000). Transcriptional activation of estrogen receptor α in human breast cancer cells by histone deacetylase inhibition. *Cancer Res.* 60, 6890–6894. Available online at: http://cancerres.aacrjournals.org/content/60/24/6890.long

Zavarzin, I. V., Antonov, Y. S., Chernoburova, E. I., Shchetinina, M. A., Kolotyrkina, N. G., and Shashkov, A. S. (2013). Interaction of 16-hydroxymethylidene derivatives of androstane and estrone with thiohydrazides of oxamic acids. *Russ. Chem. Bull.* 62, 2603–2608. doi: 10.1007/s11172-013-0379-4

3

Estrone-3-Sulfate Stimulates the Proliferation of T47D Breast Cancer Cells Stably Transfected with the Sodium-Dependent Organic Anion Transporter SOAT (SLC10A6)

*Emre Karakus[1], Daniel Zahner[1], Gary Grosser[1], Regina Leidolf[1], Cemal Gundogdu[2], Alberto Sánchez-Guijo[3], Stefan A. Wudy[3] and Joachim Geyer[1]**

[1] Institute of Pharmacology and Toxicology, Faculty of Veterinary Medicine, Justus Liebig University Giessen, Giessen, Germany, [2] Department of Pathology, Private Practitioner of Medicine, Erzurum, Turkey, [3] Steroid Research and Mass Spectrometry Unit, Pediatric Endocrinology and Diabetology, Center of Child and Adolescent Medicine, Justus Liebig University Giessen, Giessen, Germany

***Correspondence:**
Joachim Geyer
Joachim.M.Geyer@vetmed.uni-giessen.de

Estrogens play a pivotal role in the development and proliferation of hormone-dependent breast cancer. Apart from free estrogens, which can directly activate the estrogen receptor (ER) of tumor cells, sulfo-conjugated steroids, which maintain high plasma concentrations even after menopause, first have to be imported into tumor cells by carrier-mediated uptake and then can be cleaved by the steroid sulfatase to finally activate ERs and cell proliferation. In the present study, expression of the sodium-dependent organic anion transporter SOAT was analyzed in breast cancer and its role for hormone-dependent proliferation of T47D breast cancer cells was elucidated. The SOAT protein was localized to the ductal epithelium of the mammary gland by immunohistochemistry. SOAT showed high expression in different pathologies of the breast with a clear ductal localization, including ductal hyperplasia, intraductal papilloma, and intraductal carcinoma. In a larger breast cancer cDNA array, SOAT mRNA expression was high in almost all adenocarcinoma specimen, but expression did not correlate with either the ER, progesterone receptor, or human epidermal growth factor receptor 2 status. Furthermore, SOAT expression did not correlate with tumor stage or grade, indicating widespread SOAT expression in breast cancer. To analyze the role of SOAT for breast cancer cell proliferation, T47D cells were stably transfected with SOAT and incubated under increasing concentrations of estrone-3-sulfate (E_1S) and estradiol at physiologically relevant concentrations. Cell proliferation was significantly increased by 10^{-9} M estradiol as well as by E_1S with EC_{50} of 2.2 nM. In contrast, T47D control cells showed 10-fold lower sensitivity to E_1S stimulation with EC_{50} of 21.7 nM. The E_1S-stimulated proliferation of SOAT-T47D cells was blocked by the SOAT inhibitor 4-sulfooxymethylpyrene. In conclusion: The present study clearly demonstrates expression of SOAT in breast cancer tissue with ductal localization. SOAT inhibition can block the E_1S-stimulated proliferation of T47D breast cancer cells, demonstrating that SOAT is an interesting novel drug target from the group of E_1S uptake carriers for anti-proliferative breast cancer therapy.

Keywords: estrone-3-sulfate, T47D, breast cancer, SOAT, transport, proliferation, SLC10A6, sulfate steroid

INTRODUCTION

Estrogens play a pivotal role in the development and proliferation of hormone-dependent breast cancer, which represents the most common type of cancer in women (Conner et al., 2008). Estrogens act via nuclear ERs (Henderson et al., 1988) and the selective ER modulator tamoxifen has been used successfully for antiestrogen breast cancer therapy for four decades (Osborne, 1998). Despite a significant decline of free estrogens after menopause, a high percentage of all hormone-dependent breast cancer cases develop in this phase of life (Kenemans and Bosman, 2003). In contrast to free estrogens (E_1 and E_2), the sulfo-conjugated steroid forms, in particular estrone-3-sulfate (E_1S) and DHEAS, persist at higher plasma concentrations even after menopause (Rémy-Martin et al., 1983; Geisler, 2003). These sulfo-conjugated steroids can be re-converted into active free estrogens in breast cancer tissue via cleavage of the sulfate group by the STS and further conversion by the enzymes 3β-hydroxysteroid dehydrogenase and aromatase in the case of DHEA (Santner et al., 1986; Pasqualini et al., 1997; Labrie et al., 1998; Suzuki et al., 2005; Sasano et al., 2006). Inhibitors of STS (STX64) and aromatase (anastrozole, letrozole) can block this intracrine formation of estrogens and, therefore, are used for clinical (aromatase inhibitors) or experimental (STS inhibitors) breast cancer therapy (Santen and Harvey, 1999; Stanway et al., 2007).

Prior to intracellular conversion of E_1S and DHEAS, these negatively charged hydrophilic molecules first have to enter breast cancer cells via carrier-mediated uptake. Several uptake transporters for sulfo-conjugated steroid hormones have been characterized so far, including members of the OATP and the OAT families (Roth et al., 2012; Müller et al., 2015). Most of these OATP/OAT carriers are multi-specific and are involved in the transport of drugs, drug conjugates, bile salts, and some other charged molecules (Burckhardt, 2012; Hagenbuch and Stieger, 2013). Some of them are even expressed in breast cancer tissue or breast cancer cell lines, including OATP1A2, OATP1B3, OATP2B1, OATP3A1, OATP4A1, and others, thus making them candidates for steroid sulfate uptake in breast cancer (Pressler et al., 2011; Obaidat et al., 2012; Nakanishi and Tamai, 2014).

In the present study, we analyzed expression of the SOAT (gene name *SLC10A6*) in breast cancer. This carrier transports all physiologically occurring sulfo-conjugated steroid hormones, including E_1S (K_m of 12 μM), DHEAS (K_m of 29 μM) and many others (Geyer et al., 2007; Fietz et al., 2013; Grosser et al., 2018). In contrast, free steroids, steroid glucuronides, or bile salts are not transported by SOAT. Therefore, this carrier can be regarded as highly specialized for sulfo-conjugated steroid hormones (Geyer et al., 2007; Grosser et al., 2018), distinguishing it from OATPs and OATs. Another difference to the OATP/OAT carriers is the fact that SOAT mediates a secondary active transport of its substrates. SOAT is highly expressed in germ cells of the testis of men and mice (Fietz et al., 2013; Grosser et al., 2013). Here, the SOAT-mediated import of sulfo-conjugated steroid hormones was suggested to participate in the overall regulation of spermatogenesis and fertility (Fietz et al., 2013; Grosser et al., 2013; Bakhaus et al., 2018). In addition, relatively high SOAT expression was detected in pancreas, placenta, and mammary gland (Geyer et al., 2007).

In the present study, high SOAT mRNA expression was found in a large set of breast cancer specimen. The SOAT protein was localized in the normal ductal epithelium of the breast and strong SOAT expression was found in breast biopsies with different pathologies. Hormone-dependent breast cancer T47D cells, stably transfected with SOAT, showed significant proliferation after incubation with E_1S at physiologically relevant concentrations. This proliferation could be blocked successfully by SOAT inhibition, demonstrating that SOAT could be regarded as an interesting new drug target from the group of E_1S uptake carriers for antiproliferative breast cancer therapy.

Abbreviations: 4-SMP, 4-sulfooxymethylpyrene; DCC, dextran-coated charcoal; DHEAS, dehydroepiandrosterone sulfate; DMEM, Dulbecco's Modified Eagle's Medium; DMSO, dimethyl sulfoxide; E_1, estrone; E_2, estradiol; E_1S, estrone-3-sulfate; ER, estrogen receptor; FCS, fetal calf serum; HER2, human epidermal growth factor receptor 2; IHC, immunohistochemistry; LC-MS-MS, liquid chromatography-tandem mass spectrometry; OAT, organic anion transporter; OATP, organic anion transporting polypeptide; PBS, phosphate buffered saline; PR, progesterone receptor; SOAT, sodium-dependent organic anion transporter; STS, steroid sulfatase; TN, triple negative.

MATERIALS AND METHODS

Materials and Chemicals

All of the chemicals, unless otherwise stated, were from Sigma-Aldrich (Taufkirchen, Germany). The compound 4-SMP was kindly provided by Prof. Dr. Hansruedi Glatt (Potsdam-Rehbrücke). [^{3}H]estrone-3-sulfate ([^{3}H]E_1S, 57 Ci/mmol) was purchased from PerkinElmer (Boston, MA, United States) and [methyl-^{3}H]thymidine (79 Ci/mmol) was obtained from GE Healthcare (Amersham, United Kingdom). TissueScan^{TM} breast cancer cDNA arrays I-IV (BCRT101-BCRT104) were obtained from OriGene (Rockville, MD, United States).

Breast Cancer cDNA Arrays

In order to analyze SOAT expression in breast cancer, the following TissueScan^{TM} cDNA arrays were commercially obtained from OriGene (Rockville, MD, United States): Breast Cancer cDNA Array I (BCRT101), Breast Cancer cDNA Array II (BCRT102), Breast Cancer cDNA Array III (BCRT103), and Breast Cancer cDNA Array IV (BCRT104). Each array contains 48 samples covering tumors of different histopathology, stages and grades. For each tumor cDNA, detailed information is available online[1], including age, gender and ethnicity of the patient, as well as diagnosis, pathology report, histologic type, tissue images, tumor grade (based on the Nottingham grading system, Elston and Ellis, 1991) and tumor stage (according to the American Joint Committee on Cancer, 2002). In addition, the receptor status is provided for the ER, PR, and HER2.

[1]https://www.origene.com/products/tissues/tissuescan

Stable Transfection of T47D Cells With the SOAT Construct

The human breast cancer cell line T47D (obtained from Dr. Bernhard Ugele, Department of Gynecology and Obstetrics, University Hospital Munich, Germany) was maintained in a 1:1 mixture of DMEM and Ham's F12 nutrient mixture (Invitrogen, Karlsruhe, Germany) supplemented with 10% FCS, L-glutamine (4 mM), penicillin (100 units/ml), and streptomycin (100 g/ml) at 37°C, 5% CO_2, and 95% humidity. For stable transfection of T47D cells, the full length SOAT coding sequence (Geyer et al., 2007) was subcloned into the pcDNA3.1 vector (Invitrogen) using *Hin*dIII and *Xba*I restriction sites. The SOAT-pcDNA3 vector was verified by DNA sequencing and used for stable transfection of T47D cells by electroporation. Briefly, subconfluent T47D cells were trypsinized and resuspended in PBS containing 137 mM NaCl, 2.7 mM KCl, 1.5 mM KH_2PO_4, and 7.3 mM Na_2HPO_4 at pH 7.4. Approximately 10^6 cells were transferred to a 4 mm Gene Pulser Cuvette (Bio-Rad Laboratories, Munich, Germany), mixed with 20 μg plasmid and incubated for 10 min on ice. The electroporation was performed on the Gene Pulser Xcell System (Bio-Rad Laboratories) using a single electrical pulse with initial field strength of 120 V, discharged from the 960 μF capacitor and time constant of 10 ms. After an additional 10 min of incubation on ice, cells were plated onto 10 cm culture dishes. After 24 h, selection medium was added containing 750 μg/ml G418 sulfate and cells were further incubated, changing the medium every 3 days. After 12 days, several cell clones were pooled from the culture dishes (T47D-SOAT) and SOAT expression was analyzed by real-time PCR analysis. For control, T47D cells were also transfected with an empty pcDNA3.1 vector. These T47D-control cells were processed in the same manner as the T47D-SOAT cells.

Expression Analysis by Real-Time PCR

TissueScan^{TM} breast cancer cDNA arrays were directly used for expression analysis of SOAT by real-time PCR. Symplekin (SYMPK, Uniprot Q92797) that showed particularly low expression variability in breast cancer tissue and cell lines (Tilli et al., 2016) was used as endogenous control. RNA was isolated from T47D-SOAT and T47D-control cells grown in 10 cm petri dishes under DMEM/F12 medium. Cells were seeded at 10^6 cells per well for each cell type and RNA was isolated following 72 h of growth. The medium and any detached cells were removed from the wells. Total RNA isolation was performed by using the peqGOLD RNAPure reagent (PeqLab, Erlangen, Germany) according to the manufacturer's instructions. The isolated RNA was dissolved in diethylpyrocarbonate-treated water and stored at −80°C until use. The RNA concentration was determined by measuring absorbance at 260 nm with a Beckmann spectrophotometer DU-640 (Beckmann, Munich, Germany). Complementary cDNA was synthesized from the RNA samples using the Advantage RT-for-PCR kit (BD Clontech, Heidelberg, Germany) according to the manufacturer's instructions. For real-time PCR expression analysis of T47D cells, beta-actin was used as endogenous control. Relative gene expression analysis was performed by real-time PCR amplification on an ABI PRISM 7300 thermal cycler (Applied Biosystems, Darmstadt, Germany) using the TaqMan Gene Expression Assays (Applied Biosystems, Darmstadt, Germany) Hs01399354_m1 for SOAT, Hs00165853_m1 for STS, Hs00174860_m1 for ERα, Hs99999903_m1 for beta-actin, and Hs00191361_m1 for SYMPK. Real-time amplification was performed in 96-well optical plates using 5 μl cDNA, 1.25 μl TaqMan Gene Expression Assay, 12.5 μl TaqMan Universal PCR Master Mix and 6.25 μl water in each 25 μl reaction. The plates were heated for 10 min at 95°C, and 45 cycles of 15 s at 95°C and 60 s at 60°C were applied. Relative expression (ΔC_T) was calculated by subtracting the signal threshold cycle (C_T) of the endogenous control from the C_T value of the respective target.

Transport Assays in T47D Cells

For transport studies, 12-well plates were coated with poly-L-lysine for better attachment of the cells. Twenty thousand cells/well were plated and grown under DMEM/F12 medium for 3 days. Before starting the transport experiments, T47D cells were washed three times with PBS and incubated with sodium transport buffer containing 142.9 mM NaCl, 4.7 mM KCl, 1.2 mM KH_2PO_4, 1.2 mM $MgSO_4$, 1.8 mM $CaCl_2$, and 20 mM HEPES (pH 7.4). When transport assays were performed in sodium-free transport buffer, sodium chloride was substituted with equimolar concentrations of choline chloride. T47D-SOAT and T47D-control cells were incubated with 250 μl of transport buffer containing radiolabeled [^{3}H]estrone-3-sulfate ([^{3}H]E_1S) at 37°C for 30 min. Transport assays were terminated by removing the transport buffer and washing five times with ice-cold PBS. Cell monolayers were lysed in 1 N NaOH with 0.1% SDS, and the cell-associated radioactivity was determined in a Wallac 1409 liquid scintillation counter (Pharmacia, Freiburg, Germany). The protein content was determined according to Lowry et al. (1951) using aliquots of the lysed cells with bovine serum albumin as a standard. LC-MS/MS was used to measure E_1S concentrations in the cell culture medium at the end of the uptake phase as described before (Galuska et al., 2013).

Cell Proliferation Assays in T47D Cells

T47D cells were grown for at least 1 week in DMEM/F12 supplemented with 10% FCS. Then, for proliferation assays, the cells were starved for 4 days in steroid-free phenol red-free DMEM/F12 medium supplemented with 5% dextran-coated charcoal-treated FCS (DCC-FCS). DCC-FCS was prepared by incubating 0.5 g DCC in 100 ml FCS over 24 h at 4°C, followed by filtration (pleated filter MN 615 ¼, Macherey-Nagel, Düren, Germany). T47D cells were plated at a density of 10,000 or 20,000 cells/well in 24-well plates. Twenty four hour after seeding, E_2 (final concentration 10^{-9} M) or E_1S (final concentrations 10^{-12} to 10^{-4} M) were added from stock solutions containing DMSO, considering that the final DMSO concentration in the medium was below 0.1%, and cells were incubated at 37°C, 5% CO_2, and 95% humidity. The negative control included solvent alone. Seven days after seeding, cells were treated with [methyl-^{3}H]thymidine with final concentrations of 1 μCi/ml at 37°C for 2 h as reported (Chalbos et al., 1982). After incubation, the medium was removed and cells were washed five times with ice-cold PBS. Then, cell lysis was performed with 500 μl of 1 N NaOH and the radioactivity of the lysates was determined by liquid scintillation counting.

Detection of SOAT in Breast Tissues by Immunohistochemistry

Immunohistochemistry was performed on breast biopsies of different pathologies, i.e., intraductal papilloma, atypical ductal hyperplasia, intraductal carcinoma, and invasive ductal carcinoma. Paraffin-embedded tissue slides were prepared at the Department of Pathology at Atatürk University. Use of human tissue was approved by the ethics committee of Atatürk University, School of Medicine, No: 4/22, 02.06.2015. Tissue sections were incubated with the primary antibody SLC10A6 (C-13) (sc-136875, Santa Cruz, Dallas, TX, United States) at 1:100 dilution, followed by incubation with biotinylated goat anti-rabbit E0432 secondary antibody (Dako, Glostrup, Denmark) at 1:200 dilution in tris-buffered saline. Afterward, sections were incubated with the avidin-biotin complex (ABC Vectastain, Vector, Burlingame, CA, United States) and developed with 3-amino-9-ethylcarbazole (AEC, Biologo, Kronshagen, Germany). Counterstaining was performed with hematoxylin and slides were mounted with Kaiser's glycerol gelatin (Merck, Darmstadt, Germany). Validation of the SLC10A6 C-13 antibody and the IHC protocol has been previously performed for human placenta (Schweigmann et al., 2014).

Statistical Methods

Unless otherwise indicated, values are represented as means ± SD. All graphs and calculations were prepared using the GraphPad Prism software 6.07 (GraphPad Software, La Jolla, CA, United States). Student's unpaired *t*-test and one-way ANOVA with Tukey's multiple comparisons test was performed to determine statistical significance. Differences were considered significant at $p < 0.05$. The EC_{50} values were calculated by non-linear regression analysis from sigmoidal dose-response curves.

RESULTS

SOAT mRNA Expression in Breast Cancer Specimen

In order to analyze SOAT expression in different types of breast cancer, the OriGene TissueScan^{TM} Breast Cancer cDNA Arrays I-IV were screened for SOAT expression by real-time PCR. The arrays included 192 cDNAs from breast cancer samples of different pathology, stages, grades, and receptor status. All samples with pathology verification were included in the data analysis shown in **Figure 1**. Samples without pathology (array classification: within normal limits) were excluded from the analysis. SOAT mRNA expression was normalized by SYMPK expression, which has previously demonstrated particularly low variability of expression in breast cancer tissue and cell lines (Tilli et al., 2016). SOAT expression was undetectable only in very few samples and showed large variability in the tumor samples ranging from ΔC_T of 0.83 (very high expression) up to ΔC_T of 10 (very low expression). Nearly all tumor samples were classified as breast adenocarcinoma, with the vast majority being ductal. Only three cDNAs derived from ductal carcinoma *in situ* and one sample was from a squamous cell carcinoma of the breast. Interestingly, this squamous cell carcinoma showed extremely high SOAT expression that was even higher than in human testis, representing the organ with the highest physiological SOAT expression in man (Geyer et al., 2007; Fietz et al., 2013). In order to determine if SOAT mRNA expression correlates with tumor grade, stage, or receptor status, sub-analyses were performed. As indicated in **Figure 1A**, SOAT expression was not significantly different between tumors with grades G1, G2, or G3, or between tumors of different stages (I-IV). Furthermore, there was no difference in SOAT expression in tumors with different ER, PR, or HER2 status. Even in TN breast cancer samples, SOAT expression was not different from the other groups (**Figure 1B**). Further sub-analyses were performed in the adenocarcinoma samples including age and ethnos (**Figure 1C**). No effect of age on the SOAT mRNA expression of breast adenocarcinomas was detected and SOAT expression was comparable between Caucasians and African Americans.

SOAT expression was also analyzed in individual breast cancer samples at the protein level with the SLC10A6 (SOAT) C-13 antibody by IHC. Whereas SOAT expression was relatively low in the ductal epithelium of normal breast tissue (**Figure 2A**), strong SOAT immunoreactivity was detected in ductal hyperplasia (**Figure 2B**), intraductal papilloma (**Figure 2C**), atypical ductal hyperplasia (**Figure 2D**), intraductal carcinoma (**Figure 2E**), and invasive ductal carcinoma (**Figure 2F**).

Generation of Stably Transfected T47D-SOAT Cells

In order to investigate the role of the carrier-mediated import of E_1S by SOAT for the proliferation of breast cancer cells, we chose the breast cancer cell line T47D as an *in vitro* model. T47D cells have previously been described as ER expressing and they showed estrogen dependent proliferation after incubation with E_2 and E_1S at physiologically relevant concentrations (Nozawa et al., 2004). However, compared to breast cancer tissue (see **Figure 1**), where SOAT expression could be readily detected and quantified in nearly all specimen, SOAT expression was very low in T47D-control cells and was at the border of detectability (C_T~37.9) in the real-time PCR expression analysis. Therefore, in the present study, T47D cells were stably transfected with the SOAT-pcDNA3 construct in order to increase SOAT expression and mimic the situation *in vivo*. Different cell clones were pooled from the culture dishes (further referred to as T47D-SOAT). As control, T47D cells were transfected with an empty pcDNA3 vector (T47D-control). SOAT expression was analyzed by real-time PCR and revealed significantly higher mRNA expression levels in the T47D-SOAT cells compared with the T47D-control cells ($\Delta C_T = 5.4 \pm 0.3$ vs. $\Delta C_T = 18.0 \pm 0.5$). In contrast, mRNA

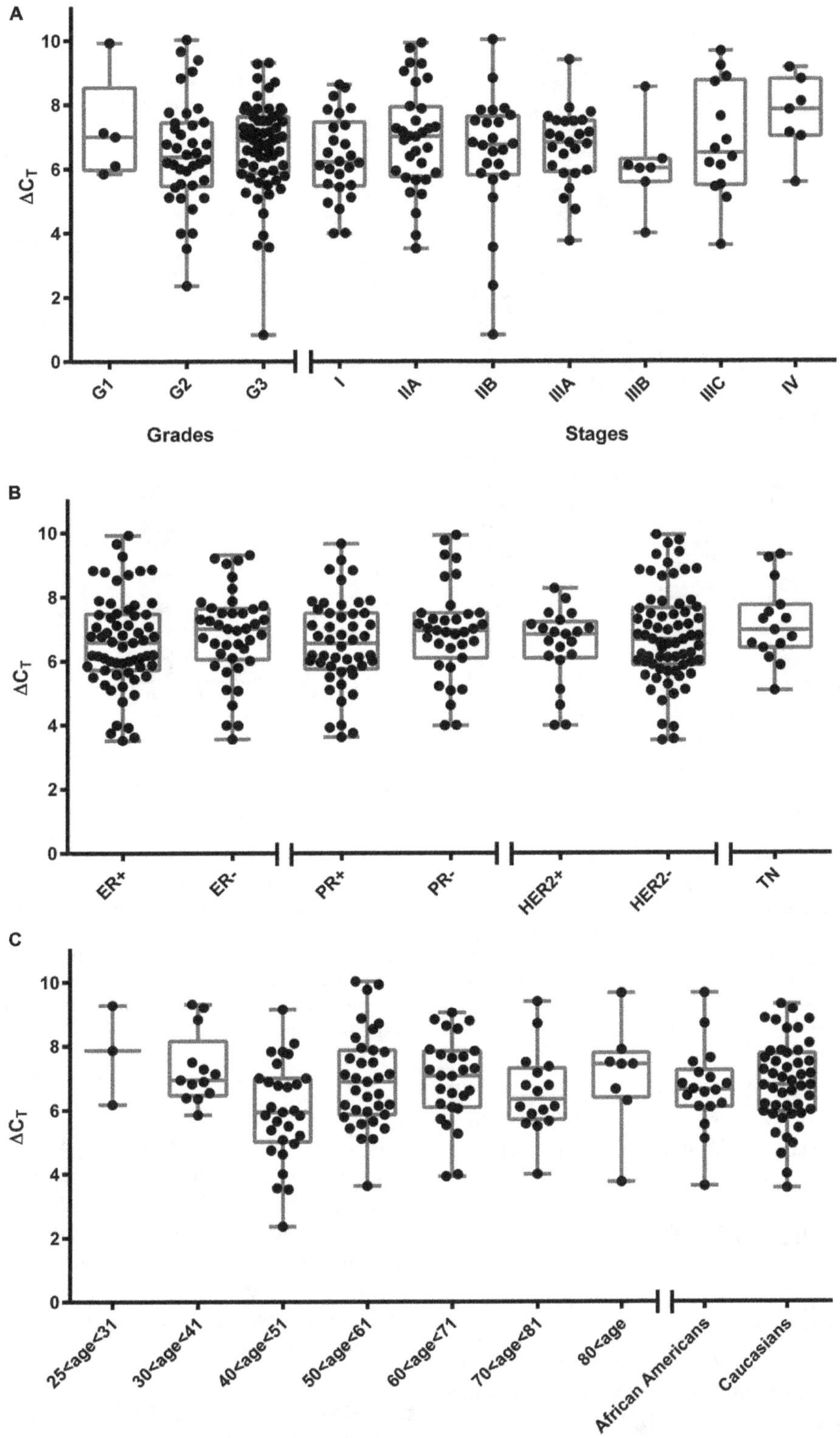

FIGURE 1 | SOAT mRNA expression in breast cancer. SOAT mRNA expression was analyzed in the TissueScan^{TM} Breast Cancer cDNA Arrays I-IV, including 176 tumor cDNAs with different classifications (histopathology, grade, stage, and receptor status). Expression of SYMPK was used as endogenous control and ΔC_T values are depicted at the *y*-axis. A cut-off was set at C_T of 40. Sub-analyses were performed, including **(A)** tumor grade and stage, **(B)** receptor status for ER, PR, HER2 and triple negative breast cancer (TN), and **(C)** age and ethnos. As the cDNA arrays were not equally distributed for the analyzed subgroups, every single value is depicted for better clarity and additional box-whiskers-plots are given. For analysis of statistical significance, one-way ANOVA with Tukey's multiple comparisons test was performed. Differences with $p < 0.05$ were not detected.

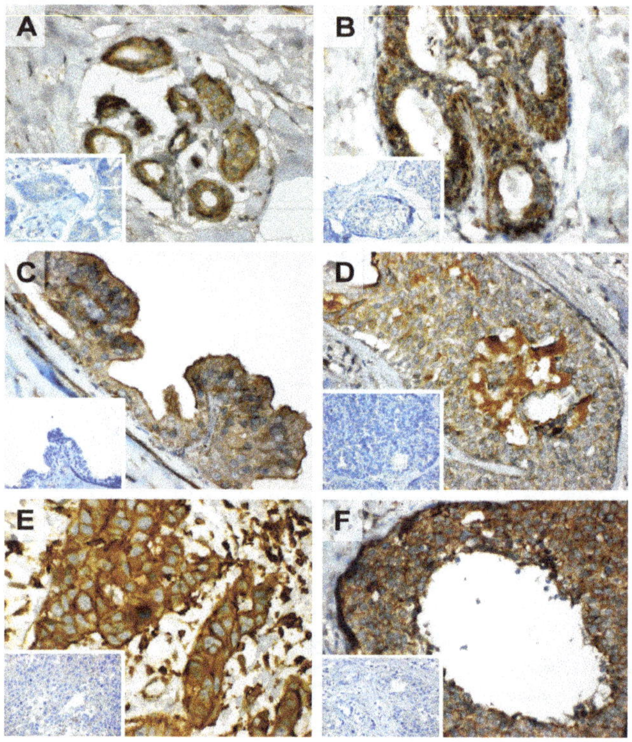

FIGURE 2 | Expression of the SOAT protein in breast cancer specimen. Expression of the SOAT protein was analyzed in different breast cancer specimen by IHC with the SOAT C-13 antibody (1:100 dilution, AEC staining, hematoxylin counter stain), primary magnification × 40. Insets: Negative control without the primary antibody, primary magnification × 40. **(A)** SOAT expression in the ductal epithelium of normal breast tissue. **(B)** Strong SOAT immunoreactivity of the ductal epithelium in usual ductal hyperplasia. **(C)** Expression of SOAT in intraductal papilloma and expression along the ductal epithelium with strong apical lining. **(D)** Strong SOAT immunoreactivity in atypical ductal hyperplasia. **(E)** Severe immunolabeling with the SOAT antibody in intraductal carcinoma. **(F)** Invasive ductal carcinoma with strong and widespread SOAT expression.

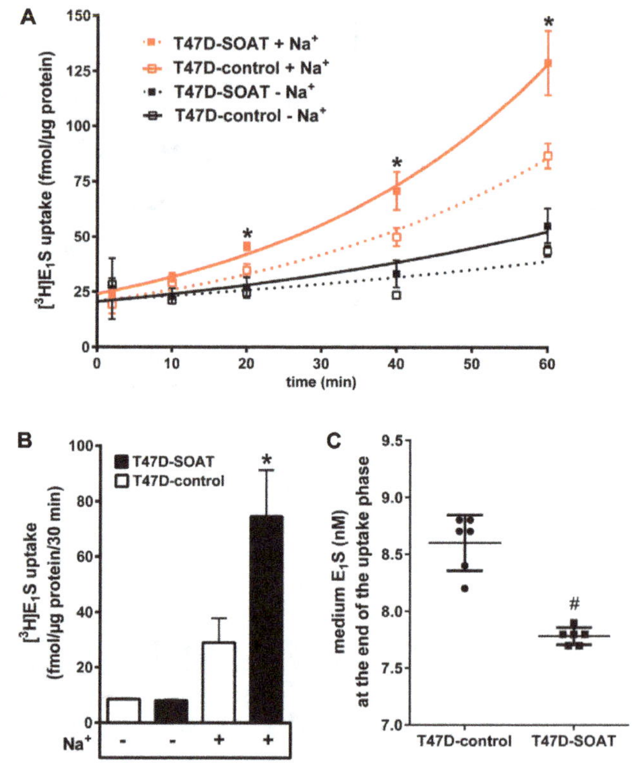

FIGURE 3 | Sodium-dependent uptake of E_1S into T47D-SOAT cells. **(A)** T47D-SOAT and T47D-control cells were incubated with 100 nM [^{3}H]E_1S at 37°C in transport buffer containing Na^+ or without Na^+ (sodium-free control). Cell-associated radioactivity was analyzed at the indicated time points. **(B)** Transport of [^{3}H]E_1S at 10 nM over 30 min. Data in **(A,B)** represent means ± SD of triplicate determinations. *Significantly higher transport compared with T47D-control cells and the sodium-free controls (one-way ANOVA with Tukey's multiple comparisons test with $p < 0.05$). **(C)** Determination of E_1S concentrations by LC-MS/MS in the cell culture medium at the end of the uptake phase. Data represent means ± SD of two independent experiments, each with triplicate determinations. #Significantly different between T47D-SOAT and T47D-control cells (unpaired t-test with $p < 0.05$).

expression levels of STS ($\Delta C_T = 10.4 \pm 0.4$ vs. $\Delta C_T = 9.7 \pm 1.2$) and ERα ($\Delta C_T = 5.2 \pm 0.3$ vs. $\Delta C_T = 5.5 \pm 0.7$) were not significantly different between T47D-SOAT and T47D-control cells.

Transport Studies in SOAT-Transfected T47D Cells

In order to verify functional SOAT carrier expression in the cell membrane of the T47D-SOAT cells, we performed transport experiments with [^{3}H]E_1S as substrate under both sodium and sodium-free conditions. The uptake of 100 nM E_1S significantly increased over time in the T47D-SOAT cells only in the presence of sodium, demonstrating significant sodium-dependent uptake, which is a clear characteristic of SOAT. T47D-control cell showed slightly higher E_1S uptake in the presence of sodium compared to sodium-free conditions, but without reaching the level of significance (**Figure 3A**). At a physiologically relevant concentration of 10 nM, T47D-SOAT cells also showed significantly higher sodium-dependent uptake of E_1S compared with T47D-control cells (**Figure 3B**). In order to verify that under incubation with 10 nM E_1S, this compound is indeed taken up into the cells, an additional medium depletion assay was performed and the E_1S concentration was determined from the medium at the end of incubation by means of LC-MS/MS. As expected, the medium of the T47D-SOAT cells contained significantly lower residue concentrations of E_1S compared to the medium of the T47D-control cells (**Figure 3C**).

E_1S-Stimulated Proliferation of T47D-SOAT Cells

In order to analyze the estrogen-dependent proliferation of the transfected cell lines, T47D-SOAT and T47D-control cells were grown in DCC-FCS medium supplemented with 10^{-9} M E_2 (positive control), increasing concentrations of E_1S ranging from 10^{-12} M to 10^{-4} M, or solvent alone (negative control). Both cell lines showed significantly increased proliferation

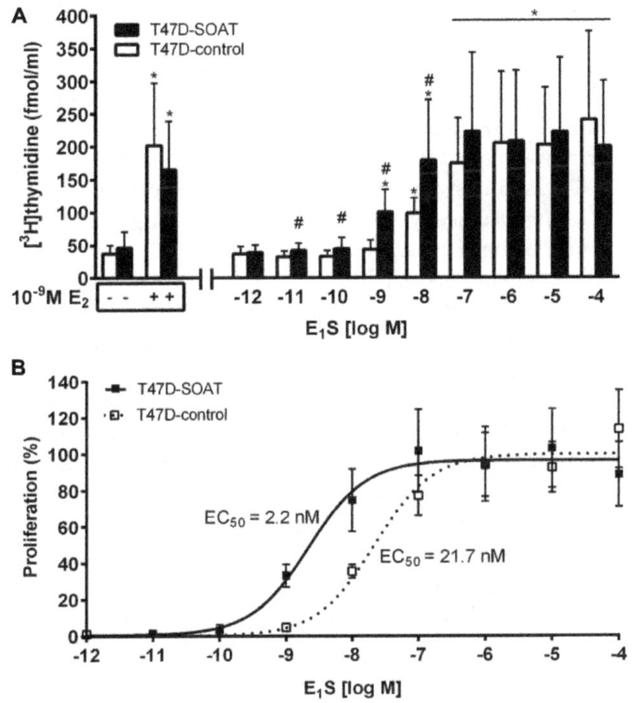

FIGURE 4 | E_1S-dependent proliferation of T47D-SOAT cells. SOAT-transfected T47D cells (T47D-SOAT, filled bars in **A**, black squares in **B**) and mock-transfected T47D cells (T47D-control, open bars in **A**, open squares in **B**) were plated at 10,000 cells/well in 24-well plates and were cultured in phenol red-free DMEM/F12 containing 5% DCC-FCS over 7 days. The culturing medium was supplemented with 10^{-9} M E_2 for positive control or increasing concentrations of E_1S ranging from 10^{-12} M to 10^{-4} M. For negative control, cells were treated with solvent alone. Seven days after seeding, the cells were incubated with 1 μCi/ml [^{3}H]thymidine for 2 h at 37°C, 5% CO_2, and 95% humidity. After five cycles of washing with PBS, cells were subjected to liquid scintillation counting. Data represent the means ± SD of quadruplicate determinations of three independent experiments (n = 12). **(A)** *Significantly higher [^{3}H]thymidine incorporation compared with negative control (one-way ANOVA with Tukey's multiple comparisons test with $p < 0.05$). #Significantly higher [^{3}H]thymidine incorporation in T47D-SOAT compared with T47D-control cells ($p < 0.05$, unpaired t-test). **(B)** Values were fitted to concentration response curves by non-linear regression analysis. Proliferation was determined relative to the top (100%) and bottom (0%) values that were derived from the sigmoidal dose response calculation. The EC_{50} values were 2.2 ± 0.3 nM and 21.7 ± 2.1 nM for the T47D-SOAT and T47D-control cells, respectively. Data represent means ± SEM.

under E_2 treatment and this proliferation occurred at equal levels for the SOAT-T47D and SOAT-control cells (**Figure 4A**). After treatment with E_1S at increasing concentrations, both cell lines showed increased proliferation, but with different profiles. Beginning at 10^{-11} M E_1S, T47D-SOAT cells showed significantly enhanced proliferation compared to T47D-control cells with a maximum proliferation at 10^{-7} M. In contrast, T47D-control cells did not start to proliferate until 10^{-9} M E_1S and required 10^{-6} M E_1S for maximum proliferation (**Figure 4A**). Within the concentration range of 10^{-11} to 10^{-8} M E_1S, T47D-SOAT showed significantly higher proliferation compared to T47D-control cells. Half-maximal stimulation (ED_{50}) of the E_1S-stimulated proliferation occurred at concentrations of 2.2 nM and

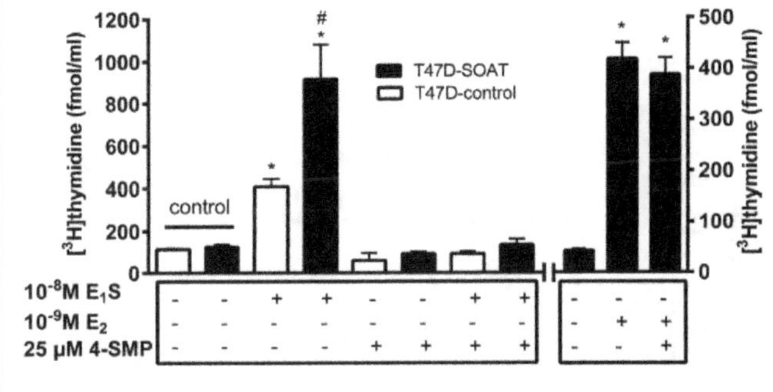

FIGURE 5 | Inhibition of the E_1S-dependent proliferation of T47D-SOAT cells. Stably SOAT-transfected T47D cells (T47D-SOAT) and mock-transfected T47D cells (T47D-control) were plated at 20,000 cells/well in 24-well plates and were cultured in phenol red-free DMEM/F12 containing 5% DCC-FCS. The culturing medium was supplemented with 10^{-8} M E_1S, 10^{-9} M E_2 or solvent alone (control). Additionally, 25 μM of the SOAT inhibitor 4-SMP were added to the culturing medium as indicated. After 6 days of cultivation, the cells were incubated with 1 μCi/ml [^{3}H]thymidine for 2 h at 37°C, 5% CO_2, and 95% humidity. After five cycles of washing with PBS, cells were subjected to liquid scintillation counting. Data represent means ± SD of quadruplicate determinations of a representative experiment. *Significantly different from solvent control (one-way ANOVA with Tukey's multiple comparisons test with $p < 0.05$). #Significantly higher [^{3}H]thymidine incorporation in T47D-SOAT compared with T47D-control cells ($p < 0.05$, unpaired t-test).

21.7 nM for the T47D-SOAT and T47D-control cells, respectively (**Figure 4B**). This indicates that SOAT-mediated transport of E_1S at physiologically relevant concentrations significantly stimulated the proliferation of T47D cells.

In order to block this increased proliferation via SOAT, 4-SMP was used as an inhibitor. 4-SMP proved to be one of the most potent inhibitors of SOAT in a previous study (Geyer et al., 2007). Indeed, incubation of T47D-SOAT cells with 25 μM 4-SMP completely blocked cell proliferation by E_1S (**Figure 5**), while 4-SMP alone had no effect on the cell proliferation of T47D-SOAT and T47D-control cells. Furthermore, 4-SMP had no effect on the E_2-stimulated cell proliferation of T47D-SOAT cells, which occurs independent from SOAT-mediated transport (**Figure 5**, right panel).

In further experiments, the time course of E_1S-stimulated T47D cell proliferation was analyzed in further detail with and without 4-SMP as inhibitor of SOAT. Both cell lines, T47D-SOAT and T47D-control, significantly increased their proliferation from days 4 to 6 under incubation with 10 nM E_1S, but at day 6, T47D-SOAT cells showed significantly higher [^{3}H]thymidine incorporation compared with the T47D-control cells. In cells additionally incubated with 4-SMP, proliferation was blocked and was not different from the control groups without E_1S incubation (**Figure 6**). Again, 4-SMP alone had no effect on cell proliferation.

DISCUSSION

As has been known for a long time, breast tumor tissue is able to metabolize steroids from sulfated precursors, which are available even after menopause, to biologically active estrogens

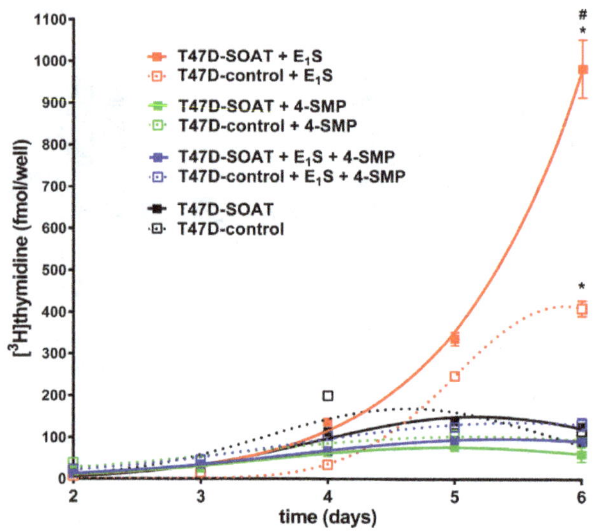

FIGURE 6 | Time course of the E_1S-dependent proliferation of T47D-SOAT cells. T47D-SOAT and T47D-control cells were plated at 20,000 cells/well in 24-well plates and were cultured in phenol red-free DMEM/F12 containing 5% DCC-FCS. The culturing medium was supplemented with 10^{-8} M E_1S, 25 µM 4-SMP or solvent alone. Additionally, 10^{-8} M E_1S were incubated together with the SOAT inhibitor 4-SMP at 25 µM. After 2, 3, 4, 5, and 6 days of cultivation, the cells were incubated with 1 µCi/ml [^{3}H]thymidine for 2 h at 37°C, 5% CO_2, and 95% humidity. After five cycles of washing with PBS, cells were subjected to liquid scintillation counting. Data represent the means ± SD of quadruplicate determinations of a representative experiment. *Significant increase compared to day 2 ($p < 0.05$, one-way ANOVA with Tukey's multiple comparisons test). #Significantly higher [^{3}H]thymidine incorporation in T47D-SOAT compared to T47D-control cells ($p < 0.05$, unpaired t-test).

(Adams and Wong, 1968; Miller and Forrest, 1976). Most studies in this field focus on the metabolic steps involved in estrogen formation, and simply presume intracellular availability of the mostly sulfated precursors (Labrie et al., 2001). However, sulfo-conjugated steroids are negatively charged molecules and can only enter target cells via carrier-mediated uptake (Müller et al., 2015). Therefore, several previous studies have investigated the expression of uptake carriers for sulfated steroids in the normal mammary gland and breast cancer tissue, including OATP1A2, OATP2B1, OATP3A1, OATP4A1, and OATP1B3 (Pizzagalli et al., 2003; Miki et al., 2006; Meyer zu Schwabedissen et al., 2008; Wlcek et al., 2008; Kindla et al., 2011; Banerjee et al., 2014). Furthermore, E_1S uptake carrier expression was demonstrated in different hormone-dependent breast cancer cell lines, such as OATP1A2, OATP3A1, and OATP4A1 in T47D cells (Nozawa et al., 2004, 2005; Meyer zu Schwabedissen et al., 2008) as well as OATP1A2, OATP2B1, OATP3A1, and OATP4A1 in MCF7 cells (Nozawa et al., 2005; Meyer zu Schwabedissen et al., 2008; Wlcek et al., 2008; Maeda et al., 2010; Stute et al., 2012; Banerjee et al., 2012, 2013, 2015; Matsumoto et al., 2015). Overall these studies demonstrated that carrier-mediated import of E_1S in breast cancer cells can stimulate their proliferation and thus these carriers were suggested as potential drug targets (Obaidat et al., 2012; Nakanishi and Tamai, 2014).

In the present study, we only focused on the expression of SOAT in breast cancer and aimed to analyze its role for hormone-dependent proliferation. SOAT was first cloned from rat adrenal gland and demonstrated significant transport of E_1S and DHEAS (Geyer et al., 2004). Later, the human SOAT transcript was cloned (Geyer et al., 2007). The substrate spectrum of SOAT was intensively analyzed and revealed specific transport of all physiologically occurring sulfo-conjugated steroid hormones, being E_1S, 17β-estradiol-3-sulfate, 17β-estradiol-17-sulfate, pregnenolone sulfate, 17α-OH-pregnenolone sulfate, androsterone sulfate, epiandrosterone sulfate, testosterone sulfate, epitestosterone sulfate, 5α-dihydrotestosterone sulfate, androstenediol sulfate, DHEAS, and 16α-OH-DHEAS (Geyer et al., 2007; Fietz et al., 2013; Schweigmann et al., 2014; Grosser et al., 2018). Sulfo-conjugated bile salts, bromosulfophthalein (BSP, a dye used in liver function tests), and the sulfooxymethylpyrenes 2-SMP and 4-SMP were identified as effective SOAT inhibitors (Geyer et al., 2007). Apart from high SOAT expression in the testis, placenta, lung and skin, SOAT also showed relatively high mRNA expression in the mammary gland (Geyer et al., 2007). Here, in the present study the SOAT protein was localized to the ductal epithelium (**Figure 2**). Based on this data, it was not surprising that SOAT showed high expression in different pathologies of the breast with a clear ductal staining pattern in IHC, including ductal hyperplasia, intraductal papilloma and intraductal carcinoma (**Figure 2**). It can be supposed that, in addition to other E_1S carriers from the OATP family, SOAT expression in ductal hyperplasia and intraductal carcinoma contributes to the import of E_1S (and probably also E_2S) and therefore provides the precursors for the intracrine formation of pro-proliferative E_2. Based on this mechanism, SOAT can be regarded as an additional drug target for anti-proliferative breast cancer therapy from the group of E_1S uptake carriers. Against this background, it is interesting to note that SOAT expression was detected in a wide range of breast cancer specimen. Most of them represent adenocarcinoma of the breast with ductal localization (**Figure 1**). SOAT expression does not correlate with tumor stage, grade or receptor status. Therefore, SOAT might be an interesting drug target in a wide variety of breast tumors.

In order to verify the role of SOAT for the E_1S-dependent proliferation of breast cancer cells, we intended to generate an *in vitro* model that mimics the *in vivo* situation as near as possible. Different ER positive breast cancer cell lines such as T47D and MCF7 have emerged as *in vitro* models for proliferation studies in the past (MacIndoe, 1988; Pasqualini et al., 1990; Evans et al., 1993; Billich et al., 2000; Schmitt et al., 2001; Maggiolini et al., 2001, 2002). Of those, we used T47D cells, as their intracrine estrogen synthesis is well characterized and E_1S uptake carrier expression has been investigated previously on these cells (Pizzagalli et al., 2003; Nozawa et al., 2004; Miki et al., 2006). However, as demonstrated by real-time PCR, SOAT expression seems to be down-regulated in T47D cells compared to breast cancer tissue. Therefore, we generated a SOAT-transfected T47D-SOAT cell line as well as a mock-transfected T47D-control cell line for proliferation assays. In the T47D-SOAT cells, high SOAT mRNA expression was confirmed by real-time PCR at the transcriptional level as well as by significant sodium-dependent transport of $[^3H]E_1S$ at the level of the active transporter protein (**Figure 3**). For proliferation studies, these T47D-SOAT cells were incubated under increasing concentrations of E_1S at 10^{-12} to 10^{-4} M. As previously described (Nozawa et al., 2004), proliferation of T47D cells can be stimulated not only by E_2, but also by E_1S at higher concentrations. In the present study, we obtained a sigmoidal dose-response curve with an effective concentration (EC_{50}) of 21.7 nM for the T47D-control cells, which is very close to previous data, being 17.1 nM (Nozawa et al., 2004). Interestingly, proliferation of the SOAT-expressing T47D-SOAT cells was stimulated already at much lower E_1S concentrations and the dose-response curve revealed an EC_{50} of 2.2 nM, meaning a 10-fold increased sensitivity to E_1S exposure. At physiological E_1S concentrations, being in the order 10^{-8} to 10^{-9} M (Pasqualini, 2004), the differences between the proliferations of T47D-SOAT vs. T47D-control cells were most pronounced (**Figure 4**). To ensure that this increased proliferation is indeed induced by SOAT-mediated import of E_1S, the cells were co-incubated with E_1S and the SOAT inhibitor 4-SMP (Geyer et al., 2007). In these experiments, E_1S was added at 10 nM to stimulate cell proliferation, representing a concentration at which T47D-SOAT cells showed significant sodium-dependent transport activity for $[^3H]E_1S$. Interestingly, 4-SMP completely blocked the E_1S-mediated proliferation of T47D-SOAT cells and likewise that of T47D-control cells. To verify that 4-SMP itself does not cause inhibition of proliferation by any other effect than by inhibiting the E_1S uptake, 4-SMP was additionally co-incubated with E_2. In these experiments, the E_2-stimulated proliferation of the T47D-SOAT cells was not affected by 4-SMP, indicating that 4-SMP had no effect on the direct estrogenic effect of E_2, but only on the transport of E_1S. The inhibiting effect of 4-SMP on the T47D-control cells could mean that here, residue E_1S transport activity is inhibited even if SOAT is expressed at very low levels in the T47D-control cells. Another explanation would be that 4-SMP inhibits other E_1S uptake transporters, such as OATP1A2, OATP2B1, OATP3A1, and OATP4A1, which have been detected previously in T47D cells (Pizzagalli et al., 2003; Nozawa et al., 2004; Miki et al., 2006). At least in the case of OAT3, 4-SMP has been described as inhibitor (Bakhiya et al., 2006), indicating that 4-SMP is not selective for SOAT. However, if 4-SMP does interfere with the E_1S transport via one of the mentioned OATPs must be elucidated.

CONCLUSION

The present study demonstrates expression of SOAT in breast cancer tissue with ductal localization. SOAT inhibition can block the E_1S-stimulated proliferation of T47D breast cancer cells and, therefore, in addition to the carriers of the OATP carrier family, can be regarded as a novel potential drug target for anti-proliferative breast cancer therapy. Very recently, novel inhibitors of SOAT were identified by pharmacophore modeling (Grosser et al., 2016). After optimization, these compounds are interesting candidates for further breast cancer proliferation studies *in vitro* and *in vivo*. These studies should also include comparative transport inhibition of SOAT and carriers of the OATP and OAT families in order to find at best an inhibitor for E_1S transport covering all uptake carriers in breast cancer cells.

AUTHOR CONTRIBUTIONS

EK, GG, RL, CG, and AS-G acquired and analyzed the data. DZ, SW, and JG interpreted the data and wrote the manuscript. DZ and JG conceived, designed, and supervised the study.

ACKNOWLEDGMENTS

The authors want to acknowledge Dr. Kerstin Funk for technical help with the real-time PCR amplification, Prof. Dr. Hansruedi Glatt for kindly providing 4-SMP, and Dr. Bernhard Ugele for kindly providing T47D cells. Michael Kirstgen and Massimo Palatini are acknowledged for their technical help with data presentation.

REFERENCES

Adams, J. B., and Wong, M. S. F. (1968). Paraendocrine behaviour of human breast carcinoma: in vitro transformation of steroids to physiologically active hormones. *J. Endocr.* 41, 41–52. doi: 10.1677/joe.0.0410041

American Joint Committee on Cancer (2002). in *Cancer Staging Manual*, 6th Edn, eds F. L. Greene, D. L. Page, I. D. Fleming, A. G. Fritz, C. M. Balch, D. G. Haller, et al. (New York, NY: Springer-Verlag). doi: 10.1007/978-1-4757-3656-4

Bakhaus, K., Bennien, J., Fietz, D., Sánchez-Guijo, A., Hartmann, M., Serafini, R., et al. (2018). Sodium-dependent organic anion transporter (Slc10a6−/−) knockout mice show normal spermatogenesis and reproduction, but elevated serum levels for cholesterol sulfate. *J. Steroid Biochem. Mol. Biol.* 179, 45–54. doi: 10.1016/j.jsbmb.2017.07.019

Bakhiya, N., Stephani, M., Bahn, A., Ugele, B., Seidel, A., Burckhardt, G., et al. (2006). Uptake of chemically reactive, DNA-damaging sulfuric acid esters into renal cells by human organic anion transporters. *J. Am. Soc. Nephrol.* 17, 1414–1421. doi: 10.1681/ASN.2005080801

Banerjee, N., Allen, C., and Bendayan, R. (2012). Differential role of organic anion-transporting polypeptides in estrone-3-sulphate uptake by breast epithelial cells and breast cancer cells. *J. Pharmacol. Exp. Ther.* 342, 510–519. doi: 10.1124/jpet.112.192344

Banerjee, N., Fonge, H., Mikhail, A., Reilly, R. M., Bendayan, R., and Allen, C. (2013). Estrone-3-sulphate, a potential novel ligand for targeting breast cancers. *PLoS One* 8:e64069. doi: 10.1371/journal.pone.0064069

Banerjee, N., Miller, N., Allen, C., and Bendayan, R. (2014). Expression of membrane transporters and metabolic enzymes involved in estrone-3-sulphate disposition in human breast tumour tissues. *Breast Cancer Res. Treat.* 145, 647–661. doi: 10.1007/s10549-014-2990-y

Banerjee, N., Wu, T. R., Chio, J., Kelly, R., Stephenson, K. A., Forbes, J., et al. (2015). 125I-Labelled 2-Iodoestrone-3-sulfate: synthesis, characterization and OATP mediated transport studies in hormone dependent and independent breast cancer cells. *Nucl. Med. Biol.* 42, 274–282. doi: 10.1016/j.nucmedbio.2014.10.011

Billich, A., Nussbaumer, P., and Lehr, P. (2000). Stimulation of MCF-7 breast cancer cell proliferation by estrone sulfate and dehydroepiandrosterone sulfate: inhibition by novel non-steroidal steroid sulfatase inhibitors. *J. Steroid Biochem. Mol. Biol.* 73, 225–235. doi: 10.1016/S0960-0760(00)00077-7

Burckhardt, G. (2012). Drug transport by organic anion transporters (OATs). *Pharmacol. Ther.* 136, 106–130. doi: 10.1016/j.pharmthera.2012.07.010

Chalbos, D., Vignon, F., Keydar, I., and Rochefort, H. (1982). Estrogens stimulate cell proliferation and induce secretory proteins in a human breast cancer cell line (T47D). *J. Clin. Endocrinol. Metab.* 55, 276–283. doi: 10.1210/jcem-55-2-276

Conner, P., Lundström, E., and von Schoultz, B. (2008). Breast cancer and hormonal therapy. *Clin. Obstet. Gynecol.* 51, 592–606. doi: 10.1097/GRF.0b013e318180b8ed

Elston, C. W., and Ellis, I. O. (1991). Pathological prognostic factors in breast cancer. I. The value of histological grade in breast cancer: experience from a large study with long-term follow-up. *Histopathol* 19, 403–410. doi: 10.1111/j.1365-2559.1991.tb00229.x

Evans, T. R., Rowlands, M. G., Luqmani, Y. A., Chander, S. K., and Coombes, R. C. (1993). Detection of breast cancer-associated estrone sulfatase in breast cancer biopsies and cell lines using polymerase chain reaction. *J. Steroid Biochem. Mol. Biol.* 46, 195–201. doi: 10.1016/0960-0760(93)90294-7

Fietz, D., Bakhaus, K., Wapelhorst, B., Grosser, G., Günther, S., Alber, J., et al. (2013). Membrane transporters for sulfated steroids in the human testis - Cellular localization, expression pattern and functional analysis. *PLoS One* 8:e62638. doi: 10.1371/journal.pone.0062638

Galuska, C. E., Hartmann, M. F., Sánchez-Guijo, A., Bakhaus, K., Geyer, J., Schuler, G., et al. (2013). Profiling intact steroid sulfates and unconjugated steroids in biological fluids by liquid chromatography-tandem mass spectrometry (LC-MS-MS). *Analyst* 138, 3792–3801. doi: 10.1039/c3an36817c

Geisler, J. (2003). Breast cancer tissue estrogens and their manipulation with aromatase inhibitors and inactivators. *J. Steroid Biochem. Mol. Biol.* 86, 245–253. doi: 10.1016/S0960-0760(03)00364-9

Geyer, J., Döring, B., Meerkamp, K., Ugele, B., Bakhiya, N., Fernandes, C. F., et al. (2007). Cloning and functional characterization of human sodium-dependent organic anion transporter (SLC10A6). *J. Biol. Chem.* 282, 19728–19741. doi: 10.1074/jbc.M702663200

Geyer, J., Godoy, J. R., and Petzinger, E. (2004). Identification of a sodium-dependent organic anion transporter from rat adrenal gland. *Biochem. Biophys. Res. Commun.* 316, 300–306. doi: 10.1016/j.bbrc.2004.02.048

Grosser, G., Baringhaus, K. H., Döring, B., Kramer, W., Petzinger, E., and Geyer, J. (2016). Identification of novel inhibitors of the steroid sulfate carrier sodium-dependent organic anion transporter SOAT (SLC10A6) by pharmacophore modelling. *Mol. Cell. Endocrinol.* 428, 133–141. doi: 10.1016/j.mce.2016.03.028

Grosser, G., Bennien, J., Sánchez-Guijo, A., Bakhaus, K., Döring, B., Hartmann, M., et al. (2018). Transport of steroid 3-sulfates and steroid 17-sulfates by the sodium-dependent organic anion transporter SOAT (SLC10A6). *J. Steroid Biochem. Mol. Biol.* 179, 20–25. doi: 10.1016/j.jsbmb.2017.09.013

Grosser, G., Fietz, D., Günther, S., Bakhaus, K., Schweigmann, H., Ugele, B., et al. (2013). Cloning and functional characterization of the mouse sodium-dependent organic anion transporter Soat (Slc10a6). *J. Steroid Biochem. Mol. Biol.* 138, 90–99. doi: 10.1016/j.jsbmb.2013.03.009

Hagenbuch, B., and Stieger, B. (2013). The SLCO (former SLC21) superfamily of transporters. *Mol. Aspects Med.* 34, 396–412. doi: 10.1016/j.mam.2012.10.009

Henderson, B. E., Ross, R., and Bernstein, L. (1988). Estrogens as a cause of human cancer: the Richard and Hinda Rosenthal foundation award lecture. *Cancer Res.* 48, 246–253.

Kenemans, P., and Bosman, A. (2003). Breast cancer and post-menopausal hormone therapy. *Best Pract. Res. Clin. Endocrinol. Metab.* 17, 123–137.

Kindla, J., Rau, T. T., Jung, R., Fasching, P. A., Strick, R., Stoehr, R., et al. (2011). Expression and localization of the uptake transporters OATP2B1, OATP3A1 and OATP5A1 in non-malignant and malignant breast tissue. *Cancer Biol. Ther.* 11, 584–591. doi: 10.4161/cbt.11.6.14533

Labrie, F., Belanger, A., Luu-The, V., Labrie, C., Simard, J., Cusan, L., et al. (1998). DHEA and the intracrine formation of androgens and estrogens in peripheral target tissues: its role during aging. *Steroids* 63, 322–328. doi: 10.1016/S0039-128X(98)00007-5

Labrie, F., Luu-The, V., Labrie, C., and Simard, J. (2001). DHEA and its transformation into androgens and estrogens in peripheral target tissues: intracrinology. *Front. Neuroendocrinol.* 22, 185–212. doi: 10.1006/frne.2001.0216

Lowry, O. H., Rosebrough, N. J., Farr, A. L., and Randall, R. J. (1951). Protein measurement with the folin phenol reagent. *J. Biol. Chem.* 193, 265–275.

MacIndoe, J. H. (1988). The hydrolysis of estrone sulfate and dehydroepiandrosterone sulfate by MCF-7 human breast cancer cells. *Endocrinology* 123, 1281–1287. doi: 10.1210/endo-123-3-1281

Maeda, T., Irokawa, M., Arakawa, H., Kuraoka, E., Nozawa, T., Tateoka, R., et al. (2010). Uptake transporter organic anion transporting polypeptide 1B3 contributes to the growth of estrogen-dependent breast cancer. *J. Steroid Biochem. Mol. Biol.* 122, 180–185. doi: 10.1016/j.jsbmb.2010.06.014

Maggiolini, M., Bonofiglio, D., Pezzi, V., Carpino, A., Marsico, S., Rago, V., et al. (2002). Aromatase overexpression enhances the stimulatory effects of adrenal androgens on MCF7 breast cancer cells. *Mol. Cell. Endocrinol.* 193, 13–18. doi: 10.1016/S0303-7207(02)00091-6

Maggiolini, M., Carpino, A., Bonofiglio, D., Pezzi, V., Rago, V., Marsico, S., et al. (2001). The direct proliferative stimulus of dehydroepiandrosterone on MCF7 breast cancer cells is potentiated by overexpression of aromatase. *Mol. Cell. Endocrinol.* 184, 163–171. doi: 10.1016/S0303-7207(01)00563-9

Matsumoto, J., Ariyoshi, N., Sakakibara, M., Nakanishi, T., Okubo, Y., Shiina, N., et al. (2015). Organic anion transporting polypeptide 2B1 expression correlates with uptake of estrone-3-sulfate and cell proliferation in estrogen receptor-positive breast cancer cells. *Drug Metab. Pharmacokinet.* 30, 133–141. doi: 10.1016/j.dmpk.2014.10.005

Meyer zu Schwabedissen, H. E., Tirona, R. G., Yip, C. S., Ho, R. H., and Kim, R. B. (2008). Interplay between the nuclear receptor pregnane X receptor and the uptake transporter organic anion transporter polypeptide 1A2 selectively enhances estrogen effects in breast cancer. *Cancer Res.* 68, 9338–9347. doi: 10.1158/0008-5472.CAN-08-0265

Miki, Y., Suzuki, T., Kitada, K., Yabuki, N., Shibuya, R., Moriya, T., et al. (2006). Expression of the steroid and xenobiotic receptor and its possible target gene, organic anion transporting polypeptide-A, in human breast carcinoma. *Cancer Res.* 66, 535–542. doi: 10.1158/0008-5472.CAN-05-1070

Miller, W. R., and Forrest, A. P. (1976). Oestradiol synthesis from C19 steroids by human breast cancers. *Br. J. Cancer* 33, 116–118. doi: 10.1038/bjc.1976.13

Müller, J. W., Gilligan, L. C., Idkowiak, J., Arlt, W., and Foster, P. A. (2015). The regulation of steroid action by sulfation and desulfation. *Endocr. Rev.* 36, 526–563. doi: 10.1210/er.2015-1036

Nakanishi, T., and Tamai, T. (2014). Putative roles of organic anion transporting polypeptides (OATPs) in cell survival and progression of human cancers. *Biopharm. Drug Dispos.* 35, 463–484. doi: 10.1002/bdd.1915

Nozawa, T., Suzuki, M., Takahashi, K., Yabuuchi, H., Maeda, T., Tsuji, A., et al. (2004). Involvement of estrone-3-sulfate transporters in proliferation of hormone-dependent breast cancer cells. *J. Pharmacol. Exp. Ther.* 311, 1032–1037. doi: 10.1124/jpet.104.071522

Nozawa, T., Suzuki, M., Yabuuchi, H., Irokawa, M., Tsuji, A., and Tamai, I. (2005). Suppression of cell proliferation by inhibition of estrone-3-sulfate transporter in estrogen-dependent breast cancer cells. *Pharm. Res.* 22, 1634–1641. doi: 10.1007/s11095-005-7096-0

Obaidat, A., Roth, M., and Hagenbuch, B. (2012). The expression and function of organic anion transporting polypeptides in normal tissue and in cancer. *Annu. Rev. Pharmacol. Toxicol.* 52, 135–151. doi: 10.1146/annurev-pharmtox-010510-100556

Osborne, C. K. (1998). Tamoxifen in the treatment of breast cancer. *N. Engl. J. Med.* 339, 1609–1618. doi: 10.1056/NEJM199811263392207

Pasqualini, J. R. (2004). The selective estrogen enzyme modulators in breast cancer: a review. *Biochim. Biophys. Acta* 1654, 123–143. doi: 10.1016/j.bbcan.2004.03.001

Pasqualini, J. R., Cortes-Prieto, J., Chetrite, G., Talbi, M., and Ruiz, A. (1997). Concentrations of estrone, estradiol and their sulfates, and evaluation of sulfatase and aromatase activities in patients with breast fibroadenoma. *Int. J. Cancer* 70, 639–643. doi: 10.1002/(SICI)1097-0215(19970317)70:6<639::AID-IJC2>3.0.CO;2-W

Pasqualini, J. R., Gelly, C., and Nguyen, B. L. (1990). Metabolism and biologic response of estrogen sulfates in hormone-dependent and hormone-independent mammary cancer cell lines. Effect of antiestrogens. *Ann. N. Y. Acad. Sci.* 595, 106–116. doi: 10.1111/j.1749-6632.1990.tb34286.x

Pizzagalli, F., Varga, Z., Huber, R. D., Folkers, G., Meier, P. J., and St-Pierre, M. V. (2003). Identification of steroid sulfate transport processes in the human mammary gland. *J. Clin. Endocrinol. Metab.* 88, 3902–3912. doi: 10.1210/jc.2003-030174

Pressler, H., Sissung, T. M., Venzon, D., Price, D. K., and Figg, W. D. (2011). Expression of OATP family members in hormone-related cancers: potential markers of progression. *PLoS One* 6:e20372. doi: 10.1371/journal.pone.0020372

Rémy-Martin, A., Prost, O., Nicollier, M., Burnod, J., and Adessi, G. L. (1983). Estrone sulfate concentrations in plasma of normal individuals, postmenopausal women with breast cancer, and men with cirrhosis. *Clin. Chem.* 29, 86–89.

Roth, M., Obaidat, A., and Hagenbuch, B. (2012). OATPs, OATs and OCTs: the organic anion and cation transporters of the SLCO and SLC22A gene superfamilies. *Br. J. Pharmacol.* 165, 1260–1287. doi: 10.1111/j.1476-5381.2011.01724.x

Santen, R. J., and Harvey, H. A. (1999). Use of aromatase inhibitors in breast carcinoma. *Endocr. Relat. Cancer* 6, 75–92. doi: 10.1677/erc.0.0060075

Santner, S. J., Leszczynski, D., Wright, C., Manni, A., Feil, P. D., and Santen, R. J. (1986). Estrone sulfate: a potential source of estradiol in human breast cancer tissues. *Breast Cancer Res. Treat.* 7, 35–44. doi: 10.1007/BF01886734

Sasano, H., Suzuki, T., Nakata, T., and Moriya, T. (2006). New development in intracrinology of breast carcinoma. *Breast Cancer* 13, 129–136. doi: 10.2325/jbcs.13.129

Schmitt, M., Klinga, K., Schnarr, B., Morfin, R., and Mayer, D. (2001). Dehydroepiandrosterone stimulates proliferation and gene expression in MCF-7 cells after conversion to estradiol. *Mol. Cell. Endocrinol.* 173, 1–13. doi: 10.1016/S0303-7207(00)00442-1

Schweigmann, H., Sánchez-Guijo, A., Ugele, B., Hartmann, K., Hartmann, M. F., Bergmann, M., et al. (2014). Transport of the placental estriol precursor 16α-hydroxy-dehydroepiandrosterone sulfate (16α-OH-DHEAS) by stably transfected OAT4-, SOAT-, and NTCP-HEK293 cells. *J. Steroid Biochem. Mol. Biol.* 143, 259–265. doi: 10.1016/j.jsbmb.2014.03.013

Stanway, S. J., Delavault, P., Purohit, A., Woo, L. W., Thurieau, C., Potter, B. V., et al. (2007). Steroid sulfatase: a new target for the endocrine therapy of breast cancer. *Oncologist* 12, 370–374. doi: 10.1634/theoncologist.12-4-370

Stute, P., Reichenbach, A., Szuwart, T., Kiesel, L., and Götte, M. (2012). Impact of testosterone on the expression of organic anion transporting polypeptides (OATP-1A2, OATP-2B1, OATP-3A1) in malignant and non-malignant human breast cells in vitro. *Maturitas* 71, 376–384. doi: 10.1016/j.maturitas.2011.12.020

Suzuki, T., Miki, Y., Nakamura, Y., Moriya, T., Ito, K., Ohuchi, N., et al. (2005). Sex steroid-producing enzymes in human breast cancer. *Endocr. Relat. Cancer* 12, 701–720. doi: 10.1677/erc.1.00834

Tilli, T. M., Castro, C. S., Tuszynski, J. A., and Carels, N. (2016). A strategy to identify housekeeping genes suitable for analysis in breast cancer diseases. *BMC Genomics* 17:639. doi: 10.1186/s12864-016-2946-1

Wlcek, K., Svoboda, M., Thalhammer, T., Sellner, F., Krupitza, G., and Jaeger, W. (2008). Altered expression of organic anion transporter polypeptide (OATP) genes in human breast carcinoma. *Cancer Biol. Ther.* 7, 1450–1455. doi: 10.4161/cbt.7.9.6282

4

Intracrine Regulation of Estrogen and Other Sex Steroid Levels in Endometrium and Non-Gynecological Tissues: Pathology, Physiology, and Drug Discovery

Gonda Konings [1,2†], Linda Brentjens [1,2†], Bert Delvoux [1,2], Tero Linnanen [3], Karlijn Cornel [1,2], Pasi Koskimies [3], Marlies Bongers [1,2], Roy Kruitwagen [1,2], Sofia Xanthoulea [1,2] and Andrea Romano [1,2*]

[1] GROW–School for Oncology and Developmental Biology, Maastricht University, Maastricht, Netherlands, [2] Department of Obstetrics and Gynaecology, Maastricht University Medical Centre, Maastricht, Netherlands, [3] Forendo Pharma Ltd., Turku, Finland

***Correspondence:**
Andrea Romano
a.romano@maastrichtuniversity.nl

† These authors have contributed equally to this work

Our understanding of the intracrine (or local) regulation of estrogen and other steroid synthesis and degradation expanded in the last decades, also thanks to recent technological advances in chromatography mass-spectrometry. Estrogen responsive tissues and organs are not passive receivers of the pool of steroids present in the blood but they can actively modify the intra-tissue steroid concentrations. This allows fine-tuning the exposure of responsive tissues and organs to estrogens and other steroids in order to best respond to the physiological needs of each specific organ. Deviations in such intracrine control can lead to unbalanced steroid hormone exposure and disturbances. Through a systematic bibliographic search on the expression of the intracrine enzymes in various tissues, this review gives an up-to-date view of the intracrine estrogen metabolisms, and to a lesser extent that of progestogens and androgens, in the lower female genital tract, including the physiological control of endometrial functions, receptivity, menopausal status and related pathological conditions. An overview of the intracrine regulation in extra gynecological tissues such as the lungs, gastrointestinal tract, brain, colon and bone is given. Current therapeutic approaches aimed at interfering with these metabolisms and future perspectives are discussed.

Keywords: intracrinology, endometrium, estrogens, lungs, gastrointestinal tract, central nervous system, bone

INTRODUCTION

The term "intracrinology," coined in 1988 by prof Labrie, refers to the ability of peripheral tissues to use blood precursors and generate steroids (Labrie, 1991). Several studies have been published but several controversies still exist and relate to the following technical and biological aspects: (a) some intracrine enzymes in peripheral tissues have low expression (300–50,000-times lower than in endocrine glands Stoffel-Wagner, 2001; Murakami et al., 2006, close to the detection limit of standard methods like western blotting and immunohistochemistry -IHC); (b) the technology to robustly quantify steroids (liquid-/gas-chromatography tandem mass-spectrometry -LC-MS or GC-MS), became available during the last 5–10 years only (Rosner et al., 2013); (c) intracrine pathways are highly complex.

This review summarizes our knowledge of intracrinology in peripheral tissues like the endometrium, lungs, gastrointestinal tract (GIT), bone and central nervous system (CNS), with special attention to the metabolism of estrogens. Drug development and potential therapeutic approaches are discussed. In this review, the enzymes involved in steroid deactivation/clearance (Rižner, 2013, 2016; with the exclusion of steroid sulphotransferases) and those involved in the transport of conjugated steroids through the plasma membrane (Rižner et al., 2017) are not described. Studies on serum/tissue steroid levels are reported and discussed only if based on gold standard GC/LC-MS.

FROM OVARIAN ESTROGEN SYNTHESIS TO INTRACRINOLOGY

Local steroid metabolism is possible because those enzymes responsible for steroid synthesis in classical glands (ovaries, adrenals, testes) are expressed in peripheral tissues, where additional and alternative routes for metabolizing steroids are present and make intracrine networks intricate and flexible (**Figures 1, 2, Tables 1, 2**). In particular, several compounds generated through these pathways, although not being estrogens, can have estrogenic action, because able to bind and activate the estrogen receptors. The biologic activity of the various compounds is given in **Table 1**, and in **Figure 2**, by the color codes.

Ovarian Steroidogenesis

Transformation of cholesterol to 17β-estradiol (E2) involves first the production of dehydroepiandrosterone (DHEA) in theca cells through the action of steroidogenic acute regulatory protein (StAR) that facilitates the transport of cholesterol into mitochondria, followed by CYP11A1 (rate-limiting) and CYP17A1 (**Figure 2**); the ovarian pathway is indicated by the yellow background; reviewed by (Miller and Auchus, 2011; Andersen and Ezcurra, 2014). CYP11A1 is a type I CYP localized in mitochondria that uses nicotine-adenine-dinucleotide-phosphate (NADPH) and ferredoxin (Fdx)/ferredoxin reductase (FdR) to cleave the cholesterol side chain and produce pregnenolone (P5). Type II CYP17A1, localized in the endoplasmic reticulum (EndRet), has both 17α-hydroxylase and 17,20-lyase activities. It uses NADPH and P450 oxidoreductase (POR) to first hydroxylate P5 to 17α-hydroxypregnenolone (17OHP5) (17α-hydroxylase action), followed by 17,20-lyase action to release DHEA. Gonad specific type 2 3β-hydroxysteroid dehydrogenase (3βHSD2) has 3β-dehydrogenase and Δ^5 to Δ^4 isomerase activities and converts DHEA to androstenedione (A4). Next, CYP19A1 catalyzes the oxidative demethylation of C_{19} androgens to C_{18} estrogens, with A-ring aromatisation; hence A4 is converted to estrone (E1). The final conversion of E1 (with low affinity for the estrogen-receptors -ERs) to E2 (high affinity for ERs and high estrogenic potency) is catalyzed by 17βHSD1 that reduces 17-keto to 17β-hydroxyl steroids. In the ovary, the 17-keto group of A4 can be reduced to 17β-hydroxyl by AKR1C3/17βHSD5 yielding testosterone (T) that is converted to E2 by CYP19A1. Upon ovulation, high 3βHSD2 levels in the corpus luteum lead to high progesterone (P) generation from P5.

Intracrine Steroidogenesis

The expression of StAR, CYP11A1 and CYP17A1 is demonstrated in a limited number of peripheral tissues (see later and **Tables 6–8**). However, pregnenes, pregnanes, androstenes and androstanes generated from these initial steps (but also abundantly available as circulating precursors) can be further metabolized locally thus generating a plethora of compounds with various biological activities (estrogenic, androgenic, progestogenic and neuroactive; **Tables 1, 2** and **Figure 2**). The Δ^5 to Δ^4 isomerization of androstenes (DHEA, androstenediol -A5- and 17αA5) and pregnenes (P5, 17OHP5) is catalyzed by 3βHSD1, which is the peripheral counterpart of ovarian 3βHSD2. Also 3βHSD2, whose expression was initially considered to be restricted to endocrine tissues, is detected peripherally in recent reports (Stoffel-Wagner, 2001; Tsai et al., 2001; Attar et al., 2009; Huhtinen et al., 2014; Osinski et al., 2018). Due to the high concentration of DHEA (both in blood and tissues), its conversion to A4 by 3βHSDs is relevant to the formation of downstream androgens and of estrogens. Additionally, 3βHSDs convert A5 and the isomer 17αA5 to T and epitestosterone (EpiT). Although minor, in the context of women's health, these pathways are relevant. A5, together with 3α and 3βDIOL (generated by AKR1Cs from DHT and AN, see below) activate both ERs and have estrogenic action (especially 3βDIOL, a potent ERβ binder). A5 possesses immune stimulatory activity whereas its 17α isomer (17αA5) has androgenic, antitumor and neuroactivity.

Abbreviations: [3H], tritiated hydrogen; [14C], radioactive carbon; AD, Alzheimer disease; ADHD, attention deficit hyperactivity disorder; AI, aromatase inhibitor; AKR, aldo-ketoreductase; AR, androgen-receptor; ART, assisted reproduction technology; BMD, bone mineral density; BMP-2, bone morphogenetic protein 2; COPD, chronic obstructive pulmonary disease; COUP-TFII, chicken-ovalbumin-upstream-promoter-transcription-factor II; CNS, central nervous system; CRC, colorectal cancer; CX43, connexin 43; DS, digestive system; Ed, embryonic day; EC, endometrial cancer; EndRet, endoplasmic reticulum; ER, estrogen-receptor; Fdx, ferredoxin; FdR, ferredoxin reductase; GC-MS, gas-chromatography tandem mass-spectrometry; GnRH, gonadotropin releasing hormone; GH, growth hormone; GIT, gastrointestinal tract; GPER, G protein-coupled estrogen-receptor; HPLC, high performance liquid-chromatography; HRT, hormone-replacement-therapy; hCG, human chorionic gonadotropin; IGF1, insulin-like growth factor 1; IHC, immunohistochemistry; IL-1, interleukin-1; IL-6, interleukin-6; KO, knock-out; LC-MS, liquid-chromatography tandem mass-spectrometry; mTOR, mammalian target of rapamycin; NAPDH, nicotine-adenine-dinucleotide-phosphate; NSCLC, non-small cell lung cancer; PAIN, phenomena of pan-assay interfering compounds; PAP, bis-phospho-nucleotide-3′-phospho-adenosine-5′-phosphate; PCOC, poly cystic ovarian syndrome; POR, P450 oxidoreductase; RT-qPCR, reverse-transcriptase quantitative polymerase-chain-reaction; SF1, steroidogenic factor 1; SHBG, sex hormone binding globulin; SNP, single nucleotide polymorphism; SRD, short-chain dehydrogenase; Th, T-helper; TNF, tumor necrosis factor; VEGF, vascular endothelial growth factor; WB, western blot/blotting; WOI, window of implantation.

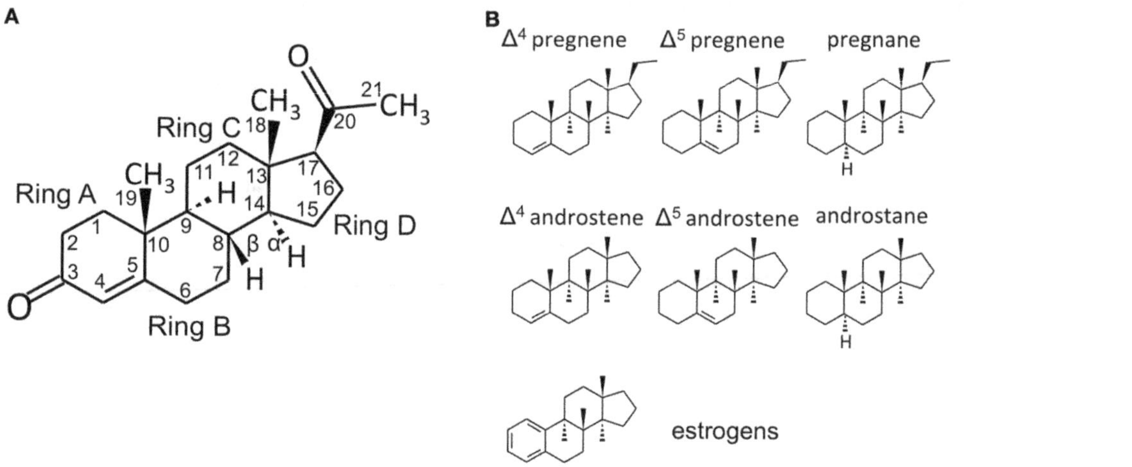

FIGURE 1 | Steroid structure. **(A)** structure of the C21 steroid progesterone (P, used as an example), with carbon numbering and steroid ring numbering. In the storied graphics in **Figures 1B** and **2**, the H groups and the relative bonds will be omitted (with the exclusion of the H in 5α-reduced steroids - androstanes and pregnanes). Methyl groups will be indicated by the bonds only without the CH_3 group. **(B)** structures of C21 pregnene (Δ^4 and Δ^5, i.e., double bond between C4 and C5 or between C5 and C6, respectively), pregnane (5α-reduced steroid), C19 androstene (Δ^4, Δ^5) and androstane and C18 (A-ring)-aromatic estrogens. Chemical structures were designed with the aid of Sketcher V2.4 (Ihlenfeldt et al., 2009), available online at PubChem (www.ncbi.nlm.nih.gov; pubchem.ncbi.nlm.nih.gov) (Kim et al., 2016).

Additionally, EpiT is a weak AR binder and a strong endogenous inhibitor of SRD5As (Loria and Graf, 2012). The endogenous occurrence of 17αA5 is demonstrated in humans (Laatikainen et al., 1971) but its route of synthesis is unclear (Shimizu, 1979). A 17αHSD able to convert A4 to EpiT and DHEA to 17αA5 is characterized in mice (Bellemare et al., 2005) but no human homologous is described yet. Similarly to the ovaries, androgen to estrogen conversion is catalyzed by CYP19A1.

A particularly important reaction is controlled by oxidative and reductive 17βHSDs, which interconvert 17-keto and 17β-hydroxysteroids. Since 17β-hydroxysteroids (T and E2) have higher affinity for the receptors than the keto-steroids (A4 and E1), this balance determines the final androgenic/estrogenic activity. Fourteen 17βHSDs exist, whose specificity is determined by tissue distribution, intracellular localization and biochemistry (**Table 2**); reviewed thoroughly in (Mindnich et al., 2004; Moeller and Adamski, 2006, 2009; Prehn et al., 2009; Miller and Auchus, 2011). Unpublished data also refer to a 15th 17βHSD (see **Table 2**; reported in Luu-The et al., 2008) with a putative role in androgen metabolism. With the exclusion of 17βHSD5 (AKR1C3, see below), all other 17βHSDs belong to the short-chain dehydrogenase (SRD) family.

Although all 17βHSDs have been postulated to use steroids as substrates based on cell-free or *in vitro* assays, recent investigations based on substrate specificity (Laplante et al., 2009) and knock-out (KO) models (**Table 4**) better clarified their roles. Type 1 17βHSD is the estrogenic enzyme and coverts E1 to E2 both in the ovary and in peripheral tissue. Type 2 17βHSD oxidizes 17-hydroxyl groups (E2 and T) to the 17-keto forms (E1 and A4), and possesses also a 20α-hydroxyl oxidative action, through which this enzyme generates P from 20αDHP. Type 6 17βHSD uses 5α-reduced androgens and has 17-hydroxyl oxidative activity (converting androsterone -AN- to androstanedione) and 3-hydroxyl oxidative activity (converting 3αDIOL to the most potent androgen dihydrotestosterone - DHT). Additional catalytic actions for 17βHSD6 (epimerase or 17-hydroxydehydrogenase) are demonstrated *in vitro* (**Table 2**). Type 14 17βHSD is postulated to have 17β-hydroxyl oxidative action on various steroids, type 7 is involved in cholesterol metabolism as indicated by KO mice (**Table 4**), whereas there is apparently little/no *in vivo* role of types 8, 9, 10, 11 and 12 17βHSDs on steroid metabolism (**Table 2** and indicated by KO mice, **Table 4**). Recently, a novel SRD, DHRS11, was shown to possess *in vitro* 17-keto to 17β-hydroxyl reductive action (able to use E1, Δ^5 or Δ^4 androstenes, androstanes), plus reductive 3βHSD activity toward Δ^4 pregnenes and other compounds (5β-steroids, bile acids; **Table 2** and **Figure 2**; Endo et al., 2016).

Androgens and progestogens can be further metabolized by aldo-ketoreductases (AKRs) and 5α-reductases (SRD5As; **Figure 2**). Cytoplasmic AKRs (AKR1C1, 1C2, 1C3/17βHSD5 and 1C4) have broad substrate specificity with non-stereo-selective 3α/3βHSD, 17- and 20-ketosteroid reductase activities (**Table 2**; Penning et al., 2004; Steckelbroeck et al., 2010). Together with the fact that they have wide tissue distribution (only AKR1C4 is restricted), AKR1Cs contribute to make intracrine networks flexible and intricate (Rižner and Penning, 2014; Sinreih et al., 2014).

SRD5As convert 3-keto Δ^4 androstene and pregnene to 5α-reduced steroids (androstanes and pregnanes), hence they are important in progestogen, androgen (DHT production) and neurosteroid metabolism (Di Costanzo et al., 2009). SRD5A1 and 3 are widely expressed, in contrast to SRD5A2. Human 5β-reductase activity, catalyzed by AKR1D1, is restricted to the liver, where 5β-steroids are directed to clearance/catabolism. However, some 5β-compounds are neuroactive and recent studies indicate

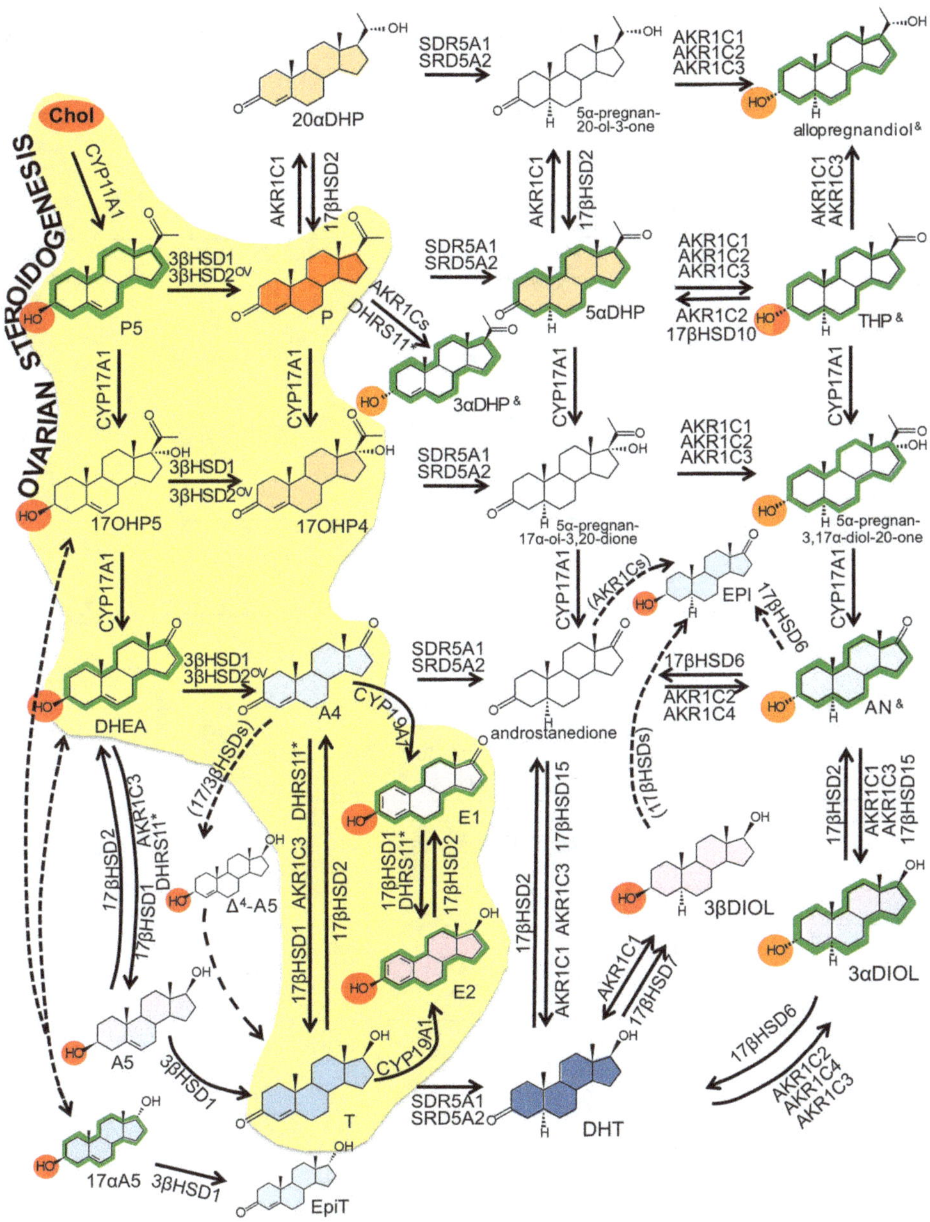

FIGURE 2 | Intracrine networks. Major intracrine networks metabolizing steroids. In this figure, each reaction reports the catalyzing enzymes whose role in that specific reaction is established based on robust evidences (*in vitro*, *ex vivo*, *in vivo*). Additional enzymes whose involvement in the same reactions is less robustly demonstrated or based only on *in silico* or cell-free assay are reported in **Table 2**. The role of 17βHSD3 is disregarded in this figure because restricted to tissues that are not assessed in the present review (testes, prostate, **Table 2**).

Color codes:

Yellow Background: Ovarian classic steroidogenesis.

Red circles: 3β-sulphated hydroxyl groups.

Orange circles: 3α-sulphated hydroxyl groups.

Biological activity (weak – strong)

- progesterone receptor activation (PRA/B)
- androgen receptor activation (AR)
- estrogen receptor activation (ERα/β)
- $GABA_A$ receptor allosteric modulator

OV ovarian specific referring to 3β-HSD2 (see text); – dotted arrows indicate reactions that are not fully demonstrated to occur or for which the responsible enzyme is not identified yet; (enzyme name) enzymes indicated by brackets are supposed to catalyze the indicated reaction based on the theoretical assumptions, no experimental proof is yet available; & these compounds (THP, 3αDHP and allopregnandiol) exist as various hydroxyl α/β isomers (3, 5, 17) with no activity, classic action or neuroactivity (see **Table 2**); * the role of DHRS11 in steroid metabolism is reported only recently by one publication (Endo et al., 2016).

TABLE 1 | Major steroidal compounds.

1. Abbreviation (used here) **2. Common name** **3. Chemical name**		**Blood concentration ** (nM)**	**Biologic activity*****	**Entries***
1. *none* 2. *none* 3. 5α-pregnan-20-ol-3-one[1]	PREGNANES	n.d.		CAS:516-59-6 HMDB:60408 CB:0504265 ChEBI:81469
1. *none* 2. allopregnandiol (4 isomers) 3 a. 5α-pregnane-3α,20α-diol ^ b. 5α-pregnane-3β,20β-diol c. 5α-pregnane-3β,20β-diol d. 5α-pregnane-3β,20α-diol		3a. M *S*: 28–49[10] 3a. F: 0.2–0.7[10]; *S*: 13–20[10]	3a. $GABA_A$+	a.CAS:566-58-5 b.CAS:516-53-0 c.CAS:516-53-0 d.CAS:516-53-0
1. 5αDHP 2. allopregnanedione 3. 5α-pregnane-3,20-dione		F: 0.2–1.1[5,10]	PR+ $GABA_A$+	CAS:566-65-4 HMDB:0003759 ChEBI:28952
1. *none* 2. *none* 3. 5α-pregnan-17α-ol-3,20-dione		n.d.		CAS:570-59-2 CB:4441841
1. *none* 2. *none* 3. 5α-pregnan-3,17α-diol-20-one [2^]		n.d.		CAS:6890-65-9 CB:7269033
1. THP (isomer 1/4) 2. allopregnanolone[3] 3. 3α-hydoxy-5α-pregnan-20-one		All: 0.2–10[6] M: 0.1–0.2[10]; *S*: 3.6–10[10] F: 0.1–0.2[10]; *S*: 4.0–6.7[10]	$GABA_A$+	CAS:516-54-1 HMDB:0001449 PC:262961
1. THP (isomer 2/4) 2. pregnanolone[3] 3. 3α-hydroxy-5β-pregnan-20-one		M *S*: 8.6–18[10] F: 0.06–0.1[10]; *S*: 5.5–10[10]	$GABA_A$+	CAS:128-20-1 HMDB:0062782 CHEBI:1712 PC:31402
1. THP (isomer 3/4) 2. isopregnanolone[3] 3. 3β-hydoxy-5α-pregnan-20-one		M *S*: 7.8–10[10] F: 0.08–0.2[10]; *S*: 3.7–7.1[10]	$GABA_A$− (THP-S)	CAS:516-55-2 HMDB:0001455 PC:92787
1. THP (isomer 4/4) 2. epipregnanolone[3] 3. 3β-hydoxy-5β-pregnan-20-one		All: 0.3–3[6] M *S*: 0.4–0.6[10] F: 0.02–0.04[10]; *S*: 1.5–2.5[10]	$GABA_A$− (THP-S)	CAS:128-21-2 HMDB:0001471 PC:228491
1. 3αDHP 2. 3α-dihydroprogesterone 3. 4-pregnen-3α-ol-20-one	PREGNENES	n.d.	$GABA_A$+	CAS:25680-68-6 PC:121951
1. 3βDHP[4] 2. 3β-dihydroprogesterone 3. 4-pregnen-3β-ol-20-one		n.d.		PC:121951
1. P 2. progesterone 3. 4-pregnene-3,20-dione		M: 0–0.4[6] Fpre: 0–80[6] Fpost: 0–0.4[6]	PR+	HMDB:01830
1. 17OHP 2. 17α-hydroxyprogesterone 3. 17-hydroxypregn-4-en-3,20-dione		M: 0.61–7.0[6] F: 0.21–2.3[6]	PR+	CAS:68-96-2 HMDB:0000374 CHEBI:17252 PC:6238

(Continued)

TABLE 1 | Continued

1. Abbreviation (used here) **2. Common name** **3. Chemical name**	Class	**Blood concentration ** (nM)**	**Biologic activity*****	**Entries***
1. 20αDHP 2. 20α-dihydroprogesterone 3. 20α-hydroxypreg-4-en-3-one	PREGNENES	Fpre: 0.8–11.7[6]	PR+	CAS:145-14-2 HMDB:0003069 PC:8956
1. 17OHP5 2. 17-hydroxypregnenolone 3. 5-Pregnen-3β,17α-diol-20-one	PREGNENES	M: 1.0–12 [6] F: 0–6.0[6]		CAS:387-79-1 HMDB:0000363 CHEBI:28750 PC:3032570
1. P5 2. pregnenolone 3. pregn-5-en-3β-ol-20-one	PREGNENES	M: 1–15[6]; *S*: 200–1,000[6] Fpre: 1.0–15[6]; *S*: 100–1,000[6] Fpost: 1.0–15[6]; *S*: 10–500[6]	$GABA_A$– (P5-S)	CAS:145-13-1 HMDB:0000253 CHEBI:16581 PC:8955
1. *none* 2. androstanedione 3. 5α-androstane-3,17-dione	ANDROSTANES	M: 0.3[7]		HMDB:0000899 CHEBI:22542
1. AN 2. androsterone 3. 3α-hydroxy-5α-androstan-17-one	ANDROSTANES	All: 0.5–0.9[7] M: 0.4–4.0[6,10]; *S*: 617–1,080[10] F: 0.3–0.6[10]; *S*: 359–1,070[10]	AR+ weak $GABA_A$+	HMDB:0000031
1. 5βAN 2. etiocholanolone 3. 3α-hydroxy-5β-androstan-17-one	ANDROSTANES	M: 0.09–0.2[10]; *S*: 32–70[10] F: 0.1–0.4 [10]; *S*: 34–88[10]	$GABA_A$+	CAS:53-42-9 HMDB:00490 CHEBI:28195 PC:5880
1. 3αDIOL 2. androstanediol 3. 5α-androstane-3α,17β-diol	ANDROSTANES	M: 0.4–0.5[9,10]; *S*: 35–121[10] F: 0.03–0.06 [10]; *S*: 2.4–4.8[10]	ERβ+ weak $GABA_A$+	HMDB:0000495
1. 3βDIOL 2. 3β-androstanediol 3. 5α-androstane-3β,17β-diol	ANDROSTANES	All: 0.15[7] M *S*: 34–103[10] F *S*: 8.7–18[10]	ERβ+	HMDB:0000493
1. EPI 2. epiandrosterone 3. 3β-hydroxy-17-oxo-5α-androstane	ANDROSTANES	M: 0.3–0.7[9,10]; *S*: 211–532[10] F: 0.3–0.7[10]; *S*: 172–350[10]	AR+ weak	CAS:481-29-8 HMDB:0000365 CHEBI:541975 PC:441302
1. DHT 2. dihydrotestosterone 3. 17β-hydroxy-5α-androstan-3-one	ANDROSTANES	M: 0/85–3.5 (50–100)[6] Fpre: 0.08–1.3[6] Fpost: 0.03–1.65[6]	AR+	HMDB:0002961 CHEBI:16330 PC:10635
1. EpiT[8] 2. epitestosterone 3. 17α-hydroxy-4-androsten-3-one	ANDROSTENES	M: 1.3–2.9[7]	AR+ weak[9]	CAS:481-30-1 HMDB:0000628 CHEBI:42534 CB:10204
1. A5 2. androstenediol 3. androst-5-ene-3β,17β-diol	ANDROSTENES	M: 2.6–3.7[9,10]; *S*: 243–494[10] F: 0.8–1.1[10,11]; *S*: 85–302[10]	AR+ weak	CAS 521-17-5 HMDB:0003818 CHEBI:2710 PC:10634
1. 17αA5 2. 17α- androstenediol 3. androst-5-ene-3β,17α-diol	ANDROSTENES	n.d.	AR+ weak GAB A_A–	CAS:521-17-5 HMDB:0003818 CHEBI:2710 PC:10634
1. Δ^4-A5 2. 4-androstenediol 3. androst-4-ene-3β,17β-diol	ANDROSTENES	n.d.		CAS:1156-92-9 HMDB:0005849 PC:12476620
1. DHEA 2. dehydroepiandrosterone 3. (3β)-3-hydroxyandrost-5-en-17-one	ANDROSTENES	M: 10–25[6]; *S*: 2K-10K[6] Fpre: 3.0–30[6]; *S*: 1K-8K[6] Fpost: 2.0–20[6]; *S*: 1K-6K[6]	$GABA_A$– (DHEA and DHEA-S)	HMDB:0000077

(Continued)

TABLE 1 | Continued

1. Abbreviation (used here) 2. Common name 3. Chemical name		Blood concentration ** (nM)	Biologic activity***	Entries*
1. A4 2. androstenedione 3. 4-Androstene-3,17-dione	ANDROSTENES	All: 3.1–5.9[7]	AR+	CAS:63-05-8 HMDB:0000053 CHEBI:16422
1. T 2. testosterone 3. 17β-hydroxyandrost-4-ene-3-one	ANDROSTENES	M: 5–25[6] Fpre: 0.2–2.0[6] Fpost: 0.2–1.0[6]	AR+	CAS:55-22-0 HMDB:0000234 CHEBI:17347
1. E2 2. 17β-estradiol 3. (17β)-estra-1,3,5(10)-triene-3,17-diol	ESTROGENS	M: 0.02–0.04[6] Fpre: 0.005–1.0[6] Fpost: 0.005–0.08[6]	ER+	CAS:50-28-2 HMDB:0000151 CHEBI:16469
1. E1 2. estrone 3. 3-hydroxy-1,3,5(10)-estratrien-17-one	ESTROGENS	M: 0.033–0.1[6]; *S*: 2.0–4.0[6] Fpre: 0.015–0.5; *S*: 2.0–5.0[6] Fpost: 0.01–0.12; *S*: 5–20(X10^{-3}) [6]	ER+	CAS:53-16-7 HMDB:0000145 CHEBI:17263

List of the steroids discussed in the present review with the major features. Nomenclature of these compounds is variable and aliases are given as ***Supplemental Materials****.*
**CAS: Chemical Abstracts Service, a division of the American Chemical Society (www.cas.org. Accessed on date: February 2018); HMDB: Human Metabolome Data Base (www.hmdb.ca. Accessed on date: February 2018) (Wishart et al., 2013); CB: Chemical Book (www.chemicalbook.com. Accessed on date: February 2018); ChEBI (www.ebi.ac.uk/chebi. Accessed on date: February 2018) (Morgat et al., 2015); PC: PubChem (www.ncbi.nlm.nih.gov; pubchem.ncbi.nlm.nih.gov. Accessed on date: February 2018) (Kim et al., 2016).*
***M: male subjects; F: female subjects; Fpre: female premenopausal subjects; Fpost: female postmenopausal subjects; -S: sulphated compounds.*
****PR, ER, AR: compound activates the indicated steroid receptor; $GABA_A$ allosteric positive (+) or negative (–) modulator.*
^This isomer is shown in ***Figure 2****.*
n.d.: not determined.
[1] 20β-/5β-isomers exist (CB8678436, Chemical Book - www.chemicalbook.com. Accessed on date: February 2018); [2]Isomer 5α-pregnan-3β,17α-diol-20-one exists (CB:0291774, Chemical Book - www.chemicalbook.com. Accessed on date: February 2018); [3]In general, 5α-reduced and 3α-hydroxysteroids are positive allosteric modulator of $GABA_A$, whereas 3α- and 3β-sulphated hydroxysteroids and 5β-reduced steroids are negative allosteric modulator of $GABA_A$. The 3β-hydroxy isomers of THP are inactive (Belelli and Lambert, 2005; Gibbs et al., 2006; [4]This compound is $GABA_A$ receptor inactive; [5]Pearson Murphy et al., 2001; [6]Mueller et al., 2015), [7]Data extracted from the Human Metabolome Data Base-HMDB (www.hmdb.ca. Accessed on date: February 2018) (Wishart et al., 2013); [8]This compound is strong inhibitor of SRD5As. [9]Kancheva et al. (2007) and [10]Bicikova et al. (2013).

the presence of AKR1D1 in placenta and myometrium (Jin et al., 2011). With the exclusion of their neuroactivity (Paragraph 4.6), 5β-steroids will not be further considered.

The sulphatase pathway is finally responsible for the balance between sulpho-conjugated and free steroids. Sulpho-conjugated steroids (-S) possess higher water solubility, increased stability and longer half-life than unconjugated compounds (e.g., 10–12 h *vs.* 20–30 min for estrogens), and although they cannot bind steroid-receptors, they serve as a reservoir for the formation of biologically active steroids (Reed et al., 2005). Sulphotransferases (SULTs) are phase-I detoxifying enzymes that use bis-phospho-nucleotide 3′-phospho-adenosine-5′-phosphate- (PAP)-sulfate as donor to conjugate 3β-hydroxyl steroids (e.g., estrogens, DHEA, P5, cholesterol; red circles in **Figure 2**) with a sulfate group (Strott, 2002; Rižner, 2016). Distinct SULTs have different specificities toward substrates, with SULT1E1 being the major estrogen sulphating enzyme (with little contribution of SULT1A1), and SULT2A1 being specific for DHEA (but also for P5, 17OHP5 and A5) (**Table 2**). Steroid sulphatase (STS) is a membrane-bound microsomal enzyme that catalyzes the hydrolysis of sulfate ester bonds from sulphated-steroids (cholesterol-S, P5-S, 17OHP5-S, DHEA-S, E1-S) (Mueller et al., 2015; Rižner, 2016), thus releasing unconjugated compounds.

Although sulphated-3α-hydroxysteroids are not thoroughly studied, they are detected in biospecimens (AN-S, 3αDIOL-S; **Table 1** and orange circles in **Figure 2**). They are most likely produced by SULT2A1 (active on 3α-hydroxy bile acids) (Strott, 2002; Rižner, 2016) but no 3α-stereo specific sulphatase is known to date. Some intracellular sulphated-steroids are converted to other compounds without prior desulphation (Sánchez-Guijo et al., 2016).

In conclusions, intracrinology presents redundant and complex pathways, which generate compounds with various activities. Genetic variants in intracrine genes are associated with various diseases (classically endocrine and not; **Table 5**). Even in the absence of the enzymatic machinery to metabolize cholesterol (StAR, steroidogenic factor, CYP17A1 and CYP11A1), DHEA, P5 and especially their sulphated-conjugates have high blood concentrations (**Table 1**), and are used to generate all other steroids in peripheral tissues.

DRUG DEVELOPMENT

Natural hormones have been historically used as drugs, and depending on definitions, approximately 90 marketed drugs share a steroidal core (see https://www.drugbank.ca). Steroids (T, E2, cortisol, DHEA), simple derivatives (ethinylestrogen, prednisolone) or more complex analogs (abiraterone, fulvestrant) are used in various conditions. This old-and-proven steroidal chemistry based approach is used even in modern era.

TABLE 2 | Major enzymes involved in steroidogenesis.

1. Abbr. **2. Gene ID** **3. *Gene name(s)***	**Chromosome** **Gene size*** **mRNA size*** **Exons (no)**	**Protein (aa)**** **Dalton** **Localization (L)*****	**1. Name** / **2. Family** **3. Catalysis** / **4. Substrates****** **5. Distribution** / **6. Cofactor**
1. StAR **2.** 6770 **3.** *STAR, STARD1*	**Chr:** 8p11.23 **gene:** 8.6 **mRNA:** 1.6 **Exons:** 8	**aa:** 285 **Dalton:** 31,914 **L:** mitochon	**1.** steroidogenic acute regulatory protein **2.** cytochrome P450 **3.** facilitate transport of cholesterol to mitochondria **4.** cholesterol **5.** restricted (adrenal, testis, ovary, placenta)
1. CYP11A1 **2.** 1583 **3.** *CYP11A1; CYP11A; CYPXIA1; P450SCC*	**Chr:** 15q24.1 **Gene:** 30.0 **mRNA:** 2.0 **Exons:** 9	**aa:** 521 **Dalton:** 60,102 **L:** mitochon	**1.** cytochrome P450 side-chain cleavage enzyme **2.** cytochrome P450, type I **3.** cleavage of cholesterol side-chain **4.** cholesterol→P5 **5.** restricted (adrenal, testis, ovary, placenta) **6.** NADP/NADPH
1. CYP17A1 **2.** 1586 **3.** *CYP17A1; CPT7; CYP17; S17AH; P450C17*	**Chr:** 10q24.32 **Gene:** 6.6 **mRNA:** 1.9 **Exons:** 8	**aa:** 508 **Dalton:** 57,371 **L:** EndRet	**1.** steroid 17α-hydroxylase/17,20-lyase **2.** cytochrome P450, type II **3.** 17α-hydroxylase and 17,20-lyase activities **4.** P5→DHEA; P→A4[$]; 5αDHP→androstanedione; THP→ 5α-pregnan-3,17α-diol-20-one **5.** restricted (adrenal, testis, ovary, placenta) **6.** NADP/NADPH
1. CYP19A1 **2.** 1588 **3.** *CYP19A1; ARO; ARO1; CPV1; CYAR; CYP19; CYPXIX; P-450AROM*	**Chr:** 15q21.1 **Gene:** 130.6 **mRNA:** 1.5–4.5 **Exons:** 10	**aa:** 503 **Dalton:** 57,883 **L:** EndRet	**1.** cytochrome P450 aromatase **2.** cytochrome P450, type II **3.** oxidative demethylation of C_{19} to C_{18} (aromatisation) **4.** A → E1; T → E2 **5.** restricted (adrenal, testis, ovary, placenta) **6.** NADP/NADPH
1. 3βHSD1 **2.** 3283 **3.** *HSD3B1; HSD3B; HSDB3; SDB3A; (more^^)*	**Chr:** 1p11–12 **Gene:** 8.1 **mRNA:** 1.7 **Exons:** 4	**aa:** 373 **Dalton:** 42,252 **L:** membrane	**1.** 3β-hydroxysteroid dehydrogenase/$\Delta^{5\to4}$ isomerase type I **2.** short chain dehydrogenase/reductase superfamily **3.** oxidative conversion of Δ^5 3β-hydroxyl to Δ^4 keto-steroids **4.** P5→P; 17OHP5→17OHP4; DHEA→A4; A5→T; 17αA5→EpiT **5.** selectively distributed (placenta, periphery) **6.** NADP/NADPH or NAD/NADH
1. 3βHSD2 **2.** 3284 **3.** *HSD3B2; HSDB; HSD3B; SDR11E2*	**Chr:** 1p11–13 **Gene:** 8.1 **mRNA:** 1.7 **Exons:** 4	**aa:** 372 **Dalton:** 42,052 **L:** mitochon	**1.** 3β-hydroxysteroid dehydrogenase/$\Delta^{5:4}$ isomerase type II **2.** short chain dehydrogenase/reductase superfamily **3.** oxidative conversion of Δ^5-3β-hydroxyl to Δ^4-ketosteroids **4.** P5→P; 17OHP5→17OHP4; DHEA→A4 **5.** restricted (adrenal, testis, ovary) **6.** NADP/NADPH or NAD/NADH
1. 17βHSD1 **2.** 3,292 **3.** *HSD17B1 E2DH; HSD17; EDHB17; EDH17B2; SDR28C1; (more^^)*	**Chr:** 17q11–21 **Gene:** 6.0 **mRNA:** 1–2.4 **Exons:** 6	**aa:** 328 **Dalton:** 34,950 **L:** cytoplasm	**1.** 17β-hydroxysteroid dehydrogenase type 1 **2.** short chain dehydrogenase/reductase superfamily **3.** reduction of 17-keto to 17β-hydroxyl (estrogens) **4.** **(established)** E1→E2; (A4→T in rodents) **(postulated)** DHEA→A5[1]; P→20αDHP[2]; DHT→3βDIOL[11]; DHT→ androstanedione[11] **5.** selectively distributed (ovary, placenta (low in endometrium, breast)[14,15] **6.** NADP/NADPH
1. 17βHSD2 **2.** 3294 **3.** *HSD17B2 HSD17; SDR9C2; EDH17B2*	**Chr:** 16q24.1–2 **Gene:** 63 **mRNA:** 1.5	**aa:** 387 **Dalton:** 42,785	**1.** 17β-hydroxysteroid dehydrogenase type 2 **2.** short chain dehydrogenase/reductase superfamily **3.** oxidation of 17β-hydroxyl to 17-keto (estrogens & androgens)

(Continued)

TABLE 2 | Continued

1. Abbr. **2. Gene ID** **3. *Gene name(s)***	**Chromosome** **Gene size*** **mRNA size*** **Exons (no)**	**Protein (aa)**** **Dalton** **Localization (L)*****	**1. Name** **2. Family** **3. Catalysis** **4. Substrates****** **5. Distribution** **6. Cofactor**
	Exons: 5	**L:** EndRet	**4. (established)** E2→E1; T→A4; DHT→androstanedione[1,10]; 20αDHP→P[16]; 5α-pregnan-20-ol -3-one→5αDHP[16]; A5→DHEA[1]; 3αDIOL→AN[5] **(postulated)** 3αDIOL→AN[(1,10)]; DHT→androstanedione[1]; A5→DHEA[1]; allopregnandiol→ THP[16] **5.** selectively distributed (liver, intestine, endometrium, placenta, pancreas, prostate, colon, kidney. *Negative* in heart, brain, skeletal muscle, spleen, thymus, ovary, or testis)[(14,17)] **6.** NAD/NADH
1. 17βHSD3[&&] **2.** 3293 **3.** *HSD17B3* *EDH17B3;*	**Chr:** 9q22 **Gene:** 67 **mRNA:** 1.2 **Exons:** 11	**aa:** 310 **Dalton:** 34,516 **L:** EndRet	**1.** 17β-hydroxysteroid dehydrogenase type 3 **2.** short chain dehydrogenase/reductase superfamily **3.** reduction of 17-keto to 17β-hydroxyl (androgens) **4. (established)** A4→T **(postulated)** AN→3αDIOL[(1,3,10)]; androstanedione→DHT[(1,9,10)] **5.** restricted (testis; low in brain, blood, skin, adipose tissue)[14] **6.** NADP/NADPH
1. 17βHSD4 **2.** 3295 **3.** *HSD17B4* *DBP; MFE-2; MPF-2; PRLTS1; SDR8C1*	**Chr:** 5q23.1 **Gene:** 184 **mRNA:** 2.9 **Exons:** 28	**aa:** 736 **Dalton:** 79,686 **L:** Peroxisome mitochon	**1.** 17β-hydroxysteroid dehydrogenase type 4 **2.** short chain dehydrogenase/reductase superfamily **3.** fatty acid β-oxidation (steroids in pigs) **4. (established)** very long chain branched fatty acids, bile acids **(postulated)** A5→DHEA[1]; E2→E1[14] **5.** ubiquitous (liver, heart, prostate, testis, lung, skeletal muscle, kidney, pancreas, thymus, ovary, intestine, placenta, brain, spleen, colon, lymphocytes)[14] **6.** NAD/NADH
1. 17βHSD6 **2.** 8630 **3.** *HSD17B6* *HSE; RODH; SDR9C6*	**Chr:** 12q13 **Gene:** 24.5 **mRNA:** 1.6 **Exons:** 8	**aa:** 317 **Dalton:** 35,966 **L:** EndRet microsomes	**1.** 17β-hydroxysteroid dehydrogenase type 6 **2.** short chain dehydrogenase/reductase superfamily **3.** 3α-3β-epimerase; 17β-hydroxyl oxidation (5α-reduced steroids); retinoids **4. (established)** 3αDIOL→DHT[10]; AN→androstanedione[5]; AN→EPI **(postulated)** 3αDIOL→AN[5]; E2→E1[5] **5.** selectively distributed (liver, testis, lung, spleen, brain, ovary, kidney, adrenal, prostate)[14] **6.** NAD/NADP
1. 17βHSD7 **2.** 51478 **3.** *HSD17B7* *PRAP; SDR37C1*	**Chr:** 1q23 **Gene:** 22.1 **mRNA:** 1.5 **Exons:** 9	**aa:** 341 **Dalton:** 38,206 **L:** EndRet	**1.** 17β-hydroxysteroid dehydrogenase type 7 **2.** short chain dehydrogenase/reductase superfamily **3.** 3-ketosteroid reductase of sterols **4. (established)** Sterols/cholesterol biosynthesis; DHT→3βDIOL[1] **5.** widely distributed (ovary, uterus, placenta, liver, breast, testis, neuronal tissue, adrenal gland, small intestine, prostate, adipose tissue lung, and thymus)[(14,18)] **6.** NADP/NADPH
1. 17βHSD8 **2.** 7923 **3.** *HSD17B8* *KE6; FABG; HKE6; FABGL; RING2; H2-KE6; (more^^)*	**Chr:** 6p21.3 **Gene:** 2.2 **mRNA:** 1.0 **Exons:** 9	**aa:** 261 **Dalton:** 26,974 **L:** mitochon	**1.** 17β-hydroxysteroid dehydrogenase type 8 **2.** short chain dehydrogenase/reductase superfamily **3.** fatty acid elongation; steroid 17βHSD action (rodents). **4. (established)** fatty acids **(postulated)** E2→E1 **5.** widely distributed (prostate, placenta, kidney, brain, cerebellum, heart, lung, small intestine, ovary, testis, adrenal, stomach, liver, adrenals)[14–19] **6.** NAD/NADP
1. 17βHSD9 **2.** 5959 **3.** *HSD17B9* *RDH5; (more^^)*	**Chr:** 12q23 **Gene:** 4.4 **mRNA:** 1.4 **Exons:** 4	**aa:** 318 **Dalton:** 34,979 **L:** EndRet	**1.** 17β-hydroxysteroid dehydrogenase type 9 **2.** short chain dehydrogenase/reductase superfamily **3.** retinoid metabolism (steroid metabolism in rodents) **4. (established)** retinoids **(postulated)** AN→3αDIOL[1]; androstanedione→DHT[1]
1. 17βHSD10 **2.** 3028	**Chr:** Xp11.2 **Gene:** 3.1	**aa:** 261	**1.** 17β-hydroxysteroid dehydrogenase type 10 **2.** short chain dehydrogenase/reductase superfamily

(Continued)

TABLE 2 | Continued

1. Abbr. **2. Gene ID** **3. *Gene name(s)***	**Chromosome** **Gene size*** **mRNA size*** **Exons (no)**	**Protein (aa)**** **Dalton** **Localization (L)*****	**1. Name** **2. Family** **3. Catalysis** **4. Substrates****** **5. Distribution** **6. Cofactor**
3. *HSD17B10* *ABAD; CAMR; ERAB; HCD2; MHBD; HADH2; MRPP2; MRX17; MRX31; (more^^)*	**mRNA:** 0.9 **Exons:** 6	**Dalton:** 26,923 **L:** mitochon	**3.** fatty acids & steroid oxidation; tRNA maturation **4. (established)** Isoleucine, fatty acid, bile acid metabolism, THP→5αDHP[(20,34)] **(postulated)** 3αDIOL→AN[1,9]; DHT→androstanedione[1,9]; T→A4[1] **5.** nearly ubiquitous (liver, small intestine, colon, kidney, heart, brain, placenta, lung, ovary, testis, spleen, thymus, prostate, leukocyte)[14] **6.** NAD/NADH
1. 17βHSD11 **2.** 51170 **3.** *HSD17B11* *DHRS8; PAN1B; RETSDR2; SDR16C2; (more^^)*	**Chr:** 4q22.1 **Gene:** 54.9 **mRNA:** 1.9 **Exons:** 7	**aa:** 300 **Dalton:** 32,936 **L:** EndRet	**1.** 17β-hydroxysteroid dehydrogenase type 11 **2.** short chain dehydrogenase/reductase superfamily **3.** Short-chain alcohol dehydrogenases **4. (established)** lipids, sec. alcohols/ketones **(postulated)** 3αDIOL→AN[1,9] **5.** nearly ubiquitous (liver, intestine, kidney, adrenal gland, heart, lung, testis, ovary, placenta, sebaceous gland and pancreas)[14,21] **6.** NAD/NADH
1. 17βHSD12 **2.** 51144 **3.** *HSD17B12* *KAR; SDR12C1*	**Chr:** 11p11.2 **Gene:** 170.1 **mRNA:** 2.6 **Exons:** 11	**aa:** 312 **Dalton:** 34,324 **L:** EndRet	**1.** 17β-hydroxysteroid dehydrogenase type 12 **2.** short chain dehydrogenase/reductase superfamily **3.** fatty acid elongation, steroid 17βHSD reductive action (rodents) **4. (established)** branched/long chain fatty acids **(postulated)** E1→E2 **5.** ubiquitous (heart, skeletal muscle, liver, kidney, adrenal gland, testis, placenta, brain, pancreas, GIT, trachea, lung, thyroid, prostate, aorta, bladder, spleen, skin, ovary, breast, uterus, vagina)[(14,22)] **6.** NADP/NADPH
1. 17βHSD13 **2.** 345275 **3.** *HSD17B13* *SCDR9; NIIL497; (more^^)*	**Chr:** 4q22.1 **Gene:** 19.1 **mRNA:** 2.3 **Exons:** 6	**aa:** 300 **Dalton:** 33,655 **L:** extracell/EndRet	**1.** 17β-hydroxysteroid dehydrogenase type 13 **2.** short chain dehydrogenase/reductase superfamily **3. and 4.** unknown **5.** restricted (liver; low in bone marrow, lung, ovary, testis, kidney, skeletal muscle brain, bladder)[14]
1. 17βHSD14 **2.** 51171 **3.** *HSD17B14* *DHRS10; SDR47C1; retSDR3*	**Chr:** 19q13.33 **Gene:** 23.7 **mRNA:** 1.3 **Exons:** 8	**aa:** 270 **Dalton:** 28,317 **L:** cytoplasm	**1.** 17β-hydroxysteroid dehydrogenase type 14 **2.** short chain dehydrogenase/reductase superfamily **3.** fatty acid & prostaglandin metabolism; 17βHSD activity **4. (established)** fatty acids **(postulated)** 3αDIOL→AN[1,9]; E2→E1[4]; T→A4[4]; A5→DHEA[5] **5.** widely distributed (brain, liver, placenta, breast)[14] **6.** NAD/NADH
1. 17βHSD15 **2.** 51109 **3.** *RDH11; PSDR1; ARSDR1; (more^^)*	**Chr:** 14q24.1 **Gene:** 19.0 **mRNA:** 1.8 **Exons:** 9	**aa:** 318 **Dalton:** 35,386 **L:** cytoplasm	**1.** retinol dehydrogenase 11 **2.** short chain dehydrogenase/reductase superfamily **3.** dehydrogenase activity of retinoid and steroids **4. (established)** retinoids **(post.)** AN→3αDIOL[1,9]; androstanedione→DHT[1,9] **5.** widely distributed **6.** NADP/NADPH
1. DHRS11[23] **2.** 79154 **3.** *DHRS11* *ARPG836; SDR24C1; spDHRS11*	**Chr:** 17q12 **Gene:** 9.0 **mRNA:** 1.6 **Exons:** 7	**aa:** 260 **Dalton:** 28,308 **L:** extracell	**1.** dehydrogenase/reductase 11 **2.** short chain dehydrogenase/reductase superfamily **3.** steroid 17HSD & 3βHSD activities; bile acids metabolism **4.** E1→E2; A4→T; DHEA→A5; androstanedione→DHT; AN→3αDIOL; P→3αDHP[23] **5.** nearly ubiquitous (testis, small intestine, colon, kidney)[23] **6.** NADP/NADPH
1. AKR1C1 **2.** 1645 **3.** *AKR1C1*	**Chr:** 10p14–15 **Gene:** 20.0 **mRNA:** 12	**aa:** 323 **Dalton:** 36,788	**1.** aldo-ketoreductase family 1 member C1 **2.** aldo-ketoreductase family **3.** 20αHSD (strong) and 17βHSD (weak) activities; moderate 3-keto reduction to 3β-hydroxyl (> 3α)

(Continued)

TABLE 2 | Continued

1. Abbr. **2. Gene ID** ***3. Gene name(s)***	**Chromosome** **Gene size*** **mRNA size*** **Exons (no)**	**Protein (aa)**** **Dalton** **Localization (L)*****	**1. Name** **2. Family** **3. Catalysis** **4. Substrates****** **5. Distribution** **6. Cofactor**
C9, DDH, DDH1, DD1, H-37, HBAB, MBAB HAKRC; DD1/DD2; 2-ALPHA-HSD; 20-ALPHA-HSD	**Exons:** 9	**L:** cytoplasm	**4. (established)** P→20αDHP[6]; 5αDHP→5α-pregnan-20-ol-3-one[6]; THP→allopregnandiol[6]; DHT→3βDIOL[7]; androstanedione→DHT[7]; 5α-pregnan-20-ol-3-one→allopregnandiol[16]; 5αDHP→THP[16] **(post.)** DHT→3αDIOL[7]; A4↔T[7]; E1→E2[7]; 3αDIOL→AN[7]; 20αDHP→ P[7]; DHT→3βDIOL[24]; 5α-pregnan-17α-ol-3,20-dione→5α-pregnan-3,17α-diol-20-one[16] **5.** ubiquitous **6.** NADP/NADPH or NAD/NADH
1. AKR1C2 **2.** 1646 **3.** *AKR1C2 DD; DD2; TDD; BABP; DD-2; DDH2; HBAB; HAKRD; MCDR2; SRXY8; DD/BABP; AKR1C-pseudo*	**Chr:** 10p14–15 **Gene:** 30.6 **mRNA:** 1.3 **Exons:** 9	**aa:** 323 **Dalton:** 36,735 **L:** cytoplasm	**1.** aldo-ketoreductase family 1 member C2 **2.** aldo-ketoreductase family **3.** 20αHSD (weak) and 17βHSD activities; 3-keto reduction to 3α- hydroxyl; bile-acid binding protein activity **4. (established)** DHT→3αDIOL[7,12]; 5αDHP↔THP[7]; androstanedione→AN[25]; 5α-pregnan-20-ol-3-one→ allopregnandiol[16]; 5αDHP→THP[16]; 5α-pregnan-17α-ol-3,20-dione→5α-pregnan-3,17α-diol-20-one[16] **(postulated)** A4→ T[7]; E1↔E2[7]; P↔20αDHP[7]; 3αDIOL→ DHT[7]; T→A4[7] **5.** ubiquitous **6.** NADP/NADPH or NAD/NADH
1. AKR1C3 **2.** 8644 **3.** *HSD17B5 AKR1C3 DD3; DDX; PGFS; HAKRB; HAKRe; HA1753; HSD17B5; hluPGFS*	**Chr:** 10p14–15 **Gene:** 13 **mRNA:** 1.2 **Exons:** 9	**aa:** 323 **Dalton:** 36,853 **L:** cytoplasm	**1.** aldo-ketoreductase family 1 member C3 **2.** aldo-ketoreductase family **3.** 20αHSD (weak) and 17βHSD activities (androgens); 3-keto reduction to 3α-/β-hydroxyl (weak); 11-ketoprostaglandin reductase[3] **4. (established)** A4→T[7]; DHT→3αDIOL[7]; 3αDIOL→AN[7]; 5αDHP→ THP[7]; 5α-pregnan-20-ol-3-one→ allopregnandiol[16]; 5αDHP→THP[16]; DHEA→A5[7]; 5α-pregnan-17α-ol-3,20-dione→5α-pregnan-3,17α-diol-20-one[16]; androstanedione→DHT[24] **(postulated)** E1↔E2[7];T→A4[7]; 20αDHP↔ P[7] **5.** nearly ubiquitous (prostate, mammary gland, liver, kidney, lung, heart, uterus, testis, brain, skeletal muscle, adipose tissue, pancreas, hearth, skeletal muscle, thymus, ovary, small intestine and colon)[14,26] **6.** NADP/NADPH or NAD/NADH
1. AKR1C4 **2.** 1109 **3.** *AKR1C4 C11; CDR; DD4; CHDR; DD-4; HAKRA;*	**Chr:** 10p15.1 **Gene:** 25.2 **mRNA:** 1.2 **Exons:** 9	**aa:** 323 **Dalton:** 37,067 **L:** cytoplasm	**1.** aldo-ketoreductase family 1 member C4 **2.** aldo-ketoreductase family **3.** 20αHSD (weak) and 17βHSD activities; 3-keto reduction to 3α-hydroxyl (>3β). **4. (established)** DHT→3αDIOL[7,10]; androstanedione→AN[7,8]; other[$$$] **(postulated)** A4↔ T[7]; E1,↔E2[7]; P↔20αDHP[7]; 3αDIOL→DHT[7] **5.** restricted (liver) **6.** NADP/NADPH or NAD/NADH
1. SRD5A1 **2.** 6715 **3.** *SRD5A1 S5AR 1*	**Chr:** 5p15.31 **Gene:** 41.0 **mRNA:** 2.3 **Exons:** 5(7)	**aa:** 259 **Dalton:** 29,459 **L:** EndRet	**1.** steroid 5α-reductase 1 **2.** steroid 5α reductase family **3.** androgen and pregnene metabolism **4.** T→DHT; A4→androstanedione; 17OHP4→5α-pregnan-17α-ol-3,20-dione; P→5αDHP; 20αDHP→5α-pregnan-20-ol-3-one **5.** ubiquitous
1. SRD5A2 **2.** 6716 **3.** *SRD5A2*	**Chr:** 2p23.1 **Gene:** 178.3 **mRNA:** 2.5 **Exons:** 5	**aa:** 254 **Dalton:** 28,393 **L:** microsomes	**1.** steroid 5α-reductase 2 **2.** steroid 5α reductase family **3.** androgen and pregnene metabolism **4.** T→DHT; A4→androstanedione **5.** restricted (prostate and androgen sensitive tissues)
1. SRD5A3 **2.** 79644 **3.** *SRD5A3 CDG1P; CDG1Q; KRIZI; SRD5A2L; SRD5A2L1*	**Chr:** 4q12 **Gene:** ..... **mRNA:** 4.1 **Exons:** 6	**aa:** 318 **Da:** 36,521 **L:** EndRet	**1.** steroid 5α-reductase 3 **2.** steroid 5α reductase AND polyprenol reductase subfamily **3.** androgen and pregnene metabolism **4.** T→DHT; A4→androstanedione; 17OHP4→5α-pregnan-17α-ol-3,20-dione; P→5αDHP; 20αDHP→5α-pregnan-20-ol-3-one **5.** ubiquitous

(Continued)

TABLE 2 | Continued

1. Abbr. 2. Gene ID 3. *Gene name(s)*	Chromosome Gene size* mRNA size* Exons (no)	Protein (aa)** Dalton Localization (L)***	1. Name 2. Family 3. Catalysis 4. Substrates**** 5. Distribution 6. Cofactor
1. STS **2.** 412 **3.** *STS* *ES; ASC; XLI; ARSC; SSDD; ARSC1*	**Chr:** Xp22.31 **Gene:** 208.3 **mRNA:** 6.4 **Exons:** 16	**aa:** 583 **Dalton:** 65,492 **L:** microsomes EndRet	**1.** steroid sulphatase **2.** sulphatase **3.** hydrolyses several 3β-hydroxysteroid sulfates **4.** sulpho conjugated cholesterol, E1, E2, DHEA, P5, 17OHP5S, A5, EPI **5.** ubiquitous (lung, aorta, thyroid, uterus, liver and testis)[27–30]
1. SULT1E1 **2.** 6783 **3.** *SULT1E1* *EST; STE; EST-1; ST1E1; (more^^)*	**Chr:** 4q13.3 **Gene:** 50.0 **mRNA:** 1.8 **Exons:** 9	**aa:** 35126 **Dalton:** 35,126 **L:** cytoplasm	**1.** estrogen sulphotransferase **2.** sulphotransferase 1 **3.** sulpho-conjugation of steroids **4.** E1, DHEA (low affinity for E2) **5.** moderately distributed (liver, adrenal, small intestine; low in brain, lung, testis, leukocytes, placenta, salivary gland, stomach, thymus, trachea, uterus, kidney)[(30,31)]
1. SULT2A1 **2.** 6822 **3.** *SULT2A1* *HST; ST2; STD; hSTa; DHEAS; ST2A1;*	**Chr:** 19q13.3 **Gene:** 15.9 **mRNA:** 2.0 **Exons:** 6	**aa:** 285 **Dalton:** 33,780 **L:** cytoplasm	**1.** dehydroepiandrosterone sulphotransferase **2.** sulphotransferase 1 **3.** sulpho-conjugation of steroids, bile acids **4.** DHEA, P5, AN, 17OHP5[32], A5[32], AN[33], EPI, bile acids **5.** restricted (liver, adrenal, small intestine (low in colon, hearth, prostate, stomach, testis, thyroid)[30]
1. SULT2B1 **2.** 6820 **3.** *SULT2B1* *HSST2; ARCI14*	**Chr:** 19q13.33 **Gene:** 48.5 **mRNA:** 1.3 **Exons:** 7	**aa:** 365 **Dalton:** 41,308 **L:** cytoplasm	**1.** alcohol sulphotransferase **2.** sulphotransferase 1 **3.** sulpho-conjugation of steroids **4.** cholesterol, DHEA **5.** moderately distributed (placenta, prostate, lung (low in kidney, salivary gland, small intestine, trachea)[30]
1. SULT1A1 **2.** 6817 **3.** *SULT1A1* *PST; STP; STP1; P-PST; ST1A1; ST1A3; TSPST1; HAST1/HAST2*	**Chr:** 16p11.2 **Gene:** 18.4 **mRNA:** 1.3 **Exons:** 13	**aa:** 295 **Dalton:** 34,165 **L:** cytoplasm	**1.** phenol sulphotransferase 1 **2.** sulphotransferase 1 **3.** sulpho-conjugation of steroids **4.** E2 **5.** nearly ubiquitous (adrenal, bone marrow, brain, colon, hearth, kidney, liver, lung, pancreas, leukocytes, placenta, prostate, salivary gland, skeletal muscle, small intestine, spinal cord, spleen, stomach, testis, thymus, thyroid, trachea, uterus)[30]

List of all enzymes discussed in the present review with the major features. Gene and gene product nomenclature is complex and variable and alias are given as ***Supplemental Materials****. Gene structure (chromosome location, gene length), transcript features (length, exons) and protein characteristics (amino-acid length, molecular weigh and cell localization) were obtained from GeneCards (www.genecards.org. Accessed on date: February 2018) (Stelzer et al., 2016).*

**Length in kilo nucleotides.*

***number of amino-acids.*

****Abbreviations: EndRet: endoplasmic reticulum; extracell: extracellular; mitochon: mitochondria.*

*****For some enzymes, substrate specificity based on robust evidences are indicated as 'established', whereas other reactions whose catalyzes is supported by less robust experimental evidences (mostly using recombinant proteins in vitro/cell-free assays) are indicated as "postulated."*

$ This reaction of CYP17A1 does not occur in vivo in humans (Miller and Auchus, 2011).

$$$ AKR1C4 has an important detoxifying function in the liver and converts chlordecone into chlordecone alcohol.

&& 17βHSD3 is testis specific and the reactions catalyzed by this enzyme are not reported in ***Figure 2****.*

^^For this gene, additional gene names exist, for details see NCBI database (https://www.ncbi.nlm.nih.gov/).

[1] Luu-The and Labrie (2010), Labrie and Labrie (2013), and Labrie (2015); [2] Smuc and Rizner (2009), [3] Miller et al. (2012b), [4] Sivik (2012); [5] GeneCards (www.genecards.org. Accessed on date: February, 2018) Stelzer et al. (2016), [6] Smuc and Rizner (2009), [7] Penning et al. (2004), Steckelbroeck et al. (2010); [8] Jin et al. (2011), [9] Manenda et al. (2016), [10] Balk and Knudsen (2008), [11] Gangloff et al. (2003), [12] Bélanger et al. (2002), [13] Perez Carrion et al. (1994), [14] Möller et al. (1999), Moeller and Adamski (2009), [15] Cornel et al. (2017), [16] Sinreih et al. (2017b), [17] Casey et al. (1994), [18] Törn et al. (2003), [19] Ohno et al. (2008), [20] Yang et al. (2016), [21] Chai et al. (2003), [22] Sakurai et al. (2006), [23] Endo et al. (2016). [24] Rižner and Penning (2014), [25] Manenda et al. (2016), [26] Lin et al. (1997), [27] Miki et al. (2002), [28] Foster et al. (2008a), [29] Purohit and Foster (2012), [30] Mueller et al. (2015), [31] Marchais-Oberwinkler et al. (2011), Mueller et al. (2015), [32] Rege et al. (2016), [33] Strott (2002), and [34] Yang et al. (2016).

By targeting steroid intracrine metabolism, the effects of steroids can be modulated locally. **Table 3** overviews the available drugs targeting intracrine enzymes and their developmental status. CYP19A1 (aromatase) inhibitors, currently at their third generation, started to be used for breast cancer during the 80's of last century (Lønning and Eikesdal, 2013), and was followed by drugs able to target other enzymes (CYP11A1, CYP17A1, SRD5As; **Table 3**).

More recently, there is a re-emerging interest in developing novel intracrine drugs. A number of compounds are in their clinical phases, like STS inhibitors (Maltais and Poirier, 2011; Woo et al., 2011; Purohit and Foster, 2012; Pohl et al., 2014; Pautier et al., 2017) or inhibitors of AKR1C3/17βHSD5, which are of particular interest because this enzyme has crucial role in androgen/estrogen and prostaglandin biosynthesis (Penning, 2017). Bayer's AKR1C3/17βHSD5 inhibitor BAY 1128688 has a modified estrogen core, it interferes with both pathways, and is in phase II clinical trial for endometriosis (Bothe et al., 2017). Astellas Pharma potent and selective AKR1C3/17βHSD5 inhibitor ASP-9521 had only modest effect in a phase II study on prostate cancer as single drug, but combination therapy approaches remain to be studied (Kikuchi et al., 2014; Loriot et al., 2014).

HSD inhibitors are being studied in the area of hormone-dependent diseases, with 11βHSD inhibitors being in clinical trials for metabolic disorders (Ye et al., 2017) and 17βHSD inhibitors approaching the clinical phase for a number of gynecological indications (**Table 3**; Abdelsamie et al., 2017).

INTRACRINOLOGY IN PERIPHERAL TISSUES

In this paragraph, intracrinology of endometrium, GIT, bone, lungs, and CNS is reviewed. To comprehensively understand the ability of these tissues and systems to generate estrogens and other steroids, we have performed a systematic search of all original papers published in English until June 2018 that described the levels of intracrine enzymes (those indicated in **Table 2**-mRNA, protein or activity) in healthy tissues. In total 177 if the four extra ref are allowed papers were reviewed, and for details of this search, see **Supplemental panel**: "Systematic Review." The results of this systematic review are summarized in **Tables 6–8** and are briefly overviewed in each section dedicated to the distinct tissues or systems. Reports describing the enzymes in cultured cells or cell lines were excluded (may have been discussed elsewhere, though). Each section follows then with a non-systematic overview of the role of intracrinology in pathophysiology. A brief non-systematic description of the intracrinology of the skin, immune system and adipose tissue is also given. We will not describe the intracrinology of breast, prostate and liver (where steroid catabolism is the most relevant aspect), and we redirect the reader to recent reviews (Foster et al., 2008a; Luu-The et al., 2008; Luu-The and Labrie, 2010; Labrie and Labrie, 2013; Labrie, 2015; Mueller et al., 2015; Zhao et al., 2016; Hilborn et al., 2017; Penning, 2017).

Endometrium

The actions of steroid hormones in the endometrium are mediated by hormone-receptors *via* the classical mechanisms, although non-genomic and rapid signaling are also present (Groothuis et al., 2007; Zwart et al., 2011; Flach and Zwart, 2016; Hewitt et al., 2016). Estrogens and P control the menstrual cycle (Groothuis et al., 2007; Andersen and Ezcurra, 2014) and the endometrium during the window of implantation (WOI), occurring in the mid-luteal phase (Wang and Dey, 2006).

In rats, the WOI is characterized by high E2 plasma levels, and endometrial ERα and PR expression shows specific and varying cytosolic/nuclear patterns (Singh et al., 1996). ERα and PR expression decreases after ovulation and in preimplantation stages in both mice (Vasquez and DeMayo, 2013) and primates (*Macaca mulatta*) (Ghosh et al., 1999).

Rodent genetic models unraveled some molecular mechanisms underlying the estrogen-dependency of these processes. ERα-KO mice are infertile, no implantation occurs, endometrium is hypoplastic and estrogen response is absent (Couse and Korach, 1999; Walker and Korach, 2004). Not only its absence, but also sustained estrogen signaling has deleterious effects on endometrial receptivity, as recapitulated by mice with uterine COUP-TFII ablation. These mice exhibit increased estrogen signaling and asynchrony between embryo competency and uterine receptivity with consequent implantation defects. This effect is rescued by treatment with the antiestrogen ICI-182780 (Lee et al., 2010). Additionally, the duration of E2 exposure and its dosage affect endometrial receptivity and WOI length in mice (Ma et al., 2003).

Available human data, mostly obtained in the context of assisted reproduction technologies (ART), also indicate that steroid stimulation retards or shortens the luteal phase, the WOI, causes shifts in the appearance of pinopodes (a classical WOI marker) and causes asynchrony between ovarian and menstrual cycles (Devroey et al., 2004).

Intracrinology in Healthy Endometrium–Systematic Search

Initial studies on steroid hormone metabolism in the endometrium date back to 1965 with first demonstration of the STS activity, followed by investigation on the oxidative and reductive 17βHSD activities (**Table 6**).

Both pre and postmenopausal tissues possess oxidative and reductive 17βHSD activities and the expression of 17βHSD1, 2, 4, 6, 7, 8, 10, 12, 14, and AKR1C3/17βHSD5 was detected at the mRNA or protein levels. Sulphatase pathway (STS and SULT1E1; recently reviewed by Rižner, 2016), CYP19A1, 3βHSDs, SRD5As and AKR1Cs are also present, indicating that human endometrium can metabolize sulphated-compounds and DHEA to form androgens and estrogens.

Few 17βHSDs have been characterized by IHC. The low expression of 17βHSD1 poses sensitivity problems using standard detection methods (Cornel et al., 2017), and few authors reported endometrial absence of 17βHSD1 (**Table 6**). Type 1 17βHSD localizes in the cytoplasm of epithelial cells (Dassen et al., 2007; Colette et al., 2013; Mori et al., 2015; Sinreih et al., 2017a) and it is also detected in primary stroma cells cultured *in vitro* (Aghajanova et al., 2009; Mori et al., 2015). Type 2 17βHSD, AKR1C3/17βHSD5 and 3βHSD1 give strong reactivity in the glandular epithelium (Rhee et al., 2003; Ito et al., 2006; Dassen et al., 2007; Vani et al., 2007; Smuc and Rizner, 2009; Zakharov et al., 2010; Colette et al., 2013; Mori et al., 2015; Sinreih et al., 2017a).

TABLE 3 | Drugs targeting intracrine enzymes.

	Inhibitor name (if known); (Drug Bank ID[#])				
	Developmental phase[&]			Approved drugs	
Name	**Discovery**	**Preclinical indication**	**Clinical indication**	**Inhibitor name**	**Indication**
CYP11A1	✓	✓	✓	Aminoglutethimide (DB00357[##])	Cushing's syndrome Breast cancer
CYP17A1	✓	✓	✓	Abiraterone (DB05812)	Prostate cancer, metastatic, castration-resistant
CYP19A1	✓	✓	Letrozole (DB01006)[19,22,24] Anastrozole (DB01217)[20,23] Exemestane (DB00990)[21] Advanced stage endometrial cancer, NSCLC^, LAM^^	Anastrozole (DB01217) Letrozole (DB01006) Exemestane (DB00990) Formestane[1] Testolactone* (DB00894)	Breast cancer: adjuvant treatment, metastatic Breast cancer, palliative
3βHSD1	✓	✓	✓	Trilostane* (DB01108)	Cushing's syndrome (veterinary use)
3βHSD2	✓	✓	✓	Trilostane* (DB01108)	Cushing's syndrome (veterinary use)
17βHSD1	✓	Endometriosis[2,3] Endometrial cancer[4] Breast cancer[5,6] Endometrial hyperplasia[7]			
17βHSD2	8,9				
17βHSD3[&&]	✓	Prostate cancer[10]			
17βHSD7	11				
AKR1C1	12				
AKR1C2	12				
AKR1C3	✓	✓	ASP-9521[13] Prostate cancer** BAY 1128688 Endometriosis***		
AKR1C4	12				
SRD5A1	✓	✓	✓	Dutasteride (DB01126)	Prostatic hyperplasia (benign)
SRD5A2	✓	✓	✓	Finasteride (DB01216) Dutasteride (DB01126)	Prostatic hyperplasia (benign)
SRD5A3	✓	✓	✓	Dutasteride (DB01216)	Prostatic hyperplasia (benign)
STS	✓	✓	Irosustat (DB02292) Endometrial cancer[14,15] Breast cancer[14–17] E2MATE/PLG2001 Endometriosis[18]		
SULT1E1	✓	✓	✓	Cyclizine (DB01176)	antistaminic for nausea/vomiting

[&] *'Clinical phase', i.e., in phase I, II or III trial; 'Preclinical phase' refers to in vivo testing; 'Discovery phase' any previous phase with some candidate compounds.*

[#] *Drug Bank ID if the compound is deposited in Drug Bank database (www.drugbank.ca/drugs. Accessed on date: February 2018) (Wishart et al., 2018).*

[##] *Aminoglutethimide (ID: DB00357) is an important inhibitor of CYP11A1 with inhibitory activity on CYP19A1 as well.*

* *No longer on the market.*

[&&] *17βHSD3 is testis specific and the reactions catalyzed by this enzyme are not reported in* ***Figure 2****.*

** *This trial for prostate cancer was prematurely terminated (www.clinicaltrials.gov, NCT01352208).*

*** *Phase I trial is concluded (www.clinicaltrials.gov, NCT02434640. Accessed on date: February 2018) and a phase II trial started 2016*

^NSCLC: non-small cell lung cancer

^^LAM: lymphangioleiomyomatosis

[1]Perez Carrion et al. (1994), [2]Arnold and Einspanier (2013), [3]Delvoux et al. (2014), [4]Konings et al. (2017), [5]Järvensivu et al. (2018), [6]Husen et al. (2006), [7]Saloniemi et al. (2010), [8]Gargano et al. (2015), [9]Soubhye et al. (2015) [10]Day et al. (2013), [11] Wang et al. (2017), [12]BroŽic et al. (2011), [13] Kikuchi et al. (2014), [14]Purohit and Foster (2012), [15]Pautier et al. (2017), [16]Palmieri et al. (2017a), [17]Palmieri et al. (2017b), [18]Pohl et al. (2014), [19]Ma et al. (2004), [20]Rose et al. (2000), [21]Lindemann et al. (2014), [22]Slomovitz et al. (2015), [23] NCT00932152; [25]Lu et al. (2017).

TABLE 4 | Mouse models (knockouts - KO or transgenic-TG, i.e., ubiquitous expression of the gene, unless specified) for intracrine enzymes.

Gene^	Modification MGI ID$	Phenotype
SatAR	Null/KO[1] MGI: 2388706	**Endocrine (steroids) & reproductive endocrinology** - abnormal endocrine organs (adrenal, ovaries, prostate, testis). - decreased steroids and increased adrenocorticotropin level. - adrenocortical insufficiency. - loss of negative feedback regulation at hypothalamic-pituitary levels. **Additional** Growth retardation neo/post natal lethality (incomplete penetrance). ***Reproductive system***: abnormal uterus; incomplete spermatogenesis; abnormal genitalia.
CYP11A1	Null/KO[2] MGI:5464022 Null/KO[3] MGI: 2183813	**Endocrine (steroids) and reproductive endocrinology** - abnormal adrenal gland morphology. - increased circulating adrenocorticotropin level. - lack of steroid production. - decreased corticosterone and aldosterone levels. **Additional** Neonatal lethality (rescued by steroid supplementation); abnormal mitochondrion morphology; abnormal lipid level. ***Reproductive system***: abnormal genitalia, prostate, testis morphology and spermatogenesis; ***Nervous system***: abnormal adrenaline and noradrenaline level; abnormal food intake, hypoactivity; postnatal growth retardation.
CYP17A1	Null/KO[4] MGI:3722780 Null/KO[5] MGI:3047328 Null/KO MGI:5605834	**Endocrine (steroids) & reproductive endocrinology** - increased circulating cholesterol level. - decreased T level. - early reproductive senescence. **Additional** Homozygous embryonic lethality (Ed7, between implantation and somite formation). ***Reproductive system***: abnormal sperm flagellum morphology/asthenozoospermia; reduced male fertility. ***Bone:*** abnormal bone structure, mineral content and density. ***Metabolism:*** increased total body fat; decreased lean body mass; increased circulating creatinine level; increased fasted circulating glucose level. ***Nervous system***: abnormal sexual interaction.
CYP19A1	Null/KO[6] MGI:2179439 Null/KO[7] MGI:2154536 Null/KO[8] MGI:2389548	**Endocrine (steroids) and reproductive endocrinology** - increased circulating cholesterol, T, DHT, FSH, LH and prolactin. - decreased circulating E2 level. - abnormal endometrium (thin, decreased uterus weight). - abnormal ovary (absence of follicles and corpus luteum, anovulation). **Additional** ***Reproductive system***: ovary hemorrhage and cysts; increased seminal vesicle weight and abnormal seminiferous tubule epithelium and oligozoospermia; female infertility and reduced male fertility. ***Metabolism:*** increased fat; obesity and susceptibility to weight gain. ***Bone:*** decreased bone mineral density and bone mass; increased bone resorption, osteoclast cell number; abnormal compact and trabecular bone morphology. ***Metabolism:*** increased circulating glucose and triglyceride levels; impaired glucose tolerance; insulin resistance; hepatic steatosis; abnormal liver physiology. ***Nervous system***: abnormal short term spatial reference memory; abnormal emotion/affect behavior; abnormal barbering behavior; increased grooming behavior; abnormal locomotor activation, bradykinesia; abnormal mating frequency.
17βHSD1	Null/KO[9] MGI:5576042 and 3799948	**Endocrine (steroids) & reproductive endocrinology** - abnormal corpus luteum morphology and decreased number. - increased ovarian E1:E2 and A4:T ratios. - increased LH level. - reduced P level. **Additional** Increased circulating alkaline phosphatase level, pigmentation, abnormal retinal pigmentation, abnormal lens morphology, abnormal retina morphology, abnormal retinal pigmentation. ***Reproductive system***: increased ovary weight; reduced female fertility. ***Metabolism:*** decreased circulating glucose level. ***Nervous system***: abnormal behavior, response to light, sleep behavior, decreased exploration in new environment; abnormal motor coordination/balance.

(Continued)

TABLE 4 | Continued

Gene^	Modification MGI ID$	Phenotype
17bHSD1	TG[10]	**Reproductive endocrinology** - female have increased T levels. - increased E1➔E2 conversion. - masculinization in females. - develop benign/malignant breast, ovarian and endometrial conditions.
17βHSD2	Null/KO[11] MGI:3773836	**No clear reproductive endocrinology phenotype** **Additional** Heterozygous mice: growth retardation at birth ant postnatal; premature death; renal degeneration. ***Reproductive system***: 70% embryonic lethality (Ed11.5) due to placental defects (homozygous); small and abnormal placenta morphology; ***Nervous system***: brain phenotype with enlarged ventricles; abnormal cortex morphology; impaired balance, coordination, abnormal sleep pattern, megacephaly.
	TG[12]	**Reproductive endocrinology** - low T level. **Additional** Growth retardation; delayed eye opening; impaired retinoic signaling. ***Reproductive system***: disrupted spermatogenesis. ***Bone:*** decreased bone formation (pre-pubertal age); decreased IGF-I and osteocalcin levels.
17βHSD4	Null/KO[13]	**No clear reproductive endocrinology phenotype** **Additional** Neonatal and postnatal lethality; postnatal growth retardation; abnormal mitochondrion morphology; abnormal bile salt level; hepatic steatosis. ***Reproductive system***: abnormal testis and spermatid morphology; seminiferous tubule degeneration; small testis; abnormal gametogenesis; reduced male fertility. ***Nervous system***: microgliosis; Purkinje cell degeneration; astrocytosis; axon degeneration; abnormal suckling behavior; increased anxiety-related response, tremors, ataxia, impaired coordination, hypoactivity, lethargy; abnormal gait. ***GIT:*** abnormal intestinal absorption. ***Metabolism:*** decreased body weight; abnormal lipid homeostasis and decreased fatty acid level.
17βHSD7	Null/KO[14] MGI:3811923	**Endocrine (steroids)** Cholesterol biosynthesis.
	Null/KO[15] MGI:4456868	**Additional** Decreased embryo size; embryo lethality due to heart malformations (Ed10.5); abnormal blood vessel and capillary morphology. ***Nervous system***: brain malformations; forebrain hypoplasia; increased neural tube apoptosis.
17βHSD9	Null/KO[16] MGI: 2446073	**No clear reproductive endocrinology phenotype**
	Null/KO[17] MGI:2388375	**Additional** Visual defects; abnormal eye electrophysiology, delayed dark adaptation.
17βHSD10	Null/KO[18]	**No clear reproductive endocrinology phenotype** **Additional** Mitochondria dysfunction; reduced plasma glucose and increase insulin levels. ***Nervous system***: neuronal damage.
	TG (brain specific)[19]	**No clear reproductive endocrinology phenotype** **Additional** ***Nervous system***: Protect against ischemia, Parkinson, Alzheimer disease model
17βHSD11	Null/KO[20] MGI:5581418	**No clear reproductive endocrinology phenotype** **Additional** Increased total circulating protein level. ***Nervous system***: hyperactivity.
17βHSD12	Null/KO[21]	**No clear reproductive endocrinology phenotype** **Additional** Embryo lethality Ed 9.5; impaired organogenesis; reduced arachidonic acid synthesis. ***Reproductive system***: ovarian dysfunction, fertility problems, smaller litters, significantly fewer numbers of ductal branches than wild type female mammary glands; ovulation problems. ***Nervous system***: high embryo expression in neuronal structures.
17βHSD13	Null/KO[22] MGI:5007180	No clear phenotype associated.

(Continued)

TABLE 4 | Continued

Gene^	Modification MGI ID$	Phenotype
17βHSD14	Null/KO[23] MGI:5007181	**No clear reproductive endocrinology phenotype** **Additional** Increased IgG2a level. ***Reproductive system***: oligozoospermia, testis degeneration, male infertility. ***Nervous system***: increased response to stress-induced hyperthermia.
17βHSD15	Null/KO[24] MGI:3526658 & 3586379	**No clear reproductive endocrinology phenotype** **Additional** Abnormal eye electrophysiology, delayed dark adaptation
AKR1C3/ 17βHSD5*	Null/KO[25] MGI:3527218 Null/KO[26] MGI:3774264	**Reproductive endocrinology** - long gestation, parturition failure. - increased levels of P. - prolonged estrous and diestrous. **Additional** Small litter size, the number of pups, especially live pups, was markedly decreased hematopoietic system phenotype. ***Nervous system***: Some behavioral phonotype,
SRD5A1	Null/KO[27] MGI:1857454	**Reproductive endocrinology** - parturition defects, rescued by 3α-DIOL supplementation. **Additional** Decreased litter size; small prostate.
SRD5A2	Null/KO[28] MGI:2178039	**Reproductive endocrinology** - T accumulation in reproductive tissues. - impaired androgen-dependent gene expression. - parturition defects, rescued by 3α-DIOL supplementation. **Additional** Decreased litter size; small prostate.
SRD5A3	Null/KO[29] MGI:5520177	***Mouse not thoroughly characterized*** Embryonic lethality, abnormal heart morphology, abnormal neural tube closure
SULT1E1	Null/KO[30] MGI:3529586	**Reproductive endocrinology** - elevated circulating estrogen levels. **Additional** Disturbed platelet physiology. ***Reproductive system***: leyding cell hyperplasia and abnormal morphology; abnormal testis morphology; abnormal placentation and amniotic fluid composition.
SULT2B1	Null/KO MGI:5432568 (unpublished)	**Endocrine (steroids)** disturbed cholesterol metabolism and levels.

^No report/references was found for 17βHSD3, 17βHSD6, 17βHSD8, 3βHSD1, 3βHSD2, DHRS11, STS, SULT2A1, SULT1A1.
**The human AKR1C3/17βHSD5 KO refers to mice with disrupted AKR1C18, however, functional conservation between the four human AKR1Cs and the eight mouse AKR1Cs in unclear (Sudeshna et al., 2013).*
$Reference ID refers to the Mouse Genome Informatics (MGI; www.informatics.jax.org. Accessed on date: February 2018) (Blake et al., 2017).
[1]Caron et al. (1997), [2]Huang et al. (2012), [3]Hu et al. (2002), [4]Liu et al. (2005), [5]Bair and Mellon (2004), [6]Nemoto et al. (2000), [7] Fisher et al. (1998), [8]Honda et al. (1998), [9]Hakkarainen et al. (2015), [10]Saloniemi et al. (2010) and Järvensivu et al. (2018), [11]Rantakari et al. (2008), [12]Zhongyi et al. (2007), [13]Baes et al. (2000), [14]Shehu et al. (2008), [15]Jokela et al. (2010), [16]Shang et al. (2002), [17]Driessen et al. (2000) and Sahu et al. (2015); [18]Li et al. (2010) and Rauschenberger et al. (2010); [19]Li et al. (2010); Rauschenberger et al. (2010), [20]Dickinson et al. (2016), [21]Rantakari et al. (2010); Kemilainen et al. (2016); [22]Tang et al. (2010), [23]Tang et al. (2010), [24]Kim et al. (2005), [25]Piekorz et al. (2005), [26]Ishida et al. (2007), [27]Mahendroo et al. (1996), [28]Mahendroo et al. (2001), [29]Dickinson et al. (2016), [30]Qian et al. (2001) and Tong et al. (2005).

CYP19A1 as well has low expression and some authors detected this enzyme only in association with diseases (see below and recently reviewed by Rižner, 2013). Although CYP19A1 immunoreactivity was initially associated with stroma cells (Watanabe et al., 1995), subsequent investigations showed also glandular expression (Kitawaki et al., 1999; Hudelist et al., 2007) and laser-capture-microdissected stroma/epithelial components detected CYP19A1 mRNA in both cell types (Matsuzaki et al., 2006).

The mRNA of those enzymes converting cholesterol to DHEA (CYP11A1, CYP17A1, StAR) and (ovarian) 3βHSD2 was reported in recent studies, suggesting that the endometrium can produce steroids from cholesterol (**Table 6**).

TABLE 5 | Diseases associated with gene variants in intracrine enzymes.

Name	Affected system or tissue *Disease*	Phenotype	OMIM ID# References
StAR	**Endocrine system** *Lipoid adrenal hyperplasia*	Deficiency of adrenal or gonadal steroids All individuals are phenotypic females Infant mortality (mineral- & glucocorticoid deficiency	OMIM: 201710[1]
CYP11A1	**Endocrine system** *Congenital adrenal insufficiency, with 46XY sex reversal*	Acute adrenal insufficiency in infancy or childhood Abnormality of cholesterol metabolism Absence of secondary sex characteristics	OMIM: 613743[1]
	Reproductive *(ass^)*	SNPs^^ associated with endometrial cancer	2
	Bone *(ass^)*	SNPs associated with skeletal adverse events to AI	3
	CNV *(ass^)*	SNPs associated with neurological disturbances	4
CYP17A1	**Endocrine system** *Congenital adrenal insufficiency (17α-hydroxyl. deficiency)*	Excessive corticosteroids leading to hypertension Low aldosterone synthesis Abnormal sex determination and secondary sex characteristics, amenorrhea	OMIM: 202110[1]
	GIT *(ass^)*	SNPs associated with risk of cancer in the CRC##	5
	Reproductive *(ass^)*	SNPs associated with endometrial cancer	6
CYP19A1	**Reprod Endocrin**** *Aromatase deficiency*	Pseudo hermaphroditism in female Cystic ovaries, delayed bone maturation, adiposity	OMIM: 613546
	Aromatase excess syndrome	Heterosexual precocity and gynecomastia in males Isosexual precocity in females	OMIM: 139300
	Reproductive *(ass^)*	SNPs associated with endometrial cancer and ovarian cancer risks, endometriosis risk and risk to develop preeclampsia	6–14
	Bone *(ass^)*	SNPs associated with osteoporosis and fracture risk	15,16
	Lung *(ass^)*	SNPs associated with lung cancer	17
	GIT *(ass^)*	SNPs associated with gastric cancer	18
3βHSD1	**Endocr syst*** *(ass^)*	SNPs associated with hypertension	19
	Skin *(ass^)*	SNPs associated with acne susceptibility	20
3βHSD2	**Endocrine system & Reprod Endocrin** *Congenital adrenal insufficiency (3β-HSD2 deficiency)*	Impaired steroid biosynthesis Low cortisol, aldosterone, P androgens, estrogens. Male new-borns exhibit pseudo hermaphroditism Incomplete masculinization of the external genitalia Affected females can have partial verification	OMIM: 201810[1]
	Urogenital *(ass^)*	SNPs associated with bladder cancer	21
17βHSD1	**Reproductive** *(ass^)*	SNPs associated with E2 levels and with endometriosis, cancer risk, abortion	22–25
17βHSD3	**Reprod Endocrin** *ketosteroidreductase deficiency of testis*	Males: pseudo hermaphroditism, gynecomastia Infertility	OMIM: 264300[1]
17βHSD4	**CNS and Reprod Endocrin** *Perrault syndrome 1*	Ovarian dysgenesis, amenorrhea, low estrogens Sensorineural deafness, Neurologic manifestations (mild mental retardation)	OMIM: 233400
	CNS *D-bifunctional protein deficiency*	Abnormal peroxisomal fatty acid beta-oxidation Deterioration of nervous system functions Infantile-onset of hypotonia, seizures, and abnormal facial features, death before the age of 2 years	OMIM: 261515

(Continued)

TABLE 5 | Continued

Name	Affected system or tissue *Disease*	Phenotype	OMIM ID# References
17βHSD6	**Reproductive** *(ass^)*	SNPs associated with PCOS***	26
17βHSD9	**Eye** *Fundus albipunctatus*	Fleck retina disease, night blindness, delayed cone and rod photopigment regeneration.	OMIM: 136880
17βHSD10	**CNS** *HSD10 mitochondrial disease*	X-linked neurodegenerative disorder	OMIM: 300438
		Multisystemic features, mitochondrial dysfunction	
	Turner type X-linked mental retardation	Moderate to profound mental retardation Macrocephaly and variable skeletal features	OMIM: 300706
17βHSD12	**Reproductive** *(ass^)*	(Male) SNPs associated with prostate cancer	27
	Lung *(ass^)*	SNPs associated with pulmonary function	28
17βHSD15	**Eye and CNS** *Retinal dystrophy, juvenile cataracts, short stature*	Decreased visual acuity, retinitis pigmentosa	OMIM: 616108
		Psychomotor delays from early childhood, lack of fine motor skills and coordination, learning difficulties, facial dysmorphism	
AKR1C1	**Lymphocytes** *(ass^)*	SNPs associated with non-Hodgkin lymphoma	29
	Lung *(ass^)*	SNPs associated with lung cancer	29
	CNS *(ass^)*	SNPs associated with panic disorders	29
AKR1C2	**Reprod Endocrin** *46XY sex reversal 8*	Males: ambiguous external genitalia, cryptorchidism	OMIM: 614279
		Disturbed endocrine features	
	Endocr. syst. *(ass^)*	SNPs associated with weight-gain predisposition	29
	Lung *(ass^)*	SNPs associated with lung cancer	29
AKR1C3	**Reproductive** *(ass^)*	SNPs associated with T levels and PCOS	29,30
	Lymphocytes *(ass^)*	SNPs associated with large B cell lymphoma	29
	Lung *(ass^)*	SNPs associated with lung cancer	29
	Leukocytes *(ass^)*	SNPs associated with lung childhood leukemia	29
	Urogenital *(ass^)*	SNPs associated with bladder cancer	29
	CNS *(ass^)*	SNPs associated with amyotrophic lateral sclerosis	29
AKR1C4	**Reprod Endocrin** *46XY sex reversal 8*	Males: ambiguous external genitalia, cryptorchidism	OMIM 614279
		Disturbed endocrine features	
	– *(ass^)*	SNPs associated with responses to anthracycline	29
	CNS *(ass^)*	SNPs associated with paranoia risk	29
SRD5A1	**Reproductive** *(ass^)*	Haplotypes associated with PCOS and hirsutum	31
SRD5A2	**Reprod Endocrin** *Pseudovaginal perineoscrotal hypospadias*	Males: pseudo hermaphroditism, ambiguous genitalia, cryptorchidism, small prostate	OMIM: 264600
		No Mullerian structures, masculinization at puberty	
		No breast development or menstruation at puberty	
		Abnormal plasma DHT (and T) level	
	Reproductive *(ass^)*	Haplotypes associated with PCOS	31
	Bone *(ass^)*	SNPs associated with low bone mineral density	32
SRD5A3	**CNS** *Type Iq congenital glycosylation disorder*	Developmental delay, midline brain malformations	OMIM: 612379
		Variable extents of visual loss	
	CNS *Kahrizi syndrome*	Mental retardation, delayed motor development, speech impairment, coarse facial features	OMIM: 612713

(Continued)

TABLE 5 | Continued

Name	Affected system or tissue *Disease*	Phenotype	OMIM ID# References
STS	**Skin** *X-linked ichthyosis*	Cutaneous manifestations: dark brown, polygonal scales and generalized dryness	OMIM: 308100[40]
	Bone *bone dysplasia*	Chondrodysplasia punctata and bone dysplasia	33
SULT1E1	**Reproductive** *(ass^)*	SNP associated with estrogen dependent diseases	34
SULT2A1	**Reproductive** *(ass^)*	SNP associated with DHEA-S, androgens and PCOS	40,35
SULT2B1	**Skin** *congenital autosomal recessive ichthyosis*	Generalized desquamation, dry scaly skin, hyperkeratosis, erythema	OMIM: 604125
SULT1A1	**Reproductive** *(ass^)*	SNPs associated with endometrial cancer	11,36
	Bone *(ass^)*	SNPs associated with low bone mineral density	32
	GIT *(ass^)*	SNPs associated with risk of cancer in the GIT	37–38
	- *(ass^)*	SNPs associated with activity and termostability	37,39

Selected papers reporting association between SNPs and diseases are reported. Association studies with enzymes involved in steroid signaling but not discusses in the present review exist (for some references, see Doherty et al., 2005; Freedman et al., 2009; Miller and Auchus, 2011; Mueller et al., 2015).
Endocr syst: Endocrine system.
**Reprod Endocrin: Reproductive endocrinology.*
***PCOS: polycystic ovarian syndrome.*
^ass: association studies, case controls.
^^SNP: single nucleotide polymorphism.
#OMIM: Online Mendelian Inheritance in Man. McKusick-Nathans Institute of Genetic Medicine, Johns Hopkins University (Baltimore, MD). (https://omim.org/. Accessed on date: February 2018).
##CRC: colorectal cancer.
[1]Miller and Auchus (2011), [2]Terry et al. (2010), [3]Rodríguez-Sanz et al. (2015), [4]Deng et al. (2016), [5]Zeng et al. (2016), [6]Olson et al. (2007), [7]Berstein et al. (2006), [8]Kitawaki et al. (2002), [9]Lundin et al. (2012), [10]Thompson et al. (2016), [11]Gulyaeva et al. (2008), [12]Setiawan et al. (2009), [13]Zacher et al. (2016), [14]Shimodaira et al. (2012), [15]Fontein et al. (2014), [16]Masi et al. (2001), [17]Zhang et al. (2013), [18]Cho et al. (2012), [19]Shimodaira et al. (2010), [20]Yang et al. (2013), [21]Andrew et al. (2012), [22]Tsuchiya et al. (2005), [23]Huber et al. (2005), [24]Setiawan et al. (2004), [25]Shi et al. (2016), [26]Jones et al. (2009), [27]Audet-Walsh et al. (2012), [28]Loth et al. (2014), [29]Alshogran (2017), [30]Qin et al. (2006), [31]Goodarzi et al. (2006), [32]Zarrabeitia et al. (2007), [33]Wöhrle et al. (1990), [34]Adjei et al. (2003), [35]Goodarzi et al. (2007), [36]Ashton et al. (2010), [37]Lilla et al. (2007), [38]Xiao et al. (2014), [39]Sun et al. (2005), and [40]Mueller et al. (2015).
Bold text indicates the system affected, italics text indicates the name of the disease.

Intratissue Steroid Levels

Endometrial steroid levels were recently profiled by LC-MS. E2 levels differ between tissue and serum during the menstrual cycle, being up to five-times higher in tissue than in serum during the proliferative phase and 1.5-fold higher in the luteal period (Huhtinen et al., 2012a, 2014). T levels were lower in tissue than in serum with no cyclic changes. The levels P and P5 (and their 17-hydroxy derivatives) did not vary between serum and tissue, indicating that, contrarily to estrogens, progestogen intra-tissue levels are determined by passive diffusion from the blood (Huhtinen et al., 2014).

Intracrinology and Reproduction

Animal models show not only that intracrine enzymes are expressed in the endometrium, but also they vary the expression levels during the endometrial phases and during implantation, as shown already during the 80's in rhesus monkeys for the oxidizing 17βHSD activity (Kreitmann et al., 1979).

In rodents, STS activity measured with [3H]E1-S in 6-days pregnant rats was lower around the implantation site compared with non-implantation sites (Loza, 1995). *In situ* hybridisation signal of 17βHSD7 mRNA varied spatio-temporally throughout implantation and early gestation, being initially detected on luminal epithelium around the implantation site and absent in decidua (embryonic day, Ed5.5). At Ed8 and Ed9.5, 17βHSD7 expression increased in the decidua capsularis (the part that interacts with the trophoblast) and later (after E9) in the junctional zone of the developing placenta and in the spongiotrophoblasts (Nokelainen et al., 2000).

A brilliant study in mice showed that decidualization is dependent on local E2 produced through CYP19A1. CYP19A1 expression increased during pregnancy and decidualization was unaffected by ovariectomy. In contrast, treatment with the aromatase inhibitor (AI) letrozole impaired decidualization and decreased decidual marker expression (e.g., PRP, BMP2 and CX43) (Das et al., 2009).

In human endometrium, 17βHSD2 and SULT1E1 are induced by P as their expression peaks in the luteal phase (Rubin et al., 1999; Tseng and Mazella, 2002; Utsunomiya et al., 2004; Dassen et al., 2007; Huhtinen et al., 2012a; Colette et al., 2013; Piccinato et al., 2016b). Since both enzymes decrease intra-tissue estrogen levels, their up-regulation is one of the mechanisms of the uterine antiestrogenic effects of P. The P-dependency of 17βHSD2 and SULT1E1 was recapitulated *in vitro* using explant cultures and

TABLE 6 | Expression of intracrine enzymes in endometrium–results of the systematic search.

Name			Menopausal status		
		Technique[#]	Pre	Post	References
StAR	mRNA	RT-PCR	yes	yes	Bukulmez et al., 2008a; Attar et al., 2009; Sinreih et al., 2017b[&]
CYP11A1	mRNA	RT-PCR	yes	n.d.	Tsai et al., 2001; Rhee et al., 2003; Attar et al., 2009; Sinreih et al., 2013; Huhtinen et al., 2014
		RT-PCR	no	n.d.	Rhee et al., 2003
CYP17A1	mRNA	RT-PCR	yes	n.d.	Tsai et al., 2001; Attar et al., 2009; Huhtinen et al., 2014
		RT-PCR	no	n.d.	Rhee et al., 2003
		IHC	no	no	Watanabe et al., 1995
CYP19A1	mRNA	RT-PCR	yes	yes	Dheenadayalu et al., 2002; Brosens et al., 2004; Matsuzaki et al., 2006; Pathirage et al., 2006; Smuc et al., 2006, 2009; Dassen et al., 2007; Bukulmez et al., 2008b; Attar et al., 2009; Smuc and Rizner, 2009; Lépine et al., 2010; Cornel et al., 2012; Huhtinen et al., 2012a; Delvoux et al., 2014; Sinreih et al., 2017a
		RT-PCR	no	no	Bulun et al., 1993, 1994; Watanabe et al., 1995; Noble et al., 1996, 1997; Kitawaki et al., 1999; Bacallao et al., 2008; Colette et al., 2009
		ISH	no	n.d.	Watanabe et al., 1995
	Protein	IHC	yes	yes	Maentausta et al., 1990; Kitaoka et al., 2004; Maia et al., 2006, 2007; Hudelist et al., 2007; Vouk et al., 2011; Miller et al., 2012a
		IHC	no	no	Watanabe et al., 1995; Kitawaki et al., 1999; Velasco et al., 2006; Acién et al., 2007; Jeon et al., 2007; Bukulmez et al., 2008b; Colette et al., 2009
		WB	N.d.	yes	Knapp et al., 2013
		activity	no	no	Bulun et al., 1993; Watanabe et al., 1995; Noble et al., 1997
		activity	yes	yes	Tseng et al., 1982; Yamaki et al., 1985; Taga et al., 1990; Yamamoto et al., 1990a,b, 1993a,b; Jongen et al., 2005; Purohit et al., 2008
3βHSD1	mRNA	RT-PCR	yes	yes	Rhee et al., 2003; Vani et al., 2007; Attar et al., 2009; Smuc et al., 2009; Gibson et al., 2013; Sinreih et al., 2013
	Protein*	IHC	yes	n.d.	Rhee et al., 2003; Vani et al., 2007
		IHC	no	no	Watanabe et al., 1995
3βHSD2	mRNA	RT-PCR	yes	yes	Tsai et al., 2001; Attar et al., 2009; Huhtinen et al., 2014; Osinski et al., 2018
17βHSDs					
oxidative activity			yes	yes	Tseng and Gurpide, 1974; Pollow et al., 1975a,b, 1976; Polow et al., 1975; Tseng et al., 1977; Lane, 1990; Kitawaki et al., 2000; Utsunomiya et al., 2001; Delvoux et al., 2007, 2009; Cornel et al., 2012
reductive activity			yes	yes	Maentausta et al., 1990; Delvoux et al., 2007, 2009, 2014; Bacallao et al., 2008
			no	no	Utsunomiya et al., 2001
17βHSD1	mRNA	RT-PCR	yes	yes	Zeitoun et al., 1998; Dassen et al., 2007; Smuc et al., 2007, 2009; Bacallao et al., 2008; Huhtinen et al., 2012a; Colette et al., 2013; Delvoux et al., 2014; Sinreih et al., 2017a; Osinski et al., 2018
		NB	yes	n.d.	Zeitoun et al., 1998
		RT-PCR	no	no	Casey et al., 1994; Utsunomiya et al., 2001
	Protein	IHC	yes	yes	Maentausta et al., 1990[&]; Mäentausta et al., 1991; Li et al., 2003; Dassen et al., 2007; Colette et al., 2013; Mori et al., 2015; He et al., 2016; Sinreih et al., 2017a
		IHC	no	no	Utsunomiya et al., 2001
17βHSD2	mRNA	RT-PCR	yes	yes	Mäentausta et al., 1991; Zeitoun et al., 1998; Kitawaki et al., 2000, 2002; Utsunomiya et al., 2001; Matsuzaki et al., 2006; Smuc et al., 2006, 2007, 2009; Carneiro et al., 2007; Dassen et al., 2007; Vani et al., 2007; Bacallao et al., 2008; Hevir et al., 2011b; Huhtinen et al., 2012a; Colette et al., 2013; Delvoux et al., 2014; Sinreih et al., 2017a; Osinski et al., 2018
		NB	yes	n.d.	Zeitoun et al., 1998
	Protein	IHC	yes	yes	Scublinsky et al., 1976; Ciuffi et al., 1982; Utsunomiya et al., 2001; Dassen et al., 2007; Colette et al., 2013; Cornel et al., 2017; Sinreih et al., 2017a
17βHSD4	mRNA	RT-PCR	yes	yes	Dassen et al., 2007; Smuc et al., 2009; Huhtinen et al., 2012a; Delvoux et al., 2014
		NB	yes	n.d.	Möller et al., 1999
17βHSD6	mRNA	RT-PCR	yes	n.d.	Huang and Luu-The, 2000; Huhtinen et al., 2012a
17βHSD7	mRNA	RT-PCR	yes	yes	Smuc et al., 2007, 2009; Smuc and Rizner, 2009; Lépine et al., 2010; Cornel et al., 2012; Huhtinen et al., 2012a; Delvoux et al., 2014

(Continued)

TABLE 6 | Continued

Name		Technique[#]	Menopausal status Pre	Post	References
17βHSD8	mRNA	RT-PCR	yes	yes	Smuc and Rizner, 2009; Smuc et al., 2009
17βHSD10	mRNA	RT-PCR	yes	n.d.	Huhtinen et al., 2012a
17βHSD12	mRNA	RT-PCR	yes	yes	Smuc and Rizner, 2009; Smuc et al., 2009; Lépine et al., 2010; Cornel et al., 2012; Huhtinen et al., 2012a; Delvoux et al., 2014
17βHSD14	mRNA	RT-PCR	yes	n.d.	Huhtinen et al., 2012a; Sinreih et al., 2017a
AKR1Cs					
AKR1C1	mRNA	RT-PCR	yes	yes	Rizner et al., 2006; Smuc and Rizner, 2009; Smuc et al., 2009; Hevir et al., 2011b; Sinreih et al., 2013
AKR1C2	mRNA	RT-PCR	yes	yes	Hevir et al., 2011b; Sinreih et al., 2013
AKR1C3/17 βHSD5	mRNA	RT-PCR	yes	yes	Penning et al., 2000; Rizner et al., 2006; Vani et al., 2007; Smuc and Rizner, 2009; Smuc et al., 2009; Hevir et al., 2011b; Cornel et al., 2012; Huhtinen et al., 2012a; Sinreih et al., 2013; Delvoux et al., 2014
	Protein	IHC	yes	yes	Pelletier et al., 1999; Ito et al., 2006; Vani et al., 2007; Smuc and Rizner, 2009; Zakharov et al., 2010
SRD5As					
SRD5A1	mRNA	RT-PCR	yes	yes	Carneiro et al., 2008; Hevir et al., 2011b; Sinreih et al., 2013; Huhtinen et al., 2014
	Protein	IHC	yes	yes	Ito et al., 2002; Carneiro et al., 2008; Tanaka et al., 2015
SRD5A2	mRNA	RT-PCR	yes	yes	Carneiro et al., 2008; Hevir et al., 2011b; Sinreih et al., 2013; Huhtinen et al., 2014
	Protein	IHC	yes	yes	Ito et al., 2002; Carneiro et al., 2008; Tanaka et al., 2015
SRD5A3		RT-PCR	yes	n.d.	Huhtinen et al., 2014
Sulphatase pathway					
STS	mRNA	RT-PCR	yes	yes	Tanaka et al., 2003; Utsunomiya et al., 2004; Smuc et al., 2006, 2007, 2009; Dalla Valle et al., 2007; Dassen et al., 2007; Bacallao et al., 2008; Smuc and Rizner, 2009; Lépine et al., 2010; Colette et al., 2013; Huhtinen et al., 2014; Piccinato et al., 2016b; Sinreih et al., 2017a
		RT-PCR	no	no	Miki et al., 2002
		Comp-RT	yes	n.d.	Yanaihara et al., 2001
	Protein	IHC	yes	yes	Yanaihara et al., 2001; Utsunomiya et al., 2004; Dassen et al., 2007; Cornel et al., 2017; Sinreih et al., 2017a
		IHC	no	no	Miki et al., 2002
		activity	yes	yes	Warren and French, 1965; Prost and Adessi, 1983; Adessi et al., 1984; Platia et al., 1984; Yamamoto et al., 1990a, 1993a; Tanaka et al., 2003; Bacallao et al., 2008; Purohit et al., 2008; Delvoux et al., 2009
		IHC	no	no	Utsunomiya et al., 2004
SULT1E1	mRNA	RT-PCR	yes	yes	Yamamoto et al., 1993a; Miki et al., 2002; Tanaka et al., 2003; Utsunomiya et al., 2004; Smuc et al., 2006, 2007; Dassen et al., 2007; Bacallao et al., 2008; Smuc and Rizner, 2009; Lépine et al., 2010; Hevir et al., 2011a, 2013; Colette et al., 2013; Piccinato et al., 2016b; Sinreih et al., 2017a
		NB	yes	n.d.	Rubin et al., 1999
	Protein	IHC	yes	yes	Miki et al., 2002; Utsunomiya et al., 2004; Hudelist et al., 2007; Cornel et al., 2017; Sinreih et al., 2017a
		activity	yes	yes	Tanaka et al., 2003; Utsunomiya et al., 2004; Bacallao et al., 2008; Purohit et al., 2008
SULT1A1	mRNA	RT-PCR	yes	yes	Hevir et al., 2011a, 2013
SULT1A1		NB	yes	n.d.	Rubin et al., 1999***
SULT2A1		NB	no	n.d.	Rubin et al., 1999
SULT2B1	mRNA	RT-PCR	yes	yes	Hevir et al., 2011a, 2013

*Primary/original references were analyzed and reviews were excluded (and are cited ad hoc in the text). The table report only the enzymes whose expression was assessed in reviewed studies**.*

[#]Technique abbreviations. For mRNA detection, NB: northern blot; ISH: in situ hybridisation; RT-PCR: reverse transcription semi or quantitative PCR; Comp-RT: competitive RT-PCR. For protein detection: IHC: immunohistochemistry; WB: western blotting. For enzyme activity measurement: activity.

[*]Most commercially available antibodies do not distinguish between 3βHSD1 and 3βHSD1.

[**]No publication was found describing the expression of 17βHSD9, 11, 13, 15, DHRS11 and AKR1C4.

[***]The same study also detected expression of SULT1A3 (Rubin et al., 1999).

n.d.: not determined.

[&]Protein level was measured by radioimmunoassay.

primary cells (Tseng and Mazella, 2002; Dassen et al., 2007; Piccinato et al., 2016b). Luteal peak expression of other SULTs (1A1 and 2B1) was also reported (Rubin et al., 1999; Koizumi et al., 2010). Some reports also suggested that STS expression increased in the luteal phase (Tanaka et al., 2003; Piccinato et al., 2016b) with a potential role during decidualization (Tseng and Mazella, 2002). Mid-luteal phase endometrium shows also peaking expression of 3βHSD1 (mRNA and protein) (Rhee et al., 2003; Vani et al., 2007).

Two studies on human ectopic pregnancies explored the endometrium around the implanted blastocyst. Expression of 3βHSD1 (mRNA and protein) was highest in decidua obtained from ectopic pregnancies (Rhee et al., 2003) and in a study on 23 tubal pregnancies, 17βHSD1 showed highest immunoreactivity at the fetal-maternal interface (Li et al., 2003), suggestive for a role of these enzymes in the nidation site.

Endometriosis

Endometriosis, an estrogen-dependent benign disorder affecting up to 10% of reproductive-aged women, is associated with pelvic pain, infertility, decreased life-quality and important health care/social costs (Simoens et al., 2011, 2012; De Graaff et al., 2013, 2015, 2016; Vercellini et al., 2014). Endometriosis is characterized by the growth of endometrium-like tissue outside the uterus (ectopic locations), beside the ovaries (endometrioma), as peritoneal implants, or as deep-lesions infiltrating peritoneal organs (deep endometriosis).

The expression of intracrine enzymes in endometriosis was reviewed in 2012, (Huhtinen et al., 2012b) and among other studies, 20 papers published between 1996 and 2009 specifically described the levels of intracrine enzymes in eutopic and ectopic endometrium from patients and control women. With the exclusion of one study that included over 100 patients (Colette et al., 2009), the rest included small study populations, and in most cases, the various endometriosis types (ovarian, peritoneal and deep infiltrating) were pooled together. Various techniques were used (RT-qPCR, immunohistochemistry, enzyme activity assay). Overall, no clear conclusion could be drawn from these studies. Comparing endometriosis with controls, CYP19A1 was up-regulated (six studies), unchanged (three studies) and one study found no expression of this gene. With respect to oxidative and reductive 17βHSDs, 17βHSD1 was reported up-regulated (three studies), 17βHSD2 was reported down-regulated or unchanged and two studies reported an up-regulation of 17βHSD7 and 12 in endometriosis vs. controls (Huhtinen et al., 2012b).

Subsequent investigations also continued to report inconsistent results. No change in mRNA (Delvoux et al., 2014) or increased expression of CYP19A1 in ovarian endometriosis vs. controls (Huhtinen et al., 2012a) were reported. An increased expression of CYP19A1 was also described using *in vitro* spheroids derived from endometrial stroma cells from patients compared with controls (Mori et al., 2015).

The mRNA expression of 17βHSD1 was higher in endometriosis compared with normal tissue using patient biopsies as well as spheroid cultures derived from endometrial stroma cells of patients and controls (Delvoux et al., 2014; Mori et al., 2015). One study assessing the three endometriosis types separately (60 patients in total) described that the increased 17βHSD1 level was restricted to endometrioma during the secretory phase of the menstrual cycle (Huhtinen et al., 2012a), whereas a second study on 79 patients and 41 controls, found no change in 17βHSD1 level, but described an increased 17βHSD1/2 ratio (Colette et al., 2013).

Regarding 17βHSD2, recent investigations reported both unchanged (Delvoux et al., 2014) and down-regulated mRNA in patient biopsies compared with controls (Huhtinen et al., 2012a; Colette et al., 2013). No variations were found in 17βHSD4, 5, 7 and 12 (Smuc et al., 2009; Delvoux et al., 2014) but an increased level of 17βHSD6 mRNA was detected in endometriosis compared with controls (Huhtinen et al., 2012a).

A few studies reported detectable levels of the enzymes involved in the generation of DHEA from cholesterol (StAR, CYP11A1 and CYP17A1) in endometriosis (Tsai et al., 2001; Rhee et al., 2003; Bukulmez et al., 2008a; Attar et al., 2009; Sinreih et al., 2013, 2017b; Huhtinen et al., 2014), suggesting that, in contrast to eutopic endometrium, endometriosis is able to produce steroids from cholesterol. However, it has also been argued that the presence of paracrine confounders of ovarian origin in studies using endometriomas could bias the results (Noël et al., 2011).

The contribution of STS, SULT1E1 and other SULTs was investigated by numerous studies and also in this case, conclusions are unclear (recently reviewed, Rižner, 2016). A recent investigation using 78 specimens described increased STS levels in endometriosis vs. control samples and found that the overall balance between STS and SULT1E1 differed between eutopic and ectopic tissue, implying an unbalanced flux of sulpho-conjugated estrogens in this disease (Piccinato et al., 2016b). The same research group also described an aberrant regulation of the enzymes involved in the estrogen oxidative metabolism in endometriosis (Piccinato et al., 2016a).

Although the level of the single enzymes in the intracrine machinery varies with apparently no clear association with the disease condition, the intracrinological nature of endometriosis was recently proven by comparison between serum and tissue levels of steroids in 60 patients (eutopic and ectopic endometrium) and 16 controls. Although E2 changed cyclically in eutopic tissue, E2 levels remained constant in the lesions and inversely correlated with the mRNA level of 17βHSD2 and 17βHSD6 suggesting an impairment in E2 deactivation to E1. P levels were equal in serum and control tissues, but resulted higher in patients and correlated with high 3βHSD2 mRNA. T, low in the tissue of controls, was over 13-times more concentrated at ectopic locations and correlated with low expression of SRD5A3 (Huhtinen et al., 2012a, 2014).

Endometrial Cancer (EC)

EC is the most common gynecological malignancy in western society and 80% of all cases are estrogen-driven (Amant et al., 2005; Morice et al., 2015). Major serum steroids are increased in patients with EC, including several substrates for intracrine E2 synthesis (Lépine et al., 2010; Audet-Walsh et al., 2011). In addition, tissue-steroid levels differ between cancer, normal tissue and serum and correlate with the levels of specific intracrine enzymes (see below) (Tanaka et al., 2015).

A systematic review recently explored all studies published between 1990 and 2017 assessing the expression of 17βHSD1, 2, STS, SULT1E1, and CYP19A1, with results that describe unbalanced intracrine regulation and important inter-patient variability (Cornel et al., 2018). Most studies compared cases with controls or tumor tissue with adjacent normal endometrium. Compared with normal tissue (from controls or adjacent to tumor), 17βHSD1 was found increased in EC (Cornel et al., 2012), decreased (Smuc and Rizner, 2009; Lépine et al., 2010) and undetected (Utsunomiya et al., 2001, 2003); 17βHSD2 was found decreased (Utsunomiya et al., 2003, 2004) or increased (Lépine et al., 2010; Cornel et al., 2012; Sinreih et al., 2013); AKR1C3/17βHSD5 was found unchanged (Cornel et al., 2012; Sinreih et al., 2013), increased (Ito et al., 2016) and decreased (Zakharov et al., 2010); 17βHSD7 both decreased (Smuc and Rizner, 2009) and unchanged (Lépine et al., 2010; Cornel et al., 2012) and 17βHSD12 was unchanged (Smuc and Rizner, 2009; Cornel et al., 2012) or increased in tumors vs. controls (Lépine et al., 2010). One recent report described decreased 17βHSD14 levels in tumor compared with adjacent tissue (Sinreih et al., 2017a). Controversial results apply to CYP19A1, described as increased (Watanabe et al., 1995; Utsunomiya et al., 2001, 2004; Smuc and Rizner, 2009) and unchanged (Jongen et al., 2005; Pathirage et al., 2006; Cornel et al., 2012). STS/SULT1E1 expression is also inconsistent in different studies (recently reviewed in Mueller et al., 2015; Rižner, 2016).

Recent studies exploring the association between enzyme levels and tumor characteristics found a correlation between STS with tumor grade and lymphovascular invasion (Sinreih et al., 2017a) and described an association between high CYP19A1 or 17βHSD1 and poor patient prognosis (Segawa et al., 2005; Cornel et al., 2017).

Other investigations emphasized the potential antiestrogenic and protective roles of androgens and P. Formation of DHT (via conversion of A4 to T by AKR1C3/17βHSD5 and of T to DHT by SRD5As) has potential antiestrogenic action because it devoids tissue from T (substrate of CYP19A1 yielding E2) and because it has direct endometrial antiproliferative effects via AR (Ito et al., 2016). Similar to the AKR1C3/17βHSD5 data reported earlier, results on SDR5A expression are inconclusive as SRD5A2 was down-regulated in a study on 47 tumor specimens compared with adjacent normal tissue (Sinreih et al., 2013), but both SRD5A1 and SRD5A2 resulted unchanged in another study on 122 tumors (although only five controls were studied) (Tanaka et al., 2015). This last study found however increased androgen levels (T and DHT) in tissue vs. blood. High DHT levels were restricted to samples with high SRD5A1 immunohistochemical staining. In addition, AR and SRD5A1 positivity was associated with good patient prognosis (Tanaka et al., 2015). The prognostic value of AR is confirmed by independent investigations (Tangen et al., 2016).

P is well-known for its antiestrogenic action, PR positivity is a good prognostic marker (Tangen et al., 2014) and P synthesis and metabolism are disturbed in EC (Sinreih et al., 2013). Interestingly, in a study on 47 tumors and adjacent normal tissues, EC had decreased StAR and CYP11A1 mRNA levels, indicative of diminished *de novo* steroid synthesis (Sinreih et al., 2013, 2017b). At the same time, EC showed decreased SRD5A2 and increased 17βHSD2 indicative of a diminished rate of conversion of P to 5αDHP and of 20αDHP to 5α-pregnan-20-ol-3-one, but increased conversion of 20αDHP to P (see **Figure 2**).

Other Endometrial/Gynecological Disorders

Although literature is scarce, a potential role of intracrinology is postulated for ovarian cancer (Ito et al., 2016), for adenomyosis and fibroids (Rižner, 2016), for sarcoma, where CYP19A1 expression may have prognostic significance (Kitaoka et al., 2004) and among infertile women (Brosens et al., 2004).

Intracrine Drug Targets

Endometriosis: blocking the systemic estrogen signaling via P, or GnRH agonist is standard care (Vercellini et al., 2014). Blocking the intracrine E2 generation is the future approach with on-going preclinical/clinical research.

STS inhibition showed promising results. Irosustat (**Table 3**) inhibited up to 100% the formation of free steroids using *ex-vivo* material from 27 patients (Purohit et al., 2008) and STS inhibition showed good results in a mouse model of endometriosis, where decreased size and weight of the lesions was observed (Colette et al., 2011). A phase-I clinical trial on 24 volunteers proved the safety of the STS inhibitor E2MATE (PLG2001), which reduced STS activity by over 90% and induced changes in endometrial markers (both alone or co-administered with norethindrone acetate) (Pohl et al., 2014).

Inhibitors of 17βHSD1 are in preclinical phase, and promising results are described using a primate model of endometriosis, where decreased behavior/pain symptoms were reported (Arnold and Einspanier, 2013) and using *ex-vivo* material from endometriosis patient (over 70% of the patients showed over 80% of enzyme inhibition) (Delvoux et al., 2014).

AKR1C3/17βHSD5 inhibition can interfere with E2, androgen synthesis, and reduce prostaglandin-associated inflammation/proliferation and an inhibitor has recently entered a phase II trial for endometriosis (**Table 3**). Overall, AIs have limited efficacy for endometriosis (Ferrero et al., 2011; Dunselman et al., 2014),

EC: only in case of advanced stage/metastatic disease hormonal care is given (progestogen, tamoxifen or AIs). AIs alone have limited efficacy with low response rates (Rose et al., 2000; Ma et al., 2004; Lindemann et al., 2014). Promising data were obtained using dual regimen (AI and mTOR inhibitor; Slomovitz et al., 2015) and additional trials on combinatory regimen are on-going. STS inhibitors showed promising results in a mouse subcutaneous model of EC, with decreased tumor growth by 48–67% (Foster et al., 2008b). However, a phase II trial on advanced stage EC was stopped because of the absence of added benefit compared with progestogen treatment (Purohit and Foster, 2012; Pautier et al., 2017).

Preclinical studies on 17βHSD1 inhibitors showed promising results in a mouse model of endometrial hyperplasia (Saloniemi et al., 2010; Järvensivu et al., 2015) and in various models of EC (Konings et al., 2018).

Endometrium: Conclusions

The ability to synthesize DHEA from cholesterol (reported by few studies) needs confirmation. However, the endometrium possesses the enzymatic machinery to metabolize sulphated-compounds and DHEA and form androgens and estrogens, (although this contention is wrangled by other authors: Labrie and Labrie, 2013; Labrie, 2015). Further, the endometrium can metabolize androgens and progestogens via AKR1Cs and SRD5As to produce a wide range of compounds, including estrogens (**Table 6** and **Figure 3**). The morphological changes during the menstrual cycle are accompanied by cyclic changes in intracrine steroid and enzyme levels, indicating that steroid exposure needs to be cyclically regulated to support endometrial physiology.

Gastrointestinal Tract (GIT) and Digestive System (DS)

ERα and ERβ are expressed throughout the GIT and DS (esophagus, stomach, colon, gallbladder, pancreas) and epidemiological studies show important influence of sex hormones in DS physiology and disturbances, with a clear gender-dependency. In the duodenum, estrogens regulate bicarbonate secretion (Nayeb-Hashemi and Kaunitz, 2009; Tuo et al., 2011). This is an important defense mechanism of the mucosa against acids discharged from the stomach, and men develop duodenal ulcer two/three-times more often than premenopausal women (Wu et al., 2008). Such estrogen protective effect is recapitulated in animal studies exposed to estrogens and anti-estrogens, and is mediated by a rapid action (i.e., non genomic) of ERα on membrane ion channels (Smith et al., 2008).

ERα, ERβ and GPER mediate important effects on the pancreatic beta-cells during adaptation to insulin resistance periods (e.g., pregnancy, puberty, obesity; Nadal et al., 2011). In mice, ERα signaling regulates proliferation of beta-cell during development and after injury (Yuchi et al., 2015).

Men are also more likely than women to develop cancer in the esophagus, stomach and colon. Accordingly, estrogen treatment for prostate cancer decreases the incidence of gastric cancer and menopausal status in women is associated with colorectal cancer CRC risk (Freedman et al., 2007; Kennelly et al., 2008; Hogan et al., 2009; Duell et al., 2010). ERβ results oncoprotective at several GIT sites (Kennelly et al., 2008; Barzi et al., 2013; Caiazza et al., 2015) and low expression correlate with high CRC stage in mice and with poor differentiated gallbladder cancer in humans (Hogan et al., 2009).

The association between estrogens and DS cancer risk is however controversial. The Women's Health Initiative and other large studies showed that combined estrogens plus P hormone replacement therapy (HRT) decreases CRC risk, but increases that of gallbladder. In addition, CRC during HRT has a higher grade (Kennelly et al., 2008; Hogan et al., 2009; Rennert et al., 2009; Foster, 2013; Mueller et al., 2015). However, a recent randomized, placebo-controlled trial enrolling over 10,000 women receiving estrogens alone vs. placebo found no difference in CRC incidence (Lavasani et al., 2015). Such complexity is recapitulated in animal studies where estrogens and androgens can have distinct and opposite effects on colitis and CRC (Amos-Landgraf et al., 2014; Heijmans et al., 2014). Overall, the association between DS disturbances/cancers with estrogens depends on the moment in life, extent and nature (endogenous or exogenous) of exposure and is influenced by the relative balance of the receptors (Foster, 2013). Similarly, androgens influence DS pathophysiology via complex and unclear mechanisms involving classical, membrane signaling, level of free and SHBG bound T (Roshan et al., 2016).

The lack of clear conclusion and the fact that the levels of circulating endogenous estrogens in women do not influence CRC risk indicates that intracrine steroids may have a predominant role irrespective of their circulating levels (Sato et al., 2009; Falk et al., 2015).

Intracrinology in Healthy GIT–Systematic Search

In total, 29 original papers were retrieved that described the levels of the intracrine enzymes in the GIT, published from the late 80's (**Table 7** and **Supplemental panel**: "Systematic Review").

Stomach intracrinology.

The stomach is an endocrine tissue, and in rodents it produces steroids starting at birth and throughout adulthood (Kobayashi et al., 2013). Human gastric mucosa expresses 17βHSD1, 2, 12 and AKR1C3/17βHSD5 (**Table 7**). The mRNA for 17βHSD2 in mucosa surface and glandular epithelium inversely correlates with age in both genders (Oduwole et al., 2003a). Luminal gastric mucosa has strong AKR1C3/17βHSD5 immunoreactivity that decreases toward the gastric pits (Chang et al., 2013). Weak immunoreactivity for 17βHSD12 localizes in the fundic glands and in the squamous epithelium of the esophagus (Sakurai et al., 2006).

Sulphatases in parietal cells of the gastric glands have a protective role in detoxification. Estrogenic SULT1E1 is not expressed whereas data for SULT2A1 are inconsistent. SULT2A1 was detected in the gastric mucosa in a study on seven subjects (Tashiro et al., 2000), but it was low/absent in other studies on 39 (Teubner et al., 2007) and 23 subjects (Chen et al., 2003).

Small intestine: duodenum–jejunum–ileum.

Due to its high exposure to food components and harmful xenobiotics, the duodenum expresses several phase I/II enzymes including DHEA/estrogenic SULT1E1, 2A1, 1A1 (**Table 7**). Protein and enzyme activity of SULT1E1 and 2A1 are present in human jejunum and ileum but absent in duodenum (Teubner et al., 2007), mRNA and protein levels vary with no relation either with age or gender (Her et al., 1996; Nishimura and Naito, 2006). In a study on 23 subjects, SULT1E1 and 2A1 varied inter-individually and between different intestine tracts (Chen et al., 2003). The duodenal mucosa expresses 17βHSD2, but not 17βHSD1 (Casey et al., 1994; Oduwole et al., 2003a) and shows strong luminal AKR1C3/17βHSD5 (Chang et al., 2013) and weak 17βHSD12 immunoreactivity (Sakurai et al., 2006) that decreases toward the Brunner's gland (Chang et al., 2013).

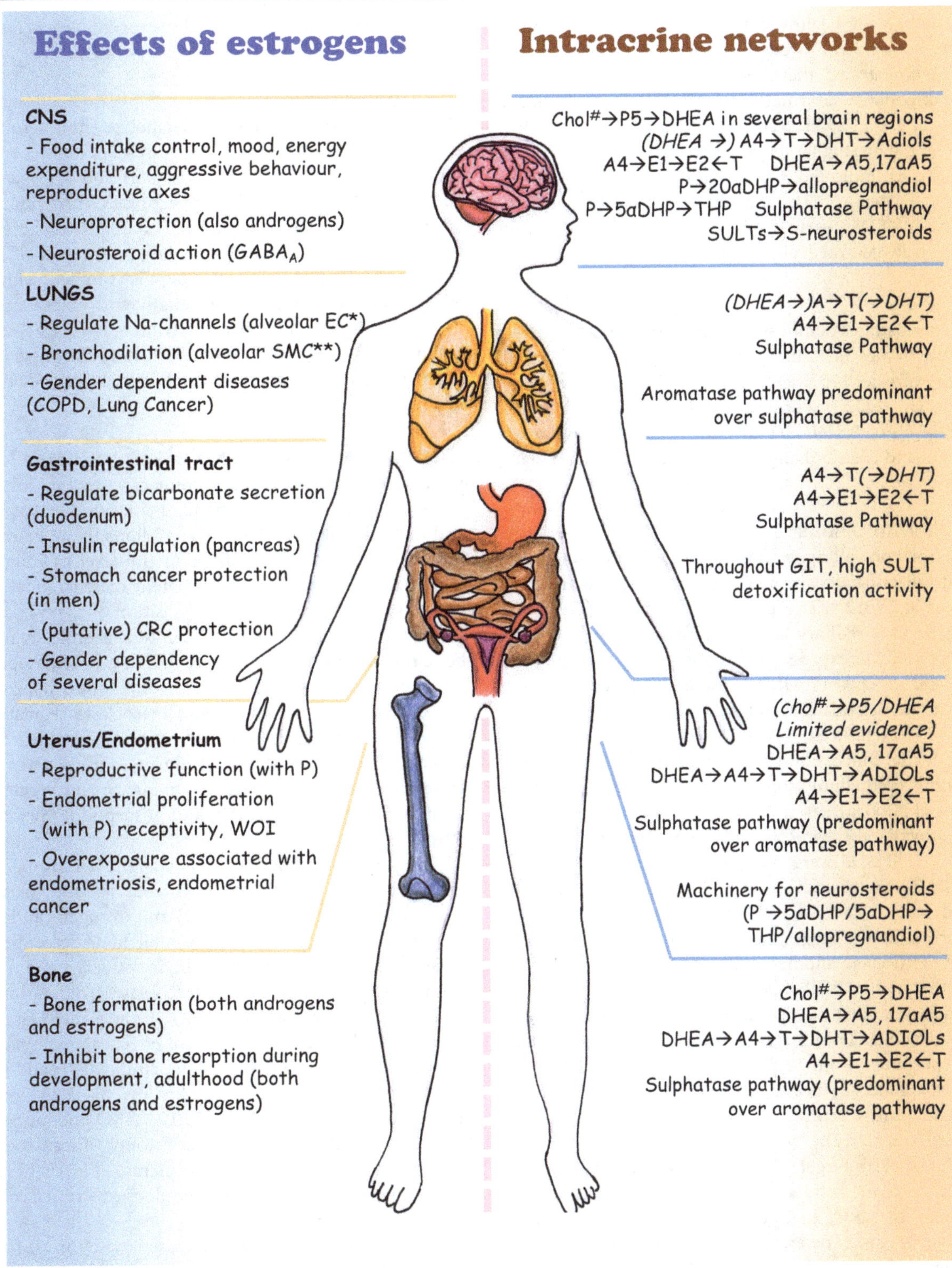

FIGURE 3 | Effect of steroids (mainly estrogens) and intracrine networks in central nervous system, lungs, digestive system, uterus and bone. Italics and by brackets are those metabolism/reactions that need conformation by independent authors (because validated at the mRNA level only or in few studies). * EC, epithelial cells; **SMC, smooth muscle cells; #Chol, cholesterol. The drawing was kindly generated by Dr. Margaretha A. Skowron (Department of Urology, University Düsseldorf, Germany) for this review.

Large intestine: Colon, Cecum, Rectum

The intracrinology of healthy colon mucosa and its relation to CRC was recently reviewed (Foster, 2013). Studies dating from 1987 demonstrated the presence of CYP19A1, 17βHSD reductive and oxidative enzymatic activities, plus the expression of 17βHSD1, 2, 4, CYP19A1, STS and SULT1E1 (**Table 7**). Most 17βHSDs tend to have higher levels at the surface than in cryptal epithelial cells as indicated for 17βHSD2 mRNA (Oduwole et al., 2002; Foster, 2013), and for the immunoreactivity of AKR1C3/17βHSD5 (very strong; Chang et al., 2013) and 17βHSD12 (weak; Sakurai et al., 2006).

Pancreas

Radiolabelled substrates demonstrated the presence of CYP19A1 and SRD5A activities in human pancreatic tissue (Iqbal et al., 1983), which expresses 17βHSD2, 12, STS, SULT1E1 (Casey et al., 1994; Miki et al., 2002; Sakurai et al., 2006; Dalla Valle et al., 2007). High levels of AKR1C3/17βHSD5 localized in pancreatic ductules (acini and islets of Langerhans resulted negative; Chang et al., 2013).

Association With Diseases

SNPs in genes controlling estrogen synthesis, response and deactivation are associated with GIT cancers (Freedman et al., 2009; Cho et al., 2012; Zeng et al., 2016) and AKR1C4 is a candidate gene in hereditary CRC (Gylfe et al., 2013; **Table 5**). Also variations in the expression of these genes associate with GIT disturbances. Low 17βHSD10 levels are associated with aberrant butyrate β-oxidation and ulcerative colitis (De Preter et al., 2012). The epithelial 17βHSD2 level is low in case of stomach, duodenal cancer and chronic gastritis, though it is high in regenerating epithelium close to active gastritis and ulcers (Oduwole et al., 2003a). In a study on 34 gastric tumors and adjacent healthy tissue, the mRNA and protein levels of 17βHSD2 and AKR1C3/17βHSD5 were down-regulated in cancer (Frycz et al., 2015, 2016). Some studies showed lower oxidative 17βHSD activity and mRNA level of 17βHSD2 (and 4) in CRC vs. adjacent normal tissue, suggesting a protective role of estrogen deactivation. However, another study on 35 women and 39 men found that high 17βHSD2 levels were associated with poor prognosis in female patients with distal CRC (reviewed in Foster, 2013). Also 17βHSD1 level measured by RT-qPCR and western blotting in specimens from 52 patients was lower in CRC than adjacent normal mucosa (Rawłuszko et al., 2011). CRC show also higher CYP19A1 mRNA compared with adjacent normal mucosa ($n = 31$) (Sato et al., 2012).

Although no clear target for drugs has been identified in the intracrine network, intracrine enzymes showed some values as biomarkers. In CRC, high STS/SULT1E1 ratio correlates with poor prognosis (Foster, 2013) and AKR1C3/17βHSD5 expression with lymph-node metastasis (Nakarai et al., 2015). In addition, AKR1C1 and AKR1C3/17βHSD5 associate with cisplatin resistance in CRC, hence inhibitors of these AKR1Cs may be used to re-sensitize patients to chemotherapy (Matsunaga et al., 2013). In a study were the levels of E1, E2 and DHEA-S were measured in CRC specimens and adjacent normal mucosa of men and women by LC-MS, intra-tumor estrogens were elevated and (in particular E1) correlated with poor prognosis. In line with an unfavorable role of intra-tissue estrogens, absence on STS was associated with long survival (Sato et al., 2009).

GIT: Conclusions

Human GIT/DS is unable to metabolize cholesterol and there is no clear evidence that it expresses 3βHSDs, hence DHEA cannot be used to generate androgens and estrogens (**Table 7** and **Figure 3**). Several SULTs are expressed throughout GIT and involved in detoxification and STS is regulated by estrogen *in vitro* via non-classical GPER signaling (Gilligan et al., 2017).

The role of steroids in pathology is complex, with divergent effects that depend on time, length and extent of exposure. In line with this, intracrine networks have unclear roles in pathogenesis. In the GIT these networks are strongly involved in the metabolisms of fatty acids and bile acids (outside the scope of this review).

Bone Tissue and Skeletal System

Bones consist of mineralized connective tissue with structural and supportive functions. The hard exterior part (cortical bone) and the trabecular and spongy cancellous tissue filling the bone interior are identical but differ in the level of mineralization. Osteoblasts, derived from multipotent mesenchymal stem cells, build the bone tissue through deposition of Type-I collagen and through the release of ions that combine chemically forming the bone mineral. Osteoclasts differentiate from hematopoietic stem cells and cause resorption of the mineralized bone mass. The balance between osteoblasts and osteoclasts regulates mineral deposition and resorption. Sex steroid hormones contribute to control bone development during puberty, contribute to bone physiology, bone mass maintenance and regulate the rate of mineral bone deposition and resorption (Svoboda et al., 2010).

The presence of the ERs as well as other hormone-receptors in normal osteoblastic cells, osteoclasts and osteoblasts is documented (Gruber et al., 2002) and estrogens and androgens stimulate bone formation and inhibit bone resorption in both males and females. During human puberty and throughout adulthood, E2 and T induce osteoblast proliferation (Kassem et al., 1998), which is mediated by IGF and GH (Riggs et al., 2002; Svoboda et al., 2010). Such human effects are well recapitulated in animal models. ERα-KO (Vidal et al., 2000) and CYP19A1-KO mice (Oz et al., 2000) exhibit low BMD in both genders and E2 treatment rescues the CYP19A1-KO phenotype (Miyaura et al., 2001). Additionally, ovariectomy stimulates osteoclast differentiation through (indirect) increased levels of IL-1, 6 and TNF in osteoblasts and other bone-derived stromal cells (Gruber et al., 2002; Svoboda et al., 2010).

Accelerated bone loss and increased osteoporotic fractures are associated with postmenopausal estrogen deficiency and low sex steroid levels elicit similar manifestations in men (Compston, 2001; Riggs et al., 2002; Syed and Khosla, 2005). Free E2 levels are associated with low lumbar spine and femoral neck bone mineral density (BMD) in both genders (Zarrabeitia et al., 2007) and estrogen therapy reduces bone loss and the risk of fracture in women with osteoporosis (Gruber et al., 2002).

TABLE 7 | Expression of intracrine enzymes in the gastrointestinal tract (GIT)-results of the systematic search.

Gene	Detection		Gastrointestinal tract					
	Molecule	Technique#	St*	References	S.I.*	References	L.I.*	References
CYP11A1	Protein	IHC	no	Saitoh et al., 1992	n.d.		n.d.	
CYP19A1	Protein	Activity	n.d.		n.d.		yes	English et al., 2000
CYP19A1	Protein	IHC	no	Saitoh et al., 1992	n.d.		yes	English et al., 2000
		WB	no	Saitoh et al., 1992	n.d.		n.d.	
HSD17B oxidative activity			n.d.		n.d.		yes	English et al., 1999
HSD17B reductive activity			n.d.		n.d.		yes	English et al., 1999
17βHSD1	mRNA	RT-PCR	no	Oduwole et al., 2003a	n.d.		yes	Rawłuszko et al., 2011
		NB	n.d.		no	Casey et al., 1994	no	Casey et al., 1994
		ISH	n.d.		no	Oduwole et al., 2002	no	Oduwole et al., 2002
	Protein	WB	n.d.		n.d.		yes	Rawłuszko et al., 2011
17βHSD2	mRNA	RT-PCR	yes	Oduwole et al., 2003a; Frycz et al., 2015	n.d.		n.d.	
		NB	n.d.		yes	Casey et al., 1994	yes	Casey et al., 1994
		ISH	n.d.		yes	Oduwole et al., 2002	yes	Oduwole et al., 2002, 2003b
	Protein	IHC	n.d.		n.d.		yes	English et al., 2000; Mueller et al., 2015
		WB	yes	Frycz et al., 2015	n.d.		yes	English et al., 2000; Mueller et al., 2015
17βHSD4	mRNA	NB	n.d.		yes	Möller et al., 1999	yes	Möller et al., 1999
	Protein	IHC	n.d.		n.d.		yes	English et al., 2000; Mueller et al., 2015
		WB	n.d.		n.d.		yes	English et al., 2000; Mueller et al., 2015
17βHSD10	mRNA	RT-PCR	n.d.		n.d.		yes	De Preter et al., 2012
17βHSD12	mRNA	RT-PCR	n.d.		yes	Sakurai et al., 2006	n.d.	
		NB	n.d.		yes	Sakurai et al., 2006	no	Sakurai et al., 2006
	Protein	IHC	yes	Sakurai et al., 2006	yes	Sakurai et al., 2006	yes	Sakurai et al., 2006
AKR1C3	mRNA	Comp-RT	yes	Frycz et al., 2016	n.d.		n.d.	
		NB	yes	Frycz et al., 2016	yes	Lin et al., 1997	yes	Lin et al., 1997
	Protein	IHC	yes	Miller et al., 2012b; Chang et al., 2013	yes	Chang et al., 2013	yes	Chang et al., 2013
SRD5A1	Protein	IHC	yes	Aumüller et al., 1996	yes	Aumüller et al., 1996	yes	Aumüller et al., 1996
SRD5A2	Protein	IHC	yes	Aumüller et al., 1996	yes	Aumüller et al., 1996	yes	Aumüller et al., 1996
STS	mRNA	RT-PCR	n.d.		no	Miki et al., 2002	yes	Dalla Valle et al., 2007
		RT-PCR	–		–		no	Miki et al., 2002
	Protein	IHC	n.d.		no	Miki et al., 2002	no	Miki et al., 2002; Sato et al., 2009
	Protein	Activity	n.d.		n.d.		yes	Munroe and Chang, 1987
SULT1E1	mRNA	RT-PCR	no	Nishimura and Naito, 2006	yes	Miki et al., 2002; Nishimura and Naito, 2006	yes	Miki et al., 2002; Teubner et al., 2007; Riches et al., 2009
			–		–		no	Nishimura and Naito, 2006
		NB	n.d.		yes	Her et al., 1996	n.d.	
	Protein	IHC	no	Chen et al., 2003; Teubner et al., 2007	yes	Miki et al., 2002; Teubner et al., 2007	yes	Miki et al., 2002; Teubner et al., 2007; Sato et al., 2009
		WB	n.d.		yes	Her et al., 1996; Chen et al., 2003; Teubner et al., 2007; Riches et al., 2009	no	Chen et al., 2003
		Activity	no	Chen et al., 2003; Teubner et al., 2007	yes	Teubner et al., 2007	yes	Teubner et al., 2007

(Continued)

TABLE 7 | Continued

Gene	Detection		Gastrointestinal tract					
	Molecule	Technique#	St*	References	S.I.*	References	L.I.*	References
SULT2A1	mRNA	RT-PCR	no	Nishimura and Naito, 2006	yes	Nishimura and Naito, 2006	no	Nishimura and Naito, 2006
		ISH	yes	Tashiro et al., 2000	n.d.		n.d.	
		NB	n.d.		yes	Her et al., 1996	n.d.	
	Protein	IHC	no	Teubner et al., 2007	yes	Teubner et al., 2007	yes	Teubner et al., 2007
		WB	yes	Tashiro et al., 2000; Chen et al., 2003	yes	Her et al., 1996; Chen et al., 2003; Teubner et al., 2007; Riches et al., 2009	yes	Chen et al., 2003; Teubner et al., 2007; Riches et al., 2009
		WB	n.d.		n.d.		no	Chen et al., 2003
		Activity	yes	Tashiro et al., 2000	yes	Chen et al., 2003; Teubner et al., 2007	yes	Chen et al., 2003; Teubner et al., 2007
		Activity	no	Teubner et al., 2007	–		–	
SULT1A1	mRNA	RT-PCR	yes	Nishimura and Naito, 2006	yes	Nishimura and Naito, 2006	yes	Nishimura and Naito, 2006
	Protein	IHC	yes	Teubner et al., 2007	yes	Teubner et al., 2007	yes	Teubner et al., 2007
		WB	yes	Teubner et al., 2007	yes	Teubner et al., 2007; Riches et al., 2009	yes	Teubner et al., 2007; Riches et al., 2009
		Activity	yes	Teubner et al., 2007	yes	Teubner et al., 2007	yes	Teubner et al., 2007
SULT2B1	mRNA	RT-PCR	no	Nishimura and Naito, 2006	yes	Nishimura and Naito, 2006	no	Nishimura and Naito, 2006
		NB	n.d.		n.d.		no	Meloche and Falany, 2001

*Primary/original references were analyzed and reviews were excluded (and are cited ad hoc in the text). The table report only the enzymes whose expression was assessed in reviewed studies**.*

**St: stomach; S.I.: small intestine; L.I.: large intestine.*

 # Technique abbreviations. For mRNA detection, NB: northern blot; ISH: in situ hybridisation; RT-PCR: reverse transcription quantitative (or semi-quantitative) PCR; Comp-RT: competitive RT-PCR assay; NB: northern blotting. For protein detection: IHC: immunohistochemistry; WB; western blotting; activity: enzyme activity measurement.

***No publication was found describing the expression of StAR, 3βHSD1, 3βHSD2, 17βHSD6, 7, 8, 9, 11, 13, 14 15, DHRS11, AKR1C1 AKR1C2 and AKR1C4.*

n.d.: not determined.

Intracrinology in Healthy Bone–Systematic Search

Bone expresses CYP19A1 and 17βHSD1, and mRNA *in situ* hybridisation and immunohistochemistry signals were seen in lining cells, osteoblasts, chondrocytes of articular cartilage, and adipocytes adjacent to bone trabeculae in both male and female tibiae. CYP19A1 mRNA was also widely present in various bones (ribs, femurs) with inter-individual variability, but no relation with gender or age (Sasano et al., 1997). STS and 17βHSD activities were demonstrated by recovery of [3H]E1 and [3H]E2 after incubating femur-head fragments with [3H]E1-S (15 women and 12 men with osteoarthritis indicated for hip replacement). No gender-related differences were observed and E2 formation from androgens was lower than that from E1-S, indicating a predominant role of the sulphatase pathway in bone estrogen supply (Muir et al., 2004). Subsequent studies also demonstrated the presence of CYP11A1, CYP17A1, 17βHSD reductive and oxidative activity in bone tissues (**Table 8**). Overall, however, only six papers describing the level of intracrine enzymes in bone tissues were retrieved by the systemic search (**Table 8**) and most studies on bone intracrinology used *in vitro* cell cultures. *In vitro* studies were not included in our systematic review, but those on bone are briefly described in the next paragraph. These studies demonstrate the presence of a complex intracrine networks.

Bone Intracrinology: *In vitro* and *in vivo*

From early '90s, various isotopic techniques demonstrated the presence of CYP19A1, 17βHSD reductive/oxidative, 3βHSD and STS activities and the mRNA expression of 17βHSD1, 2, 4, STS, SULT1E1, CYP19A1 and SDR5A in human osteoblastic (e.g., HOS, U20S, HTB-96 and MG63) and osteosarcoma cell lines like CRL-1543 (Purohit et al., 1992; Fujikawa et al., 1997; Jakob et al., 1997; Dong et al., 1998; Saito and Yanaihara, 1998; Janssen et al., 1999; Muir et al., 2004; Svoboda et al., 2007; Dias and Selcer, 2014).

In vitro evidence using osteoblastic cells show that E2 has mitogenic effects, which is blocked by the ERα antagonist fulvestrant. Since both E1-S and DHEA-S elicit effects similar to E2, which are blocked by STS inhibition (Selcer and Difrancesca, 2012; Dias and Selcer, 2014), these studies demonstrate that conjugated steroids are activated and that DHEA is converted to E2. Studies in rat osteoblast with [14C]T demonstrated that T is converted by SRD5As and AKR1Cs to 3α/3βDIOLs, which induce proliferation via activation of ER (and not AR) (Enríquez et al., 2013).

In vitro models of osteoblast differentiation showed that various differentiation stages are accompanied by declines in STS, CYP19A1 and 17βHSD1 (Janssen et al., 1999; Dias and Selcer, 2016).

In rats, during and after sexual maturation, *in situ* hybridization showed that ERα and ERβ localize in osteoblasts, osteoclasts and osteocytes covering the tibia metaphysis (responsible for elongation of long bones), and co-localize with STS. Starting at sexual maturation (e.g., 7-week-old), ERs also co-localize with CYP19A1, 17βHSD1, 2 and SRD5A1 (van der Eerden et al., 2004). In addition, male transgenic mice overexpressing 17βHSD2 show disturbed IGF-I/steroid actions in bone, with growth retardation, decreased bone formation at prepuberty and decreased serum levels of IGF-I, osteocalcin and T (Shen et al., 2008).

Diseases and Treatments

Genetic variants of estrogen and intracrine pathways are associated with bone disturbances (**Table 5**). Defects in the CYP19A1 and ERα are associated with low BMD and other skeletal disturbances (e.g., high stature, delayed bone age) and estrogen therapy ameliorates some bone abnormalities caused by CYP19A1 deficiencies in men (Smith et al., 1994; Morishima et al., 1995; Carani et al., 1997; Mullis et al., 1997; Bilezikian et al., 1998). In lumbar vertebrae, CYP19A1 levels correlate with changes in osteoporotic degree (Sasano et al., 1997).

Inhibitors of 17βHSD2 attracted attention as potential drugs to oppose the effects of low E2 on BMD, fracture and osteoporosis. Ovariectomised female macaques receiving a 17βHSD2 inhibitor display desirable bone balance, bone strength and lower bone resorption compared with untreated controls (Bagi et al., 2008). Several compounds targeting this enzyme have been developed and their use and challenges in osteoporosis were recently reviewed (Soubhye et al., 2015).

In a study on 35 chondrosarcoma biopsies (a malignant bone cancer occurring in middle aged patients), ERα (mRNA and IHC) and CYP19A1 (mRNA and activity) were demonstrated in the majority of the samples, and the AI exemestane impaired the E2- and androgen-induced proliferation of primary chondrosarcoma cells (Cleton-Jansen et al., 2005). Although AIs were proposed as novel drugs to treat this condition (Bovée et al., 2005), a pilot study on six patients with progressive disease showed no benefit of exemestane in progression-free survival compared with untreated patients (Meijer et al., 2011).

In a study of 28 osteosarcoma specimens (one of the most common bone cancers developing at young age) strong ERβ and PR immunoreactivity was seen in over 80% of the samples (and also correlated with Ki67). ERα and AR staining was seen in 30% of the samples, whereas CYP19A1 was undetected (Dohi et al., 2008). In another study, 20 osteosarcoma specimens, including 11 good responders to chemotherapy and nine poor responders, were subjected to cDNA microarray and 17βHSD10 resulted unregulated in the poor responder group. Results were further confirmed by IHC on 69 archival biopsies, hence targeting 17βHSD10 may be a valuable approach for drug (re)sensitisation (Salas et al., 2009).

Additional intracrine imbalances are described in bone diseases, such as higher androgen reducing 17βHSD activity in benign vs. malignant tumors, declines of CYP19A1 from normal bone to osteosarcoma and expression of SULT1E1 in the majority of the skeletal benign and malignant lesions, originated in bones or from primary tumors elsewhere (Svoboda et al., 2007).

Bone Tissue: Conclusions

In vitro, animal and human studies show that intracrinology controls bone development, benign and malignant conditions, and offer novel potential drug targets (**Table 8** and **Figure 3**). Steroids can be synthesized *in situ* from cholesterol (Rodríguez-Sanz et al., 2015) and can be recruited from the serum *via* the sulphatase pathway. DHEA is substrate for androgen and estrogen production. The action of androgens is partly mediated by their conversion to estrogens *via* CYP19A1 or to estrogenic 3α/βDIOLs (Vanderschueren et al., 2008).

Lungs

Sex steroids play an important role in lung development and homeostasis. Androgens, progestogens and estrogens are present and exert genomic and non-genomic actions via their hormone-receptors. Classical ERs (with ERβ as predominant form) and membrane GPER are expressed (Couse et al., 1997; Prossnitz and Barton, 2011; Konings et al., 2017). Sex steroids remain active in the lungs throughout lifetime and modulate lung function in both a beneficial or detrimental way, extensively reviewed (González-Arenas and Agramonte-Hevia, 2012; Townsend et al., 2012; Sathish et al., 2015).

E2 and P regulate epithelial sodium channel expression in alveolar epithelial cells (Luo et al., 2015). In alveolar smooth muscle cells, E2 induces bronchodilation via the reduction of intracellular Ca^{2+} (Townsend et al., 2010).

Both human and animal studies support a promoting role for estrogens and inhibitory role for androgens in lung development and maturation. During gestation and neonatal period, AR is expressed in mesenchymal and epithelial cells. Androgens inhibit the production of surfactants, which starts later in male than in female neonatal lungs (Carey et al., 2007), but also support the developing lung during branching morphogenesis (Kimura et al., 2003).

Lung Intracrinology in Lungs–Systematic Search

Adult human lungs express CYP19A1 and most 17βHSDs (1, 2, 4, 7, 8, 11, 12, 17βHSD5/AKR1C3; **Table 8**). STS, SULT and 17βHSD1, 12 and 17βHSD5/AKR1C3 immunoreactivity localizes in the bronchial epithelium (weak for types 1 and 12, strong for type 17βHSD5) and alveolar macrophages (Sakurai et al., 2006; Miller et al., 2012b; Chang et al., 2013; Konings et al., 2017).

Intracrinology controls lung development and maturation as shown in various animal models (Boucher et al., 2009) and intracrine enzymes are expressed already during fetal stages. Human fetal lungs possess StAR, CYP11A1, 3βHSD1 mRNA (Pezzi et al., 2003), SULT1E1 activity (Jones et al., 1992) and show 17βHSD1 and 2 mRNAs expression at 13 and 20 weeks of gestational age (Takeyama et al., 2000). High mRNA levels of AR, 17βHSD2 and 17βHSD5/AKR1C3 in mid-late gestation period and adult lungs indicate the present of androgen metabolism (Simard et al., 2010). Immunoreactivity for 17βHSD11 is detected in bronchioles of 14 and 31 weeks old fetuses, whereas other structures are negative (e.g., alveoli, ciliated epithelium, acini of the trachea). The expression of 17βHSD11 increases during the second half of pregnancy and maintains similar patterns in neonatal (14 days) and adult lugs (Brereton et al., 2001).

Intracrinology and Lung Diseases

Altered intracrinology is involved in lung disorders already from neonatal stages toward adulthood, and SNPs in intracrine genes are associated with the onset of diseases (Zhang et al.,

2013). Higher concentration of estrogens were measured by LC-MS in women with multiple-synchronous-lung adenocarcinoma compared with single adenocarcinoma (Ikeda et al., 2016) and in neoplastic tissue compared with adjacent normal lungs (Niikawa et al., 2008; Verma et al., 2013). Type 1 17βHSD mRNA, protein and activity are present in various non-small-cell-lung-cancer (NSCLC) cell lines where the mitogenic effect of E1 is abrogated by 17βHSD1 knockdown (Drzewiecka and Jagodzinski, 2012; Verma et al., 2013). In specimens from 48 NSCLC patients, 17βHSD1 expression was associated with squamous cell carcinoma and stage 3A disease (Drzewiecka et al., 2015). In another study on 103 NSCLC specimens, high 17βHSD1 immunoreactivity was associated with low intratumoural E1 and high E2:E1 ratio, whereas higher 17βHSD2 immunoreactivity was associated with high intratumoural E1. Multivariate regression analysis also demonstrated that increased 17βHSD1 immunoreactivity in tumors was an independent negative prognostic factor (Verma et al., 2013).

CYP19A1 is expressed in lung cancer and has potential therapeutic value (Niikawa et al., 2008; Verma et al., 2011; Siegfried and Stabile, 2014). A recent IHC study on 335 NSCLC specimens found an inverse association between CYP19A1 expression with disease specific survival (Skjefstad et al., 2016). Similar data, although restricted to women only, were confirmed in an independent study on 150 primary lung adenocarcinoma specimens, where CYP19A1 was found as the main driver of local estrogen supply (Tanaka et al., 2016). Another study on 110 lung adenocarcinoma specimens found an association between CYP19A1 mRNA (RT-qPCR) and poor prognosis in females, never-smokers and harboring EGFR mutations (Kohno et al., 2014). However, a recent mRNA study on 96 NSCLC patients showed that CYP19A1 in combination with ER is a good prognostic marker (Aresti et al., 2014).

STS and SULT1E1 immunoreactivity is detected in the majority of NSCLC cases, and STS is a good prognostic marker (Iida et al., 2013).

Lymphangioleiomyomatosis (LAM) is a rare, potentially fatal disease affecting predominantly young women. It is strongly hormone sensitive and it is hypothesized to originate from the uterus as lung metastasis (Prizant and Hammes, 2016). The levels of ERs, PR, AR, CYP19A1, STS, 17βHSD1 and SRD5A2 were recently assessed among 30 LAM biopsies. CYP19A1 expression resulted a useful classification marker with implication for potential therapy (Adachi et al., 2015). A recent study on specimens from 73 patients with chronic obstructive pulmonary disease (COPD) and 48 controls described an association between both CYP19A1 and 17βHSD1 with COPD (Konings et al., 2017). CYP19A1 is also implicated in interstitial pneumonia interstitial pneumonia, where local E2 concentration and CYP19A1 activity and immunoreactivity were elevated in diseased compared with normal tissue (Taniuchi et al., 2014).

Potential Novel Treatments

Blocking the estrogen signaling showed promising preclinical results in animal models of lung cancer (Verma et al., 2011). In humans, antiestrogen treatments (ER antagonists, GnRH, oophorectomy, P) have been used in LAM (Taveira-DaSilva and Moss, 2014) and lung cancer patients (Verma et al., 2011; Kohno et al., 2014). A phase II study on advanced NSCLC patients non-responsive to platinum-based drugs tested the dual-regimen mTOR/CYP19A1 inhibitors. Unfortunately, this study was prematurely terminated due to high toxicity (Singhal et al., 2015) and one additional trial using ER antagonist plus AI (fulvestrant and anastrozole) as consolidation therapy in postmenopausal women with advanced NSCLC (NCT00932152) was terminated due to poor recruitment.

Better results were obtained using the AI letrozole as single agent or in combination with rapamycin in a phase II trial on 17 postmenopausal women with LAM (NCT01353209). AI treatment was safe and well tolerated also in the dual drug regimen (Lu et al., 2017).

Lungs: Conclusions

Steroids are involved in lung maturation, development and in susceptibility to diseases. Most 17βHSDs, STS/SULT1E1, CYP19A1 are expressed indicating the lung's ability to metabolize androgens, estrogens and progestogens. Evidence of 3βHSDs is limited to fetal tissues (**Table 8** and **Figure 3**). Approaches aimed at decreasing local estrogens may offer future novel treatments for various lung diseases.

Brain and Central Nervous System (CNS)

One of the first CNS actions of sex steroids to be described is the hypothalamus-pituitary-gonadal axes control (Andersen and Ezcurra, 2014). The identification of steroid-receptors outside the hypothalamus, like hippocampus (controlling memory), prefrontal cortex, cerebellum and dopaminergic system regulation indicated that sex steroids have complex and widespread effects in the CNS. They control aggressive behavior, cognitive functions, mood, food intake, appetite, addiction, blood pressure, fine motor skills, motor coordination, pain circuit and both estrogens and androgens are neuroprotective (López and Tena-Sempere, 2015; Soma et al., 2015; McEwen and Milner, 2017). Estrogen deprivation in animals and humans is associated with development of metabolic disorders and estrogen administration has a general catabolic effect (López and Tena-Sempere, 2015). Animal experiments and KO models show that ERα mediates the major actions of estrogens in the CNS, like the metabolic control functions (Musatov et al., 2007) and the negative-feedback on the hypothalamus-pituitary-gonadal axes (Couse et al., 2003). However, both nuclear and non-nuclear ERs are relevant in distinct CNS regions (Almey et al., 2015; López and Tena-Sempere, 2015; McEwen and Milner, 2017).

Local steroid synthesis in the CNS is demonstrated in animal studies. CYP19A1-KO mice have increased ischemic damages compared with ovariectomised wild-type mice, indicating a local action of CYP19A1 (McEwen and Milner, 2017). Similar conclusions were drawn for the estrogen protective effects on stroke, Alzheimer (AD), Parkinson diseases, aggressive behavior (Soma et al., 2015; McEwen and Milner, 2017) and mice with ablation in various 17βHSDs show neuronal defects (**Table 4**). In rodents, CNS regions like the hippocampus and the hypothalamus express the enzymes involved in the local generation of steroids, like StAR, CYP11A1, CYP17A1, 3βHSD1,

TABLE 8 | Expression of intracrine enzymes in bone, lungs and central nervous system (CNS) – results of the systematic search.

Gene	Detection		Bone	References	Lung	References	CNS	References
	Molecule	**Technique#**						
StAR	mRNA	RT-PCR	n.d.		yes^	Pezzi et al., 2003	n.d.	
CYP11A1	mRNA	RT-PCR	yes	Rodríguez-Sanz et al., 2015	yes^	Pezzi et al., 2003	yes	Stoffel-Wagner, 2001
		Comp-RT	n.d.		n.d.		yes	Beyenburg et al., 1999; Watzka et al., 1999
	Protein	WB	yes*	Rodríguez-Sanz et al., 2015			n.d.	
CYP17A1	mRNA	RT-PCR	yes	Rodríguez-Sanz et al., 2015	no^	Pezzi et al., 2003	yes	Stoffel-Wagner, 2001
		RT-PCR	–		–		no	Steckelbroeck et al., 2004b
	Protein	WB	yes*	Rodríguez-Sanz et al., 2015	n.d.		n.d.	
		IHC	n.d.		n.d.		no	Steckelbroeck et al., 2004b
		Activity	n.d.		n.d.		no	Steckelbroeck et al., 2004b
CYP19A1	mRNA	RT-PCR	yes	Oz et al., 2001	yes	Pezzi et al., 2003; Aresti et al., 2014; Kohno et al., 2014; Konings et al., 2017	yes	Sasano et al., 1998; Stoffel-Wagner et al., 1998a; Stoffel-Wagner, 2001; Yague et al., 2006
		Comp-RT	n.d.		n.d.		yes	Stoffel-Wagner et al., 1999a
		ISH	yes	Sasano et al., 1997	n.d.		n.d.	
	Protein	IHC	yes	Sasano et al., 1997; Oz et al., 2001	yes	Verma et al., 2013; Siegfried and Stabile, 2014; Taniuchi et al., 2014; Konings et al., 2017	yes	Naftolin et al., 1996; Yague et al., 2006, 2010
		ELISA	n.d.		yes	Aresti et al., 2014; Skjefstad et al., 2016; Tanaka et al., 2016	n.d.	
		Activity	yes	Schweikert et al., 1995	yes	Taniuchi et al., 2014	yes	Naftolin and MacLusky, 1982; Stoffel-Wagner, 2001
3βHSD1	mRNA	RT-PCR	n.d.		yes^	Pezzi et al., 2003	no	Stoffel-Wagner, 2001
3βHSD2	mRNA	RT-PCR	n.d.		no^	Pezzi et al., 2003	no	Stoffel-Wagner, 2001
17βHSDs								
HSD17B oxidative activity			yes	Muir et al., 2004	n.d.		yes	Steckelbroeck et al., 1999, 2003; Stoffel-Wagner, 2001
HSD17B reductive activity			yes	Muir et al., 2004	n.d.	Tsai et al., 2001; Attar et al., 2009; Huhtinen et al., 2014	yes	Steckelbroeck et al., 1999, 2003; Stoffel-Wagner, 2001
17βHSD1	mRNA	RT-PCR	n.d.		yes	Takeyama et al., 2000; Drzewiecka et al., 2015; Konings et al., 2017)	yes	Stoffel-Wagner et al., 1999a; Stoffel-Wagner, 2001
		Comp-RT	n.d.		n.d.		yes	Beyenburg et al., 2000
	mRNA	ISH	yes	Sasano et al., 1997	n.d.		n.d.	
17βHSD1	Protein	Comp-RT	n.d.		n.d.		yes	Stoffel-Wagner et al., 1999b; Beyenburg et al., 2000
		IHC	yes	Sasano et al., 1997	yes	Verma et al., 2013; Drzewiecka et al., 2015; Konings et al., 2017	n.d.	
		WB	n.d.		yes	Drzewiecka et al., 2015	n.d.	
17βHSD2	mRNA	RT-PCR	n.d.		yes	Takeyama et al., 2000; Simard et al., 2010; Konings et al., 2017	no	Stoffel-Wagner, 2001
		Comp-RT	n.d.		n.d.		n.d.	Stoffel-Wagner et al., 1999b; Beyenburg et al., 2000
		NB	n.d.		n.d.		no	Casey et al., 1994
	Protein	IHC	n.d.		yes	Verma et al., 2013	n.d.	
		WB			n.d.		n.d.	

(Continued)

TABLE 8 | Continued

Gene	Detection		Bone	References	Lung	References	CNS	References
	Molecule	Technique#						
17βHSD3	mRNA	RT-PCR	n.d.		n.d.		yes	Stoffel-Wagner, 2001
		Comp-RT	n.d.		n.d.		yes	Stoffel-Wagner et al., 1999b; Beyenburg et al., 2000
17βHSD4	mRNA	RT-PCR	n.d.		yes	Konings et al., 2017	yes	Stoffel-Wagner et al., 1999a; Stoffel-Wagner, 2001; Steckelbroeck et al., 2003
		Comp-RT	n.d.		n.d.		yes	Stoffel-Wagner et al., 1999b; Beyenburg et al., 2000
		NB	n.d.		yes	Möller et al., 1999	yes	Möller et al., 1999
17βHSD6	mRNA	RT-PCR	n.d.				yes	Huang and Luu-The, 2000; Steckelbroeck et al., 2003
17βHSD7	mRNA	RT-PCR	n.d.		yes	Törn et al., 2003; Konings et al., 2017	yes	Steckelbroeck et al., 2003
17βHSD8	mRNA	RT-PCR	n.d.		yes	Ohno et al., 2008	yes	Steckelbroeck et al., 2003
17βHSD9	mRNA	RT-PCR	n.d.		n.d.		yes	Steckelbroeck et al., 2003
17βHSD10	mRNA	RT-PCR	n.d.		n.d.		yes	Steckelbroeck et al., 2003; He and Yang, 2006; Hovorkova et al., 2008
	Protein	IHC	n.d.		n.d.		yes	He et al., 2005b
		C-ELISA	n.d.		n.d.		yes	Hovorkova et al., 2008
17βHSD11	mRNA	RT-PCR	n.d.		yes	Chai et al., 2003	yes	Steckelbroeck et al., 2003
	mRNA	NB	n.d.		yes	Chai et al., 2003	n.d.	
	Protein	IHC	n.d.		yes	Brereton et al., 2001	n.d.	
17βHSD12	mRNA	RT-PCR	n.d.		yes	Sakurai et al., 2006; Konings et al., 2017	yes	Sakurai et al., 2006
	mRNA	NB	n.d.		yes	Sakurai et al., 2006	yes	Sakurai et al., 2006
	mRNA	NB	n.d.		n.d.		no	Casey et al., 1994
	Protein	IHC	n.d.		Yes$	Sakurai et al., 2006	n.d.	
AKR1C activity			n.d.		n.d.		yes	Steckelbroeck et al., 2010
AKR1C1	mRNA	RT-PCR	n.d.		n.d.		yes	Penning et al., 2000; Stoffel-Wagner et al., 2003; Steckelbroeck et al., 2010
AKR1C2	mRNA	RT PCR	n.d.		n.d.		yes	Penning et al., 2000
		Comp-RT	n.d.		n.d.		yes	Stoffel-Wagner et al., 2003; Steckelbroeck et al., 2004a, 2010
AKR1C3	mRNA	RT PCR	n.d.		yes	Simard et al., 2010; Konings et al., 2017	n.d.	
		Comp-RT	n.d.		n.d.		yes	Stoffel-Wagner et al., 2000, 2003; Steckelbroeck et al., 2001, 2004a; Stoffel-Wagner, 2001
		NB	n.d.		n.d.	Lin et al., 1997	n.d.	
	Protein	IHC	n.d.		yes	Miller et al., 2012b; Chang et al., 2013	n.d.	
AKR1C4	mRNA	RT-PCR	n.d.		n.d.		no	Steckelbroeck et al., 2010
		Comp-RT	n.d.		n.d.		no	Stoffel-Wagner et al., 2000, 2003; Steckelbroeck et al., 2004a

(Continued)

TABLE 8 | Continued

Gene	Detection		Bone	Reference	Lung	Reference	CNS	Reference
	molecule	technique#						
SRD5A1	mRNA	Comp-RT	n.d.		n.d.		yes	Stoffel-Wagner et al., 1998b, 2000, 2003
	Protein	IHC	n.d.		yes	Aumüller et al., 1996	yes	Aumüller et al., 1996
		activity	n.d.		n.d.		yes	Stoffel-Wagner et al., 1998b; Steckelbroeck et al., 2001
SRD5A2	mRNA	Comp-RT	n.d.		n.d.		no	Stoffel-Wagner et al., 1998b, 2000
	Protein	IHC	n.d.		yes	Aumüller et al., 1996	yes	Aumüller et al., 1996
STS	mRNA	RT-PCR	n.d.		yes	Konings et al., 2017	yes	Steckelbroeck et al., 2004b
		RT-PCR	–		no	Miki et al., 2002	no	Miki et al., 2002
	Protein	IHC	n.d.		yes	Iida et al., 2013	yes	Steckelbroeck et al., 2004b
		IHC	–		no	Miki et al., 2002	no	Miki et al., 2002
		Activity	yes	Muir et al., 2004	yes	Milewich et al., 1983; Munroe and Chang, 1987	yes	Platia et al., 1984
SULT1E1	mRNA	RT-PCR	yes	Svoboda et al., 2007	yes	Miki et al., 2002; Konings et al., 2017	yes	Miki et al., 2002; Nishimura and Naito, 2006
		RT-PCR	n.d.		n.d.		no	Salman et al., 2011
		NB	n.d.		n.d.		n.d.	
	Protein	IHC	n.d.		yes	Miki et al., 2002; Iida et al., 2013	yes	Miki et al., 2002
		IHC	n.d.		–		no	Salman et al., 2011
		WB	n.d.		yes	Riches et al., 2009	n.d.	
		Activity	n.d.		yes	Jones et al., 1992	no	Miki et al., 2002
SULT2A1	mRNA	RT-PCR	n.d.		n.d.		no	Nishimura and Naito, 2006; Salman et al., 2011 3/4 *Table VII continues*
	Protein	IHC	n.d.		yes	Riches et al., 2009	no	Steckelbroeck et al., 2004b; Salman et al., 2011
		Activity	n.d.		n.d.		no	Steckelbroeck et al., 2004b.
SULT1A1	mRNA	RT-PCR	n.d.		n.d.		yes	Nishimura and Naito, 2006; Salman et al., 2011
	Protein	IHC	n.d.		n.d.		yes	Nishimura and Naito, 2006; Salman et al., 2011
		WB	n.d.		yes	Riches et al., 2009	n.d.	
SULT2B1	mRNA	RT-PCR	n.d.		yes	He et al., 2004, 2005a	yes	Nishimura and Naito, 2006; Salman et al., 2011
		NB	n.d.		yes	He et al., 2004, 2005a	no	Meloche and Falany, 2001
		NB	–		no	Meloche and Falany, 2001	–	
	Protein	IHC	n.d.		yes	He et al., 2004, 2005a	yes	Nishimura and Naito, 2006; Salman et al., 2011

*Primary/original references were analyzed and reviews were excluded (and are cited ad hoc in the text). The table report only the enzymes whose expression was assessed in reviewed studies**.*

 # Technique abbreviations. For mRNA detection, NB: northern blot; ISH: in situ hybridisation; RT-PCR: reverse transcription quantitative (or semi-quantitative) PCR; Comp-RT: competitive RT-PCR assay; NB: northern blotting. For protein detection: IHC: immunohistochemistry; C-ELISA: competitive ELISA assay; WB: western blotting; activity: enzyme activity measurement.

** CYP11A1 and CYP17A1 activities were detected in primary cells of bone.*

*** No publication was found describing the expression of 17βHSD13, 14, 15 and DHRS11.*

^ Detected in fetal lung tissue.

$ IHC signal in bronchial epithelium.

CYP19A1, 17βHSD1, SRD5A1 and 2 (mRNA and protein by immunohistochemistry or western blot), and can produce pregnenolone, DHEA, androgens and estrogens from cholesterol, as confirmed by HPLC using radiolabelled substrates and tissue cultures of brain slices (Mukai et al., 2006; Murakami et al., 2006). CYP enzymes of rat hippocampus co-localize in pyramidal neurons (CA1–CA3 regions) and granule cells (dentate gyrus) (Mukai et al., 2006; Murakami et al., 2006).

Regulation of intracrine enzymes varies during development and sexual maturation, as indicated by mRNA expression (RT-qPCR) of 20 intracrine enzymes analyzed in rat hippocampus post-natal and throughout early (1 week) development (Kimoto et al., 2010).

Intracrinology in the CNS is particularly relevant because, beside the traditional pathway *via* the receptors, several steroids have neuroactivity and are allosteric modulators of $GABA_A$ receptors (**Figure 2**). Such actions are possessed also by steroids that are unable to activate the steroid hormone receptors, such as 3β- and 3α-hydroxyl sulpho-conjugates (P5-S and DHEA-S), 5β-reduced steroids (5βAN, etiocholanolone and 5β-THP isomers; **Table 1**), which are all $GABA_A$ negative modulators (in contrast to unconjugated 3α-hydroxysteroids) (Stoffel-Wagner, 2001; Belelli and Lambert, 2005; Agís-Balboa et al., 2006; Gibbs et al., 2006; Reddy, 2010; Steckelbroeck et al., 2010).

Intracrinology in CNS–Systematic Search

Intracrine enzymes are widely expressed in human CNS (**Table 8**) and intratissue concentrations of steroids in distinct regions differ between regions and from the levels in the blood (Mukai et al., 2006; Murakami et al., 2006; Jäntti et al., 2010). In contrast to rodents, however, the presence of the complete steroid biosynthetic pathway is not clearly demonstrated in the human CNS and contrasting data were reported (**Table 8**). CYP11A1 mRNA was detected in the temporal, frontal neocortex and subcortical white matter of men, women and children (Stoffel-Wagner, 2001). Low mRNA levels of CYP17A1 were detected in the hippocampus, amygdala, caudate nucleus, cerebellum, corpus callosum, spinal cord and thalamus (Stoffel-Wagner, 2001; Yu et al., 2002), but other authors found no expression of this enzyme (Steckelbroeck et al., 2004b, 2010; MacKenzie et al., 2008). No 3βHSD1 or 2 was detected in temporal lobes, hippocampus, thalamus and amygdala (Stoffel-Wagner, 2001; Steckelbroeck et al., 2010), although other authors detected low levels in amygdala, caudate nucleus, cerebellum, corpus callosum, hippocampus, spinal cord and thalamus (Yu et al., 2002).

The temporal lobes (both neocortex and white matter) have 17βHSD oxidative and reductive activities, CYP19A1 mRNA expression and activity, which is also present in hippocampus (Stoffel-Wagner et al., 1999a; Stoffel-Wagner, 2001). Temporal lobe specimens from 10 men to 12 women indicated that 17βHSD estrogen-oxidative and DHEA-reductive metabolisms are predominant, thus producing E1 and A5, respectively (Stoffel-Wagner, 2001). Regarding the different 17βHSDs, type 1, 3, and 4 mRNAs (but not type 2) were demonstrated by competitive reverse transcription-PCR in specimens from 34 women, 32 men and 10 children (Casey et al., 1994; Beyenburg et al., 2000). Subsequent studies confirmed the expression of types 4, 7, 8, 10, 11 17βHSD and AKR1C3/17βHSD5 in temporal lobes and hippocampus (Stoffel-Wagner, 2001; Steckelbroeck et al., 2003). In particular 17βHSD10 is involved in the deactivation of THP to 5αDHP, and it is an important regulator of neurological functions (Yang et al., 2016).

Production of 5α-androstane and pregnane neurosteroids is mediated by the action of SRD5As and AKR1Cs (**Figure 2**). SRD5A1 (not type 2) mRNA and enzyme activity were demonstrated in temporal neocortex and subcortical white matter, hippocampus, cerebellum, hypothalamus (Steckelbroeck et al., 2001; Stoffel-Wagner, 2001), and AKR1C4 mRNA was detected in both hippocampus and temporal lobe (Stoffel-Wagner, 2001). AKR1C1 and AKR1C2 are widely expressed in CNS and since no specific inhibitors directed against AKR1C1 to 4 could completely inhibit AKR1C brain activity, the involvement of an unidentified enzyme is suggested (Steckelbroeck et al., 2010). Isomeric 5β-neurosteroids require the action of AKR1D1, and it is unknown whether AKR1D1 is expressed in CNS, or liver 5β-steroids reach peripheral regions via the circulation (Jin et al., 2011).

The sulphatase pathway in the CNS is relevant because (although recent studies are revisiting this paradigm; Qaiser et al., 2017), sulphated-steroids do not cross the blood-brain barrier. Therefore, sulphated neurosteroids like DHEA-S and P5-S need to be generated locally, and in line with this, their level in the CNS is independent from the level in the blood (Rajkowski et al., 1997) and varies throughout distinct brain regions (especially hippocampus and hypothalamus) (Jäntti et al., 2010).

STS and SULTs are widely expressed, with no gender-related differences (**Table 8**) (Kríz et al., 2008a,b; Mueller et al., 2015). SULT1A1 has high expression especially in specimens isolated from cerebellum, occipital and frontal lobes (Salman et al., 2009). No brain region expresses SULT2A1, whereas contrasting data exist for SULT2B1 and SULT1E1 (**Table 8**).

Diseases and Treatments

Steroid metabolism is deviated in schizophrenia (Bicikova et al., 2013) and aberrations and unbalances of intracrine enzymes are associated with neurological disorders (Luchetti et al., 2011 and see **Table 5**). In a study of 49 patients with AD, prefrontal cortex mRNA levels of 17βHSD1, CYP19A1 and AKR1C2 increased at late stages (Luchetti et al., 2011). STS and SULT activities, measured by radioimmunoassay and GC-MS in 55 human brain tumor specimens, varied between tumor types (Kríz et al., 2008b). Immunoreactivity for AKR1C3/17βHSD5 was low in medulloblastomas ($n = 10$ analyzed), high in 37 glial neoplasms and 18 meningiomas and was absent in intracranial schwannoma ($n = 7$) (Park et al., 2010). A recent screening of a chemical library of steroid inhibitors using three low grade pediatric glioma cell lines found that inhibition of 17βHSD3 blocked cell growth and induced apoptosis *in vitro* (Ajeawung et al., 2013)

Type 10 17βHSD is associated with AD and is a potential target in diseases like AD, Parkinson, and an X-linked mental retardation, that may arise from the impaired degradation of branched chain fatty acid, isoleucine or aberrant neurosteroid (THP) metabolism (Lim et al., 2011; Yang et al., 2016).

STS has been implicated in ADHD and a recent mouse study indicates that genetic and pharmacological manipulations of the STS axis influence the inhibitory processes and give rise to improvements in response control (Davies et al., 2014). A recent animal experiment using a model of autoimmune encephalomyelitis showed high SULT1A1 mRNA expression in laser-captured-micro-dissected white matter astrocytes, suggesting that deactivation of estrogens (and other phenolic substrates) may be responsible for the resistance to anti-neuro-inflammatory treatments in these cells and could be possibly used as new treatments to protect CNS from inflammatory injuries (Guillot et al., 2015).

CNS: Conclusions

CNS can synthesize steroids from cholesterol, although this is restricted to few brain regions. Steroid metabolism in the CNS is particular complex due to the formation of both 5α-/β-reduced and sulpho-conjugated neurosteroids (**Table 8** and **Figure 3**).

Intracrinology in Other Tissues and Systems

Steroid metabolism is also important in the immune system, skin and adipose tissue. A thorough review of these systems is outside the scope of this study, however, a brief mention is given below.

Immune System and Inflammation

Beside corticosteroids, several other steroids affect the immune system and inflammation. A5 induces white blood cells and platelets production in bone marrow (Chen et al., 2004); estrogens and androgens control B-lymphocyte development in a sex-dependent way and modulate autoimmune diseases (McCarthy, 2000; Calippe et al., 2010; Sakiani et al., 2013).

Lipopolysaccharide-mediated proinflammatory pathway in macrophages and NF-κB activation are blocked by estrogens, which induce T-helper (Th) type 2 responses, whereas androgens stimulate type 1 responses (Iwasa et al., 2015). DHEA and DHEA-S also regulate the maturation of Th1 or Th2 cells. It was shown that plasma Th2 lymphocytes and its major secreted cytokine IL6 increase with age, and this is reversed in mice upon administration of DHEA or DHEA-S (Reed et al., 2005). Such effect was recapitulated *in vitro* by DHEA but not DHEA-S implicating the involvement of macrophage STS in lymphoid tissues where Th cell maturation occurs. In line with this, the effect of DHEA-S, but not DHEA, was impaired *in vivo* by an STS inhibitor (Reed et al., 2005). These data prompted to propose STS inhibition as a therapeutic approach for diseases associated with inappropriate immune responses and excess Th1 cytokines such as rheumatoid arthritis (Reed et al., 2005). Whether the action of DHEA is secondary to its conversion to androgens or estrogens is currently unclear. STS activity of peripheral blood leukocytes is higher in women during the follicular phase of the menstrual cycle than in women in the luteal phase or in men and it becomes highest during pregnancy, suggesting a role for P in regulating STS activity (Reed et al., 2005; Mueller et al., 2015). *In vitro* studies also demonstrated that STS activity is induced by cytokines such as IL6 and TNF (Mueller et al., 2015).

Opposite deregulation of the sulphatase pathway is seen in other chronic inflammatory diseases/cell types. Vascular smooth muscle cells show higher STS activity in women with mild atherosclerosis compared with women with severe disease (and male), whereas SULT1E1 activity is lower in women with severe disease (Mueller et al., 2015).

CYP19A1 is also expressed in macrophages (Konings et al., 2017) and KO mice have increased numbers of peripheral blood and bone marrow cells and inflammatory renal lesions (Shim et al., 2004). CYP19A1 inhibitors exacerbate the autoimmune lesions in a murine model of Sjögren syndrome and estrogen administration reverses such phenotype (Iwasa et al., 2015; Park et al., 2015). Opposite effects are observed in prostate, where elevated intracrine estrogens due to CYP19A1 overexpression induce inflammation and pre-malignant pathology (Ellem et al., 2009) as well as in adipose tissue (Reed et al., 2005).

Skin

The skin is the largest human organ and first barrier against pathogens where important immune functions interconnected with intracrine steroid metabolism take place (Slominski et al., 2013). Keratinocytes and sebocytes express ERs, intracrine enzymes, and the activity of sebaceous glands is influenced by steroids as indicated by the sebum production at andrenarche (Slominski et al., 2013). CYP17A1, CYP19A1, 17βHSD1, 2, 3, 4 (and enzymes metabolizing corticosteroid - outside the scope of this review) are detected in human skin. Some genes are under the influence of vitamin D and sebocytes can synthesize T from adrenal precursors (Hughes et al., 1997; Thiboutot et al., 1998; Slominski et al., 2013). Low 17βHSD oxidative metabolism characterizes sebaceous glands from skin areas prone to develop acne compared with other locations, suggesting a protective role of the oxidative metabolism against androgen excess (Fritsch et al., 2001). Sulphatase pathway is present in the skin (Reed et al., 2005; Simard et al., 2005), and genetic variants in STS and SULTs are associated with skin disturbances, most likely because of unbalanced steroid accumulation (**Table 5**).

Adipose Tissue

The adipose tissue is one of the most complex endocrine organs that besides secreting leptin and adiponectin, is a site of steroid metabolism, it establishes interaction with the CNS for glucose and lipid metabolism control, energy homeostasis and inflammation. The implication of sex steroids in adipose tissue is demonstrated by the different fat distribution that characterizes men and women (Mauvais-Jarvis et al., 2013; Varlamov et al., 2014; López and Tena-Sempere, 2015, 2016; Palmer and Clegg, 2015). ER-KO and CYP19A1-KO mice develop obesity with human-like phenotypes (López and Tena-Sempere, 2015). Estrogens protect against metabolic syndrome and men lacking endogenous estrogens (CYP19A1 or ER-α deficiency) develop hypertriglyceridemia, glucose intolerance and insulin resistance (Kim et al., 2014). In adipose tissue of men, 17βHSD2 levels and androgen inactivation correlate with BMI (Fouad Mansour et al., 2015). A mouse study also showed that increased unsulphated-estrogen availability due to loss of SULT1E1 improved metabolic function in a model of type 2 diabetes, which leads to speculations about a potential role of SULT1E1 inhibition for this disease - at least in women (Gao et al., 2012).

Fat consists of different tissue types (white and brown) and different regional depots with distinct physiological, intracrinological characteristics and distinct relations with pathologies and metabolic disorders (Blouin et al., 2009; Mauvais-Jarvis et al., 2013). White adipose tissue is mainly subcutaneous (abdomen) or visceral (surrounding the inner organs), this last being associated with metabolic risks. A plethora of investigations demonstrated the ability of adipose tissue to aromatise androgens into estrogens and that the intra-tissue steroid levels are higher than the levels in blood (Bélanger et al., 2002). Androgenic and estrogenic 17βHSD activity and the mRNA for 17βHSD1, 2, 3, 7, 12, AKR1C3/17βHSD5 were detected in both intra-abdominal and subcutaneous fat (Bélanger et al., 2002; Quinkler et al., 2004; Bellemare et al., 2009; Wang et al., 2013).

Both subcutaneous and visceral fat tissue of women expresses the androgenic 17βHSD3 (generally considered testis specific) indicating that adipose tissue in women is substantially androgenic. Such characteristic in the visceral depot increased with increasing BMI, suggesting a link between central obesity and metabolic diseases (Corbould et al., 2002).

Additionally, several enzymes (AKR1C2, AKR1C3/17βHSD5, CYP19A1, STS and SULT1E1) vary throughout adipocyte differentiation and maturation (Quinkler et al., 2004; Bellemare et al., 2009; Blouin et al., 2009; Mueller et al., 2015).

CONCLUSIONS AND RECOMMENDATIONS

Intracrinology consists of a complex and intricate network of alternative and redundant pathways that generate, deactivate steroids in peripheral tissues and ultimately control steroid exposure in a tissue specific manner. A number of compounds have that ability to bind and activate more than one nuclear receptors thus exerting multiple biological actions. Blood steroids represent a reservoir of substrates that support these intracrine networks. Studies retrieved by the systematic search demonstrated that most investigations rely on RT-PCR or IHC to detect enzyme and protein, and frequently without multiple-technique confirmation of the data. Since both techniques present limitations, and antibodies for IHC often perform sub-optimally (detection limit is not sufficient to detect some intracrine enzymes, crossreactivity between isoforms) these techniques are not always suitable to infer the real biological role of a reaction/enzyme.

However, the recent technological advances in steroid profiling together with an improved knowledge of intracrine enzymes and the possibility to validate data using multiple approaches (RNA, protein, activity, steroid profiling) create today unprecedented opportunities to expand our understanding of intracrinology, its relation with endocrinology and to exploit this knowledge in patient care. Improved multiplex platforms allowing to profile in peripheral tissues all steroids depicted in **Figure 2** are awaited and will elucidate the relevant tissue-specific networks. It is envisaged that novel prognostic markers and drug targets will become of clinical relevance soon.

We should however be aware that the redundant actions of intracrine enzymes, their substrate promiscuity, the existence of alternative pathways and the patient-to-patient variability might result in drug insensitivity. Dual/triple inhibitors will help solving this problem. In addition, in order to optimize research on novel drugs, the classical preclinical drug discovery pipelines (safety, pharmacokinetics and dynamics), should encompass parallel research lines to learn how to pre-select potentially responsive patients.

Finally, since we know that steroidal and intracrine drugs might have profound effects on the CNS, it is desirable to have in depth research on the neurological effects of potential novel drugs during the nonclinical phase of drug development. This will facilitate to select suitable compounds to the clinical development.

AUTHOR CONTRIBUTIONS

GK drafted the study, prepared figures, tables, intermediate versions, final version and approved final version. LB drafted part of the study, contributed to intermediate versions and approved final version. KC drafted part of the study, contributed to intermediate versions and approved final version. BD contributed to intermediate versions and approved final version. TL drafted part of the study, contributed to intermediate versions and approved final version. PK contributed to intermediate versions and approved final version. MB contributed to intermediate versions and approved final version. RK contributed to intermediate versions and approved final version. SX drafted part of the study, contributed to intermediate versions and approved final version. AR drafted the study, prepared figures, tables, intermediate versions, final version and approved final version.

ACKNOWLEDGMENTS

We are grateful to Dr. Margaretha A Skowron (Department of Urology, University Düsseldorf, Germany) for graphic arts.

We also would like to thank the management and curator of the online databases we made use of, namely: the database of chemical molecules PubChem (www.ncbi.nlm.nih.gov; pubchem.ncbi.nlm.nih.gov) maintained by the National Center for Biotechnology Information (NCBI; National Library of Medicine/United States National Institutes of Health - NIH); Chemical Abstracts Service (CAS), maintained by the American Chemical Society (www.cas.org); Human Metabolome Data Base (HMDB, www.hmdb.ca), funded and maintained by Genome Canada; Chemical Book (www.chemicalbook.com), funded by industrial partners; Chemical Entities of Biological Interest (ChEBI; www.ebi.ac.uk/chebi/init.do), curated by the European Bioinformatics Institute of the European Molecular Biology Laboratory (EMBL); drug and drug target database Drugbank (www.drugbank.ca/drugs), University of Alberta and The Metabolomics Innovation Centre; GeneCards (www.genecards.org), developed and maintained by the Crown Human Genome Center at the Weizmann Institute of Science; Online Mendelian Inheritance in Man® (OMIM®, https://omim.org/),

McKusick-Nathans Institute of Genetic Medicine, Johns Hopkins University (Baltimore, MD); Mouse Genome Informatics (MGI; www.informatics.jax.org), Mouse Genome Database at the Mouse Genome Informatics website, The Jackson Laboratory, Bar Harbor, Maine.

REFERENCES

Abdelsamie, A. S., van Koppen, C. J., Bey, E., Salah, M., Börger, C., Siebenbürger, L. et al. (2017). 17β-HSD1 inhibitor with sub-nanomolar IC50 for a proof-of-principle study. *Eur. J. Med. Chem.* 127, 944–957. doi: 10.1016/j.ejmech.2016.11.004

Acién, P., Velasco, I., Gutiérrez, M., and Martínez-Beltrán, M. (2007). Aromatase expression in endometriotic tissues and its relationship to clinical and analytical findings. *Fertil. Steril.* 88, 32–38. doi: 10.1016/j.fertnstert.2006.11.188

Adachi, K., Miki, Y., Saito, R., Hata, S., Yamauchi, M., Mikami, Y., et al. (2015). Intracrine steroid production and mammalian target of rapamycin pathways in pulmonary lymphangioleiomyomatosis. *Hum. Pathol.* 46, 1685–1693. doi: 10.1016/j.humpath.2015.02.019

Adessi, G. L., Prost, O., Agnani, G., Petitjean, A., and Burnod, J. (1984). Estrone sulfatase activity in normal and abnormal endometrium. *Arch. Gynecol.* 236, 13–18. doi: 10.1007/BF02114864

Adjei, A. A., Thomae, B. A., Prondzinski, J. L., Eckloff, B. W., Wieben, E. D., and Weinshilboum, R. M. (2003). Human estrogen sulfotransferase (SULT1E1) pharmacogenomics: Gene resequencing and functional genomics. *Br. J. Pharmacol.* 139, 1373–1382. doi: 10.1038/sj.bjp.0705369

Aghajanova, L., Hamilton, A., Kwintkiewicz, J., Vo, K. C., and Giudice, L. C. (2009). Steroidogenic enzyme and key decidualization marker dysregulation in endometrial stromal cells from women with versus without endometriosis. *Biol. Reprod.* 80, 105–114. doi: 10.1095/biolreprod.108.070300

Agís-Balboa, R. C., Pinna, G., Zhubi, A., Maloku, E., Veldic, M., Costa, E., et al. (2006). Characterization of brain neurons that express enzymes mediating neurosteroid biosynthesis. *Proc. Natl. Acad. Sci. U.S.A.* 103, 14602–14607. doi: 10.1073/pnas.0606544103

Ajeawung, N. F., Maltais, R., Jones, C., Poirier, D., and Kamnasaran, D. (2013). Viability screen on pediatric low grade glioma cell lines unveils a novel anti-cancer drug of the steroid biosynthesis inhibitor family. *Cancer Lett.* 330, 96–105. doi: 10.1016/j.canlet.2012.11.034

Almey, A., Milner, T. A., and Brake, W. G. (2015). Estrogen receptors in the central nervous system and their implication for dopamine-dependent cognition in females. *Horm. Behav.* 74, 125–138. doi: 10.1016/j.yhbeh.2015.06.010

Alshogran, O. Y. (2017). Pharmacogenetics of aldo-keto reductase 1C (AKR1C) enzymes. *Expert Opin. Drug Metab. Toxicol.* 13, 1063–1073. doi: 10.1080/17425255.2017.1376648

Amant, F., Moerman, P., Neven, P., Timmerman, D., Van Limbergen, E., and Vergote, I. (2005). Endometrial cancer. *Lancet* 366, 491–505. doi: 10.1016/S0140-6736(05)67063-8

Amos-Landgraf, J. M., Heijmans, J., Wielenga, M. C., Dunkin, E., Krentz, K. J., Clipson, L., et al. (2014). Sex disparity in colonic adenomagenesis involves promotion by male hormones, not protection by female hormones. *Proc. Natl. Acad. Sci. U.S.A.* 111, 16514–16519. doi: 10.1073/pnas.1323064111

Andersen, C. Y., and Ezcurra, D. (2014). Human steroidogenesis: implications for controlled ovarian stimulation with exogenous gonadotropins. *Reprod. Biol. Endocrinol.* 12:128. doi: 10.1186/1477-7827-12-128

Andrew, A. S., Hu, T., Gu, J., Gui, J., Ye, Y., Marsit, C. J., et al. (2012). HSD3B and gene-gene interactions in a pathway-based analysis of genetic susceptibility to bladder cancer. *PLoS ONE* 7:e51301. doi: 10.1371/journal.pone.0051301

Aresti, U., Carrera, S., Iruarrizaga, E., Fuente, N., Marrodan, I., de Lobera, A. R., et al. (2014). Estrogen receptor 1 gene expression and its combination with estrogen receptor 2 or aromatase expression predicts survival in non-small cell lung cancer. *PLoS ONE* 9:e109659. doi: 10.1371/journal.pone.0109659

Arnold, C., and Einspanier, A. (2013). Medical treatment improves social behavior in a primate endometriosis model (Callithrix jacchus). *J. Med. Primatol.* 42, 112–119. doi: 10.1111/jmp.12042

Ashton, K. A., Proietto, A., Otton, G., Symonds, I., McEvoy, M., Attia, J., et al. (2010). Polymorphisms in genes of the steroid hormone biosynthesis and metabolism pathways and endometrial cancer risk. *Cancer Epidemiol.* 34, 328–337. doi: 10.1016/j.canep.2010.03.005

Attar, E., Tokunaga, H., Imir, G., Yilmaz, M. B., Redwine, D., Putman, M., et al. (2009). Prostaglandin E2 via steroidogenic factor-1 coordinately regulates transcription of steroidogenic genes necessary for estrogen synthesis in endometriosis. *J. Clin. Endocrinol. Metab.* 94, 623–631. doi: 10.1210/jc.2008-1180

Audet-Walsh, É., Bellemare, J., Lacombe, L., Fradet, Y., Fradet, V., Douville, P., et al. (2012). The impact of germline genetic variations in hydroxysteroid (17-beta) dehydrogenases on prostate cancer outcomes after prostatectomy. *Eur. Urol.* 62, 88–96. doi: 10.1016/j.eururo.2011.12.021

Audet-Walsh, E., Lepine, J., Gregoire, J., Plante, M., Caron, P., Tetu, B., et al. (2011). Profiling of endogenous estrogens, their precursors, and metabolites in endometrial cancer patients: association with risk and relationship to clinical characteristics. *J. Clin. Endocrinol. Metab.* 96, E330–E339. doi: 10.1210/jc.2010-2050

Aumüller, G., Eicheler, W., Renneberg, H., Adermann, K., Vilja, P., and Forssmann, W. G. (1996). Immunocytochemical evidence for differential subcellular localization of 5 alpha-reductase isoenzymes in human tissues. *Acta Anat. (Basel).* 156, 241–252. doi: 10.1159/000147852

Bacallao, K., Leon, L., Gabler, F., Soto, E., Romero, C., Valladares, L., et al. (2008). In situ estrogen metabolism in proliferative endometria from untreated women with polycystic ovarian syndrome with and without endometrial hyperplasia. *J. Steroid Biochem. Mol. Biol.* 110, 163–169. doi: 10.1016/j.jsbmb.2008.03.031

Baes, M., Huyghe, S., Carmeliet, P., Declercq, P. E., Collen, D., Mannaerts, G. P., et al. (2000). Inactivation of the peroxisomal multifunctional protein-2 in mice impedes the degradation of not only 2-methyl-branched fatty acids and bile acid intermediates but also of very long chain fatty acids. *J. Biol. Chem.* 275, 16329–16336. doi: 10.1074/jbc.M001994200

Bagi, C. M., Wood, J., Wilkie, D., and Dixon, B. (2008). Effect of 17β-hydroxysteroid dehydrogenase type 2 inhibitor on bone strength in ovariectomized cynomolgus monkeys. *J. Musculoskelet. Neuronal Interact.* 8, 267–280.

Bair, S. R., and Mellon, S. H. (2004). Deletion of the mouse P450c17 gene causes early embryonic lethality. *Mol. Cell. Biol.* 24, 5383–5390. doi: 10.1128/MCB.24.12.5383-5390.2004

Balk, S. P., and Knudsen, K. E. (2008). AR, the cell cycle, and prostate cancer. *Nucl. Recept. Signal.* 6:e001.

Barzi, A., Lenz, A. M., Labonte, M. J., and Lenz, H. J. (2013). Molecular pathways: estrogen pathway in colorectal cancer. *Clin. Cancer Res.* 19, 5842–5848. doi: 10.1158/1078-0432.CCR-13-0325

Bélanger, C., Luu-The, V., Dupont, P., and Tchernof, A. (2002). Adipose tissue intracrinology: potential importance of local androgen/estrogen metabolism in the regulation of adiposity. *Horm. Metab. Res.* 34, 737–745. doi: 10.1055/s-2002-38265

Belelli, D., and Lambert, J. J. (2005). Neurosteroids: endogenous regulators of the GABA(A) receptor. *Nat. Rev. Neurosci.* 6, 565–575. doi: 10.1038/nrn1703

Bellemare, V., Faucher, F., Breton, R., and Luu-The, V. (2005). Characterization of 17α-hydroxysteroid dehydrogenase activity (17α-HSD) and its involvement in the biosynthesis of epitestosterone. *BMC Biochem.* 6:12. doi: 10.1186/1471-2091-6-12

Bellemare, V., Laberge, P., Noel, S., Tchernof, A., and Luu-The, V. (2009). Differential estrogenic 17β-hydroxysteroid dehydrogenase activity and type 12, 17β-hydroxysteroid dehydrogenase expression levels in preadipocytes and differentiated adipocytes. *J. Steroid Biochem. Mol. Biol.* 114, 129–134. doi: 10.1016/j.jsbmb.2009.01.002

Berstein, L., Zimarina, T., Imyanitov, E., Kovalevskij, A., Maximov, S., Pujol, P., et al. (2006). Hormonal imbalance in two types of endometrial cancer and genetic polymorphism of steroidogenic enzymes. *Maturitas* 54, 352–355. doi: 10.1016/j.maturitas.2006.04.017

Beyenburg, S., Stoffel-Wagner, B., Watzka, M., Blumcke, I., Bauer, J., Schramm, J., et al. (1999). Expression of cytochrome P450scc mRNA in the hippocampus of patients with temporal lobe epilepsy. *Neuroreport* 10, 3067–3070. doi: 10.1097/00001756-199909290-00035

Beyenburg, S., Watzka, M., Blumcke, I., Schramm, J., Bidlingmaier, F., Elger, C. E., et al. (2000). Expression of mRNAs encoding for 17β-hydroxisteroid dehydrogenase isozymes 1, 2, 3 and 4 in epileptic human hippocampus. *Epilepsy Res.* 41, 83–91. doi: 10.1016/S0920-1211(00)00130-3

Bicikova, M., Hill, M., Ripova, D., Mohr, P., and Hampl, R. (2013). Determination of steroid metabolome as a possible tool for laboratory diagnosis of schizophrenia. *J. Steroid Biochem. Mol. Biol.* 133, 77–83. doi: 10.1016/j.jsbmb.2012.08.009

Bilezikian, J. P., Morishima, A., Bell, J., and Grumbach, M. M. (1998). Increased bone mass as a result of estrogen therapy in a man with aromatase deficiency. *N. Engl. J. Med.* 339, 599–603. doi: 10.1056/NEJM199808273390905

Blake, J. A., Eppig, J. T., Kadin, J. A., Richardson, J. E., Smith, C. L., Bult, C. J., et al. (2017). Mouse Genome Database (MGD)-2017: community knowledge resource for the laboratory mouse. *Nucleic Acids Res.* 45, D723–D729. doi: 10.1093/nar/gkw1040

Blouin, K., Nadeau, M., Mailloux, J., Daris, M., Lebel, S., Luu-The, V., et al. (2009). Pathways of adipose tissue androgen metabolism in women: depot differences and modulation by adipogenesis. *Am. J. Physiol. Endocrinol. Metab.* 296, E244–E255. doi: 10.1152/ajpendo.00039.2008

Bothe, U., Busemann, M., Steinmeyer, A., Droescher, P., Fischer, O. M., Peters, M., et al. (2017). "First time disclosure of BAY 1128688: a novel AKR1C3 inhibitor for the treatment of endometriosis," in *254th ACS National Meeting & Exposition* (Washington, DC).

Boucher, E., Provost, P. R., Plante, J., and Tremblay, Y. (2009). Androgen receptor and 17β-HSD type 2 regulation in neonatal mouse lung development. *Mol. Cell. Endocrinol.* 311, 109–119. doi: 10.1016/j.mce.2009.06.012

Bovée, J. V., Cleton-Jansen, A. M., Taminiau, A. H., and Hogendoorn, P. C. (2005). Emerging pathways in the development of chondrosarcoma of bone and implications for targeted treatment. *Lancet Oncol.* 6, 599–607. doi: 10.1016/S1470-2045(05)70282-5

Brereton, P., Suzuki, T., Sasano, H., Li, K., Duarte, C., Obeyesekere, V., et al. (2001). Pan1b (17βHSD11)-enzymatic activity and distribution in the lung. *Mol. Cell. Endocrinol.* 171, 111–117. doi: 10.1016/S0303-7207(00)00417-2

Brosens, J., Verhoeven, H., Campo, R., Gianaroli, L., Gordts, S., Hazekamp, J., et al. (2004). High endometrial aromatase P450 mRNA expression is associated with poor IVF outcome. *Hum. Reprod.* 19, 352–356. doi: 10.1093/humrep/deh075

BroŽic, P., Turk, S., Rizner, T. L., and Gobec, S. (2011). Inhibitors of aldo-keto reductases AKR1C1-AKR1C4. *Curr. Med. Chem.* 18, 2554–2565. doi: 10.2174/092986711795933713

Bukulmez, O., Hardy, D. B., Carr, B. R., Auchus, R. J., Toloubeydokhti, T., Word, R. A., et al. (2008a). Androstenedione up-regulation of endometrial aromatase expression via local conversion to estrogen: potential relevance to the pathogenesis of endometriosis. *J. Clin. Endocrinol. Metab.* 93, 3471–3477. doi: 10.1210/jc.2008-0248

Bukulmez, O., Hardy, D. B., Carr, B. R., Word, R. A., and Mendelson, C. R. (2008b). Inflammatory status influences aromatase and steroid receptor expression in endometriosis. *Endocrinology* 149, 1190–1204. doi: 10.1210/en.2007-0665

Bulun, S. E., Economos, K., Miller, D., and Simpson, E. R. (1994). CYP19 (aromatase cytochrome P450) gene expression in human malignant endometrial tumors. *J. Clin. Endocrinol. Metab.* 79, 1831–1834.

Bulun, S. E., Mahendroo, M. S., and Simpson, E. R. (1993). Polymerase chain reaction amplification fails to detect aromatase cytochrome P450 transcripts in normal human endometrium or decidua. *J. Clin. Endocrinol. Metab.* 76, 1458–1463.

Caiazza, F., Ryan, E. J., Doherty, G., Winter, D. C., and Sheahan, K. (2015). Estrogen receptors and their implications in colorectal carcinogenesis. *Front. Oncol.* 5:19. doi: 10.3389/fonc.2015.00019

Calippe, B., Douin-Echinard, V., Delpy, L., Laffargue, M., Lelu, K., Krust, A., et al. (2010). 17β-estradiol promotes TLR4-triggered proinflammatory mediator production through direct estrogen receptor alpha signaling in macrophages *in vivo*. *J. Immunol.* 185, 1169–1176. doi: 10.4049/jimmunol.0902383

Carani, C., Qin, K., Simoni, M., Faustini-Fustini, M., Serpente, S., Boyd, J., et al. (1997). Effect of testosterone and estradiol in a man with aromatase deficiency. *N. Engl. J. Med.* 337, 91–95. doi: 10.1056/NEJM199707103370204

Carey, M. A., Card, J. W., Voltz, J. W., Arbes, S. J. Jr., Germolec, D. R., Korach, K. S., et al. (2007). It's all about sex: gender, lung development and lung disease. *Trends Endocrinol. Metab.* 18, 308–313. doi: 10.1016/j.tem.2007.08.003

Carneiro, M. M., Morsch, D. M., Camargos, A. F., Reis, F. M., and Spritzer, P. M. (2008). Androgen receptor and 5α-reductase are expressed in pelvic endometriosis. *BJOG* 115, 113–117. doi: 10.1111/j.1471-0528.2007.01521.x

Carneiro, M. M., Morsch, D. M., Camargos, A. F., Spritzer, P. M., and Reis, F. M. (2007). Expression of 17β-hydroxysteroid dehydrogenase type 2 in pelvic endometriosis. *Gynecol. Endocrinol.* 23, 188–192. doi: 10.1080/09513590701200850

Caron, K. M., Soo, S. C., Wetsel, W. C., Stocco, D. M., Clark, B. J., and Parker, K. L. (1997). Targeted disruption of the mouse gene encoding steroidogenic acute regulatory protein provides insights into congenital lipoid adrenal hyperplasia. *Proc. Natl. Acad. Sci. U.S.A.* 94, 11540–11545. doi: 10.1073/pnas.94.21.11540

Casey, M. L., MacDonald, P. C., and Andersson, S. (1994). 17 beta-Hydroxysteroid dehydrogenase type 2: chromosomal assignment and progestin regulation of gene expression in human endometrium. *J. Clin. Invest.* 94, 2135–2141. doi: 10.1172/JCI117569

Chai, Z., Brereton, P., Suzuki, T., Sasano, H., Obeyesekere, V., Escher, G., et al. (2003). 17β-hydroxysteroid dehydrogenase type XI localizes to human steroidogenic cells. *Endocrinology* 144, 2084–2091. doi: 10.1210/en.2002-221030

Chang, T. S., Lin, H. K., Rogers, K. A., Brame, L. S., Yeh, M. M., Yang, Q., et al. (2013). Expression of aldo-keto reductase family 1 member C3 (AKR1C3) in neuroendocrine tumors & adenocarcinomas of pancreas, gastrointestinal tract, and lung. *Int. J. Clin. Exp. Pathol.* 6, 2419–2429.

Chen, F., Knecht, K., Leu, C., Rutledge, S. J., Scafonas, A., Gambone, C., et al. (2004). Partial agonist/antagonist properties of androstenedione and 4-androsten-3β,17β-diol. *J. Steroid Biochem. Mol. Biol.* 91, 247–257. doi: 10.1016/j.jsbmb.2004.04.009

Chen, G., Zhang, D., Jing, N., Yin, S., Falany, C. N., and Radominska-Pandya, A. (2003). Human gastrointestinal sulfotransferases: identification and distribution. *Toxicol. Appl. Pharmacol.* 187, 186–197. doi: 10.1016/S0041-008X(02)00073-X

Cho, L. Y., Yang, J. J., Ko, K. P., Ma, S. H., Shin, A., Choi, B. Y., et al. (2012). Genetic susceptibility factors on genes involved in the steroid hormone biosynthesis pathway and progesterone receptor for gastric cancer risk. *PLoS ONE* 7:e47603. doi: 10.1371/journal.pone.0047603

Ciuffi, M., Savino, L., Santini, D., Buzzoni, P., Scarselli, G., and Mazzei, T. (1982). Estradiol and progestin receptors, 17-beta-hydroxysteroid-dehydrogenase and histopathologic grade in endometrial carcinoma. *Tumori* 68, 217–221. doi: 10.1177/030089168206800305

Cleton-Jansen, A. M., van Beerendonk, H. M., Baelde, H. J., Bovee, J. V., Karperien, M., and Hogendoorn, P. C. (2005). Estrogen signaling is active in cartilaginous tumors: implications for antiestrogen therapy as treatment option of metastasized or irresectable chondrosarcoma. *Clin. Cancer Res.* 11, 8028–8035. doi: 10.1158/1078-0432.CCR-05-1253

Colette, S., Defrere, S., Lousse, J. C., Van Langendonckt, A., Gotteland, J. P., Loumaye, E., et al. (2011). Inhibition of steroid sulfatase decreases endometriosis in an *in vivo* murine model. *Hum. Reprod.* 26, 1362–1370. doi: 10.1093/humrep/der079

Colette, S., Defrere, S., Van Kerk, O., Van Langendonckt, A., Dolmans, M. M., and Donnez, J. (2013). Differential expression of steroidogenic enzymes according to endometriosis type. *Fertil. Steril.* 100, 1642–1649. doi: 10.1016/j.fertnstert.2013.08.003

Colette, S., Lousse, J. C., Defrere, S., Curaba, M., Heilier, J. F., Van Langendonckt, A., et al. (2009). Absence of aromatase protein and mRNA expression in endometriosis. *Hum. Reprod.* 24, 2133–2141. doi: 10.1093/humrep/dep199

Compston, J. E. (2001). Sex steroids and bone. *Physiol. Rev.* 81, 419–447. doi: 10.1152/physrev.2001.81.1.419

Corbould, A. M., Bawden, M. J., Lavranos, T. C., Rodgers, R. J., and Judd, S. J. (2002). The effect of obesity on the ratio of type 3, 17β-hydroxysteroid dehydrogenase mRNA to cytochrome P450 aromatase mRNA in subcutaneous abdominal and intra-abdominal adipose tissue of women. *Int. J. Obes. Relat. Metab. Disord.* 26, 165–175. doi: 10.1038/sj.ijo.0801886

Cornel, K. M., Krakstad, C., Delvoux, B., Xanthoulea, S., Jori, B., Bongers, M. Y., et al. (2017). High mRNA levels of 17β-hydroxysteroid dehydrogenase type 1 correlate with poor prognosis in endometrial cancer. *Mol. Cell. Endocrinol.* 442, 51–57. doi: 10.1016/j.mce.2016.11.030

Cornel, K. M., Kruitwagen, R. F., Delvoux, B., Visconti, L., Van de Vijver, K. K., Day, J. M., et al. (2012). Overexpression of 17β-Hydroxysteroid Dehydrogenase Type 1 Increases the exposure of endometrial cancer to 17β-Estradiol. *J. Clin. Endocrinol. Metab.* 97, E591–E601. doi: 10.1210/jc.2011-2994

Cornel, K. M. C., Bongers M. Y., Kruitwagen, R. P. F. M., Romano, A. (2018). Local estrogen metabolism (intracrinology) in endometrial cancer: a systematic review. *Mol. Cell. Endocrinol.* Accepted for publication.

Couse, J. F., and Korach, K. S. (1999). Estrogen receptor null mice: what have we learned and where will they lead us? *Endocr. Rev.* 20, 358–417.

Couse, J. F., Lindzey, J., Grandien, K., Gustafsson, J. A., and Korach, K. S. (1997). Tissue distribution and quantitative analysis of estrogen receptor-α (ERα) and estrogen receptor-β (ERβ) messenger ribonucleic acid in the wild-type and ERα-knockout mouse. *Endocrinology* 138, 4613–4621. doi: 10.1210/endo.138.11.5496

Couse, J. F., Yates, M. M., Walker, V. R., and Korach, K. S. (2003). Characterization of the hypothalamic-pituitary-gonadal axis in estrogen receptor (ER) Null mice reveals hypergonadism and endocrine sex reversal in females lacking ERα but not ERβ. *Mol. Endocrinol.* 17, 1039–1053. doi: 10.1210/me.2002-0398

Dalla Valle, L., Toffolo, V., Nardi, A., Fiore, C., Armanini, D., Belvedere, P., et al. (2007). The expression of the human steroid sulfatase-encoding gene is driven by alternative first exons. *J. Steroid Biochem. Mol. Biol.* 107, 22–29. doi: 10.1016/j.jsbmb.2007.05.004

Das, A., Mantena, S. R., Kannan, A., Evans, D. B., Bagchi, M. K., and Bagchi, I. C. (2009). *De novo* synthesis of estrogen in pregnant uterus is critical for stromal decidualization and angiogenesis. *Proc. Natl. Acad. Sci. U.S.A.* 106, 12542–12547. doi: 10.1073/pnas.0901647106

Dassen, H., Punyadeera, C., Kamps, R., Delvoux, B., Van Langendonckt, A., Donnez, J., et al. (2007). Estrogen metabolizing enzymes in endometrium and endometriosis. *Hum. Reprod.* 22, 3148–3158. doi: 10.1093/humrep/dem310

Davies, W., Humby, T., Trent, S., Eddy, J. B., Ojarikre, O. A., and Wilkinson, L. S. (2014). Genetic and pharmacological modulation of the steroid sulfatase axis improves response control; comparison with drugs used in ADHD. *Neuropsychopharmacology* 39, 2622–2632. doi: 10.1038/npp.2014.115

Day, J. M., Foster, P. A., Tutill, H. J., Schmidlin, F., Sharland, C. M., Hargrave, J. D., et al. (2013). STX2171, a 17β-hydroxysteroid dehydrogenase type 3 inhibitor, is efficacious *in vivo* in a novel hormone-dependent prostate cancer model. *Endocr. Relat. Cancer* 20, 53–64. doi: 10.1530/ERC-12-0231

De Graaff, A. A., D'Hooghe, T. M., Dunselman, G. A., Dirksen, C. D., Hummelshoj, L., Consortium, W. E., et al. (2013). The significant effect of endometriosis on physical, mental and social wellbeing: results from an international cross-sectional survey. *Hum. Reprod.* 28, 2677–2685. doi: 10.1093/humrep/det284

De Graaff, A. A., Dirksen, C. D., Simoens, S., De Bie, B., Hummelshoj, L., D'Hooghe, T. M., et al. (2015). Quality of life outcomes in women with endometriosis are highly influenced by recruitment strategies. *Hum. Reprod.* 30, 1331–1341. doi: 10.1093/humrep/dev084

De Graaff, A. A., Van Lankveld, J., Smits, L. J., Van Beek, J. J., and Dunselman, G. A. (2016). Dyspareunia and depressive symptoms are associated with impaired sexual functioning in women with endometriosis, whereas sexual functioning in their male partners is not affected. *Hum. Reprod.* 31, 2577–2586. doi: 10.1093/humrep/dew215

De Preter, V., Arijs, I., Windey, K., Vanhove, W., Vermeire, S., Schuit, F., et al. (2012). Impaired butyrate oxidation in ulcerative colitis is due to decreased butyrate uptake and a defect in the oxidation pathway. *Inflamm. Bowel Dis.* 18, 1127–1136. doi: 10.1002/ibd.21894

Delvoux, B., D'Hooghe, T., Kyama, C., Koskimies, P., Hermans, R. J., Dunselman, G. A., et al. (2014). Inhibition of type 1, 17β-hydroxysteroid dehydrogenase impairs the synthesis of 17β-estradiol in endometriosis lesions. *J. Clin. Endocrinol. Metab.* 99, 276–284. doi: 10.1210/jc.2013-2851

Delvoux, B., Groothuis, P., D'Hooghe, T., Kyama, C., Dunselman, G., and Romano, A. (2009). Increased production of 17β-estradiol in endometriosis lesions is the result of impaired metabolism. *J. Clin. Endocrinol. Metab.* 94, 876–883. doi: 10.1210/jc.2008-2218

Delvoux, B., Husen, B., Aldenhoff, Y., Koole, L., Dunselman, G., Thole, H., et al. (2007). A sensitive HPLC method for the assessment of metabolic conversion of estrogens. *J. Steroid Biochem. Mol. Biol.* 104, 246–251. doi: 10.1016/j.jsbmb.2007.03.006

Deng, H. Z., You, C., Xing, Y., Chen, K. Y., and Zou, X. B. (2016). A Family-Based Association Study of CYP11A1 and CYP11B1 Gene Polymorphisms With Autism in Chinese Trios. *J. Child Neurol.* 31, 733–737. doi: 10.1177/0883073815620672

Devroey, P., Bourgain, C., Macklon, N. S., and Fauser, B. C. (2004). Reproductive biology and IVF: ovarian stimulation and endometrial receptivity. *Trends Endocrinol. Metab.* 15, 84–90. doi: 10.1016/j.tem.2004.01.009

Dheenadayalu, K., Mak, I., Gordts, S., Campo, R., Higham, J., Puttemans, P., et al. (2002). Aromatase P450 messenger RNA expression in eutopic endometrium is not a specific marker for pelvic endometriosis. *Fertil. Steril.* 78, 825–829. doi: 10.1016/S0015-0282(02)03324-1

Di Costanzo, L., Penning, T. M., and Christianson, D. W. (2009). Aldo-keto reductases in which the conserved catalytic histidine is substituted. *Chem. Biol. Interact.* 178, 127–133. doi: 10.1016/j.cbi.2008.10.046

Dias, N. J., and Selcer, K. W. (2014). Steroid sulfatase mediated growth Sof human MG-63 pre-osteoblastic cells. *Steroids* 88, 77–82. doi: 10.1016/j.steroids.2014.07.001

Dias, N. J., and Selcer, K. W. (2016). Steroid sulfatase in the human MG-63 preosteoblastic cell line: Antagonistic regulation by glucocorticoids and NFkappaB. *Mol. Cell. Endocrinol.* 420, 85–96. doi: 10.1016/j.mce.2015.11.029

Dickinson, M. E., Flenniken, A. M., Ji, X., Teboul, L., Wong, M. D., White, J. K., et al. (2016). High-throughput discovery of novel developmental phenotypes. *Nature* 537, 508–514. doi: 10.1038/nature19356

Doherty, J. A., Weiss, N. S., Freeman, R. J., Dightman, D. A., Thornton, P. J., Houck, J. R., et al. (2005). Genetic factors in catechol estrogen metabolism in relation to the risk of endometrial cancer. *Cancer Epidemiol. Biomarkers Prev.* 14, 357–366. doi: 10.1158/1055-9965.EPI-04-0479

Dohi, O., Hatori, M., Suzuki, T., Ono, K., Hosaka, M., Akahira, J., et al. (2008). Sex steroid receptors expression and hormone-induced cell proliferation in human osteosarcoma. *Cancer Sci.* 99, 518–523. doi: 10.1111/j.1349-7006.2007.00673.x

Dong, Y., Qiu, Q. Q., Debear, J., Lathrop, W. F., Bertolini, D. R., and Tamburini, P. P. (1998). 17β-hydroxysteroid dehydrogenases in human bone cells. *J. Bone Miner. Res.* 13, 1539–1546. doi: 10.1359/jbmr.1998.13.10.1539

Driessen, C. A., Winkens, H. J., Hoffmann, K., Kuhlmann, L. D., Janssen, B. P., Van Vugt, A. H., et al. (2000). Disruption of the 11-cis-retinol dehydrogenase gene leads to accumulation of cis-retinols and cis-retinyl esters. *Mol. Cell. Biol.* 20, 4275–4287. doi: 10.1128/MCB.20.12.4275-4287.2000

Drzewiecka, H., Galecki, B., Jarmolowska-Jurczyszyn, D., Kluk, A., Dyszkiewicz, W., and Jagodzinski, P. P. (2015). Increased expression of 17-beta-hydroxysteroid dehydrogenase type 1 in non-small cell lung cancer. *Lung Cancer* 87, 107–116. doi: 10.1016/j.lungcan.2014.12.012

Drzewiecka, H., and Jagodzinski, P. P. (2012). Conversion of estrone to 17-beta-estradiol in human non-small-cell lung cancer cells *in vitro*. *Biomed. Pharmacother.* 66, 530–534. doi: 10.1016/j.biopha.2012.02.006

Duell, E. J., Travier, N., Lujan-Barroso, L., Boutron-Ruault, M. C., Clavel-Chapelon, F., Palli, D., et al. (2010). Menstrual and reproductive factors, exogenous hormone use, and gastric cancer risk in a cohort of women from the European Prospective Investigation Into Cancer and Nutrition. *Am. J. Epidemiol.* 172, 1384–1393. doi: 10.1093/aje/kwq321

Dunselman, G. A., Vermeulen, N., Becker, C., Calhaz-Jorge, C., D'Hooghe, T., De Bie, B., et al. (2014). ESHRE guideline: management of women with endometriosis. *Hum. Reprod.* 29, 400–412. doi: 10.1093/humrep/det457

Ellem, S. J., Wang, H., Poutanen, M., and Risbridger, G. P. (2009). Increased endogenous estrogen synthesis leads to the sequential induction of prostatic inflammation (prostatitis) and prostatic pre-malignancy. *Am. J. Pathol.* 175, 1187–1199. doi: 10.2353/ajpath.2009.081107

Endo, S., Miyagi, N., Matsunaga, T., Hara, A., and Ikari, A. (2016). Human dehydrogenase/reductase (SDR family) member 11 is a novel type of 17β-hydroxysteroid dehydrogenase. *Biochem. Biophys. Res. Commun.* 472, 231–236. doi: 10.1016/j.bbrc.2016.01.190

English, M. A., Hughes, S. V., Kane, K. F., Langman, M. J., Stewart, P. M., and Hewison, M. (2000). Oestrogen inactivation in the colon: analysis of the expression and regulation of 17β-hydroxysteroid dehydrogenase isozymes in normal colon and colonic cancer. *Br. J. Cancer* 83, 550–558. doi: 10.1054/bjoc.2000.1324

English, M. A., Kane, K. F., Cruickshank, N., Langman, M. J., Stewart, P. M., and Hewison, M. (1999). Loss of estrogen inactivation in colonic cancer. *J. Clin. Endocrinol. Metab.* 84, 2080–2085. doi: 10.1210/jcem.84.6.5772

Enríquez, J., Larrea, F., Santillan, R., Hernandez, A., Herrero, B., Perez-Palacios, G., et al. (2013). Neonatal rat osteoblasts bioconvert testosterone to non-phenolic metabolites with estrogen-like effects on bone cell proliferation and differentiation. *Horm. Mol. Biol. Clin. Investig.* 13, 41–49. doi: 10.1515/hmbci-2012-0035

Falk, R. T., Dallal, C. M., Lacey, J. V. Jr., Bauer, D. C., Buist, D. S., Cauley, J. A., et al. (2015). Estrogen metabolites are not associated with colorectal cancer risk in postmenopausal women. *Cancer Epidemiol. Biomarkers Prev.* 24, 1419–1422. doi: 10.1158/1055-9965.EPI-15-0541

Ferrero, S., Gillott, D. J., Venturini, P. L., and Remorgida, V. (2011). Use of aromatase inhibitors to treat endometriosis-related pain symptoms: a systematic review. *Reprod. Biol. Endocrinol.* 9, 89. doi: 10.1186/1477-7827-9-89

Fisher, C. R., Graves, K. H., Parlow, A. F., and Simpson, E. R. (1998). Characterization of mice deficient in aromatase (ArKO) because of targeted disruption of the cyp19 gene. *Proc. Natl. Acad. Sci. U.S.A.* 95, 6965–6970. doi: 10.1073/pnas.95.12.6965

Flach, K. D., and Zwart, W. (2016). The first decade of estrogen receptor cistromics in breast cancer. *J. Endocrinol.* 229 R43–56. doi: 10.1530/JOE-16-0003

Fontein, D. B., Houtsma, D., Nortier, J. W., Baak-Pablo, R. F., Kranenbarg, E. M., van der Straaten, T. R., et al. (2014). Germline variants in the $CYP_{19}A_1$ gene are related to specific adverse events in aromatase inhibitor users: a substudy of Dutch patients in the TEAM trial. *Breast Cancer Res. Treat.* 144, 599–606. doi: 10.1007/s10549-014-2873-2

Foster, P. A. (2013). Oestrogen and colorectal cancer: mechanisms and controversies. *Int. J. Colorectal Dis.* 28, 737–749. doi: 10.1007/s00384-012-1628-y

Foster, P. A., Reed, M. J., and Purohit, A. (2008a). Recent developments of steroid sulfatase inhibitors as anti-cancer agents. *Anticancer. Agents Med. Chem.* 8, 732–738. doi: 10.2174/187152008785914815

Foster, P. A., Woo, L. W., Potter, B. V., Reed, M. J., and Purohit, A. (2008b). The use of steroid sulfatase inhibitors as a novel therapeutic strategy against hormone-dependent endometrial cancer. *Endocrinology* 149, 4035–4042. doi: 10.1210/en.2008-0223

Fouad Mansour, M., Pelletier, M., Boulet, M. M., Mayrand, D., Brochu, G., Lebel, S., et al. (2015). Oxidative activity of 17β-hydroxysteroid dehydrogenase on testosterone in male abdominal adipose tissues and cellular localization of 17β-HSD type 2. *Mol. Cell. Endocrinol.* 414, 168–176. doi: 10.1016/j.mce.2015.06.016

Freedman, N. D., Ahn, J., Hou, L., Lissowska, J., Zatonski, W., Yeager, M., et al. (2009). Polymorphisms in estrogen- and androgen-metabolizing genes and the risk of gastric cancer. *Carcinogenesis* 30, 71–77. doi: 10.1093/carcin/bgn258

Freedman, N. D., Chow, W. H., Gao, Y. T., Shu, X. O., Ji, B. T., Yang, G., et al. (2007). Menstrual and reproductive factors and gastric cancer risk in a large prospective study of women. *Gut* 56, 1671–1677. doi: 10.1136/gut.2007.129411

Fritsch, M., Orfanos, C. E., and Zouboulis, C. C. (2001). Sebocytes are the key regulators of androgen homeostasis in human skin. *J. Invest. Dermatol.* 116, 793–800. doi: 10.1046/j.1523-1747.2001.01312.x

Frycz, B. A., Murawa, D., Borejsza-Wysocki, M., Marciniak, R., Murawa, P., Drews, M., et al. (2015). Expression of 17β-hydroxysteroid dehydrogenase type 2 is associated with some clinicopathological features in gastric cancer. *Biomed. Pharmacother.* 70, 24–27. doi: 10.1016/j.biopha.2014.12.042

Frycz, B. A., Murawa, D., Borejsza-Wysocki, M., Wichtowski, M., Spychala, A., Marciniak, R., et al. (2016). Transcript level of AKR1C3 is down-regulated in gastric cancer. *Biochem. Cell Biol.* 94, 138–146. doi: 10.1139/bcb-2015-0096

Fujikawa, H., Okura, F., Kuwano, Y., Sekizawa, A., Chiba, H., Shimodaira, K., et al. (1997). Steroid sulfatase activity in osteoblast cells. *Biochem. Biophys. Res. Commun.* 231, 42–47. doi: 10.1006/bbrc.1996.6038

Gangloff, A., Shi, R., Nahoum, V., and Lin, S. X. (2003). Pseudo-symmetry of C19 steroids, alternative binding orientations, and multispecificity in human estrogenic 17β-hydroxysteroid dehydrogenase. *FASEB J.* 17, 274–276. doi: 10.1096/fj.02-0397fje

Gao, J., He, J., Shi, X., Stefanovic-Racic, M., Xu, M., O'Doherty, R. M., et al. (2012). Sex-specific effect of estrogen sulfotransferase on mouse models of type 2 diabetes. *Diabetes* 61, 1543–1551. doi: 10.2337/db11-1152

Gargano, E. M., Allegretta, G., Perspicace, E., Carotti, A., Van Koppen, C., Frotscher, M., et al. (2015). 17β-Hydroxysteroid dehydrogenase Type 2 inhibition: discovery of selective and metabolically stable compounds inhibiting both the human enzyme and its murine ortholog. *PLoS ONE* 10:e0134754. doi: 10.1371/journal.pone.0134754

Ghosh, D., Dhara, S., Kumar, A., and Sengupta, J. (1999). Immunohistochemical localization of receptors for progesterone and oestradiol-17 beta in the implantation site of the rhesus monkey. *Hum. Reprod.* 14, 505–514. doi: 10.1093/humrep/14.2.505

Gibbs, T. T., Russek, S. J., and Farb, D. H. (2006). Sulfated steroids as endogenous neuromodulators. *Pharmacol. Biochem. Behav.* 84, 555–567. doi: 10.1016/j.pbb.2006.07.031

Gibson, D. A., McInnes, K. J., Critchley, H. O., and Saunders, P. T. (2013). Endometrial Intracrinology-generation of an estrogen-dominated microenvironment in the secretory phase of women. *J. Clin. Endocrinol. Metab.* 98, E1802–E1806. doi: 10.1210/jc.2013-2140

Gilligan, L. C., Gondal, A., Tang, V., Hussain, M. T., Arvaniti, A., Hewitt, A. M., et al. (2017). Estrone sulfate transport and steroid sulfatase activity in colorectal cancer: implications for hormone replacement therapy. *Front. Pharmacol.* 8:103. doi: 10.3389/fphar.2017.00103

González-Arenas, A., and Agramonte-Hevia, J. (2012). Sex steroid hormone effects in normal and pathologic conditions in lung physiology. *Mini Rev. Med. Chem.* 12, 1055–1062. doi: 10.2174/138955712802762194

Goodarzi, M. O., Antoine, H. J., and Azziz, R. (2007). Genes for enzymes regulating dehydroepiandrosterone sulfonation are associated with levels of dehydroepiandrosterone sulfate in polycystic ovary syndrome. *J. Clin. Endocrinol. Metab.* 92, 2659–2664. doi: 10.1210/jc.2006-2600

Goodarzi, M. O., Shah, N. A., Antoine, H. J., Pall, M., Guo, X., and Azziz, R. (2006). Variants in the 5α-reductase type 1 and type 2 genes are associated with polycystic ovary syndrome and the severity of hirsutism in affected women. *J. Clin. Endocrinol. Metab.* 91, 4085–4091. doi: 10.1210/jc.2006-0227

Groothuis, P. G., Dassen, H. H., Romano, A., and Punyadeera, C. (2007). Estrogen and the endometrium: lessons learned from gene expression profiling in rodents and human. *Hum. Reprod. Update* 13, 405–417. doi: 10.1093/humupd/dmm009

Gruber, C. J., Tschugguel, W., Schneeberger, C., and Huber, J. C. (2002). Production and actions of estrogens. *N. Engl. J. Med.* 346, 340–352. doi: 10.1056/NEJMra000471

Guillot, F., Garcia, A., Salou, M., Brouard, S., Laplaud, D. A., and Nicot, A. B. (2015). Transcript analysis of laser capture microdissected white matter astrocytes and higher phenol sulfotransferase 1A1 expression during autoimmune neuroinflammation. *J. Neuroinflammation* 12, 130. doi: 10.1186/s12974-015-0348-y

Gulyaeva, L. F., Mikhailova, O. N., Pustylnyak, V. O., Kim, I. V. IV., Gerasimov, A. V., Krasilnikov, S. E., et al. (2008). Comparative analysis of SNP in estrogen-metabolizing enzymes for ovarian, endometrial, and breast cancers in Novosibirsk, Russia. *Adv. Exp. Med. Biol.* 617, 359–366. doi: 10.1007/978-0-387-69080-3_34

Gylfe, A. E., Katainen, R., Kondelin, J., Tanskanen, T., Cajuso, T., Hanninen, U., et al. (2013). Eleven candidate susceptibility genes for common familial colorectal cancer. *PLoS Genet.* 9:e1003876. doi: 10.1371/journal.pgen.1003876

Hakkarainen, J., Jokela, H., Pakarinen, P., Heikela, H., Katkanaho, L., Vandenput, L., et al. (2015). Hydroxysteroid (17β)-dehydrogenase 1-deficient female mice present with normal puberty onset but are severely subfertile due to a defect in luteinization and progesterone production. *FASEB J.* 29, 3806–3816. doi: 10.1096/fj.14-269035

He, D., Frost, A. R., and Falany, C. N. (2005a). Identification and immunohistochemical localization of Sulfotransferase 2B1b (SULT2B1b) in human lung. *Biochim Biophys Act.* 1724, 119–126. doi: 10.1016/j.bbagen.2005.03.018

He, D., Meloche, C. A., Dumas, N. A., Frost, A. R., and Falany, C. N. (2004). Different subcellular localization of sulphotransferase 2B1b in human placenta and prostate. *Biochem. J.* 379, 533–540. doi: 10.1042/bj20031524

He, W., Gauri, M., Li, T., Wang, R., and Lin, S. X. (2016). Current knowledge of the multifunctional 17β-hydroxysteroid dehydrogenase type 1 (HSD17B1). *Gene* 588, 54–61. doi: 10.1016/j.gene.2016.04.031

He, X. Y., Wegiel, J., Yang, Y. Z., Pullarkat, R., Schulz, H., and Yang, S. Y. (2005b). Type 10, 17β-hydroxysteroid dehydrogenase catalyzing the oxidation of steroid modulators of gamma-aminobutyric acid type A receptors. *Mol. Cell. Endocrinol.* 229, 111–117. doi: 10.1016/j.mce.2004.08.011

He, X. Y., and Yang, S. Y. (2006). Roles of type 10, 17β-hydroxysteroid dehydrogenase in intracrinology and metabolism of isoleucine and fatty acids. *Endocr. Metab. Immune Disord. Drug Targets* 6, 95–102. doi: 10.2174/187153006776056639

Heijmans, J., Wielenga, M. C., Rosekrans, S. L., van Lidth de Jeude, J. F., Roelofs, J., Groothuis, P., et al. (2014). Oestrogens promote tumorigenesis in a mouse model for colitis-associated cancer. *Gut* 63, 310–316. doi: 10.1136/gutjnl-2012-304216

Her, C., Szumlanski, C., Aksoy, I. A., and Weinshilboum, R. M. (1996). Human jejunal estrogen sulfotransferase and dehydroepiandrosterone sulfotransferase: immunochemical characterization of individual variation. *Drug Metab. Dispos.* 24, 1328–1335.

Hevir, N., Ribic-Pucelj, M., and Lanisnik Rizner, T. (2013). Disturbed balance between phase I and II metabolizing enzymes in ovarian endometriosis: a source of excessive hydroxy-estrogens and ROS? *Mol. Cell. Endocrinol.* 367, 74–84. doi: 10.1016/j.mce.2012.12.019

Hevir, N., Sinkovec, J., and Rizner, T. L. (2011a). Disturbed expression of phase I and phase II estrogen-metabolizing enzymes in endometrial cancer: lower levels of CYP1B1 and increased expression of S-COMT. *Mol. Cell. Endocrinol.* 331, 158–167. doi: 10.1016/j.mce.2010.09.011

Hevir, N., Vouk, K., Sinkovec, J., Ribic-Pucelj, M., and Rizner, T. L. (2011b). Aldo-keto reductases AKR1C1, AKR1C2 and AKR1C3 may enhance progesterone metabolism in ovarian endometriosis. *Chem. Biol. Interact.* 191, 217–226. doi: 10.1016/j.cbi.2011.01.003

Hewitt, S. C., Winuthayanon, W., and Korach, K. S. (2016). What's new in estrogen receptor action in the female reproductive tract. *J. Mol. Endocrinol.* 56 R55–71. doi: 10.1530/JME-15-0254

Hilborn, E., Stal, O., and Jansson, A. (2017). Estrogen and androgen-converting enzymes 17β-hydroxysteroid dehydrogenase and their involvement in cancer: with a special focus on 17β-hydroxysteroid dehydrogenase type 1, 2, and breast cancer. *Oncotarget* 8, 30552–30562. doi: 10.18632/oncotarget.15547

Hogan, A. M., Collins, D., Baird, A. W., and Winter, D. C. (2009). Estrogen and gastrointestinal malignancy. *Mol. Cell. Endocrinol.* 307, 19–24. doi: 10.1016/j.mce.2009.03.016

Honda, S., Harada, N., Ito, S., Takagi, Y., and Maeda, S. (1998). Disruption of sexual behavior in male aromatase-deficient mice lacking exons 1 and 2 of the cyp19 gene. *Biochem. Biophys. Res. Commun.* 252, 445–449. doi: 10.1006/bbrc.1998.9672

Hovorkova, P., Kristofikova, Z., Horinek, A., Ripova, D., Majer, E., Zach, P., et al. (2008). Lateralization of 17β-hydroxysteroid dehydrogenase type 10 in hippocampi of demented and psychotic people. *Dement. Geriatr. Cogn. Disord.* 26, 193–198. doi: 10.1159/000151778

Hu, M. C., Hsu, N. C., El Hadj, N. B., Pai, C. I., Chu, H. P., Wang, C. K., et al. (2002). Steroid deficiency syndromes in mice with targeted disruption of Cyp11a1. *Mol. Endocrinol.* 16, 1943–1950. doi: 10.1210/me.2002-0055

Huang, C. C., Shih, M. C., Hsu, N. C., Chien, Y., and Chung, B. C. (2012). Fetal glucocorticoid synthesis is required for development of fetal adrenal medulla and hypothalamus feedback suppression. *Endocrinology* 153, 4749–4756. doi: 10.1210/en.2012-1258

Huang, X. F., and Luu-The, V. (2000). Molecular characterization of a first human 3(α-> β)-hydroxysteroid epimerase. *J. Biol. Chem.* 275, 29452–29457. doi: 10.1074/jbc.M000562200

Huber, A., Keck, C. C., Hefler, L. A., Schneeberger, C., Huber, J. C., Bentz, E. K., et al. (2005). Ten estrogen-related polymorphisms and endometriosis: a study of multiple gene-gene interactions. *Obstet. Gynecol.* 106, 1025–1031. doi: 10.1097/01.AOG.0000185259.01648.41

Hudelist, G., Czerwenka, K., Keckstein, J., Haas, C., Fink-Retter, A., Gschwantler-Kaulich, D., et al. (2007). Expression of aromatase and estrogen sulfotransferase in eutopic and ectopic endometrium: evidence for unbalanced estradiol production in endometriosis. *Reprod. Sci.* 14, 798–805. doi: 10.1177/1933719107309120

Hughes, S. V., Robinson, E., Bland, R., Lewis, H. M., Stewart, P. M., and Hewison, M. (1997). 1,25-dihydroxyvitamin D3 regulates estrogen metabolism in cultured keratinocytes. *Endocrinology* 138, 3711–3718. doi: 10.1210/endo.138.9.5406

Huhtinen, K., Desai, R., Stahle, M., Salminen, A., Handelsman, D. J., Perheentupa, A., et al. (2012a). Endometrial and endometriotic concentrations of estrone and estradiol are determined by local metabolism rather than circulating levels. *J. Clin. Endocrinol. Metab.* 97, 4228–4235. doi: 10.1210/jc.2012-1154

Huhtinen, K., Saloniemi-Heinonen, T., Keski-Rahkonen, P., Desai, R., Laajala, D., Stahle, M., et al. (2014). Intra-tissue steroid profiling indicates differential progesterone and testosterone metabolism in the endometrium and endometriosis lesions. *J. Clin. Endocrinol. Metab.* 99 E2188–2197. doi: 10.1210/jc.2014-1913

Huhtinen, K., Stahle, M., Perheentupa, A., and Poutanen, M. (2012b). Estrogen biosynthesis and signaling in endometriosis. *Mol. Cell. Endocrinol.* 358, 146–154. doi: 10.1016/j.mce.2011.08.022

Husen, B., Huhtinen, K., Poutanen, M., Kangas, L., Messinger, J., and Thole, H. (2006). Evaluation of inhibitors for 17β-hydroxysteroid dehydrogenase type 1 *in vivo* in immunodeficient mice inoculated with MCF-7 cells stably expressing the recombinant human enzyme. *Mol. Cell. Endocrinol.* 248, 109–113. doi: 10.1016/j.mce.2005.11.042

Ihlenfeldt, W. D., Bolton, E. E., and Bryant, S. H. (2009). The PubChem chemical structure sketcher. *J. Cheminform.* 1:20. doi: 10.1186/1758-2946-1-20

Iida, S., Kakinuma, H., Miki, Y., Abe, K., Sakurai, M., Suzuki, S., et al. (2013). Steroid sulphatase and oestrogen sulphotransferase in human non-small-cell lung carcinoma. *Br. J. Cancer* 108, 1415–1424. doi: 10.1038/bjc.2013.84

Ikeda, K., Shiraishi, K., Yoshida, A., Shinchi, Y., Sanada, M., Motooka, Y., et al. (2016). Synchronous multiple lung adenocarcinomas: estrogen concentration in peripheral lung. *PLoS ONE* 11:e0160910. doi: 10.1371/journal.pone.0160910

Iqbal, M. J., Greenway, B., Wilkinson, M. L., Johnson, P. J., and Williams, R. (1983). Sex-steroid enzymes, aromatase and 5 alpha-reductase in the pancreas: a comparison of normal adult, foetal and malignant tissue. *Clin. Sci.* 65, 71–75. doi: 10.1042/cs0650071

Ishida, M., Choi, J. H., Hirabayashi, K., Matsuwaki, T., Suzuki, M., Yamanouchi, K., et al. (2007). Reproductive phenotypes in mice with targeted disruption of the 20α-hydroxysteroid dehydrogenase gene. *J. Reprod. Dev.* 53, 499–508. doi: 10.1262/jrd.18125

Ito, K., Miki, Y., Suzuki, T., McNamara, K. M., and Sasano, H. (2016). In situ androgen and estrogen biosynthesis in endometrial cancer: focus on androgen actions and intratumoral production. *Endocr. Relat. Cancer* 23 R323–335. doi: 10.1530/ERC-15-0470

Ito, K., Suzuki, T., Akahira, J., Moriya, T., Kaneko, C., Utsunomiya, H., et al. (2002). Expression of androgen receptor and 5α-reductases in the human normal endometrium and its disorders. *Int. J. Cancer* 99, 652–657. doi: 10.1002/ijc.10394

Ito, K., Utsunomiya, H., Suzuki, T., Saitou, S., Akahira, J., Okamura, K., et al. (2006). 17β-hydroxysteroid dehydrogenases in human endometrium and its disorders. *Mol. Cell. Endocrinol.* 248, 136–140. doi: 10.1016/j.mce.2005.11.038

Iwasa, A., Arakaki, R., Honma, N., Ushio, A., Yamada, A., Kondo, T., et al. (2015). Aromatase controls Sjogren syndrome-like lesions through monocyte chemotactic protein-1 in target organ and adipose tissue-associated macrophages. *Am. J. Pathol.* 185, 151–161. doi: 10.1016/j.ajpath.2014.09.006

Jakob, F., Siggelkow, H., Homann, D., Kohrle, J., Adamski, J., and Schutze, N. (1997). Local estradiol metabolism in osteoblast- and osteoclast-like cells. *J. Steroid Biochem. Mol. Biol.* 61, 167–174. doi: 10.1016/S0960-0760(97)80009-X

Janssen, J. M., Bland, R., Hewison, M., Coughtrie, M. W., Sharp, S., Arts, J., et al. (1999). Estradiol formation by human osteoblasts via multiple pathways: relation with osteoblast function. *J. Cell. Biochem.* 75, 528–537. doi: 10.1002/(SICI)1097-4644(19991201)75:3<528::AID-JCB16>3.0.CO;2-3

Jäntti, S. E., Tammimaki, A., Raattamaa, H., Piepponen, P., Kostiainen, R., and Ketola, R. A. (2010). Determination of steroids and their intact glucuronide conjugates in mouse brain by capillary liquid chromatography-tandem mass spectrometry. *Anal. Chem.* 82, 3168–3175. doi: 10.1021/ac902321z

Järvensivu, P., Heinosalo, T., Hakkarainen, J., Kronqvist, P., Saarinen, N., and Poutanen, M. (2018). HSD17B1 expression induces inflammation-aided rupture of mammary gland myoepithelium. *Endocr. Relat. Cancer* 25, 393–406. doi: 10.1530/ERC-17-0476

Järvensivu, P., Saloniemi-Heinonen, T., Awosanya, M., Koskimies, P., Saarinen, N., and Poutanen, M. (2015). HSD17B1 expression enhances estrogen signaling stimulated by the low active estrone, evidenced by an estrogen responsive element-driven reporter gene *in vivo*. *Chem. Biol. Interact.* 234, 126–134. doi: 10.1016/j.cbi.2015.01.008

Jeon, Y. T., Park, S. Y., Kim, Y. B., Kim, J. W., Park, N. H., Kang, S. B., et al. (2007). Aromatase expression was not detected by immunohistochemistry in endometrial cancer. *Ann. N. Y. Acad. Sci.* 1095, 70–75. doi: 10.1196/annals.1397.010

Jin, Y., Mesaros, A. C., Blair, I. A., and Penning, T. M. (2011). Stereospecific reduction of 5β-reduced steroids by human ketosteroid reductases of the AKR (aldo-keto reductase) superfamily: role of AKR1C1-AKR1C4 in the metabolism of testosterone and progesterone via the 5β-reductase pathway. *Biochem. J.* 437, 53–61. doi: 10.1042/BJ20101804

Jokela, H., Rantakari, P., Lamminen, T., Strauss, L., Ola, R., Mutka, A. L., et al. (2010). Hydroxysteroid (17β) dehydrogenase 7 activity is essential for fetal de novo cholesterol synthesis and for neuroectodermal survival and cardiovascular differentiation in early mouse embryos. *Endocrinology* 151, 1884–1892. doi: 10.1210/en.2009-0928

Jones, A. L., Hume, R., Bamforth, K. J., and Coughtrie, M. W. (1992). Estrogen and phenol sulfotransferase activities in human fetal lung. *Early Hum. Dev.* 28, 65–77. doi: 10.1016/0378-3782(92)90007-4

Jones, M. R., Mathur, R., Cui, J., Guo, X., Azziz, R., and Goodarzi, M. O. (2009). Independent confirmation of association between metabolic phenotypes of polycystic ovary syndrome and variation in the type 6, 17β-hydroxysteroid dehydrogenase gene. *J. Clin. Endocrinol. Metab.* 94, 5034–5038. doi: 10.1210/jc.2009-0931

Jongen, V. H., Thijssen, J. H., Hollema, H., Donker, G. H., Santema, J. G., Van der Zee, A. G., et al. (2005). Is aromatase cytochrome P450 involved in the pathogenesis of endometrioid endometrial cancer? *Int. J. Gynecol. Cancer* 15, 529–536. doi: 10.1111/j.1525-1438.2005.15320.x

Kancheva, L., Hill, M., Vcelakova, H., Vrbikova, J., Pelikanova, T., and Starka, L. (2007). The identification and simultaneous quantification of neuroactive androstane steroids and their polar conjugates in the serum of adult men, using gas chromatography-mass spectrometry. *Steroids* 72, 792–801. doi: 10.1016/j.steroids.2007.06.006

Kassem, M., Okazaki, R., Harris, S. A., Spelsberg, T. C., Conover, C. A., and Riggs, B. L. (1998). Estrogen effects on insulin-like growth factor gene expression in a human osteoblastic cell line with high levels of estrogen receptor. *Calcif. Tissue Int.* 62, 60–66. doi: 10.1007/s002239900395

Kemilainen, H., Adam, M., Maki-Jouppila, J., Damdimopoulou, P., Damdimopoulos, A. E., Kere, J., et al. (2016). The hydroxysteroid (17β) dehydrogenase family gene HSD17B12 Is involved in the prostaglandin synthesis pathway, the ovarian function, and regulation of fertility. *Endocrinology* 157, 3719–3730. doi: 10.1210/en.2016-1252

Kennelly, R., Kavanagh, D. O., Hogan, A. M., and Winter, D. C. (2008). Oestrogen and the colon: potential mechanisms for cancer prevention. *Lancet Oncol.* 9, 385–391. doi: 10.1016/S1470-2045(08)70100-1

Kikuchi, A., Furutani, T., Azami, H., Watanabe, K., Niimi, T., Kamiyama, Y., et al. (2014). *In vitro* and *in vivo* characterisation of ASP9521: a novel, selective, orally bioavailable inhibitor of 17β-hydroxysteroid dehydrogenase type 5 (17βHSD5; AKR1C3). *Invest. New Drugs* 32, 860–870. doi: 10.1007/s10637-014-0130-5

Kim, J. H., Cho, H. T., and Kim, Y. J. (2014). The role of estrogen in adipose tissue metabolism: insights into glucose homeostasis regulation. *Endocr. J.* 61, 1055–1067. doi: 10.1507/endocrj.EJ14-0262

Kim, S., Thiessen, P. A., Bolton, E. E., Chen, J., Fu, G., Gindulyte, A., et al. (2016). PubChem substance and compound databases. *Nucleic Acids Res.* 44, D1202–D1213. doi: 10.1093/nar/gkv951

Kim, T. S., Maeda, A., Maeda, T., Heinlein, C., Kedishvili, N., Palczewski, K., et al. (2005). Delayed dark adaptation in 11-cis-retinol dehydrogenase-deficient mice: a role of RDH11 in visual processes *in vivo*. *J. Biol. Chem.* 280, 8694–8704. doi: 10.1074/jbc.M413172200

Kimoto, T., Ishii, H., Higo, S., Hojo, Y., and Kawato, S. (2010). Semicomprehensive analysis of the postnatal age-related changes in the mRNA expression of sex steroidogenic enzymes and sex steroid receptors in the male rat hippocampus. *Endocrinology* 151, 5795–5806. doi: 10.1210/en.2010-0581

Kimura, Y., Suzuki, T., Kaneko, C., Darnel, A. D., Akahira, J., Ebina, M., et al. (2003). Expression of androgen receptor and 5α-reductase types 1 and 2 in early gestation fetal lung: a possible correlation with branching morphogenesis. *Clin. Sci.* 105, 709–713. doi: 10.1042/CS20030236

Kitaoka, Y., Kitawaki, J., Koshiba, H., Inoue, S., Ishihara, H., Teramoto, M., et al. (2004). Aromatase cytochrome P450 and estrogen and progesterone receptors in uterine sarcomas: correlation with clinical parameters. *J. Steroid Biochem. Mol. Biol.* 88, 183–189. doi: 10.1016/j.jsbmb.2003.11.013

Kitawaki, J., Kado, N., Ishihara, H., Koshiba, H., Kitaoka, Y., and Honjo, H. (2002). Endometriosis: the pathophysiology as an estrogen-dependent disease. *J. Steroid Biochem. Mol. Biol.* 83, 149–155. doi: 10.1016/S0960-0760(02)00260-1

Kitawaki, J., Koshiba, H., Ishihara, H., Kusuki, I., Tsukamoto, K., and Honjo, H. (2000). Progesterone induction of 17β-hydroxysteroid dehydrogenase type 2 during the secretory phase occurs in the endometrium of estrogen-dependent benign diseases but not in normal endometrium. *J. Clin. Endocrinol. Metab.* 85, 3292–3296. doi: 10.1210/jcem.85.9.6829

Kitawaki, J., Kusuki, I., Koshiba, H., Tsukamoto, K., Fushiki, S., and Honjo, H. (1999). Detection of aromatase cytochrome P-450 in endometrial biopsy specimens as a diagnostic test for endometriosis. *Fertil. Steril.* 72, 1100–1106. doi: 10.1016/S0015-0282(99)00424-0

Knapp, P., Chabowski, A., Blachnio-Zabielska, A., Walentowicz-Sadlecka, M., Grabiec, M., and Knapp, P. A. (2013). Expression of estrogen receptors (alpha, beta), cyclooxygenase-2 and aromatase in normal endometrium and endometrioid cancer of uterus. *Adv. Med. Sci.* 58, 96–103. doi: 10.2478/v10039-012-0055-1

Kobayashi, H., Yoshida, S., Sun, Y. J., Shirasawa, N., and Naito, A. (2013). Postnatal development of gastric aromatase and portal venous estradiol-17β levels in male rats. *J. Endocrinol.* 218, 117–124. doi: 10.1530/JOE-13-0074

Kohno, M., Okamoto, T., Suda, K., Shimokawa, M., Kitahara, H., Shimamatsu, S., et al. (2014). Prognostic and therapeutic implications of aromatase expression in lung adenocarcinomas with EGFR mutations. *Clin. Cancer Res.* 20, 3613–3622. doi: 10.1158/1078-0432.CCR-13-2683

Koizumi, M., Momoeda, M., Hiroi, H., Hosokawa, Y., Tsutsumi, R., Osuga, Y., et al. (2010). Expression and regulation of cholesterol sulfotransferase (SULT2B1b) in human endometrium. *Fertil. Steril.* 93, 1538–1544. doi: 10.1016/j.fertnstert.2009.01.075

Konings, G. F., Cornel, K. M., Xanthoulea, S., Delvoux, B., Skowron, M. A., Kooreman, L., et al. (2018). Blocking 17β-hydroxysteroid dehydrogenase type 1 in endometrial cancer: a potential novel endocrine therapeutic approach. *J. Pathol.* 244, 203–214. doi: 10.1002/path.5004

Konings, G. F., Reynaert, N. L., Delvoux, B., Verhamme, F. M., Bracke, K. R., Brusselle, G. G., et al. (2017). Increased levels of enzymes involved in local estradiol synthesis in chronic obstructive pulmonary disease. *Mol. Cell. Endocrinol.* 443, 23–31. doi: 10.1016/j.mce.2016.12.001

Kreitmann, O., Kreitmann-Gimbal, B., Bayard, F., and Hodgen, G. D. (1979). 17 beta-hydroxysteroid dehydrogenase in monkey endometrium: characterization of enzyme activity, and effects of estradiol alone or in combination with progesterone. *Steroids* 34, 693–703. doi: 10.1016/0039-128X(79)90139-9

Kríz, L., Bicikova, M., and Hampl, R. (2008a). Roles of steroid sulfatase in brain and other tissues. *Physiol. Res.* 57, 657–668.

Kríz, L., Bicikova, M., Mohapl, M., Hill, M., Cerny, I., and Hampl, R. (2008b). Steroid sulfatase and sulfuryl transferase activities in human brain tumors. *J. Steroid Biochem. Mol. Biol.* 109, 31–39. doi: 10.1016/j.jsbmb.2007.12.004

Laatikainen, T., Laitinen, E. A., and Vihko, R. (1971). Secretion of free and sulfate-conjugated neutral steroids by the human testis. Effect of administration of human chorionic gonadotropin. *J. Clin. Endocrinol. Metab.* 32, 59–64. doi: 10.1210/jcem-32-1-59

Labrie, F. (1991). Intracrinology. *Mol. Cell. Endocrinol.* 78, C113–C118. doi: 10.1016/0303-7207(91)90116-A

Labrie, F. (2015). All sex steroids are made intracellularly in peripheral tissues by the mechanisms of intracrinology after menopause. *J. Steroid Biochem. Mol. Biol.* 145, 133–138. doi: 10.1016/j.jsbmb.2014.06.001

Labrie, F., and Labrie, C. (2013). DHEA and intracrinology at menopause, a positive choice for evolution of the human species. *Climacteric* 16, 205–213. doi: 10.3109/13697137.2012.733983

Lane, G. (1990). The histochemistry of isocitric and oestradiol-17 beta dehydrogenases in the endometrium of postmenopausal women treated with oestrogens and progestogens. *Histochem. J.* 22, 45–50. doi: 10.1007/BF01962878

Laplante, Y., Rancourt, C., and Poirier, D. (2009). Relative involvement of three 17β-hydroxysteroid dehydrogenases (types 1, 7 and 12) in the formation of estradiol in various breast cancer cell lines using selective inhibitors. *Mol. Cell. Endocrinol.* 301, 146–153. doi: 10.1016/j.mce.2008.08.026

Lavasani, S., Chlebowski, R. T., Prentice, R. L., Kato, I., Wactawski-Wende, J., Johnson, K. C., et al. (2015). Estrogen and colorectal cancer incidence and mortality. *Cancer* 121, 3261–3271. doi: 10.1002/cncr.29464

Lee, D. K., Kurihara, I., Jeong, J. W., Lydon, J. P., DeMayo, F. J., Tsai, M. J., et al. (2010). Suppression of ERα activity by COUP-TFII is essential for successful implantation and decidualization. *Mol. Endocrinol.* 24, 930–940. doi: 10.1210/me.2009-0531

Lépine, J., Audet-Walsh, E., Gregoire, J., Tetu, B., Plante, M., Menard, V., et al. (2010). Circulating estrogens in endometrial cancer cases and their relationship with tissular expression of key estrogen biosynthesis and metabolic pathways. *J. Clin. Endocrinol. Metab.* 95, 2689–2698. doi: 10.1210/jc.2010-2648

Li, C., Chen, P., Palladino, A., Narayan, S., Russell, L. K., Sayed, S., et al. (2010). Mechanism of hyperinsulinism in short-chain 3-hydroxyacyl-CoA dehydrogenase deficiency involves activation of glutamate dehydrogenase. *J. Biol. Chem.* 285, 31806–31818. doi: 10.1074/jbc.M110.123638

Li, Y., Qin, L., Xiao, Z. J., Wang, Y. L., Herva, R., Leng, J. H., et al. (2003). Expression of P450 aromatase and 17β-hydroxysteroid dehydrogenase type 1 at fetal-maternal interface during tubal pregnancy. *J. Steroid Biochem. Mol. Biol.* 87, 241–246. doi: 10.1016/j.jsbmb.2003.09.013

Lilla, C., Risch, A., Verla-Tebit, E., Hoffmeister, M., Brenner, H., and Chang-Claude, J. (2007). SULT1A1 genotype and susceptibility to colorectal cancer. *Int. J. Cancer* 120, 201–206. doi: 10.1002/ijc.22156

Lim, Y. A., Grimm, A., Giese, M., Mensah-Nyagan, A. G., Villafranca, J. E., Ittner, L. M., et al. (2011). Inhibition of the mitochondrial enzyme ABAD restores the amyloid-beta-mediated deregulation of estradiol. *PLoS ONE* 6:e28887. doi: 10.1371/journal.pone.0028887

Lin, H. K., Jez, J. M., Schlegel, B. P., Peehl, D. M., Pachter, J. A., and Penning, T. M. (1997). Expression and characterization of recombinant type 2, 3 α-hydroxysteroid dehydrogenase (HSD) from human prostate: demonstration of bifunctional 3α/17β-HSD activity and cellular distribution. *Mol. Endocrinol.* 11, 1971–1984.

Lindemann, K., Malander, S., Christensen, R. D., Mirza, M. R., Kristensen, G. B., Aavall-Lundqvist, E., et al. (2014). Examestane in advanced or recurrent endometrial carcinoma: a prospective phase II study by the Nordic Society of Gynecologic Oncology (NSGO). *BMC Cancer* 14:68. doi: 10.1186/1471-2407-14-68

Liu, Y., Yao, Z. X., Bendavid, C., Borgmeyer, C., Han, Z., Cavalli, L. R., et al. (2005). Haploinsufficiency of cytochrome P450, 17β-hydroxylase/17,20 lyase (CYP17) causes infertility in male mice. *Mol. Endocrinol.* 19, 2380–2389. doi: 10.1210/me.2004-0418

Lønning, P. E., and Eikesdal, H. P. (2013). Aromatase inhibition 2013: clinical state of the art and questions that remain to be solved. *Endocr. Relat. Cancer* 20, R183–R201. doi: 10.1530/ERC-13-0099

López, M., and Tena-Sempere, M. (2015). Estrogens and the control of energy homeostasis: a brain perspective. *Trends Endocrinol. Metab.* 26, 411–421. doi: 10.1016/j.tem.2015.06.003

López, M., and Tena-Sempere, M. (2016). Estradiol and brown fat. *Best Pract. Res. Clin. Endocrinol. Metab.* 30, 527–536. doi: 10.1016/j.beem.2016.08.004

Loria, R. M., and Graf, M. R. (2012). 17α-androstenediol-mediated oncophagy of tumor cells by different mechanisms is determined by the target tumor. *Ann. N. Y. Acad. Sci.* 1262, 127–133. doi: 10.1111/j.1749-6632.2012.06602.x

Loriot, Y., Fizazi, K., Jones, R. J., Van den Brande, J., Molife, R. L., Omlin, A., et al. (2014). Safety, tolerability and anti-tumour activity of the androgen biosynthesis inhibitor ASP9521 in patients with metastatic castration-resistant prostate cancer: multi-centre phase I/II study. *Invest. New Drugs* 32, 995–1004. doi: 10.1007/s10637-014-0101-x

Loth, D. W., Soler Artigas, M., Gharib, S. A., Wain, L. V., Franceschini, N., Koch, B., et al. (2014). Genome-wide association analysis identifies six new loci associated with forced vital capacity. *Nat. Genet.* 46, 669–677. doi: 10.1038/ng.3011

Loza, M. C. (1995). Hydrolysis of estrone sulfate in uterine minces of the 6-days pregnant rat. *J. Steroid Biochem. Mol. Biol.* 52, 277–280. doi: 10.1016/0960-0760(94)00177-N

Lu, C., Lee, H. S., Pappas, G. P., Dilling, D. F., Burger, C. D., Shifren, A., et al. (2017). A Phase II Clinical Trial of an Aromatase Inhibitor for Postmenopausal Women with Lymphangioleiomyomatosis. *Ann. Am. Thorac. Soc.* 14, 919–928. doi: 10.1513/AnnalsATS.201610-824OC

Luchetti, S., Bossers, K., Van de Bilt, S., Agrapart, V., Morales, R. R., Frajese, G. V., et al. (2011). Neurosteroid biosynthetic pathways changes in prefrontal cortex in Alzheimer's disease. *Neurobiol. Aging* 32, 1964–1976. doi: 10.1016/j.neurobiolaging.2009.12.014

Lundin, E., Wirgin, I., Lukanova, A., Afanasyeva, Y., Krogh, V., Axelsson, T., et al. (2012). Selected polymorphisms in sex hormone-related genes, circulating sex hormones and risk of endometrial cancer. *Cancer Epidemiol.* 36, 445–452. doi: 10.1016/j.canep.2012.04.006

Luo, L., Deng, J., Wang, D. X., He, J., and Deng, W. (2015). Regulation of epithelial sodium channel expression by oestradiol and progestogen in alveolar epithelial cells. *Respir. Physiol. Neurobiol.* 216, 52–62. doi: 10.1016/j.resp.2015.06.001

Luu-The, V., Belanger, A., and Labrie, F. (2008). Androgen biosynthetic pathways in the human prostate. *Best Pract. Res. Clin. Endocrinol. Metab.* 22, 207–221. doi: 10.1016/j.beem.2008.01.008

Luu-The, V., and Labrie, F. (2010). The intracrine sex steroid biosynthesis pathways. *Prog. Brain Res.* 181, 177–192. doi: 10.1016/S0079-6123(08)81010-2

Ma, B. B., Oza, A., Eisenhauer, E., Stanimir, G., Carey, M., Chapman, W., et al. (2004). The activity of letrozole in patients with advanced or recurrent endometrial cancer and correlation with biological markers–a study of the National Cancer Institute of Canada Clinical Trials Group. *Int. J. Gynecol. Cancer* 14, 650–658. doi: 10.1111/j.1048-891X.2004.14419.x

Ma, W. G., Song, H., Das, S. K., Paria, B. C., and Dey, S. K. (2003). Estrogen is a critical determinant that specifies the duration of the window of uterine receptivity for implantation. *Proc. Natl. Acad. Sci. U.S.A.* 100, 2963–2968. doi: 10.1073/pnas.0530162100

MacKenzie, S. M., Dewar, D., Stewart, W., Fraser, R., Connell, J. M., and Davies, E. (2008). The transcription of steroidogenic genes in the human cerebellum and hippocampus: a comparative survey of normal and Alzheimer's tissue. *J. Endocrinol.* 196, 123–130. doi: 10.1677/JOE-07-0427

Maentausta, O., Peltoketo, H., Isomaa, V., Jouppila, P., and Vihko, R. (1990). Immunological measurement of human 17β-hydroxysteroid dehydrogenase. *J. Steroid. Biochem.* 36, 673–680.

Mäentausta, O., Sormunen, R., Isomaa, V., Lehto, V. P., Jouppila, P., and Vihko, R. (1991). Immunohistochemical localization of 17 beta-hydroxysteroid dehydrogenase in the human endometrium during the menstrual cycle. *Lab. Invest.* 65, 582–587.

Mahendroo, M. S., Cala, K. M., Hess, D. L., and Russell, D. W. (2001). Unexpected virilization in male mice lacking steroid 5 alpha-reductase enzymes. *Endocrinology* 142, 4652–4662. doi: 10.1210/endo.142.11.8510

Mahendroo, M. S., Cala, K. M., and Russell, D. W. (1996). 5 alpha-reduced androgens play a key role in murine parturition. *Mol. Endocrinol.* 10, 380–392.

Maia, H. Jr., Pimentel, K., Casoy, J., Correia, T., Freitas, L. A., Zausner, B., et al. (2007). Aromatase expression in the eutopic endometrium of myomatous uteri: the influence of the menstrual cycle and oral contraceptive use. *Gynecol. Endocrinol.* 23, 320–324. doi: 10.1080/09513590701321565

Maia, H. Jr., Pimentel, K., Silva, T. M., Freitas, L. A., Zausner, B., Athayde, C., et al. (2006). Aromatase and cyclooxygenase-2 expression in endometrial polyps during the menstrual cycle. *Gynecol. Endocrinol.* 22, 219–224. doi: 10.1080/09513590600585955

Maltais, R., and Poirier, D. (2011). Steroid sulfatase inhibitors: a review covering the promising 2000-2010 decade. *Steroids* 76, 929–948. doi: 10.1016/j.steroids.2011.03.010

Manenda, M. S., Hamel, C. J., Masselot-Joubert, L., Picard, M. E., and Shi, R. (2016). Androgen-metabolizing enzymes: A structural perspective. *J. Steroid Biochem. Mol. Biol.* 161, 54–72. doi: 10.1016/j.jsbmb.2016.02.021

Marchais-Oberwinkler, S., Wetzel, M., Ziegler, E., Kruchten, P., Werth, R., Henn, C., et al. (2011). New drug-like hydroxyphenylnaphthol steroidomimetics as potent and selective 17β-hydroxysteroid dehydrogenase type 1 inhibitors for the treatment of estrogen-dependent diseases. *J. Med. Chem.* 54, 534–547. doi: 10.1021/jm1009082

Masi, L., Becherini, L., Gennari, L., Amedei, A., Colli, E., Falchetti, A., et al. (2001). Polymorphism of the aromatase gene in postmenopausal Italian women: distribution and correlation with bone mass and fracture risk. *J. Clin. Endocrinol. Metab.* 86, 2263–2269. doi: 10.1210/jc.86.5.2263

Matsunaga, T., Hojo, A., Yamane, Y., Endo, S., El-Kabbani, O., and Hara, A. (2013). Pathophysiological roles of aldo-keto reductases (AKR1C1 and AKR1C3) in development of cisplatin resistance in human colon cancers. *Chem. Biol. Interact.* 202, 234–242. doi: 10.1016/j.cbi.2012.09.024

Matsuzaki, S., Canis, M., Pouly, J. L., Dechelotte, P. J., and Mage, G. (2006). Analysis of aromatase and 17β-hydroxysteroid dehydrogenase type 2 messenger ribonucleic acid expression in deep endometriosis and eutopic endometrium using laser capture microdissection. *Fertil. Steril.* 85, 308–313. doi: 10.1016/j.fertnstert.2005.08.017

Mauvais-Jarvis, F., Clegg, D. J., and Hevener, A. L. (2013). The role of estrogens in control of energy balance and glucose homeostasis. *Endocr. Rev.* 34, 309–338. doi: 10.1210/er.2012-1055

McCarthy, M. (2000). The "gender gap" in autoimmune disease. *Lancet* 356, 1088. doi: 10.1016/S0140-6736(05)74535-9

McEwen, B. S., and Milner, T. A. (2017). Understanding the broad influence of sex hormones and sex differences in the brain. *J. Neurosci. Res.* 95, 24–39. doi: 10.1002/jnr.23809

Meijer, D., Gelderblom, H., Karperien, M., Cleton-Jansen, A. M., Hogendoorn, P. C., and Bovee, J. V. (2011). Expression of aromatase and estrogen receptor alpha in chondrosarcoma, but no beneficial effect of inhibiting estrogen signaling both *in vitro* and *in vivo*. *Clin. Sarcoma Res.* 1:5. doi: 10.1186/2045-3329-1-5

Meloche, C. A., and Falany, C. N. (2001). Expression and characterization of the human 3 beta-hydroxysteroid sulfotransferases (SULT2B1a and SULT2B1b). *J. Steroid Biochem. Mol. Biol.* 77, 261–269. doi: 10.1016/S0960-0760(01)00064-4

Miki, Y., Nakata, T., Suzuki, T., Darnel, A. D., Moriya, T., Kaneko, C., et al. (2002). Systemic distribution of steroid sulfatase and estrogen sulfotransferase in human adult and fetal tissues. *J. Clin. Endocrinol. Metab.* 87, 5760–5768. doi: 10.1210/jc.2002-020670

Milewich, L., Garcia, R. L., and Johnson, A. R. (1983). Steroid sulfatase activity in human lung tissue and in endothelial pulmonary cells in culture. *J. Clin. Endocrinol. Metab.* 57, 8–14. doi: 10.1210/jcem-57-1-8

Miller, P. B., Parnell, B. A., Bushnell, G., Tallman, N., Forstein, D. A., Higdon, H. L III., et al. (2012a). Endometrial receptivity defects during IVF cycles with and without letrozole. *Hum. Reprod.* 27, 881–888. doi: 10.1093/humrep/der452

Miller, V. L., Lin, H. K., Murugan, P., Fan, M., Penning, T. M., Brame, L. S., et al. (2012b). Aldo-keto reductase family 1 member C3 (AKR1C3) is expressed in adenocarcinoma and squamous cell carcinoma but not small cell carcinoma. *Int. J. Clin. Exp. Pathol.* 5, 278–289.

Miller, W. L., and Auchus, R. J. (2011). The molecular biology, biochemistry, and physiology of human steroidogenesis and its disorders. *Endocr. Rev.* 32, 81–151. doi: 10.1210/er.2010-0013

Mindnich, R., Moller, G., and Adamski, J. (2004). The role of 17 beta-hydroxysteroid dehydrogenases. *Mol. Cell. Endocrinol.* 218, 7–20. doi: 10.1016/j.mce.2003.12.006

Miyaura, C., Toda, K., Inada, M., Ohshiba, T., Matsumoto, C., Okada, T., et al. (2001). Sex- and age-related response to aromatase deficiency in bone. *Biochem. Biophys. Res. Commun.* 280, 1062–1068. doi: 10.1006/bbrc.2001.4246

Moeller, G., and Adamski, J. (2006). Multifunctionality of human 17β-hydroxysteroid dehydrogenases. *Mol. Cell. Endocrinol.* 248, 47–55. doi: 10.1016/j.mce.2005.11.031

Moeller, G., and Adamski, J. (2009). Integrated view on 17β-hydroxysteroid dehydrogenases. *Mol. Cell. Endocrinol.* 301, 7–19. doi: 10.1016/j.mce.2008.10.040

Möller, G., Leenders, F., van Grunsven, E. G., Dolez, V., Qualmann, B., Kessels, M. M., et al. (1999). Characterization of the HSD17B4 gene: D-specific multifunctional protein 2/17β-hydroxysteroid dehydrogenase IV. *J. Steroid Biochem. Mol. Biol.* 69, 441–446. doi: 10.1016/S0960-0760(99)00066-7

Morgat, A., Axelsen, K. B., Lombardot, T., Alcantara, R., Aimo, L., Zerara, M., et al. (2015). Updates in Rhea–a manually curated resource of biochemical reactions. *Nucleic Acids Res.* 43, D459–D464. doi: 10.1093/nar/gku961

Mori, T., Ito, F., Matsushima, H., Takaoka, O., Koshiba, A., Tanaka, Y., et al. (2015). Dienogest reduces HSD17β1 expression and activity in endometriosis. *J. Endocrinol.* 225, 69–76. doi: 10.1530/JOE-15-0052

Morice, P., Leary, A., Creutzberg, C., Abu-Rustum, N., and Darai, E. (2015). Endometrial cancer. *Lancet* 387, 1094–1108. doi: 10.1016/S0140-6736(15)00130-0

Morishima, A., Grumbach, M. M., Simpson, E. R., Fisher, C., and Qin, K. (1995). Aromatase deficiency in male and female siblings caused by a novel mutation and the physiological role of estrogens. *J. Clin. Endocrinol. Metab.* 80, 3689–3698.

Mueller, J. W., Gilligan, L. C., Idkowiak, J., Arlt, W., and Foster, P. A. (2015). The regulation of steroid action by sulfation and desulfation. *Endocr. Rev.* 36, 526–563. doi: 10.1210/er.2015-1036

Muir, M., Romalo, G., Wolf, L., Elger, W., and Schweikert, H. U. (2004). Estrone sulfate is a major source of local estrogen formation in human bone. *J. Clin. Endocrinol. Metab.* 89, 4685–4692. doi: 10.1210/jc.2004-0049

Mukai, H., Tsurugizawa, T., Ogiue-Ikeda, M., Murakami, G., Hojo, Y., Ishii, H., et al. (2006). Local neurosteroid production in the hippocampus: influence on synaptic plasticity of memory. *Neuroendocrinology* 84, 255–263. doi: 10.1159/000097747

Mullis, P. E., Yoshimura, N., Kuhlmann, B., Lippuner, K., Jaeger, P., and Harada, H. (1997). Aromatase deficiency in a female who is compound heterozygote for two new point mutations in the P450arom gene: impact of estrogens on hypergonadotropic hypogonadism, multicystic ovaries, and bone densitometry in childhood. *J. Clin. Endocrinol. Metab.* 82, 1739–1745. doi: 10.1210/jc.82.6.1739

Munroe, D. G., and Chang, P. L. (1987). Tissue-specific expression of human arylsulfatase-C isozymes and steroid sulfatase. *Am. J. Hum. Genet.* 40, 102–114.

Murakami, G., Tanabe, N., Ishii, H. T., Ogiue-Ikeda, M., Tsurugizawa, T., Mukai, H., et al. (2006). Role of cytochrome p450 in synaptocrinology: endogenous estrogen synthesis in the brain hippocampus. *Drug Metab. Rev.* 38, 353–369. doi: 10.1080/03602530600724068

Musatov, S., Chen, W., Pfaff, D. W., Mobbs, C. V., Yang, X. J., Clegg, D. J., et al. (2007). Silencing of estrogen receptor alpha in the ventromedial nucleus of hypothalamus leads to metabolic syndrome. *Proc. Natl. Acad. Sci. U.S.A.* 104, 2501–2506. doi: 10.1073/pnas.0610787104

Nadal, A., Alonso-Magdalena, P., Soriano, S., Ripoll, C., Fuentes, E., Quesada, I., et al. (2011). Role of estrogen receptors alpha, beta and GPER1/GPR30 in pancreatic beta-cells. *Front Biosci (Landmark Ed)* 16, 251–260. doi: 10.2741/3686

Naftolin, F., Horvath, T. L., Jakab, R. L., Leranth, C., Harada, N., and Balthazart, J. (1996). Aromatase immunoreactivity in axon terminals of the vertebrate brain. An immunocytochemical study on quail, rat, monkey and human tissues. *Neuroendocrinology* 63, 149–155. doi: 10.1159/000126951

Naftolin, F., and MacLusky, N. J. (1982). Aromatase in the central nervous system. *Cancer Res* 42, 3274s—3276s.

Nakarai, C., Osawa, K., Akiyama, M., Matsubara, N., Ikeuchi, H., Yamano, T., et al. (2015). Expression of AKR1C3 and CNN3 as markers for detection of lymph node metastases in colorectal cancer. *Clin. Exp. Med.* 15, 333–341. doi: 10.1007/s10238-014-0298-1

Nayeb-Hashemi, H., and Kaunitz, J. D. (2009). Gastroduodenal mucosal defense. *Curr. Opin. Gastroenterol.* 25, 537–543. doi: 10.1097/MOG.0b013e328330da7b

Nemoto, Y., Toda, K., Ono, M., Fujikawa-Adachi, K., Saibara, T., Onishi, S., et al. (2000). Altered expression of fatty acid-metabolizing enzymes in aromatase-deficient mice. *J. Clin. Invest.* 105, 1819–1825. doi: 10.1172/JCI9575

Niikawa, H., Suzuki, T., Miki, Y., Suzuki, S., Nagasaki, S., Akahira, J., et al. (2008). Intratumoral estrogens and estrogen receptors in human non-small cell lung carcinoma. *Clin. Cancer Res.* 14, 4417–4426. doi: 10.1158/1078-0432.CCR-07-1950

Nishimura, M., and Naito, S. (2006). Tissue-specific mRNA expression profiles of human phase I metabolizing enzymes except for cytochrome P450 and phase II metabolizing enzymes. *Drug Metab. Pharmacokinet.* 21, 357–374. doi: 10.2133/dmpk.21.357

Noble, L. S., Simpson, E. R., Johns, A., and Bulun, S. E. (1996). Aromatase expression in endometriosis. *J. Clin. Endocrinol. Metab.* 81, 174–179.

Noble, L. S., Takayama, K., Zeitoun, K. M., Putman, J. M., Johns, D. A., Hinshelwood, M. M., et al. (1997). Prostaglandin E2 stimulates aromatase expression in endometriosis-derived stromal cells. *J. Clin. Endocrinol. Metab.* 82, 600–606. doi: 10.1210/jc.82.2.600

Noël, J. C., Anaf, V., Borghese, B., Vaiman, D., Fayt, I., and Chapron, C. (2011). The steroidogenic factor-1 protein is not expressed in various forms of endometriosis but is strongly present in ovarian cortical or medullary mesenchymatous cells adjacent to endometriotic foci. *Fertil. Steril.* 95, 2655–2657. doi: 10.1016/j.fertnstert.2011.01.131

Nokelainen, P., Peltoketo, H., Mustonen, M., and Vihko, P. (2000). Expression of mouse 17β-hydroxysteroid dehydrogenase/17-ketosteroid reductase type 7 in the ovary, uterus, and placenta: localization from implantation to late pregnancy. *Endocrinology* 141, 772–778. doi: 10.1210/endo.141.2.7309

Oduwole, O. O., Isomaa, V. V., Nokelainen, P. A., Stenback, F., and Vihko, P. T. (2002). Downregulation of estrogen-metabolizing 17 beta-hydroxysteroid dehydrogenase type 2 expression correlates inversely with Ki67 proliferation marker in colon-cancer development. *Int. J. Cancer* 97, 1–6. doi: 10.1002/ijc.1567

Oduwole, O. O., Makinen, J. M., Isomaa, V. V., Karttunen, T. J., and Vihko, P. T. (2003a). Sex steroid metabolism in human gastric mucosa: 17 beta-hydroxysteroid dehydrogenase type 2 in normal, inflamed and neoplastic gastric tissues. *Anticancer Res.* 23, 3889–3897.

Oduwole, O. O., Makinen, M. J., Isomaa, V. V., Pulkka, A., Jernvall, P., Karttunen, T. J., et al. (2003b). 17β-hydroxysteroid dehydrogenase type 2: independent prognostic significance and evidence of estrogen protection in female patients with colon cancer. *J. Steroid Biochem. Mol. Biol.* 87, 133–140. doi: 10.1016/j.jsbmb.2003.08.008

Ohno, S., Nishikawa, K., Honda, Y., and Nakajin, S. (2008). Expression in *E. coli* and tissue distribution of the human homologue of the mouse Ke 6 gene, 17β-hydroxysteroid dehydrogenase type 8. *Mol. Cell. Biochem.* 309, 209–215. doi: 10.1007/s11010-007-9637-9

Olson, S. H., Bandera, E. V., and Orlow, I. (2007). Variants in estrogen biosynthesis genes, sex steroid hormone levels, and endometrial cancer: a HuGE review. *Am. J. Epidemiol.* 165, 235–245. doi: 10.1093/aje/kwk015

Osinski, M., Wirstlein, P., Wender-Ozegowska, E., Mikolajczyk, M., Jagodzinski, P. P., and Szczepanska, M. (2018). HSD3B2, HSD17B1, HSD17B2, ESR1, ESR2 and AR expression in infertile women with endometriosis. *Ginekol. Pol.* 89, 125–134. doi: 10.5603/GP.a2018.0022

Oz, O. K., Millsaps, R., Welch, R., Birch, J., and Zerwekh, J. E. (2001). Expression of aromatase in the human growth plate. *J. Mol. Endocrinol.* 27, 249–253. doi: 10.1677/jme.0.0270249

Oz, O. K., Zerwekh, J. E., Fisher, C., Graves, K., Nanu, L., Millsaps, R., et al. (2000). Bone has a sexually dimorphic response to aromatase deficiency. *J. Bone Miner. Res.* 15, 507–514. doi: 10.1359/jbmr.2000.15.3.507

Palmer, B. F., and Clegg, D. J. (2015). The sexual dimorphism of obesity. *Mol. Cell. Endocrinol.* 402, 113–119. doi: 10.1016/j.mce.2014.11.029

Palmieri, C., Stein, R. C., Liu, X., Hudson, E., Nicholas, H., Sasano, H., et al. (2017a). IRIS study: a phase II study of the steroid sulfatase inhibitor Irosustat when added to an aromatase inhibitor in ER-positive breast cancer patients. *Breast Cancer Res. Treat.* 165, 343–353. doi: 10.1007/s10549-017-4328-z

Palmieri, C., Szydlo, R., Miller, M., Barker, L., Patel, N. H., Sasano, H., et al. (2017b). IPET study: an FLT-PET window study to assess the activity of the steroid sulfatase inhibitor irosustat in early breast cancer. *Breast Cancer Res. Treat.* 166, 527–539. doi: 10.1007/s10549-017-4427-x

Park, A. L., Lin, H. K., Yang, Q., Sing, C. W., Fan, M., Mapstone, T. B., et al. (2010). Differential expression of type 2, 3α/type 5, 17β-hydroxysteroid dehydrogenase (AKR1C3) in tumors of the central nervous system. *Int. J. Clin. Exp. Pathol.* 3, 743–754.

Park, Y. S., Gauna, A. E., and Cha, S. (2015). Mouse models of primary Sjogren's syndrome. *Curr. Pharm. Des.* 21, 2350–2364. doi: 10.2174/1381612821666150316120024

Pathirage, N., Di Nezza, L. A., Salmonsen, L. A., Jobling, T., Simpson, E. R., and Clyne, C. D. (2006). Expression of aromatase, estrogen receptors, and their coactivators in patients with endometrial cancer. *Fertil. Steril.* 86, 469–472. doi: 10.1016/j.fertnstert.2005.12.057

Pautier, P., Vergote, I., Joly, F., Melichar, B., Kutarska, E., Hall, G., et al. (2017). A Phase 2, randomized, open-label study of irosustat versus megestrol acetate in advanced endometrial cancer. *Int. J. Gynecol. Cancer* 27, 258–266. doi: 10.1097/IGC.0000000000000862

Pearson Murphy, B. E., Steinberg, S. I., Hu, F. Y., and Allison, C. M. (2001). Neuroactive ring A-reduced metabolites of progesterone in human plasma during pregnancy: elevated levels of 5 alpha-dihydroprogesterone in depressed patients during the latter half of pregnancy. *J. Clin. Endocrinol. Metab.* 86, 5981–5987. doi: 10.1210/jcem.86.12.8122

Pelletier, G., Luu-The, V., Tetu, B., and Labrie, F. (1999). Immunocytochemical localization of type 5, 17β-hydroxysteroid dehydrogenase in human reproductive tissues. *J. Histochem. Cytochem.* 47, 731–738. doi: 10.1177/002215549904700602

Penning, T. M. (2017). Aldo-Keto Reductase (AKR) 1C3 inhibitors: a patent review. *Expert Opin. Ther. Pat.* 27, 1329–1340. doi: 10.1080/13543776.2017.1379503

Penning, T. M., Burczynski, M. E., Jez, J. M., Hung, C. F., Lin, H. K., Ma, H., et al. (2000). Human 3α-hydroxysteroid dehydrogenase isoforms (AKR1C1-AKR1C4) of the aldo-keto reductase superfamily: functional plasticity and tissue distribution reveals roles in the inactivation and formation of male and female sex hormones. *Biochem. J.* 351, 67–77. doi: 10.1042/bj3510067

Penning, T. M., Jin, Y., Steckelbroeck, S., Lanisnik Rizner, T., and Lewis, M. (2004). Structure-function of human 3 alpha-hydroxysteroid dehydrogenases: genes and proteins. *Mol. Cell. Endocrinol.* 215, 63–72. doi: 10.1016/j.mce.2003.11.006

Perez Carrion, R., Alberola Candel, V., Calabresi, F., Michel, R. T., Santos, R., Delozier, T., et al. (1994). Comparison of the selective aromatase inhibitor formestane with tamoxifen as first-line hormonal therapy in postmenopausal women with advanced breast cancer. *Ann. Oncol.* 5(Suppl. 7), S19–S24.

Pezzi, V., Mathis, J. M., Rainey, W. E., and Carr, B. R. (2003). Profiling transcript levels for steroidogenic enzymes in fetal tissues. *J. Steroid Biochem. Mol. Biol.* 87, 181–189. doi: 10.1016/j.jsbmb.2003.07.006

Piccinato, C. A., Neme, R. M., Torres, N., Sanches, L. R., Cruz Derogis, P. B., Brudniewski, H. F., et al. (2016a). Increased expression of CYP1A1 and CYP1B1 in ovarian/peritoneal endometriotic lesions. *Reproduction* 151, 683–692. doi: 10.1530/REP-15-0581

Piccinato, C. A., Neme, R. M., Torres, N., Sanches, L. R., Derogis, P., Brudniewski, H. F., et al. (2016b). Effects of steroid hormone on estrogen sulfotransferase and on steroid sulfatase expression in endometriosis tissue and stromal cells. *J. Steroid Biochem. Mol. Biol.* 158, 117–126. doi: 10.1016/j.jsbmb.2015.12.025

Piekorz, R. P., Gingras, S., Hoffmeyer, A., Ihle, J. N., and Weinstein, Y. (2005). Regulation of progesterone levels during pregnancy and parturition by signal transducer and activator of transcription 5 and 20α-hydroxysteroid dehydrogenase. *Mol. Endocrinol.* 19, 431–440. doi: 10.1210/me.2004-0302

Platia, M. P., Fencl, M. D., Elkind-Hirsch, K. E., Canick, J. A., and Tulchinsky, D. (1984). Estrone sulfatase activity in the human brain and estrone sulfate levels in the normal menstrual cycle. *J. Steroid Biochem.* 21, 237–241. doi: 10.1016/0022-4731(84)90275-9

Pohl, O., Bestel, E., and Gotteland, J. P. (2014). Synergistic effects of E2MATE and norethindrone acetate on steroid sulfatase inhibition: a randomized phase I proof-of-principle clinical study in women of reproductive age. *Reprod. Sci.* 21, 1256–1265. doi: 10.1177/1933719114522526

Pollow, K., Lubbert, H., Jeske, R., and Pollow, B. (1975a). Studies on 17β-hydroxysteroid dehydrogenase in human endometrium and endometrial carcinoma. *Acta Endocrinol.* 79, 146–156.

Pollow, K., Lubbert, H., and Pollow, B. (1975b). Studies on 17 beta-hydroxysteroid dehydrogenase in human endometrium and endometrial carcinoma. III. Partial purification and characterization of the microsomal enzyme. *Acta Endocrinol (Copenh)* 80, 355-364.

Pollow, K., Lubbert, H., and Pollow, B. (1976). On the mitochondrial 17β-hydroxysteroid dehydrogenase from human endometrium and endometrial carcinoma: characterization and intramitochondrial distribution. *J. Steroid Biochem.* 7, 45–50. doi: 10.1016/0022-4731(76)90163-1

Polow, K., Lubbert, H., Boquoi, E., Kreutzer, G., Jeske, R., and Pollow, B. (1975). Studies on 17β-hydroxysteroid dehydrogenase in human endometrium and endometrial carcinoma I. Subcellular distribution and variations of specific enzyme activity. *Acta Endocrinol (Copenh)* 79, 134–145.

Prehn, C., Moller, G., and Adamski, J. (2009). Recent advances in 17β-hydroxysteroid dehydrogenases. *J. Steroid Biochem. Mol. Biol.* 114, 72–77. doi: 10.1016/j.jsbmb.2008.12.024

Prizant, H., and Hammes, S. R. (2016). Minireview: lymphangioleiomyomatosis (LAM): the "Other" steroid-sensitive cancer. *Endocrinology* 157, 3374–3383. doi: 10.1210/en.2016-1395

Prossnitz, E. R., and Barton, M. (2011). The G-protein-coupled estrogen receptor GPER in health and disease. *Nat. Rev. Endocrinol.* 7, 715–726. doi: 10.1038/nrendo.2011.122

Prost, O., and Adessi, G. L. (1983). Estrone and dehydroepiandrosterone sulfatase activities in normal and pathological human endometrium biopsies. *J. Clin. Endocrinol. Metab.* 56, 653–661. doi: 10.1210/jcem-56-4-653

Purohit, A., Flanagan, A. M., and Reed, M. J. (1992). Estrogen synthesis by osteoblast cell lines. *Endocrinology* 131, 2027–2029. doi: 10.1210/endo.131.4.1396346

Purohit, A., and Foster, P. A. (2012). Steroid sulfatase inhibitors for estrogen- and androgen-dependent cancers. *J. Endocrinol.* 212, 99–110. doi: 10.1530/JOE-11-0266

Purohit, A., Fusi, L., Brosens, J., Woo, L. W., Potter, B. V., and Reed, M. J. (2008). Inhibition of steroid sulphatase activity in endometriotic implants by 667 COUMATE: a potential new therapy. *Hum. Reprod.* 23, 290–297. doi: 10.1093/humrep/dem308

Qaiser, M. Z., Dolman, D. E. M., Begley, D. J., Abbott, N. J., Cazacu-Davidescu, M., Corol, D. I., et al. (2017). Uptake and metabolism of sulphated steroids by the blood-brain barrier in the adult male rat. *J. Neurochem.* 142, 672–685. doi: 10.1111/jnc.14117

Qian, Y. M., Sun, X. J., Tong, M. H., Li, X. P., Richa, J., and Song, W. C. (2001). Targeted disruption of the mouse estrogen sulfotransferase gene reveals a role of estrogen metabolism in intracrine and paracrine estrogen regulation. *Endocrinology* 142, 5342–5350. doi: 10.1210/endo.142.12.8540

Qin, K., Ehrmann, D. A., Cox, N., Refetoff, S., and Rosenfield, R. L. (2006). Identification of a functional polymorphism of the human type 5, 17β-hydroxysteroid dehydrogenase gene associated with polycystic ovary syndrome. *J. Clin. Endocrinol. Metab.* 91, 270–276. doi: 10.1210/jc.2005-2012

Quinkler, M., Sinha, B., Tomlinson, J. W., Bujalska, I. J., Stewart, P. M., and Arlt, W. (2004). Androgen generation in adipose tissue in women with simple obesity–a site-specific role for 17β-hydroxysteroid dehydrogenase type 5. *J. Endocrinol.* 183, 331–342. doi: 10.1677/joe.1.05762

Rajkowski, K. M., Robel, P., and Baulieu, E. E. (1997). Hydroxysteroid sulfotransferase activity in the rat brain and liver as a function of age and sex. *Steroids* 62, 427–436. doi: 10.1016/S0039-128X(97)00013-5

Rantakari, P., Lagerbohm, H., Kaimainen, M., Suomela, J. P., Strauss, L., Sainio, K., et al. (2010). Hydroxysteroid (17{beta}) dehydrogenase 12 is essential for mouse organogenesis and embryonic survival. *Endocrinology* 151, 1893–1901. doi: 10.1210/en.2009-0929

Rantakari, P., Strauss, L., Kiviranta, R., Lagerbohm, H., Paviala, J., Holopainen, I., et al. (2008). Placenta defects and embryonic lethality resulting from disruption of mouse hydroxysteroid (17-beta) dehydrogenase 2 gene. *Mol. Endocrinol.* 22, 665–675. doi: 10.1210/me.2007-0257

Rauschenberger, K., Scholer, K., Sass, J. O., Sauer, S., Djuric, Z., Rumig, C., et al. (2010). A non-enzymatic function of 17β-hydroxysteroid dehydrogenase type 10 is required for mitochondrial integrity and cell survival. *EMBO Mol. Med.* 2, 51–62. doi: 10.1002/emmm.200900055

Rawłuszko, A. A., Horbacka, K., Krokowicz, P., and Jagodzinski, P. P. (2011). Decreased expression of 17β-hydroxysteroid dehydrogenase type 1 is associated with DNA hypermethylation in colorectal cancer located in the proximal colon. *BMC Cancer* 11:522. doi: 10.1186/1471-2407-11-522

Reddy, D. S. (2010). Neurosteroids: endogenous role in the human brain and therapeutic potentials. *Prog. Brain Res.* 186, 113–137. doi: 10.1016/B978-0-444-53630-3.00008-7

Reed, M. J., Purohit, A., Woo, L. W., Newman, S. P., and Potter, B. V. (2005). Steroid sulfatase: molecular biology, regulation, and inhibition. *Endocr. Rev.* 26, 171–202. doi: 10.1210/er.2004-0003

Rege, J., Karashima, S., Lerario, A. M., Smith, J. M., Auchus, R. J., Kasa-Vubu, J. Z., et al. (2016). Age-dependent increases in adrenal cytochrome b5 and serum 5-androstenediol-3-sulfate. *J. Clin. Endocrinol. Metab.* 101, 4585–4593. doi: 10.1210/jc.2016-2864

Rennert, G., Rennert, H. S., Pinchev, M., Lavie, O., and Gruber, S. B. (2009). Use of hormone replacement therapy and the risk of colorectal cancer. *J. Clin. Oncol.* 27, 4542–4547. doi: 10.1200/JCO.2009.22.0764

Rhee, H. S., Oh, S. H., Ko, B. J., Han, D. M., Jeon, B. H., Park, H., et al. (2003). Expression of 3β-hydroxysteroid dehydrogenase and P450 side chain cleavage enzyme in the human uterine endometrium. *Exp. Mol. Med.* 35, 160–166. doi: 10.1038/emm.2003.22

Riches, Z., Stanley, E. L., Bloomer, J. C., and Coughtrie, M. W. (2009). Quantitative evaluation of the expression and activity of five major sulfotransferases (SULTs) in human tissues: the SULT "pie". *Drug Metab. Dispos.* 37, 2255–2261. doi: 10.1124/dmd.109.028399

Riggs, B. L., Khosla, S., and Melton, L. J. III. (2002). Sex steroids and the construction and conservation of the adult skeleton. *Endocr. Rev.* 23, 279–302. doi: 10.1210/edrv.23.3.0465

Rižner, T. L. (2013). Estrogen biosynthesis, phase I and phase II metabolism, and action in endometrial cancer. *Mol. Cell. Endocrinol.* 381, 124–139. doi: 10.1016/j.mce.2013.07.026

Rižner, T. L. (2016). The important roles of steroid sulfatase and sulfotransferases in gynecological diseases. *Front. Pharmacol.* 7:30. doi: 10.3389/fphar.2016.00030

Rižner, T. L., and Penning, T. M. (2014). Role of aldo-keto reductase family 1 (AKR1) enzymes in human steroid metabolism. *Steroids* 79, 49–63. doi: 10.1016/j.steroids.2013.10.012

Rizner, T. L., Smuc, T., Rupreht, R., Sinkovec, J., and Penning, T. M. (2006). AKR1C1 and AKR1C3 may determine progesterone and estrogen ratios in endometrial cancer. *Mol. Cell. Endocrinol.* 248, 126–135. doi: 10.1016/j.mce.2005.10.009

Rižner, T. L., Thalhammer, T., and Ozvegy-Laczka, C. (2017). The importance of steroid uptake and intracrine action in endometrial and ovarian cancers. *Front. Pharmacol.* 8:346. doi: 10.3389/fphar.2017.00346

Rodríguez-Sanz, M., Garcia-Giralt, N., Prieto-Alhambra, D., Servitja, S., Balcells, S., Pecorelli, R., et al. (2015). CYP11A1 expression in bone is associated with aromatase inhibitor-related bone loss. *J. Mol. Endocrinol.* 55, 69–79. doi: 10.1530/JME-15-0079

Rose, P. G., Brunetto, V. L., VanLe, L., Bell, J., Walker, J. L., and Lee, R. B. (2000). A phase II trial of anastrozole in advanced recurrent or persistent endometrial carcinoma: a Gynecologic Oncology Group study. *Gynecol. Oncol.* 78, 212–216. doi: 10.1006/gyno.2000.5865

Roshan, M. H., Tambo, A., and Pace, N. P. (2016). The role of testosterone in colorectal carcinoma: pathomechanisms and open questions. *EPMA J.* 7, 22. doi: 10.1186/s13167-016-0071-5

Rosner, W., Hankinson, S. E., Sluss, P. M., Vesper, H. W., and Wierman, M. E. (2013). Challenges to the measurement of estradiol: an endocrine society position statement. *J. Clin. Endocrinol. Metab.* 98, 1376–1387. doi: 10.1210/jc.2012-3780

Rubin, G. L., Harrold, A. J., Mills, J. A., Falany, C. N., and Coughtrie, M. W. (1999). Regulation of sulphotransferase expression in the endometrium during the menstrual cycle, by oral contraceptives and during early pregnancy. *Mol. Hum. Reprod.* 5, 995–1002. doi: 10.1093/molehr/5.11.995

Sahu, B., Sun, W., Perusek, L., Parmar, V., Le, Y. Z., Griswold, M. D., et al. (2015). Conditional ablation of retinol dehydrogenase 10 in the retinal pigmented epithelium causes delayed dark adaption in mice. *J. Biol. Chem.* 290, 27239–27247. doi: 10.1074/jbc.M115.682096

Saito, H., and Yanaihara, T. (1998). Steroid formation in osteoblast-like cells. *J. Int. Med. Res.* 26, 1–12. doi: 10.1177/030006059802600101

Saitoh, Y., Sasano, H., Naganuma, H., Ohtani, H., Sasano, N., Ohuchi, A., et al. (1992). *De novo* expression of aromatase in gastric carcinoma. Light and electron microscopic immunohistochemical and immunoblot study. *Pathol. Res. Pract.* 188, 53–60. doi: 10.1016/S0344-0338(11)81156-8

Sakiani, S., Olsen, N. J., and Kovacs, W. J. (2013). Gonadal steroids and humoral immunity. *Nat. Rev. Endocrinol.* 9, 56–62. doi: 10.1038/nrendo.2012.206

Sakurai, N., Miki, Y., Suzuki, T., Watanabe, K., Narita, T., Ando, K., et al. (2006). Systemic distribution and tissue localizations of human 17β-hydroxysteroid dehydrogenase type 12. *J. Steroid Biochem. Mol. Biol.* 99, 174–181. doi: 10.1016/j.jsbmb.2006.01.010

Salas, S., Jezequel, P., Campion, L., Deville, J. L., Chibon, F., Bartoli, C., et al. (2009). Molecular characterization of the response to chemotherapy in conventional osteosarcomas: predictive value of HSD17B10 and IFITM2. *Int. J. Cancer* 125, 851–860. doi: 10.1002/ijc.24457

Salman, E. D., Faye-Petersen, O., and Falany, C. N. (2011). Hydroxysteroid sulfotransferase 2B1b expression and localization in normal human brain. *Horm. Mol. Biol. Clin. Investig.* 8, 445–454. doi: 10.1515/HMBCI.2011.117

Salman, E. D., Kadlubar, S. A., and Falany, C. N. (2009). Expression and localization of cytosolic sulfotransferase (SULT) 1A1 and SULT1A3 in normal human brain. *Drug Metab. Dispos.* 37, 706–709. doi: 10.1124/dmd.108.025767

Saloniemi, T., Jarvensivu, P., Koskimies, P., Jokela, H., Lamminen, T., Ghaem-Maghami, S., et al. (2010). Novel hydroxysteroid (17β) dehydrogenase 1 inhibitors reverse estrogen-induced endometrial hyperplasia in transgenic mice. *Am. J. Pathol.* 176, 1443–1451. doi: 10.2353/ajpath.2010.090325

Sánchez-Guijo, A., Neunzig, J., Gerber, A., Oji, V., Hartmann, M. F., Schuppe, H. C., et al. (2016). Role of steroid sulfatase in steroid homeostasis and characterization of the sulfated steroid pathway: Evidence from steroid sulfatase deficiency. *Mol. Cell. Endocrinol.* 437, 142–153. doi: 10.1016/j.mce.2016.08.019

Sasano, H., Takashashi, K., Satoh, F., Nagura, H., and Harada, N. (1998). Aromatase in the human central nervous system. *Clin. Endocrinol. (Oxf).* 48, 325–329. doi: 10.1046/j.1365-2265.1998.00390.x

Sasano, H., Uzuki, M., Sawai, T., Nagura, H., Matsunaga, G., Kashimoto, O., et al. (1997). Aromatase in human bone tissue. *J. Bone Miner. Res.* 12, 1416–1423. doi: 10.1359/jbmr.1997.12.9.1416

Sathish, V., Martin, Y. N., and Prakash, Y. S. (2015). Sex steroid signaling: implications for lung diseases. *Pharmacol. Ther.* 150, 94–108. doi: 10.1016/j.pharmthera.2015.01.007

Sato, R., Suzuki, T., Katayose, Y., Miura, K., Shiiba, K., Miki, Y., et al. (2012). Aromatase in colon carcinoma. *Anticancer Res.* 32, 3069–3075.

Sato, R., Suzuki, T., Katayose, Y., Miura, K., Shiiba, K., Tateno, H., et al. (2009). Steroid sulfatase and estrogen sulfotransferase in colon carcinoma: regulators of intratumoral estrogen concentrations and potent prognostic factors. *Cancer Res.* 69, 914–922. doi: 10.1158/0008-5472.CAN-08-0906

Schweikert, H. U., Wolf, L., and Romalo, G. (1995). Oestrogen formation from androstenedione in human bone. *Clin. Endocrinol. (Oxf).* 43, 37–42. doi: 10.1111/j.1365-2265.1995.tb01890.x

Scublinsky, A., Marin, C., and Gurpide, E. (1976). Localization of estradiol 17β dehydrogenase in human endometrium. *J. Steroid Biochem.* 7, 745–747. doi: 10.1016/0022-4731(76)90174-6

Segawa, T., Shozu, M., Murakami, K., Kasai, T., Shinohara, K., Nomura, K., et al. (2005). Aromatase expression in stromal cells of endometrioid endometrial cancer correlates with poor survival. *Clin. Cancer Res.* 11, 2188–2194. doi: 10.1158/1078-0432.CCR-04-1859

Selcer, K. W., and Difrancesca, H. M. (2012). Characterization of steroid sulfatase in the MC3T3-E1 mouse pre-osteoblastic cell line. *Steroids* 77, 696–702. doi: 10.1016/j.steroids.2012.02.024

Setiawan, V. W., Doherty, J. A., Shu, X. O., Akbari, M. R., Chen, C., De Vivo, I., et al. (2009). Two estrogen-related variants in $CYP_{19}A_1$ and endometrial cancer risk: a pooled analysis in the epidemiology of endometrial cancer consortium. *Cancer Epidemiol. Biomarkers Prev.* 18, 242–247. doi: 10.1158/1055-9965.EPI-08-0689

Setiawan, V. W., Hankinson, S. E., Colditz, G. A., Hunter, D. J., and De Vivo, I. (2004). HSD17B1 gene polymorphisms and risk of endometrial and breast cancer. *Cancer Epidemiol. Biomarkers Prev.* 13, 213–219. doi: 10.1158/1055-9965.EPI-03-0241

Shang, E., Lai, K., Packer, A. I., Paik, J., Blaner, W. S., de Morais Vieira, M., et al. (2002). Targeted disruption of the mouse cis-retinol dehydrogenase gene: visual and nonvisual functions. *J. Lipid Res.* 43, 590–597.

Shehu, A., Mao, J., Gibori, G. B., Halperin, J., Le, J., Devi, Y. S., et al. (2008). Prolactin receptor-associated protein/17β-hydroxysteroid dehydrogenase type 7 gene (Hsd17b7) plays a crucial role in embryonic development and fetal survival. *Mol. Endocrinol.* 22, 2268–2277. doi: 10.1210/me.2008-0165

Shen, Z., Peng, Z., Sun, Y., Vaananen, H. K., and Poutanen, M. (2008). Overexpression of human hydroxysteroid (17β) dehydrogenase 2 induces disturbance in skeletal development in young male mice. *J. Bone Miner. Res.* 23, 1217–1226. doi: 10.1359/jbmr.080322

Shi, L., Yang, X., Dong, X., and Zhang, B. (2016). Polymorphism of HSD17B1 Ser312Gly with Cancer Risk: Evidence from 66,147 Subjects. *Twin Res. Hum. Genet.* 19, 136–145. doi: 10.1017/thg.2016.6

Shim, G. J., Warner, M., Kim, H. J., Andersson, S., Liu, L., Ekman, J., et al. (2004). Aromatase-deficient mice spontaneously develop a lymphoproliferative autoimmune disease resembling Sjogren's syndrome. *Proc. Natl. Acad. Sci. U.S.A.* 101, 12628–12633. doi: 10.1073/pnas.0405099101

Shimizu, K. (1979). Metabolism of [17-^{2}H]pregnenolone into 5-[17β-^{2}H, 17α-^{18}O]androstene-3β, 17α-diol and other products by incubation with the microsomal fraction of boar testis under $^{18}O_2$ atmosphere. *Biochim. Biophys. Acta* 575, 37–45. doi: 10.1016/0005-2760(79)90128-0

Shimodaira, M., Nakayama, T., Sato, I., Sato, N., Izawa, N., Mizutani, Y., et al. (2012). Estrogen synthesis genes $CYP_{19}A_1$, HSD_3B_1, and HSD_3B_2 in hypertensive disorders of pregnancy. *Endocrine* 42, 700–707. doi: 10.1007/s12020-012-9699-7

Shimodaira, M., Nakayama, T., Sato, N., Aoi, N., Sato, M., Izumi, Y., et al. (2010). Association of HSD3B1 and HSD3B2 gene polymorphisms with essential hypertension, aldosterone level, and left ventricular structure. *Eur. J. Endocrinol.* 163, 671–680. doi: 10.1530/EJE-10-0428

Siegfried, J. M., and Stabile, L. P. (2014). Estrongenic steroid hormones in lung cancer. *Semin. Oncol.* 41, 5–16. doi: 10.1053/j.seminoncol.2013.12.009

Simard, J., Ricketts, M. L., Gingras, S., Soucy, P., Feltus, F. A., and Melner, M. H. (2005). Molecular biology of the 3β-hydroxysteroid dehydrogenase/Δ^5-Δ^4 isomerase gene family. *Endocr. Rev.* 26, 525–582. doi: 10.1210/er.2002-0050

Simard, M., Plante, J., Boucher, M., Provost, P. R., and Tremblay, Y. (2010). Type 2 and 5, 17β-hydroxysteroid dehydrogenases and androgen receptor in human fetal lungs. *Mol. Cell. Endocrinol.* 319, 79–87. doi: 10.1016/j.mce.2009.12.007

Simoens, S., Dunselman, G., Dirksen, C., Hummelshoj, L., Bokor, A., Brandes, I., et al. (2012). The burden of endometriosis: costs and quality of life of women with endometriosis and treated in referral centres. *Hum. Reprod.* 27, 1292–1299. doi: 10.1093/humrep/des073

Simoens, S., Hummelshoj, L., Dunselman, G., Brandes, I., Dirksen, C., and D'Hooghe, T. (2011). Endometriosis cost assessment (the EndoCost study): a cost-of-illness study protocol. *Gynecol. Obstet. Invest.* 71, 170–176. doi: 10.1159/000316055

Singh, M. M., Trivedi, R. N., Chauhan, S. C., Srivastava, V. M., Makker, A., Chowdhury, S. R., et al. (1996). Uterine estradiol and progesterone receptor concentration, activities of certain antioxidant enzymes and dehydrogenases and histoarchitecture in relation to time of secretion of nidatory estrogen and high endometrial sensitivity in rat. *J. Steroid Biochem. Mol. Biol.* 59, 215–224. doi: 10.1016/S0960-0760(96)00102-1

Singhal, N., Vatandoust, S., and Brown, M. P. (2015). Phase II study evaluating efficacy and safety of everolimus with letrozole for management of advanced (unresectable or metastatic) non-small cell lung cancer after failure of platinum-based treatment: a preliminary analysis of toxicity. *Cancer Chemother. Pharmacol.* 75, 325–331. doi: 10.1007/s00280-014-2644-0

Sinreih, M., Anko, M., Zukunft, S., Adamski, J., and Rizner, T. L. (2014). Important roles of the AKR1C2 and SRD5A1 enzymes in progesterone metabolism in endometrial cancer model cell lines. *Chem. Biol. Interact.* 234, 297–308. doi: 10.1016/j.cbi.2014.11.012.

Sinreih, M., Hevir, N., and Rizner, T. L. (2013). Altered expression of genes involved in progesterone biosynthesis, metabolism and action in endometrial cancer. *Chem. Biol. Interact.* 202, 210–217. doi: 10.1016/j.cbi.2012.11.012

Sinreih, M., Knific, T., Anko, M., Hevir, N., Vouk, K., Jerin, A., et al. (2017a). The significance of the sulfatase pathway for local estrogen formation in endometrial cancer. *Front. Pharmacol.* 8:368. doi: 10.3389/fphar.2017.00368

Sinreih, M., Stupar, S., Cemazar, L., Verdenik, I., Frkovic Grazio, S., Smrkolj, S., et al. (2017b). STAR and AKR1B10 are down-regulated in high-grade endometrial cancer. *J. Steroid Biochem. Mol. Biol.*. doi: 10.1016/j.jsbmb.2017.02.015

Sivik, T. (2012). Elucidating the *Role* of 17β *Hydroxysteroid Dehydrogenase Type* 14 in *Normal Physiology and in Breast Cancer*. Department of Clinical and Experimental Medicine: Linköping University (Linköping).

Skjefstad, K., Grindstad, T., Khanehkenari, M. R., Richardsen, E., Donnem, T., Kilvaer, T., et al. (2016). Prognostic relevance of estrogen receptor α, β and aromatase expression in non-small cell lung cancer. *Steroids* 113, 5–13. doi: 10.1016/j.steroids.2016.05.008

Slominski, A., Zbytek, B., Nikolakis, G., Manna, P. R., Skobowiat, C., Zmijewski, M., et al. (2013). Steroidogenesis in the skin: implications for local immune functions. *J. Steroid Biochem. Mol. Biol.* 137, 107–123. doi: 10.1016/j.jsbmb.2013.02.006

Slomovitz, B. M., Jiang, Y., Yates, M. S., Soliman, P. T., Johnston, T., Nowakowski, M., et al. (2015). Phase II study of everolimus and letrozole in patients with recurrent endometrial carcinoma. *J. Clin. Oncol.* 33, 930–936. doi: 10.1200/JCO.2014.58.3401

Smith, A., Contreras, C., Ko, K. H., Chow, J., Dong, X., Tuo, B., et al. (2008). Gender-specific protection of estrogen against gastric acid-induced duodenal injury: stimulation of duodenal mucosal bicarbonate secretion. *Endocrinology* 149, 4554–4566. doi: 10.1210/en.2007-1597

Smith, E. P., Boyd, J., Frank, G. R., Takahashi, H., Cohen, R. M., Specker, B., et al. (1994). Estrogen resistance caused by a mutation in the estrogen-receptor gene in a man. *N. Engl. J. Med.* 331, 1056–1061. doi: 10.1056/NEJM199410203311604

Smuc, T., Hevir, N., Ribic-Pucelj, M., Husen, B., Thole, H., and Rizner, T. L. (2009). Disturbed estrogen and progesterone action in ovarian endometriosis. *Mol. Cell. Endocrinol.* 301, 59–64. doi: 10.1016/j.mce.2008.07.020

Smuc, T., Pucelj, M. R., Sinkovec, J., Husen, B., Thole, H., and Lanisnik Rizner, T. (2007). Expression analysis of the genes involved in estradiol and progesterone action in human ovarian endometriosis. *Gynecol. Endocrinol.* 23, 105–111. doi: 10.1080/09513590601152219

Smuc, T., and Rizner, T. L. (2009). Aberrant pre-receptor regulation of estrogen and progesterone action in endometrial cancer. *Mol. Cell. Endocrinol.* 301, 74–82. doi: 10.1016/j.mce.2008.09.019

Smuc, T., Rupreht, R., Sinkovec, J., Adamski, J., and Rizner, T. L. (2006). Expression analysis of estrogen-metabolizing enzymes in human endometrial cancer. *Mol. Cell. Endocrinol.* 248, 114–117. doi: 10.1016/j.mce.2005.10.013

Soma, K. K., Rendon, N. M., Boonstra, R., Albers, H. E., and Demas, G. E. (2015). DHEA effects on brain and behavior: insights from comparative studies of aggression. *J. Steroid Biochem. Mol. Biol.* 145, 261–272. doi: 10.1016/j.jsbmb.2014.05.011

Soubhye, J., Alard, I. C., van Antwerpen, P., and Dufrasne, F. (2015). Type 2, 17-beta hydroxysteroid dehydrogenase as a novel target for the treatment of osteoporosis. *Future Med. Chem.* 7, 1431–1456. doi: 10.4155/fmc.15.74

Steckelbroeck, S., Jin, Y., Gopishetty, S., Oyesanmi, B., and Penning, T. M. (2004a). Human cytosolic 3alpha-hydroxysteroid dehydrogenases of the aldo-keto reductase superfamily display significant 3beta-hydroxysteroid dehydrogenase activity: implications for steroid hormone metabolism and action. *J. Biol. Chem.* 279, 10784–10795. doi: 10.1074/jbc.M313308200

Steckelbroeck, S., Lutjohann, D., Bauman, D. R., Ludwig, M., Friedl, A., Hans, V. H., et al. (2010). Non-stereo-selective cytosolic human brain tissue 3-ketosteroid reductase is refractory to inhibition by AKR1C inhibitors. *Biochim. Biophys. Act.* 1801, 1221–1231. doi: 10.1016/j.bbalip.2010.07.005

Steckelbroeck, S., Nassen, A., Ugele, B., Ludwig, M., Watzka, M., Reissinger, A., et al. (2004b). Steroid sulfatase (STS) expression in the human temporal lobe: enzyme activity, mRNA expression and immunohistochemistry study. *J. Neurochem.* 89, 403–417. doi: 10.1046/j.1471-4159.2004.02336.x

Steckelbroeck, S., Stoffel-Wagner, B., Reichelt, R., Schramm, J., Bidlingmaier, F., Siekmann, L., et al. (1999). Characterization of 17β-hydroxysteroid dehydrogenase activity in brain tissue: testosterone formation in the human temporal lobe. *J. Neuroendocrinol.* 11, 457–464. doi: 10.1046/j.1365-2826.1999.00363.x

Steckelbroeck, S., Watzka, M., Reichelt, R., Hans, V. H., Stoffel-Wagner, B., Heidrich, D. D., et al. (2001). Characterization of the 5α-reductase-3α-hydroxysteroid dehydrogenase complex in the human brain. *J. Clin. Endocrinol. Metab.* 86, 1324–1331. doi: 10.1210/jcem.86.3.7325

Steckelbroeck, S., Watzka, M., Reissinger, A., Wegener-Toper, P., Bidlingmaier, F., Bliesener, N., et al. (2003). Characterisation of estrogenic 17β-hydroxysteroid dehydrogenase (17β-HSD) activity in the human brain. *J. Steroid Biochem. Mol. Biol.* 86, 79–92. doi: 10.1016/S0960-0760(03)00251-6

Stelzer, G., Rosen, N., Plaschkes, I., Zimmerman, S., Twik, M., Fishilevich, S., et al. (2016). The GeneCards suite: from gene data mining to disease genome sequence analyses. *Curr Protoc Bioinformatics* 54, 1.30, 31–31, 30, 33. doi: 10.1002/cpbi.5

Stoffel-Wagner, B. (2001). Neurosteroid metabolism in the human brain. *Eur. J. Endocrinol.* 145, 669–679. doi: 10.1530/eje.0.1450669

Stoffel-Wagner, B., Beyenburg, S., Watzka, M., Blumcke, I., Bauer, J., Schramm, J., et al. (2000). Expression of 5α-reductase and 3α-hydroxisteroid oxidoreductase in the hippocampus of patients with chronic temporal lobe epilepsy. *Epilepsia* 41, 140–147. doi: 10.1111/j.1528-1157.2000.tb00133.x

Stoffel-Wagner, B., Watzka, M., Schramm, J., Bidlingmaier, F., and Klingmuller, D. (1999a). Expression of CYP19 (aromatase) mRNA in different areas of the human brain. *J. Steroid Biochem. Mol. Biol.* 70, 237–241. doi: 10.1016/S0960-0760(99)00114-4

Stoffel-Wagner, B., Watzka, M., Steckelbroeck, S., Ludwig, M., Clusmann, H., Bidlingmaier, F., et al. (2003). Allopregnanolone serum levels and expression of 5 alpha-reductase and 3 alpha-hydroxysteroid dehydrogenase isoforms in hippocampal and temporal cortex of patients with epilepsy. *Epilepsy Res.* 54, 11–19. doi: 10.1016/S0920-1211(03)00036-6

Stoffel-Wagner, B., Watzka, M., Steckelbroeck, S., Schramm, J., Bidlingmaier, J. F., and Klingmuller, D. (1999b). Expression of 17β-hydroxysteroid dehydrogenase types 1, 2, 3 and 4 in the human temporal lobe. *J. Endocrinol.* 160, 119–126. doi: 10.1677/joe.0.1600119

Stoffel-Wagner, B., Watzka, M., Steckelbroeck, S., Schwaab, R., Schramm, J., Bidlingmaier, F., et al. (1998a). Expression of CYP19 (aromatase) mRNA in the human temporal lobe. *Biochem. Biophys. Res. Commun.* 244, 768–771. doi: 10.1006/bbrc.1998.8337

Stoffel-Wagner, B., Watzka, M., Steckelbroeck, S., Wickert, L., Schramm, J., Romalo, G., et al. (1998b). Expression of 5α-reductase in the human temporal lobe of children and adults. *J. Clin. Endocrinol. Metab.* 83, 3636–3642.

Strott, C. A. (2002). Sulfonation and molecular action. *Endocr. Rev.* 23, 703–732. doi: 10.1210/er.2001-0040

Sudeshna, T., Anand, K., and Medhamurthy, R. (2013). Analysis of 20α-hydroxysteroid dehydrogenase expression in the corpus luteum of the buffalo cow: effect of prostaglandin F2-α treatment on circulating 20α-hydroxyprogesterone levels. *Reprod. Biol. Endocrinol.* 11:111. doi: 10.1186/1477-7827-11-111

Sun, X. F., Ahmadi, A., Arbman, G., Wallin, A., Asklid, D., and Zhang, H. (2005). Polymorphisms in sulfotransferase 1A1 and glutathione S-transferase P1 genes in relation to colorectal cancer risk and patients' survival. *World J. Gastroenterol.* 11, 6875–6879. doi: 10.3748/wjg.v11.i43.6875

Svoboda, M., Hamilton, G., and Thalhammer, T. (2010). Steroid hormone metabolizing enzymes in benign and malignant human bone tumors. *Expert Opin. Drug Metab. Toxicol.* 6, 427–437. doi: 10.1517/17425251003592129

Svoboda, M., Thalhammer, T., Aust, S., Arrich, F., Assadian, O., and Toma, C. D. (2007). Estrogen sulfotransferase (SULT1E1) expression in benign and malignant human bone tumors. *J. Surg. Oncol.* 95, 572–581. doi: 10.1002/jso.20748

Syed, F., and Khosla, S. (2005). Mechanisms of sex steroid effects on bone. *Biochem. Biophys. Res. Commun.* 328, 688–696. doi: 10.1016/j.bbrc.2004.11.097

Taga, S., Yoshida, N., and Sekiba, K. (1990). Distribution and cyclic change of aromatase cytochrome P-450 activity in human uteri. *J. Steroid Biochem. Mol. Biol.* 37, 741–745. doi: 10.1016/0960-0760(90)90359-S

Takeyama, J., Suzuki, T., Hirasawa, G., Muramatsu, Y., Nagura, H., Iinuma, K., et al. (2000). 17β-hydroxysteroid dehydrogenase type 1 and 2 expression in the human fetus. *J. Clin. Endocrinol. Metab.* 85, 410–416. doi: 10.1210/jcem.85.1.6323

Tanaka, K., Kubushiro, K., Iwamori, Y., Okairi, Y., Kiguchi, K., Ishiwata, I., et al. (2003). Estrogen sulfotransferase and sulfatase: Roles in the regulation of estrogen activity in human uterine endometrial carcinomas. *Cancer Sci.* 94, 871–876. doi: 10.1111/j.1349-7006.2003.tb01369.x

Tanaka, K., Shimizu, K., Kakegawa, S., Ohtaki, Y., Nagashima, T., Kaira, K., et al. (2016). Prognostic significance of aromatase and estrogen receptor beta expression in EGFR wild-type lung adenocarcinoma. *Am. J. Transl. Res.* 8, 81–97.

Tanaka, S., Miki, Y., Hashimoto, C., Takagi, K., Doe, Z., Li, B., et al. (2015). The role of 5α-reductase type 1 associated with intratumoral dihydrotestosterone concentrations in human endometrial carcinoma. *Mol. Cell. Endocrinol.* 401, 56–64. doi: 10.1016/j.mce.2014.11.022

Tang, T., Li, L., Tang, J., Li, Y., Lin, W. Y., Martin, F., et al. (2010). A mouse knockout library for secreted and transmembrane proteins. *Nat. Biotechnol.* 28, 749–755. doi: 10.1038/nbt.1644

Tangen, I. L., Onyango, T. B., Kopperud, R., Berg, A., Halle, M. K., Oyan, A. M., et al. (2016). Androgen receptor as potential therapeutic target in metastatic endometrial cancer. *Oncotarget* 7, 49289–49298. doi: 10.18632/oncotarget.10334

Tangen, I. L., Werner, H. M., Berg, A., Halle, M. K., Kusonmano, K., Trovik, J., et al. (2014). Loss of progesterone receptor links to high proliferation and increases from primary to metastatic endometrial cancer lesions. *Eur J Cancer* 50, 3003–3010. doi: 10.1016/j.ejca.2014.09.003

Taniuchi, S., Fujishima, F., Miki, Y., Abe, K., Nakamura, Y., Sato, S., et al. (2014). Tissue concentrations of estrogens and aromatase immunolocalization in interstitial pneumonia of human lung. *Mol. Cell. Endocrinol.* 392, 136–143. doi: 10.1016/j.mce.2014.05.016

Tashiro, A., Sasano, H., Nishikawa, T., Yabuki, N., Muramatsu, Y., Coughtrie, M. W., et al. (2000). Expression and activity of dehydroepiandrosterone sulfotransferase in human gastric mucosa. *J. Steroid Biochem. Mol. Biol.* 72, 149–154. doi: 10.1016/S0960-0760(00)00020-0

Taveira-DaSilva, A. M., and Moss, J. (2014). Management of lymphangioleiomyomatosis. *F1000Prime Rep.* 6, 116. doi: 10.12703/P6-116

Terry, K., McGrath, M., Lee, I. M., Buring, J., and De Vivo, I. (2010). Genetic variation in CYP11A1 and StAR in relation to endometrial cancer risk. *Gynecol. Oncol.* 117, 255–259. doi: 10.1016/j.ygyno.2010.02.002

Teubner, W., Meinl, W., Florian, S., Kretzschmar, M., and Glatt, H. (2007). Identification and localization of soluble sulfotransferases in the human gastrointestinal tract. *Biochem. J.* 404, 207–215. doi: 10.1042/BJ20061431

Thiboutot, D., Martin, P., Volikos, L., and Gilliland, K. (1998). Oxidative activity of the type 2 isozyme of 17β-hydroxysteroid dehydrogenase (17β-HSD) predominates in human sebaceous glands. *J. Invest. Dermatol.* 111, 390–395. doi: 10.1046/j.1523-1747.1998.00322.x

Thompson, D. J., O'Mara, T. A., Glubb, D. M., Painter, J. N., Cheng, T., Folkerd, E., et al. (2016). $CYP_{19}A_1$ fine-mapping and Mendelian randomization: estradiol is causal for endometrial cancer. *Endocr. Relat. Cancer* 23, 77–91. doi: 10.1530/ERC-15-0386

Tong, M. H., Jiang, H., Liu, P., Lawson, J. A., Brass, L. F., and Song, W. C. (2005). Spontaneous fetal loss caused by placental thrombosis in estrogen sulfotransferase-deficient mice. *Nat. Med.* 11, 153–159. doi: 10.1038/nm1184

Törn, S., Nokelainen, P., Kurkela, R., Pulkka, A., Menjivar, M., Ghosh, S., et al. (2003). Production, purification, and functional analysis of recombinant human and mouse 17β-hydroxysteroid dehydrogenase type 7. *Biochem. Biophys. Res. Commun.* 305, 37–45. doi: 10.1016/S0006-291X(03)00694-6

Townsend, E. A., Miller, V. M., and Prakash, Y. S. (2012). Sex differences and sex steroids in lung health and disease. *Endocr. Rev.* 33, 1–47. doi: 10.1210/er.2010-0031

Townsend, E. A., Thompson, M. A., Pabelick, C. M., and Prakash, Y. S. (2010). Rapid effects of estrogen on intracellular Ca^{2+} regulation in human airway smooth muscle. *Am. J. Physiol. Lung Cell. Mol. Physiol.* 298 L521–530. doi: 10.1152/ajplung.00287.2009

Tsai, S. J., Wu, M. H., Lin, C. C., Sun, H. S., and Chen, H. M. (2001). Regulation of steroidogenic acute regulatory protein expression and progesterone production in endometriotic stromal cells. *J. Clin. Endocrinol. Metab.* 86, 5765–5773. doi: 10.1210/jcem.86.12.8082

Tseng, L., and Gurpide, E. (1974). Estradiol and 20α-dihydroprogesterone dehydrogenase activities in human endometrium during the menstrual cycle. *Endocrinology* 94, 419–423. doi: 10.1210/endo-94-2-419

Tseng, L., Gusberg, S. B., and Gurpide, E. (1977). Estradiol receptor and 17 beta-dehydrogenase in normal and abnormal human endometrium. *Ann. N. Y. Acad. Sci.* 286, 190–198. doi: 10.1111/j.1749-6632.1977.tb29416.x

Tseng, L., and Mazella, J. (2002). Endometrial cell specific gene activation during implantation and early pregnancy. *Front. Biosci.* 7, d1566–d1574. doi: 10.2741/A861

Tseng, L., Mazella, J., Mann, W. J., and Chumas, J. (1982). Estrogen synthesis in normal and malignant human endometrium. *J. Clin. Endocrinol. Metab.* 55, 1029–1031. doi: 10.1210/jcem-55-5-1029

Tsuchiya, M., Nakao, H., Katoh, T., Sasaki, H., Hiroshima, M., Tanaka, T., et al. (2005). Association between endometriosis and genetic polymorphisms of the estradiol-synthesizing enzyme genes HSD17B1 and CYP19. *Hum. Reprod.* 20, 974–978. doi: 10.1093/humrep/deh726

Tuo, B., Wen, G., Wei, J., Liu, X., Wang, X., Zhang, Y., et al. (2011). Estrogen regulation of duodenal bicarbonate secretion and sex-specific protection of human duodenum. *Gastroenterology* 141, 854–863. doi: 10.1053/j.gastro.2011.05.044

Utsunomiya, H., Ito, K., Suzuki, T., Kitamura, T., Kaneko, C., Nakata, T., et al. (2004). Steroid sulfatase and estrogen sulfotransferase in human endometrial carcinoma. *Clin. Cancer Res.* 10, 5850–5856. doi: 10.1158/1078-0432.CCR-04-0040

Utsunomiya, H., Suzuki, T., Ito, K., Moriya, T., Konno, R., Sato, S., et al. (2003). The correlation between the response to progestogen treatment and the expression of progesterone receptor B and 17β-hydroxysteroid dehydrogenase type 2 in human endometrial carcinoma. *Clin. Endocrinol. (Oxf).* 58, 696–703. doi: 10.1046/j.1365-2265.2003.01766.x

Utsunomiya, H., Suzuki, T., Kaneko, C., Takeyama, J., Nakamura, J., Kimura, K., et al. (2001). The analyses of 17β-hydroxysteroid dehydrogenase isozymes in human endometrial hyperplasia and carcinoma. *J. Clin. Endocrinol. Metab.* 86, 3436–3443. doi: 10.1210/jcem.86.7.7661

van der Eerden, B. C., Lowik, C. W., Wit, J. M., and Karperien, M. (2004). Expression of estrogen receptors and enzymes involved in sex steroid metabolism in the rat tibia during sexual maturation. *J. Endocrinol.* 180, 457–467. doi: 10.1677/joe.0.1800457

Vanderschueren, D., Gaytant, J., Boonen, S., and Venken, K. (2008). Androgens and bone. *Curr. Opin. Endocrinol. Diabetes Obes.* 15, 250–254. doi: 10.1097/MED.0b013e3282fe6ca9

Vani, S., McDonald, S. E., Williams, A. R., Mason, J. I., Thong, K. J., and Critchley, H. O. (2007). Mid-luteal endometrial intracrinology following controlled ovarian hyperstimulation involving use of a gonadotrophin releasing hormone antagonist. *Hum. Reprod.* 22, 2981–2991. doi: 10.1093/humrep/dem269

Varlamov, O., Bethea, C. L., and Roberts, C. T. Jr. (2014). Sex-specific differences in lipid and glucose metabolism. *Front. Endocrinol. (Lausanne).* 5:241. doi: 10.3389/fendo.2014.00241

Vasquez, Y. M., and DeMayo, F. J. (2013). Role of nuclear receptors in blastocyst implantation. *Semin. Cell Dev. Biol.* 24, 724–735. doi: 10.1016/j.semcdb.2013.08.004

Velasco, I., Rueda, J., and Acien, P. (2006). Aromatase expression in endometriotic tissues and cell cultures of patients with endometriosis. *Mol. Hum. Reprod.* 12, 377–381. doi: 10.1093/molehr/gal041

Vercellini, P., Vigano, P., Somigliana, E., and Fedele, L. (2014). Endometriosis: pathogenesis and treatment. *Nat. Rev. Endocrinol.* 10, 261–275. doi: 10.1038/nrendo.2013.255

Verma, M. K., Miki, Y., Abe, K., Suzuki, T., Niikawa, H., Suzuki, S., et al. (2013). Intratumoral localization and activity of 17β-hydroxysteroid dehydrogenase type 1 in non-small cell lung cancer: a potent prognostic factor. *J. Transl. Med.* 11, 167. doi: 10.1186/1479-5876-11-167

Verma, M. K., Miki, Y., and Sasano, H. (2011). Aromatase in human lung carcinoma. *Steroids* 76, 759–764. doi: 10.1016/j.steroids.2011.02.020

Vidal, O., Lindberg, M. K., Hollberg, K., Baylink, D. J., Andersson, G., Lubahn, D. B., et al. (2000). Estrogen receptor specificity in the regulation of skeletal growth and maturation in male mice. *Proc. Natl. Acad. Sci. U.S.A.* 97, 5474–5479. doi: 10.1073/pnas.97.10.5474

Vouk, K., Smuc, T., Guggenberger, C., Ribic-Pucelj, M., Sinkovec, J., Husen, B., et al. (2011). Novel estrogen-related genes and potential biomarkers of ovarian endometriosis identified by differential expression analysis. *J. Steroid Biochem. Mol. Biol.* 125, 231–242. doi: 10.1016/j.jsbmb.2011.03.010

Walker, V. R., and Korach, K. S. (2004). Estrogen receptor knockout mice as a model for endocrine research. *ILAR J.* 45, 455–461. doi: 10.1093/ilar.45.4.455

Wang, F., Vihma, V., Soronen, J., Turpeinen, U., Hamalainen, E., Savolainen-Peltonen, H., et al. (2013). 17β-Estradiol and estradiol fatty acyl esters and estrogen-converting enzyme expression in adipose tissue in obese men and women. *J. Clin. Endocrinol. Metab.* 98, 4923–4931. doi: 10.1210/jc.2013-2605

Wang, H., and Dey, S. K. (2006). Roadmap to embryo implantation: clues from mouse models. *Nat. Rev. Genet.* 7, 185–199. doi: 10.1038/nrg1808

Wang, X. Q., Aka, J. A., Li, T., Xu, D., Doillon, C. J., and Lin, S. X. (2017). Inhibition of 17β-hydroxysteroid dehydrogenase type 7 modulates breast cancer protein profile and enhances apoptosis by down-regulating GRP78. *J. Steroid Biochem. Mol. Biol.* 172, 188–197. doi: 10.1016/j.jsbmb.2017.06.009

Warren, J. C., and French, A. P. (1965). DISTRIBUTION OF STEROID SULFATASE IN HUMAN TISSUES. *J. Clin. Endocrinol. Metab.* 25, 278–282. doi: 10.1210/jcem-25-2-278

Watanabe, K., Sasano, H., Harada, N., Ozaki, M., Niikura, H., Sato, S., et al. (1995). Aromatase in human endometrial carcinoma and hyperplasia. Immunohistochemical, in situ hybridization, and biochemical studies. *Am. J. Pathol.* 146, 491–500.

Watzka, M., Bidlingmaier, F., Schramm, J., Klingmuller, D., and Stoffel-Wagner, B. (1999). Sex- and age-specific differences in human brain CYP11A1 mRNA expression. *J. Neuroendocrinol.* 11, 901–905. doi: 10.1046/j.1365-2826.1999.00407.x

Wishart, D. S., Feunang, Y. D., Guo, A. C., Lo, E. J., Marcu, A., Grant, J. R., et al. (2018). DrugBank 5.0: a major update to the DrugBank database for 2018. *Nucleic Acids Res.* 46, D1074–D1082. doi: 10.1093/nar/gkx1037

Wishart, D. S., Jewison, T., Guo, A. C., Wilson, M., Knox, C., Liu, Y., et al. (2013). HMDB 3.0-the human metabolome database in 2013. *Nucleic Acids Res.* 41, D801–D807. doi: 10.1093/nar/gks1065

Wöhrle, D., Barbi, G., Schulz, W., and Steinbach, P. (1990). Heterozygous expression of X-linked chondrodysplasia punctata. Complex chromosome aberration including deletion of MIC2 and STS. *Hum. Genet.* 86, 215–218. doi: 10.1007/BF00197708

Woo, L. W., Purohit, A., and Potter, B. V. (2011). Development of steroid sulfatase inhibitors. *Mol. Cell. Endocrinol.* 340, 175–185. doi: 10.1016/j.mce.2010.12.035

Wu, H. C., Tuo, B. G., Wu, W. M., Gao, Y., Xu, Q. Q., and Zhao, K. (2008). Prevalence of peptic ulcer in dyspeptic patients and the influence of age, sex, and *Helicobacter pylori* infection. *Dig. Dis. Sci.* 53, 2650–2656. doi: 10.1007/s10620-007-0177-7

Xiao, J., Zheng, Y., Zhou, Y., Zhang, P., Wang, J., Shen, F., et al. (2014). Sulfotransferase SULT1A1 Arg213His polymorphism with cancer risk: a meta-analysis of 53 case-control studies. *PLoS ONE* 9:e106774. doi: 10.1371/journal.pone.0106774

Yague, J. G., Azcoitia, I., DeFelipe, J., Garcia-Segura, L. M., and Munoz, A. (2010). Aromatase expression in the normal and epileptic human hippocampus. *Brain Res.* 1315, 41–52. doi: 10.1016/j.brainres.2009.09.111

Yague, J. G., Munoz, A., de Monasterio-Schrader, P., Defelipe, J., Garcia-Segura, L. M., and Azcoitia, I. (2006). Aromatase expression in the human temporal cortex. *Neuroscience* 138, 389–401. doi: 10.1016/j.neuroscience.2005.11.054

Yamaki, J., Yamamoto, T., and Okada, H. (1985). Aromatization of androstenedione by normal and neoplastic endometrium of the uterus. *J. Steroid Biochem.* 22, 63–66. doi: 10.1016/0022-4731(85)90142-6

Yamamoto, T., Fukuoka, M., Fujimoto, Y., Kitawaki, J., Nakakoshi, M., Yoshihama, M., et al. (1990a). Inhibitory effect of a new androstenedione derivative, 14α-hydroxy-4-androstene-3,6,17-trione (14α-OHAT) on aromatase activity of human uterine tumors. *J. Steroid Biochem.* 36, 517–21. doi: 10.1016/0022-4731(90)90167-Q

Yamamoto, T., Kitawaki, J., Urabe, M., Honjo, H., Tamura, T., Noguchi, T., et al. (1993a). Estrogen productivity of endometrium and endometrial cancer tissue; influence of aromatase on proliferation of endometrial cancer cells. *J. Steroid Biochem. Mol. Biol.* 44, 463–468. doi: 10.1016/0960-0760(93)90251-Q

Yamamoto, T., Noguchi, T., Tamura, T., Kitawaki, J., and Okada, H. (1993b). Evidence for estrogen synthesis in adenomyotic tissues. *Am. J. Obstet. Gynecol.* 169, 734–738. doi: 10.1016/0002-9378(93)90654-2

Yamamoto, T., Urabe, M., Naitoh, K., Kitawaki, J., Honjo, H., and Okada, H. (1990b). Estrone sulfatase activity in human uterine leiomyoma. *Gynecol. Oncol.* 37, 315–318. doi: 10.1016/0090-8258(90)90358-R

Yanaihara, Yanaihara, T., Toma, Y., Shimizu, Y., Saito, H., Okai, T., et al. (2001). Localization and expression of steroid sulfatase in human fallopian tubes. *Steroids* 66, 87–91. doi: 10.1016/S0039-128X(00)00204-X

Yang, W., Wu, G., Broeckel, U., Smith, C. A., Turner, V., Haidar, C. E., et al. (2016). Comparison of genome sequencing and clinical genotyping for pharmacogenes. *Clin. Pharmacol. Ther.* 100, 380–388. doi: 10.1002/cpt.411

Yang, X. Y., Wu, W. J., Yang, C., Yang, T., He, J. D., Yang, Z., et al. (2013). Association of HSD17B3 and HSD3B1 polymorphisms with acne vulgaris in Southwestern Han Chinese. *Dermatology* 227, 202–208. doi: 10.1159/000353581

Ye, X. Y., Chen, S. Y., Wu, S., Yoon, D. S., Wang, H., Hong, Z., et al. (2017). Discovery of Clinical Candidate 2-((2S,6S)-2-Phenyl-6-hydroxyadamantan-2-yl)-1-(3'-hydroxyazetidin-1-yl)ethanone [BMS-816336], an orally active novel selective 11β-Hydroxysteroid dehydrogenase type 1 inhibitor. *J. Med. Chem.* 60, 4932–4948. doi: 10.1021/acs.jmedchem.7b00211

Yu, L., Romero, D. G., Gomez-Sanchez, C. E., and Gomez-Sanchez, E. P. (2002). *Steroidogenic enzyme* gene expression in the human brain. *Mol. Cell. Endocrinol.* 190, 9–17. doi: 10.1016/S0303-7207(02)00041-2

Yuchi, Y., Cai, Y., Legein, B., De Groef, S., Leuckx, G., Coppens, V., et al. (2015). Estrogen receptor α regulates β-cell formation during pancreas development and following injury. *Diabetes* 64, 3218–3228. doi: 10.2337/db14-1798

Zacher, A., Kaulich, K., Stepanow, S., Wolter, M., Kohrer, K., Felsberg, J., et al. (2016). Molecular diagnostics of gliomas using next generation sequencing of a glioma-tailored gene panel. *Brain Pathol.* 27, 146–159. doi: 10.1111/bpa.12367

Zakharov, V., Lin, H. K., Azzarello, J., McMeekin, S., Moore, K. N., Penning, T. M., et al. (2010). Suppressed expression of type 2, 3α/type 5, 17β-hydroxysteroid dehydrogenase (AKR1C3) in endometrial hyperplasia and carcinoma. *Int. J. Clin. Exp. Pathol.* 3, 608–617.

Zarrabeitia, M. T., Hernandez, J. L., Valero, C., Zarrabeitia, A., Amado, J. A., Gonzalez-Macias, J., et al. (2007). Adiposity, estradiol, and genetic variants of steroid-metabolizing enzymes as determinants of bone mineral density. *Eur. J. Endocrinol.* 156, 117–122. doi: 10.1530/eje.1.02318

Zeitoun, K., Takayama, K., Sasano, H., Suzuki, T., Moghrabi, N., Andersson, S., et al. (1998). Deficient 17β-hydroxysteroid dehydrogenase type 2 expression in endometriosis: failure to metabolize 17β-estradiol. *J. Clin. Endocrinol. Metab.* 83, 4474–4480.

Zeng, C., Matsuda, K., Jia, W. H., Chang, J., Kweon, S. S., Xiang, Y. B., et al. (2016). Identification of susceptibility loci and genes for colorectal cancer risk. *Gastroenterology* 150, 1633–1645. doi: 10.1053/j.gastro.2016.02.076

Zhang, J., Yin, Y., Niu, X. M., Liu, Y., Garfield, D., Chen, S. F., et al. (2013). $CYP_{19}A_1$ gene polymorphisms and risk of lung cancer. *J. Int. Med. Res.* 41, 735–742. doi: 10.1177/0300060513477291

Zhao, H., Zhou, L., Shangguan, A. J., and Bulun, S. E. (2016). Aromatase expression and regulation in breast and endometrial cancer. *J. Mol. Endocrinol.* 57 R19–33. doi: 10.1530/JME-15-0310

Zhongyi, S., Rantakari, P., Lamminen, T., Toppari, J., and Poutanen, M. (2007). Transgenic male mice expressing human hydroxysteroid dehydrogenase 2 indicate a role for the enzyme independent of its action on sex steroids. *Endocrinology* 148, 3827–3836. doi: 10.1210/en.2007-0365

Zwart, W., Theodorou, V., Kok, M., Canisius, S., Linn, S., and Carroll, J. S. (2011). Oestrogen receptor-co-factor-chromatin specificity in the transcriptional regulation of breast cancer. *EMBO J.* 30, 4764–4776. doi: 10.1038/emboj.2011.368

5

Clinical Significance of Organic Anion Transporting Polypeptide Gene Expression in High-Grade Serous Ovarian Cancer

Martin Svoboda[1†], *Felicitas Mungenast*[1†], *Andreas Gleiss*[2], *Ignace Vergote*[3], *Adriaan Vanderstichele*[3], *Jalid Sehouli*[4], *Elena Braicu*[4], *Sven Mahner*[5], *Walter Jäger*[6], *Diana Mechtcheriakova*[1], *Dan Cacsire-Tong*[7], *Robert Zeillinger*[8], *Theresia Thalhammer*[1*] and *Dietmar Pils*[2,9*]

[1] Department of Pathophysiology and Allergy Research, Center for Pathophysiology, Infectiology and Immunology, Medical University of Vienna, Vienna, Austria, [2] Institute of Clinical Biometrics, Center for Medical Statistics, Informatics, and Intelligent Systems, Medical University of Vienna, Vienna, Austria, [3] Division of Gynaecological Oncology, Department of Gynaecology and Obstetrics, Leuven Cancer Institute, University Hospital Leuven, Katholieke Universiteit Leuven, Leuven, Belgium, [4] Department of Gynecology, Charité – Universitätsmedizin Berlin, Corporate Member of Freie Universität Berlin, Berlin Institute of Health, Humboldt-Universität zu Berlin, Berlin, Germany, [5] Department of Gynecology, University Medical Center Hamburg-Eppendorf, Hamburg, Germany, [6] Department of Clinical Pharmacy and Diagnostics, University of Vienna, Vienna, Austria, [7] Translational Gynecology Group, Department of Obstetrics and Gynaecology, Comprehensive Cancer Center, Medical University of Vienna, Vienna, Austria, [8] Molecular Oncology Group, Department of Obstetrics and Gynaecology, Comprehensive Cancer Center, Medical University of Vienna, Vienna, Austria, [9] Department of Surgery, Medical University of Vienna, Vienna, Austria

***Correspondence:**
Theresia Thalhammer
theresia.thalhammer@meduniwien.ac.at
Dietmar Pils
dietmar.pils@meduniwien.ac.at

† These authors have contributed equally to this work.

High-grade serous ovarian cancer (HGSOC) is considered the most deadly and frequently occurring type of ovarian cancer and is associated with various molecular compositions and growth patterns. Evaluating the mRNA expression pattern of the organic anion transporters (OATPs) encoded by *SLCO* genes may allow for improved stratification of HGSOC patients for targeted invention. The expression of *SLCO* mRNA and genes coding for putative functionally related ABC-efflux pumps, enzymes, pregnane-X-receptor, *ESR1* and *ESR2* (coding for estrogen receptors ERα and ERß) and HER-2 were assessed using RT-qPCR. The expression levels were assessed in a cohort of 135 HGSOC patients to elucidate the independent impact of the expression pattern on the overall survival (OS). For identification of putative regulatory networks, Graphical Gaussian Models were constructed from the expression data with a tuning parameter K varying between meaningful borders (Pils et al., 2012; Auer et al., 2015, 2017; Kurman and Shih le, 2016; Karam et al., 2017; Labidi-Galy et al., 2017; Salomon-Perzynski et al., 2017; Sukhbaatar et al., 2017). The final value used ($K = 4$) was determined by maximizing the proportion of explained variation of the corresponding LASSO Cox regression model for OS. The following two networks of directly correlated genes were identified: (i) *SLCO2B1* with *ABCC3* implicated in estrogen homeostasis; and (ii) two ABC-efflux pumps in the immune regulation (*ABCB2/ABCB3*) with *ABCC3* and *HER-2*. Combining LASSO Cox regression and univariate Cox regression analyses, *SLCO5A1* coding for OATP5A1, an estrogen metabolite transporter located in the cytoplasm and plasma membranes of ovarian cancer cells, was identified as significant and independent prognostic factor for OS (HR = 0.68, CI 0.49–0.93; p = 0.031). Furthermore, results indicated the benefits of patients with high expression by adding 5.1% to the 12.8% of the proportion of explained variation (PEV) for clinicopathological parameters known for prognostic significance (FIGO stage, age and residual tumor after debulking). Additionally, overlap with previously described signatures that indicated a more favorable prognosis for ovarian cancer patients was shown for *SLCO5A1*, the network *ABCB2/ABCB3/ABCC4/HER2* as well as *ESR1*. Furthermore, expression of *SLCO2A1* and *PGDH*, which are important for PGE_2 degradation, was associated with the non-miliary peritoneal tumor spreading. In conclusion, the present findings suggested that *SLCOs* and the related molecules identified as potential biomarkers in HGSOC may be useful for the development of novel therapeutic strategies.

Keywords: high-grade serous ovarian cancer, *SLCO*, OATP, transporter, overall survival, estrogens

INTRODUCTION

High-grade serous ovarian cancer (HGSOC) is the most frequent occurring and aggressive subtype of all ovarian cancer types. HGSOC is often diagnosed late and is associated with therapeutic resistance following surgical debulking and platin- and taxane-based chemotherapy as standard of care. These factors contribute to the high mortality. Since the poor overall survival (OS) of HGSOC patients has not improved greatly during the last decades, more knowledge on the characteristic of these tumors is required (Karam et al., 2017).

HGSOC develops from epithelial cells in the fimbriae region of the fallopian tubes that undergo neoplastic transformation to serous tubal intraepithelial carcinomas (STICs) to form HGSOC in the ovary (Labidi-Galy et al., 2017). In some cases, HGSOC might also develop from the less aggressive low-grade serous ovarian carcinomas (LGSOC), which arises from ovarian tissue (Auer et al., 2017; Sukhbaatar et al., 2017). Notably, mutations in *TP53* are considered important for the diagnosis of HGSOC and are observed in >95% of cases (Kurman and Shih Ie, 2016). Aside from *TP53* mutations, HGSOC can also present with variable molecular compositions and growth patterns, thus a further sub-classification based on the morphologic and molecular heterogeneity of these tumors is recommended (Pils et al., 2012; Salomon-Perzynski et al., 2017).

In contrast to other cancer types of the reproductive organs with broad lymphatic or haematogenous dissemination to distant organs, including cervix and breast, ovarian cancer cells spread predominantly in the peritoneal cavity. Of note, epithelial and mesenchymal markers are simultaneously expressed in HGSOC cells and a continuous dynamic epithelial/mesenchymal transition (EMT) can enable tumor cells to adapt for peritoneal implantation and local tumor metastasis (Auer et al., 2015). It is thought that tumor cells in the peritoneal fluid and those circulating in the blood implant in the peritoneum and omentum to form metastatic tumors, which can result in the destruction of neighboring organs (Yeung et al., 2015; Obermayr et al., 2017). A close relation between the pattern of peritoneal metastases and the putative origin of HGSOC tumor cells in the fallopian tubes (T) or the ovary (O) was previously demonstrated by a comparative transcriptome analyses (Pradeep et al., 2014; Auer et al., 2015; Bachmayr-Heyda et al., 2017). Tumor cells of ovarian origin grow in the peritoneum in a non-miliary (n-M) fashion and result in the production of large tumor nodes. Typically these n-M tumors can be removed completely, which contributes to improved prognosis of tumors with this pattern of metastasis. However, miliary (M) growing tumors form many small (millet-sized) tumor nodes, which at the time of the diagnosis are widely spread in the peritoneum. According to the signature of M tumors, they originate from the fallopian tube epithelium. Because complete removal is usually difficult to achieve and they seem to be more aggressive than other ovarian cancers, the prognosis is generally worse than that of n-M tumors (Pils et al., 2012; Torres et al., 2017).

Other classification systems to stratify HGSOC patients according to their risk for a cancer-related death were developed as molecular signatures for these tumors. Similar to breast cancer, many tumors express estrogen receptor alpha (ERα), estrogen receptor beta (ERβ) and/or other steroid hormone receptors. A subgroup of these tumors express additionally/or exclusively epidermal growth factor receptor 2 (HER-2, ERBB2); however, some tumors been demonstrated to express none of these markers. Importantly, HGSOC tumors expressing high levels of ERα are usually sensitive to estrogens and are associated with a better prognosis compared with tumors expressing HER-2, but lack expression of ERα (Voutsadakis, 2016; Rižner et al., 2017). Another risk classification system to stratify HGSOC patients into two groups (group 1 and group 2) based on molecular signature was defined by Yoshihara (Yoshihara et al., 2009). Group 1 is characterized by a better response to chemotherapy and a more favorable prognosis compared to group 2. Most prominent in this identified signature is the reduced expression of immune-response-related genes in tumors classified into group 2. Furthermore, genes coding for transport proteins in the antigen presentation pathway are downregulated. The ATP-binding cassette (ABC)-transporters ABCB2 (TAP1) and ABCB3 (TAP2), which are encoded by *ABCB2* and *ABCB3* genes, respectively, are part of the major histocompatibility complex class I restricted antigen processing machinery. Consequently, high levels of *ABCB2/ABCB3* are associated with improved survival in ovarian cancer patients, indicating the importance of transport proteins in ovarian cancer progression.

Aside from the immune system, many transmembrane transport proteins play an important role in cancer cell survival and progression in relation to their transport function in cancer cells (Thakkar et al., 2015). For uptake of drugs, xenobiotics and compound from the endogenous metabolism, eleven member of the family of organic anion transporting polypeptides (OATPs) encoded by *SLCO* genes have been identified (Hagenbuch and Gui, 2008; Obaidat et al., 2012; Stieger and Hagenbuch, 2014). Eleven members of the organic anion transporting polypeptides (OATPs) family encoded by *SLCO* genes have been described to be associated with the uptake of drugs, xenobiotics and compounds associated with endogenous metabolism (Hagenbuch and Gui, 2008; Obaidat et al., 2012; Stieger and Hagenbuch, 2014). Notably, ubiquitously expressed *SLCO2A1, SLCO2B1, SLCO3A1,* and *SLCO4A1* genes have been identified in ovarian cancer (Tamai et al., 2000). In addition, we previously detected SLCOs with a more restricted localization in normal tissue using samples from different ovarian cancer subtypes. These included the following: (i) *SLCO1B1* and liver-type *SLCO1B3* (lt-*SLCO1B3*), which are normally expressed in the liver; (ii) *SLCO4C1*, which is highly expressed in the kidney; (iii) testis-specific *SLCO6A1*; and (iv) *SLCO5A1*, which is more widely distributed in the body (Svoboda et al., 2011). Novel *SLCO1B3* variants were identified in cancerous tissues. A cancer-type variant with a distinct 5′region, termed cancer-type (ct)-*SLCO1B3* coding for the cancer-type (ct)-OATP1B3 transporter was identified as the main OATP1B3 variant in colon, lung (Sun et al., 2014) pancreatic (Thakkar et al., 2013), and also ovarian cancer (Alam et al., 2018).

Thus far, various members of the OATP family (OATP1A2, OATP1B1, lt-OATP1B3, OATP2B1, OATP3A1, OATP4A1, and OATP5A1) have been identified as transporters for the 17β-estradiol (E2) precursor, estrone sulfate (E1S) and/or dehydroepiandrosterone sulfate (DHEA-S). Subsequently, OATP-mediated uptake of precursors may influence the progression of hormone-sensitive cancer subtypes. Of note, expression of OATP2B1 and OATP1A2, two transporters for steroid hormones, has been identified as important for the progression of hormone-dependent breast cancer (Banerjee et al., 2012; Matsumoto et al., 2015) and may also be significant for HGSOC. As serous ovarian carcinomas typically arise in postmenopausal women following the termination of ovarian estrogen synthesis, expression of OATPs might be important for providing E2 to hormone-dependent tumor cells. For an optimal estrogen turnover, uptake transporters must collaborate with the ABC-efflux transporter for the excretion of estrogen metabolites (Buxhofer-Ausch et al., 2013; Mueller et al., 2015; Rižner et al., 2017). After inactivation of E2 and other estrogens, for which conjugation through to sulfate via estrogen-preferring sulfotransferase is an important step, the conjugates are excreted via ATP-dependent drug efflux pumps (ABC-transporters), such as ABCC2 and ABCC3. Therefore, the expression of *SLCOs*/OATPs and ABC-efflux pumps could be of relevance in the progression of estrogen-sensitive HGSOC (Rižner et al., 2017).

OATPs may also be considered important for the accumulation of cytotoxic drugs in tumor cells; however, ABC-efflux pumps can limit the exposure of cells to their toxic effects. This suggests an influence of transporter gene expression on the efficacy of chemotherapeutic drugs (Ween et al., 2015; Bugde et al., 2017). From all established members of the OATP family, lt-OATP1B3 has been extensively characterized for its function as an uptake transporter for several established OATP substrates and for its role in paclitaxel uptake (van de Steeg et al., 2013). Because the OATP variant has poor transport capacity compared to the lt-OATP1B3, paclitaxel uptake by ct-OATP1B3 into ovarian cancer cells is unlikely (Thakkar et al., 2013; Sun et al., 2014; Furihata et al., 2015; Sissung et al., 2017; Alam et al., 2018).

ABCB1 (P-glycoprotein), which is encoded by the *ABCB1* gene, has been found to be significant in the efflux of taxanes from cells (Szakács et al., 2006). Notably, a previous study revealed that, although reduced *ABCB1* expression levels in epithelial ovarian cancer were related to longer progression-free survival of patients (Elsnerova et al., 2016), the role of P-glycoprotein in epithelial ovarian cancer is uncertain. Similarly, the expression of a number of ABC-transporters has been related to drug resistance and has been indicated to limit the exposure of cells to cytotoxic drugs. Furthermore, following platinum- and taxane-based standard chemotherapy, the upregulation of *ABCC2, ABCC3, ABCC4,* and *ABCC10* genes, which code for their respective ABC-transporters (multidrug resistance-related proteins MRP2, 3, 4, and 10, respectively) can contribute to drug resistance (Auner et al., 2010). Previous findings have suggested that the expression of a number of genes in the OATP and ABC-transporter families can be induced by the pregnane X receptor (PXR), which can be activated by many drugs and chemicals. Therefore, a possible co-expression of PXR and transporters may influence drug resistance. Furthermore, PXR expression has been related to ovarian cancer progression in previous studies (Nymoen et al., 2015; Dong et al., 2017).

Another possible important factor regarding OATPs and ABC-efflux pumps in ovarian cancer is their role in the regulation of the pro-inflammatory prostaglandin PGE_2. After synthesis via the cytosolic PG-synthase 2 (COX2), PGE_2 is exported by ABCC4 to the extracellular space for plasma membrane receptor binding. For the degradation of PGE_2 via the prostaglandin-dehydrogenase (PGDH), a re-uptake into cells by PG transporters, including OATP2A1, is required. The collaboration between OATP and ABC-transporters together with prostaglandin-synthesizing/degrading enzymes has been proposed previously (Nomura et al., 2004; Holla et al., 2008; Kochel and Fulton, 2015).

Based on the proposed roles of individual OATPs to modify estrogen homeostasis, confer resistance to anticancer drugs and control the levels of pro-inflammatory prostaglandins, we sought to identify networks of directly correlated genes; *SLCOs* with genes coding for selected ABC-transporters, PXR, associated enzymes and the markers for HGSOC subtypes ERα/ERβ/HER-2. Providing further data on the expression of *SLCOs* and related genes to the well-established clinicopathologic prognostic parameters may allow improved risk stratification for patients with HGSOC because their specific expression pattern may reflect the heterologous nature of these tumors. The specific expression pattern may also point to the origin of the tumors and the pattern of peritoneal metastasis, which may influence the prognosis of patients. Therefore, the mRNA expression levels of SLCOs and the putative functionally-related genes were assessed in the present study using RT-qPCR in a cohort of 135 patients with late-stage HGSOC and compared with 21 benign ovarian cysts.

MATERIALS AND METHODS

Patients

Tumor samples of epithelial ovarian cancer (EOC) were collected in the course of the European Commission's 6th framework program project OVCAD (Ovarian Cancer: Diagnosis of a silent killer; grant agreement no. 018698). Contributors were: Department of Gynecology at Charité, Medical University Berlin, Germany; The Department of Obstetrics and Gynecology and Gynecologic Oncology, University Hospital Leuven, Belgium; Department of Gynecology and Obstetrics, University Medical Center Hamburg-Eppendorf, Hamburg, Germany; and The Department of Obstetrics and Gynecology, Medical University of Vienna, Austria. Benign ovarian cysts were collected at the Department of Obstetrics and Gynecology, Medical University of Vienna, Austria.

The study protocol was approved by the Ethics Committees of the participating institutions (approval nos. EK207/2003, Berlin; ML2524, Leuven; HEK190504, Hamburg; EK366/2003 and EK260/2003, Vienna). Permission to characterize new molecular prognostic factors for patients with advanced EOC was given by the Ethics committees and informed consent was obtained from all patients.

TABLE 1 | Clinicopathological characteristics of patients with high-grade serous epithelial ovarian cancer (HGSOC) and benign ovarian cysts.

HGSOC Patients	**135 (100%)**
Age at diagnosis [years]	
Median (IQR)	56 (49–67)
Overall Survival [months]	
Median (IQR)	48.0 (25.5–65.0)
Number of deaths (%)	82 (61%)
FIGO STAGE (%)	
III	109 (81%)
IV	26 (19%)
HISTOLOGICAL GRADING (%)	
G2	32 (24%)
G3	103 (76%)
RESIDUAL TUMOR AFTER DEBULKING SURGERY (%)*	
No	94 (71%)
Yes	39 (28%)
Benign Ovarian Cysts Patients	**21**
Age at diagnosis [years]	
Median (IQR)	53 (39.5–65.5)

**Data from 2 patients are missing; IQR, interquartile range.*

Information on clinic-pathological characteristics was documented by experienced clinicians and pathologists at the respective centers and the data are summarized in **Table 1** (see Chekerov et al., 2013). Only patients with advanced stage (FIGO stage III-IV) and high grade (>1) serous tumors were included in the present study. Patients with additional malignancies were excluded. For comparison, samples from benign ovarian cysts were taken from patients (median age 53 years; interquartile range 39.5–65.5 years). All patients with EOC received standard first-line chemotherapy with platinum- and taxane-based chemotherapeutics after debulking surgery. Optimal cytoreduction with absence of residual disease was defined as macroscopically complete resection of tumor material. This was achieved in 71% of cases. The median age of cancer patients at diagnosis was 56 years (interquartile range, 49–67 years). The median follow-up time was 72 months with a median survival time of 48 (25.5–65.0) months. There were 92 cases of death (61%, all related to EOC) within the follow-up period.

RNA Isolation and Reverse Transcription-Quantitative Polymerase Chain Reaction (RT-qPCR)

Tumor tissue was immediately frozen in liquid nitrogen and stored frozen until further use. For RNA isolation, approximately 100 mg of tissue was used as described previously (Svoboda et al., 2016). RNA was purified using the RNeasy Minikit (Qiagen Gmbh, Hilden, Germany) and quantified with a bioPhotometer (Eppendorf AG, Hamburg, Germany) and quality was assessed on an RNA Nano chip (Agilent Technologies Inc., Santa Clara, USA) and an Agilent 2100 Bioanalyzer.

Reverse transcription of 0.5 μg total RNA was performed using the High Capacity cDNA RT kit (ABI, Thermo Fisher Scientific, Inc., Waltham, MA, USA). To account for various cell types within the ovarian cancer tissues, out of a panel of 12 housekeeping genes (geNorm kit; Primer-Design Ltd., Southampton, UK) the following genes *ACTB, TOP1, UBC,* and *YWHAZ* were identified as the most stably expressed genes and were therefore were appropriate reference genes. Primers for genes of interest were purchased from ABI (**Supplementary Table 1**). The assay kit for ACTB was from ABI; assays for the reference house-keeping genes *TOP1, UBC,* and YWHAZ were purchased from PrimerDesign Ltd.

RT-qPCR analysis was performed on ABI 7900HT instrument equipped with SDS 2.3 software (Applied Biosystems) as described (Svoboda et al., 2016). Human Universal Reference Total RNA (Clontech Laboratories) was used for calibration.

Results were calculated according to the ΔΔCq method using the DataAssist™ v2.0 Software (ABI). Relative quantities (RQ) were normalized to the geometric mean of the four reference genes *ACTB, TOP1, UBC,* and *YWHAZ.* Values were shown relative to the mean value calculated from the calibrator samples. Samples with quantification cycle values (Cq) >35 were considered as not expressed (undetectable).

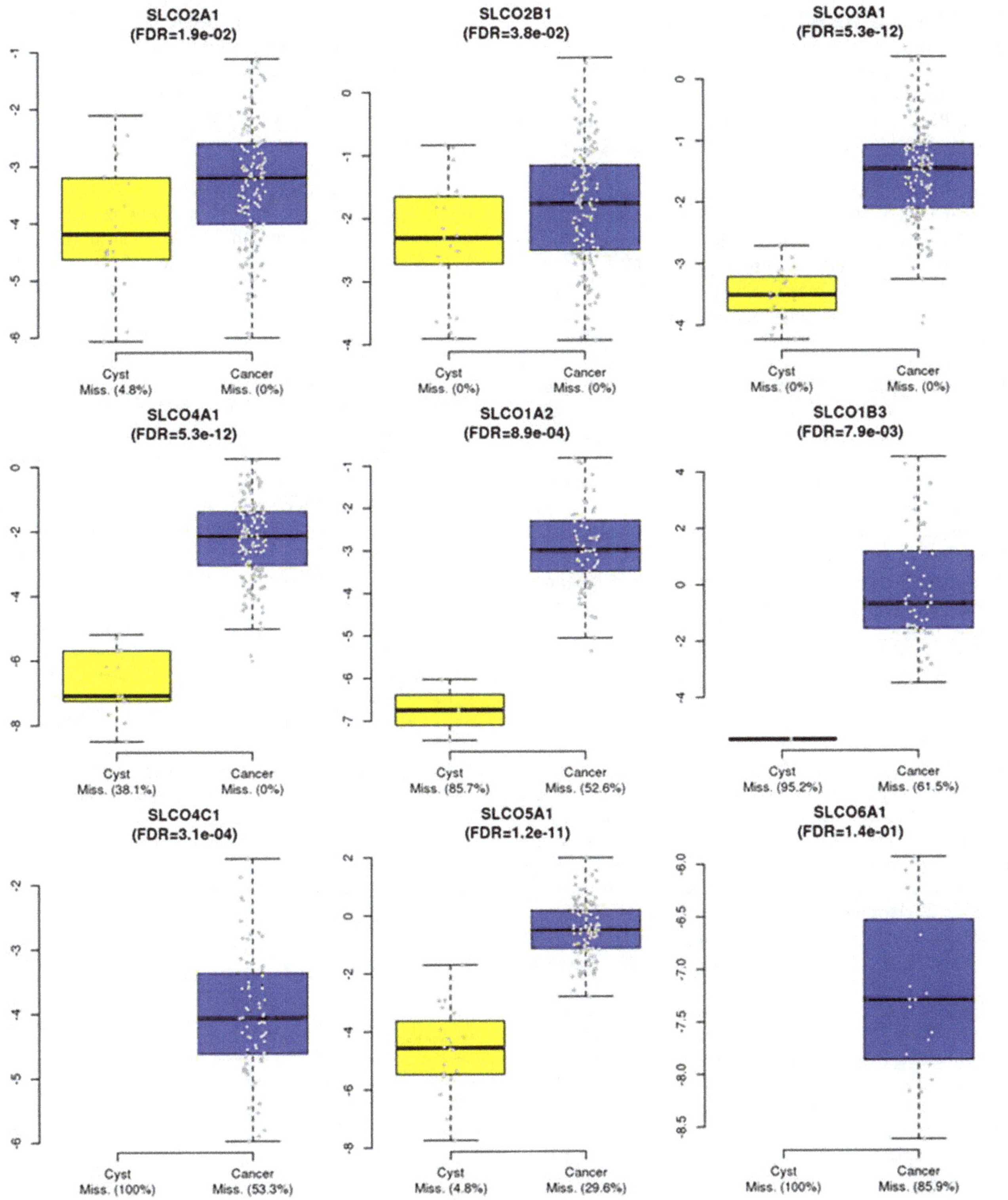

FIGURE 1 | Expression of *SLCOs* in HGSOC tissues and benign ovarian cysts. *SLCOs,* which were expressed in a significant number of the 135 HGSOC samples were also assessed by RT-qPCR in 21 tissues from benign ovarian cysts. Boxplots are shown and missing rates in cancer samples and benign cysts are indicated in the x-axis legends. For certain genes in some samples, gene expression was below detection limit. Therefore, the boxplots represent only detectable values of the corresponding expression levels in the groups (*cf.* Materials and Methods). False Discovery Rates (FDRs) of p-values were calculated using a *two-part* Wilcoxon test (combining a test for continuous values with a test comparing point-mass proportions). Corrections for multiple testing were done by the Benjamini-Hochberg procedure.

Immunohistochemical Staining of OATP5A1 on HGSOC Sections

Tissue sections (4 μm) from tumors from HGSOC patients were analyzed. Samples were collected between 2006 and 2008. For immunohistochemical staining, the polyclonal rabbit anti-OATP5A1 antibody against OATP5A1 (HPA05062, Atlas antibodies, Stockholm, SW) was used in a dilution of 1:25. After deparaffinization with the Epitope Retrieval Solution DEPP-9 pH 9 (Eubio, Vienna, AT), samples were rehydrated, and treated with 3% H_2O_2. A blocking solution (Ultra V Block; TA-015HP, Eubio) was applied for 7 min and then the primary anti-OATP5A1 antibody was added for 1 h at room temperature. A rabbit immunoglobulin was applied as negative control. For enhancement, slides were incubated with primary antibody enhancer (Primary Antibody Enhancer; TL-015-PB, Eubio) for 10 min followed by a HRP Polymer (HRP Polymer; TL-015-PH, Eubio) for 15 min. Subsequently, slides were incubated with diaminobenzidine, which acted as a chromogen, and counterstained with hematoxylin before mounting.

Immunofluorescence staining was performed as described previously (Wlcek et al., 2011). OATP5A1 antibody HPA05062 (Atlas Antibodies) was applied in the double-immunofluorescence staining experiments at a dilution of 1:50 with a monoclonal antibody against cytokeratin 19 (AP06201PU-N, Origene, Rockville, MD) at a dilution of 1:500. Anti-mouse Alexa 568 and anti-rabbit Alexa 488 antibodies (Invitrogen, Thermo Fisher Scientific, Waltham, MA) were applied. Nuclei were counterstained with DAPI.

Statistics

Normalized gene expression values were used as $\log_2$ transformed ΔΔCq values and represented with two variables if undetectable samples (Cq values >35) were present: One variable containing the continuous $\log_2$ expression values (for all Cq <35) and one variable containing the information for detectable (=1) or non-detectable (=0) information in each sample (named with a suffix "_2K") (*cf.* **Supplementary Table 2**). In all modeling approaches (Cox, logistic and linear regression) both variables were either included or excluded together. Samples with undetectable expression values were not included in the boxplots (**Figure 1**) but were always directing in the same direction (relatively more undetectable values in the group with the lower expression values, namely *SLCO2A1, SLCO4A1, SLCO1A2,* and *SLCO1B3*, but not for gene *SLCO5A1).* Statistical testing was performed with a "two part" test combining a continuous component (Wilcoxon test) plus a point-mass (undetectable samples) (Taylor and Pollard, 2009) and corrected for multiple testing according to the Benjamini-Hochberg procedure (False Discovery Rates, FDRs).

For graphical Gaussian modeling (GGM) only gene expression values with no missing values were used with R-package GGMselect (0.1–12.1) (Giraud et al., 2012). GGM, also known as "covariance selection" or "concentration graph" modeling, is used to build gene association networks from expression data. The principle behind GGM is to use partial correlations as a measure of independence of any two genes which allows for distinguishing direct from indirect interactions. Only genes with complete expression values were included, to fulfill the requirements of GGM, which provided a Gaussian distribution of the data. The tuning parameter K for the penalty function was varied between 1 and 8 and the function selectFast [family=c("C01," "LA," "EW")] was used for optimizing the model employing the C01 algorithm, the Lasso-And (LA), and the Adaptive lasso (EW) families (https://cran.r-project.org/web/packages/GGMselect/vignettes/Notice.pdf). At each K the corresponding gene-networks were summarized by the first principal components and used together with all remaining single gene expression values that were not summarized in a network and the clinicopathological parameters. The LASSO Cox regression models were determined by grouped LASSO regression with R-package grpregOverlap 2.2-0 (Zeng and Breheny, 2016) at each K, optimizing lambda by minimization of the negative log likelihood ($\alpha = 1$). The percentages of explained variation (PEV) of the Cox-regression models at each K-value were calculated by using the R-package Surev (v1.2) (Dunkler et al., 2007; Lusa et al., 2007) and maximized over K (*cf.* **Supplementary Figure 1**). PEVs given in **Table 2** were also calculated using this R-package. Hazard ratios, confidence intervals, and *p*-values of all predictive factors (from simple or multivariable models) were summarized in forest plots (R-package, forestplot 1.8). In cases of simple models where two variables have to be considered (continuous and _2K), the *p*-values of the Wald test with two degrees of freedom were shown for both variables.

To estimate the association of the single gene expression levels and gene-network principal components (calculated from

TABLE 2 | Percentages of explained variation (PEV) of factors of/ and the final LASSO Cox regression model.

Clinic/Genes	PEV	Partial PEV	Total PEV
Age	12.80%		
FIGO stage			
Residual tumor			
SLCO4C1 (categorical and continuous)		0.99%	
SLCO5A1 (categorical and continuous)		5.08%	
SLCO1B7		0.32%	
SLCO2A1		1.12%	
ABCC2		0.84%	
ESR1		1.08%	
ABCB2/ABCB3/ABCC4/HER2		0.08%	
			23.13%

The corresponding PEVs for the final multi-variable Cox model are shown (starting from 12.80% for the model including only the three clinicopathological factors). After including all seven additional predictors, a PEV of 23.13% was reached. The categorical and continuous variables for SLCO4C1 and SLCO5A1 were used together (see ***Figure 2****).*

TABLE 3 | Spearman rank correlation coefficients.

Gene/Network/Clinic	nM_M	O_T	EMT	Yoshihara
ABCB2/ABCB3/ABCC4/HER2	−0.01	0.02	0.08	−0.19
ABCC2	0.02	−0.01	−0.01	0.06
ESR1	−0.01	0.12	−0.12	−0.15
SLCO1B7	0.01	0.06	0.03	0.05
SLCO2A1	−0.16	0.02	−0.09	0.28
SLCO4C1	−0.08	0.12	0.04	−0.13
SLCO5A1	−0.09	−0.14	0.00	−0.13
Age	−0.13	0.04	0.01	0.12
FIGO	−0.01	−0.09	−0.17	0.04
Residual tumor	−0.06	0.02	0.04	0.12
ABCA1	−0.07	0.04	−0.13	0.21
ABCB1	−0.10	0.10	0.04	0.00
ABCC10	0.02	0.08	0.01	0.04
ESR2	−0.04	−0.05	−0.15	−0.26
HPGD	−0.18	0.08	−0.07	0.13
PTGS2	0.01	0.00	−0.12	0.05
PXR	−0.11	0.05	−0.02	−0.21
SLCO1A2	−0.22	−0.07	−0.10	−0.04
SLCO1B3	0.03	0.03	0.14	0.02
SLCO2B1/ABCC3	−0.05	0.11	−0.04	0.28
SLCO3A1	−0.10	0.13	−0.04	−0.08
SLCO4A1	0.07	0.10	0.19	−0.08
SLCO6A1	0.02	−0.08	−0.01	−0.03
SULT1E1	−0.06	0.11	−0.06	0.02

Data are given for (i) gene expressions, the first principal components of the co-expression networks, and clinicopathological parameters with (ii) gene signatures indicating molecular characteristics: peritoneal spread types, non-miliary or miliary (nM_M), positive value: high expression with M spreading; putative tumor origin, ovarian or fallopian tube (O_T), positive value: high expression with T origin; the epithelial-mesenchymal status (EMT), positive value: high expression with a more epithelial characteristic; and the Yoshihara (Yosh) molecular sub-classification system, high expression with subclass 2. Gray labeled are those genes, which were selected by the grouped LASSO approach predicting corresponding molecular characteristic. Bold printed are all genes/networks not present in any predictive LASSO regression model.

the GGM selected networks) with molecular characteristics known to be important in HGSC biology, which included a molecular subclassification system (Yoshihara, "Yosh") (Yoshihara et al., 2009), a signature indicating tumor spread types, non-miliary and miliary ("nM_M"; Auer et al., 2015), a signature indicating putative origin of HGSOC, either fallopian tubes or ovaries ("O_T"; Auer et al., 2017), and a signature indicating the epithelial-mesenchymal status ("EMT"; Miow et al., 2015), grouped LASSO logistic (Yoshihara subclasses 1 and 2) and linear (all other signatures) regression analyses were employed. Simple Spearman's rank correlation coefficients are shown in **Table 3**. The overlap with Yoshihara subclasses and the gene signatures were calculated from the corresponding microarray expression values that were previously determined in our lab (Pils et al., 2012). Overlapping genes related to the overall survival ("OS") and the four subclassification/gene signatures were illustrated by a Venn diagram (R-package VennDiagram, v1.6.19). All calculations were performed in R version 3.4.3 (R Core Team, 2018).

RESULTS

Analysis Outline

The expression levels of genes coding for organic anion transporting polypeptides OATPs (*SLCOs*, $n = 12$), ABC-efflux pumps related to drug resistance ($n = 8$), the nuclear receptor PXR and three enzymes with possible relevance to the putative function of the transporters in the turnover of prostaglandins and estrogens (*PTGS2, PGDH,* and *SULT1E1)* were studied in samples from serous ovarian cancer together with *ESR1* coding for ERα, *ESR2* coding for ERβ and *HER-2* (**Supplementary Tables 1, 2**). Notably, the chosen enzymes PTGS2 and PGDH were used because of the importance of PTGS2 and PGDH in regulating PGE2 levels and their potential influence on inflammatory processes in cancer (Nomura et al., 2004), whereas SULT1E1 was used because it was shown that higher SULT1E1 protein levels were associated with an improved OS rate in HGSOC (Mungenast et al., 2017).

The main aim of the analysis was to elucidate the independent impact of the expression of these genes on OS with regard being given to the typical clinicopathological parameters known to predict outcome: age, FIGO stage IV vs. III, and residual tumor mass after debulking surgery (yes vs. no). Genes, which were expressed below the detection limit in some samples were represented by two variables in all models [one categorical variable ("_2K") indicating expressed or not expressed (i.e., below detection limit) and another numerical variable for those samples where expression values were available, and both variables were forced to be included into the model either together or not at all]. To narrow down the number of predictors and to obtain biological information regarding the putative regulatory networks, we tried to use a method used to distinguish direct from indirect interactions by constructing the GGMs, from the expression data, only including genes with complete expression values (no samples below the detection limit). For GGM building, the tuning parameter K was varied between meaningful borders (Pils et al., 2012; Auer et al., 2015, 2017; Kurman and Shih Ie, 2016; Karam et al., 2017; Labidi-Galy et al., 2017; Salomon-Perzynski et al., 2017; Sukhbaatar et al., 2017) and selected according the maximized proportion of explained variation (PEV) of the corresponding LASSO Cox regression models for OS. The networks of directly correlated genes, as determined by the GGM procedure at each tuning variable value, were represented by the first principal component (PC1) of the network-gene expression values during model building (**Supplementary Figures 1, 2**).

To determine the impact of the genes or co-regulated networks (GGM networks) on the different characteristics of HGSOC tumors [related to a putative origin in T or O, molecular subclass, peritoneal tumor metastasis characteristic (nM or M) and EMT status], we used grouped LASSO logistic or linear regression modeling.

mRNA Expression in HGSOC (RT-qPCR)

Reverse transcriptase RT-qPCR was performed on total RNAs isolated from the tumor samples from 135 patients with advanced (FIGO stage III/IV) HGSOC (**Supplementary Table 1**).

Expression levels were calculated from the log2 expression values of the respective genes normalized to the geometric mean of four stably expressed genes (*ACTB, TOP1, UBC,* and *YWHAZ*) for individual samples. Data for all genes are summarized in **Supplementary Table 2**. As expected from previous findings on *SLCO* expression in various ovarian cancer subtypes (Svoboda et al., 2011), *SLCO2A1, SLCO2B1, SLCO3A1,* and *SLCO4A1* were detected in all samples, while expression of the other 8 *SLCOs* was undetectable (requiring >35 cycles in the real-time RT-PCR) in a varying number of samples within the collective. Four *SLCOs,* namely *SLCO1A2, SLCO1B3, SLCO4C1,* and *SLCO5A1* were expressed (detectable) in a larger number of samples (47.4, 38.5, 46.7 and 70.3% of samples, respectively), but no discrimination was made for *SLCO1B3* variants (*lt-SLCO1B3* and *ct-SLCO1B3*). Three *SLCOs* that demonstrated a unique expression pattern in healthy tissues (liver, testis and brain) were also detected in a small number of ovarian cancer samples: "liver-specific" *SLCO1B1* in 1.5%, "testis-specific" *SLCO6A1* in 14.1% and *SLCO1C1*, which codes for the "brain thyroid transporter," in 3% of samples.

In all samples of our cohort we detected the expression of *SLCO1B7*, which was previously considered a pseudogene but has recently been characterized for protein coding (Malagnino et al., 2018). This was a notable finding as the expression of *SLCO1B7* in normal tissues is considered to be high only in liver (https://www.ncbi.nlm.nih.gov/gene/338821).

mRNA expression levels of other genes investigated (the ABC-transporters coding *ABCA1, ABCB1, ABCB2, ABCB3, ABCC1, ABCC2, ABCC3, ABCC4,* and *ABCC10*, as well as *ESR1, ESR2, HER-2, PXR, PTGS2, PGDH,* and *SULT1E1*) were detectable in all samples (**Supplementary Table 2**).

Comparison of *SLCO* Expression Between HGSOCs and Benign Ovarian Cysts

By comparing the expression of *SLCOs* in HGSOC with that in benign ovarian cyst samples, we found that the expression values of *SLCOs* were generally higher in HGSOCs compared with benign tumors. Excluded from the calculation were *SLCO1B1* and *SLCO1C1*, which were rarely expressed in HGSOC tumor tissues (**Supplementary Table 2**) and were never observed in benign cysts (data not shown). All other data were used for estimating the differences between benign cysts and tumor tissues were presented as boxplots (**Figure 1**). Corresponding significance values (FDRs; Mann-Whitney-Wilcoxon tests corrected for multiple testing) and missing rates in benign cysts and cancer samples were shown. The data indicated that all analyzed *SLCO* genes exhibited significantly increased expression levels (and/or were more often detectable) in cancer compared with benign tissue samples (FDR ranging from 0.038 for *SLCO2B1* to 5.3×10^{-12} for SLCO3A1 and SLCO4A1, respectively). Importantly, *SLCO1B3* expression was only detected in 1/21 cysts (4.8%) and in 38.5% of HGSOC tissues (FDR = 0.0079). Although our analysis did not discriminate between lt-*SLCO1B3* and the cancer-type variant, it is most likely that ct-*SLCO1B3* might be the prominent isoform in the tumors investigated (Furihata et al., 2015; Thakkar et al., 2015; Alam et al., 2018). Both, *SLCO4C1* (FDR = 3.1×10^{-4}) and *SLCO6A1* (FDR = 0.14) were not detectable in any of the benign ovarian cysts, however, there was no significant difference between the broad range of SLCO6A1 expression in the 14.1% of HGSOC samples compared with the benign ovarian cysts.

Networks of Directly Correlated Genes

We studied the impact of all genes investigated on the OS in the present HGSOC cohort. Clinicopathological parameters (age, FIGO stage IV vs. III, and residual tumor mass after debulking surgery) were always added as independent variables. Two *SLCO* genes were excluded from further analyses because they were only expressed in a limited number of samples (*SLCO1B1* and *SLCO1C1*). Five *SLCO* genes, which were expressed below the detection limit in several samples (**Supplementary Table 2**), were represented by two variables (one with suffix "_2K") in all models (*SLCO1A2, SLCO1B3, SLCO4C1, SLCO5A1,* and *SLCO6A1*). To narrow down the number of predictors in the LASSO Cox regression models and to obtain biological information regarding putative regulatory connections, we constructed GGMs. As shown in the inset of **Supplementary Figure 1**, the tuning parameter K was varied between meaningful borders (Pils et al., 2012; Auer et al., 2015, 2017; Kurman and Shih Ie, 2016; Karam et al., 2017; Labidi-Galy et al., 2017; Salomon-Perzynski et al., 2017; Sukhbaatar et al., 2017) and the final used value determined by maximizing the PEV of the corresponding LASSO Cox regression model for OS was conducted for GGM building. The PEVs of the Cox regression models are shown for all used GGM tuning parameter values (**Table 2**). A steady increase of the PEV up to $K = 4$ was seen, with no further increase beyond 4. Therefore, the model at $K = 4$ was used for all further analyses, which yielded two putative co-regulated networks: *ABCB2/ABCB3/ABCC4/HER2* and *ABCC3/SLCO2B1* (**Supplementary Figure 1**). In **Supplementary Figure 2**, the correlation between genes within network 1 and network 2, respectively, are shown based on the model at $K = 4$.

Influence of Genes and Networks on OS

In **Figure 2** (**A**: simple, **B**: final multi-variable model), forest plots of Cox regression models for the 20 independent genes and the two networks at $K = 4$ for OS are presented. In addition to the three clinicopathological parameters age, FIGO stage and residual tumor with a statistically significant negative impact on OS, *SLCO5A1* was the only independent single gene with a significant positive impact on OS [HR, 0.44 (CI 0.27–0.73) and 0.68 (0.49–0.93) for _2K and the continuous variable, respectively; $p = 0.0031$; Wald test with two degrees of freedom]. A significant positive impact on OS was also observed for *ESR1* coding for ERα, which was as expected (**Figure 2A**; HR, 0.89; unadjusted $p = 0.0325$).

Notably, there was only *SLCO4C1* exhibited a trend for negative impact at _2K [HR, 3.74 (CI 1.02–13.71)] and at the corresponding continuous variable [HR, 1.26 (CI 0.92–1.72) $p = 0.0577$]. Similarly, a tendency for a negative impact was noted for *SLCO1A2* and *SLCO6A1*, and a positive impact on the OS for *SLCO1B3* and *SLCO1B7* was also indicated. However, because of the high variability of data and

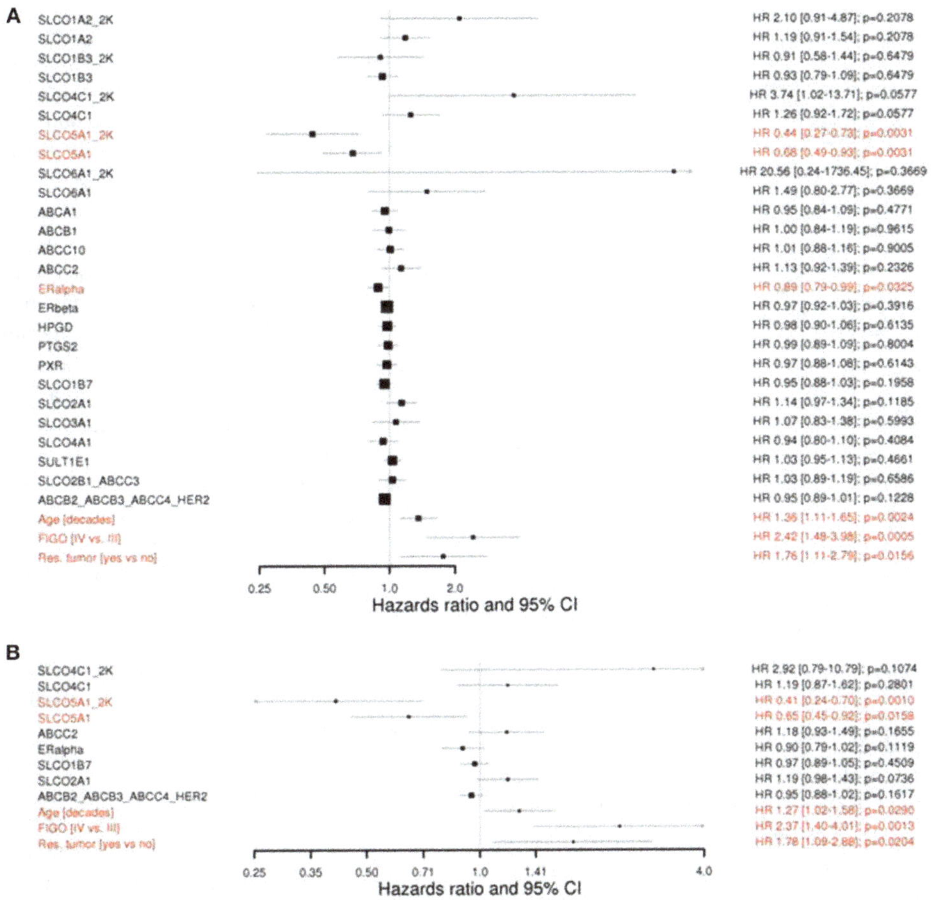

FIGURE 2 | Forest plots showing the univariate Cox regression analyses **(A)** and the LASSO COX regression model for overall survival **(B)**. Current clinicopathological factors in ovarian cancer, including age, FIGO stage and residual tumor after debulking surgery are shown. Genes in networks are indicated by "_" between their names. "_2K" demonstrates the dichotomized variable indicating either expressed or undetectable (*cf.* Methods). *P*-values were from the 2 degrees of freedom Wald test if two variables, a continuous and a "_2K" were considered together. HR, hazard ratio; CI, confidence intervals; FIGO, International Federation of Gynecology Obstetrics; OS, overall survival. Note that *SLCO5A1* expression is significantly associated with improved prognosis in both analyses.

restricted expression values, no level of significance was reached. Furthermore, no significant independent influence on the OS in the univariate and multivariate analysis was demonstrated for the two identified gene networks *ABCB2/ABCB3/ABCC4/HER2,* and SLCO2B1/ABCC3 for the remaining genes.

In the multivariable analysis (**Figure 2B**), only *SLCO5A1* but not *ESR1* exhibited a significant positive impact on OS (HR, 0.41; $p = 0.001$ and HR, 0.65; $p = 0.0158$ for _2K and the continuous variable, respectively).

Using the Cox regression model at $K = 4$, the probabilities of survival were estimated for patients categorized according to the terciles in subgroups, i.e., low-, medium- and high-risk (**Figure 3**). Five-year survival estimates were 73.5% [CI 63.5–85.0], 43.6% [CI 35.0–54.2] and 10.7% [CI 5.1–22.3], respectively.

Combining the results from both analyses (LASSO Cox regression and univariate Cox regression), we indicated that *SLCO5A1* has a significant prognostic effect on OS, with favorable outcomes associated with patients with high *SLCO5A1* expression.

The corresponding percentages of PEVs for the final multivariable Cox model were shown, starting with 12.8% for the model, including the three clinicopathological factors alone (**Table 2**). It reached 23.13% after including all seven additional genes, which were found to have a prognostic impact (the categorical and continuous variables for *SLCO4C1* and *SLCO5A1* were used together, see **Figure 2**). Remarkably, *SLCO5A1* increased the PEV by 5.08%, while the contribution of *SLCO2A1* and *ESR1* was only 1.12 and 1.08%, respectively. However, these measures of added prognostic accuracy were determined on the same data set that was used for gene network and variable selection and could therefore be over-optimistic.

Immunohistochemistry of OATP5A1 in Ovarian Cancer Tissues

To validate the OATP5A1 protein expression in ovarian cancer tissues, the localization of the transporter in paraffin-embedded sections from serous ovarian cancer tissues was analyzed by using immunohistochemistry and immunofluorescence staining

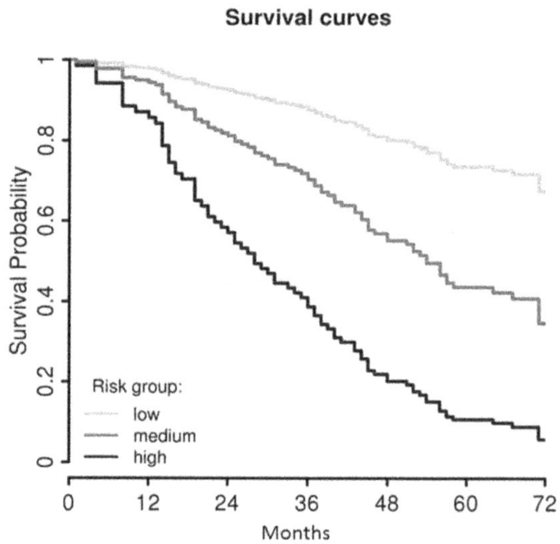

FIGURE 3 | Survival curves of the final LASSO COX regression model (*cf.* **Figure 2B**), trichotomized according the terciles of the model value in low-, medium-, and high-risk groups. As these survival curves represent a multivariable Cox model, no censored patients are indicated.

(**Figures 4A–F**). We used an antibody against OATP5A1, which was previously shown to detect the transporter by western blot analysis of OATP5A1 overexpressing Sf9 cells (Patik et al., 2015). Immunohistochemistry results indicated positive staining for OATP5A1 observed in a number of tumor cells clustered together in the tumor center, while other areas were negative for OATP5A1 (magnification 10x, **Figure 4E**). An area with OATP5A1-positive cells was also shown at a higher magnification (40x) (**Figure 4F**).

Double-immunofluorescence staining of green OATP5A1 (**Figure 4B**) and red cytokeratin-19 (**Figure 4C**), which was used as a marker for epithelial cells resulted in orange to yellow staining in some cells as a result from the overlay of green transporter with the red epithelial marker (**Figures 4A–D**). Predominately membranous staining or a more cytoplasmic staining pattern for OATP5A1 was visible in different specimens (**Figure 4B** vs. **4D**). Interestingly, OATP5A1 was more frequently detectable in tumor cells with weaker cytokeratin-19 staining compared with that in cells with strong cytokeratin-19 staining (**Figure 4A**). This was also observed in other samples ($n = 8$) from HGSOC tumors (data not shown) revealing that OATP5A1 is not restricted to tumor cells with epithelial characteristics.

Correlation With HGSOC Subclassification Systems and Gene Signatures

In the previous sections we have studied the impact of *SLCOs*, related genes and networks on OS. In this section we want to elucidate if the same genes and networks are related to published subclassification systems and gene signatures associated with specific characteristics of HGSOC (**Table 3**, **Figure 5**). Grouped LASSO logistic or linear regression modeling was used. The following characteristics were calculated from the gene expression data as described in the following references: A dichotomous molecular subclassification system published by Yoshihara et al. (Yoshihara et al., 2009) that was validated by us for OS (Auer et al., 2017); and three gene signatures correlating with (i) the EMT status (Miow et al., 2015), (ii) the putative origin of the tumors ovarian surface epithelium or fallopian tube secretory epithelial cells (O_T) (Auer et al., 2017; Sukhbaatar et al., 2017) and (iii) a signature indicating either military (M) or non-miliary (nM) tumor metastasis (nM_M) (Auer et al., 2015, 2016, 2017; Bachmayr-Heyda et al., 2016; Sukhbaatar et al., 2017). In **Figure 5**, the overlap of genes and networks used for the analysis (see also **Supplementary Figure 2**) with molecular characteristics of HGSOC (represented by these four gene signatures) was demonstrated in a Venn plot. Additionally, Spearman's rank correlation coefficients of all combinations are shown in **Table 3**.

Importantly, the positive impact of *SLCO5A1* on OS determined by the multivariate and univariate COX analyses correlated with its attribution to the Yoshihara subclass 1, which suggested a favorable OS. Consistent with our validation data (OS), within this group we identified *SLCO5A1*, *ESR1*, and the network *ABCB2/ABCB3/ABCC4/HER2*. Notably, *SLCO1B7 and ABCC2* corresponded with our own validated signature (OS).

Remarkably, *SLCO3A1* was associated with Yoshihara group 1 but also with a signature reflecting a putative origin from the ovaries rather than from the Fallopian tubes (O_T) and EMT. Notably, tumors to be considered of ovarian origin were also characterized with an improved prognosis. Since ovarian cancer cells express mesenchymal and epithelial markers simultaneously, transition from one state to another might be a continuous process in these cells (Auer et al., 2017), for which *SLCO3A1* might be a marker.

Interestingly, the genes coding for the prostaglandin transporter *SLCO2A1* and the PGE_2-inactivating enzyme *HPGD*, respectively, overlap with the Yoshihara signature and the n-M signature for peritoneal metastasis. An overlap with the n-M_M signature was also observed for *SLCO1A2*. *SLCO2A1* additionally belonged to our OS signature. It was indicated that the N-M tumor metastasis pattern and a putative ovarian origin, rather than tubular origin, are associated with a more favorable prognosis (Auer et al., 2017), which would be in line with a role of *SLCO2A1* and *HPGD* implicated in the degradation of pro-inflammatory prostaglandins.

From the 21 genes investigated, 5 genes (*SLCO1B3*, *SLCO6A1*, *ABCB1*, *ABCC10*, and *PTGS2*) did not belong to any signature in the subclassification systems used in our LASSO regression models.

DISCUSSION

The present study investigated the impact of the expression of *SLCO* and related genes coding for ABC-transporters, PXR, ESR1/2, and HER-2 in serous ovarian cancer patients treated with debulking surgery and platinium- and taxane-based chemotherapy. The results indicated that all *SLCOs* were upregulated in HGSOC compared with benign ovarian cysts

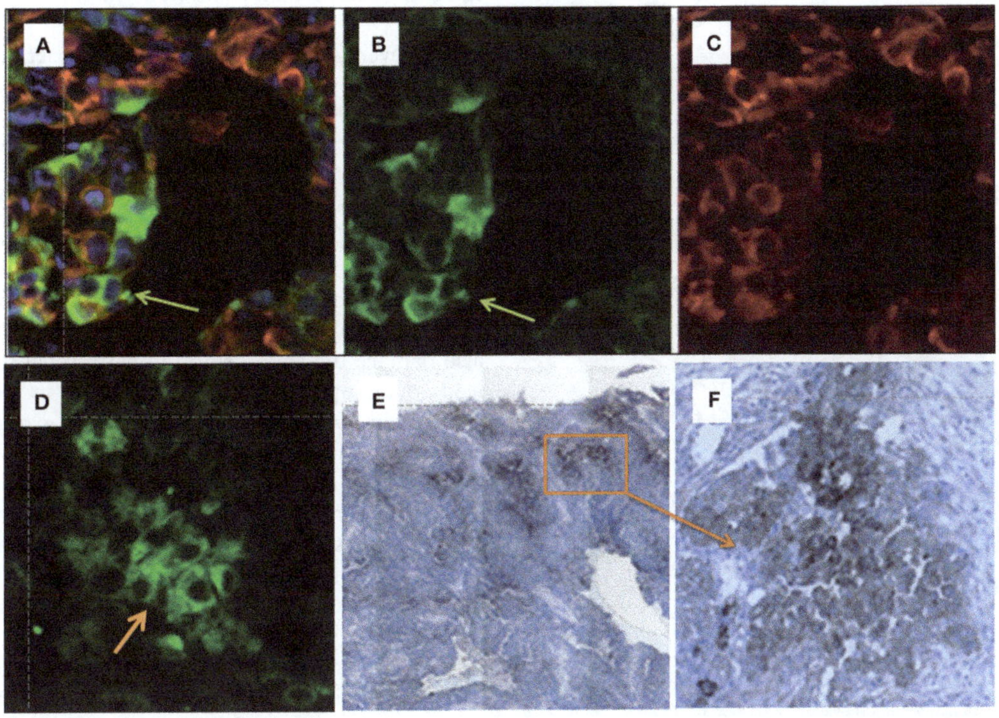

FIGURE 4 | (A–F) Immunohistochemical detection of OATP5A1 in HGSOC tissue samples. Double immunofluorescence staining of OATP5A1 (green) and cytokeratin 19 (red) in paraffin-embedded sections from serous ovarian carcinomas **(A–D)**. **(A)** Merged image of OATP5A1 **(B)** and cytokeratin-19 **(C)**. The orange overlay color for co-localized OATP5A1 and cytokeratin-19 is only visible in some cells (yellow arrow) in the tumor. Note the staining of the cytoplasm and membrane with the antibody against OATP5A1 is visible in image **(B)**, and the predominantly cytoplasmic staining of OATP5A1 in image **(D)**. Immunohistochemical staining of OATP5A1 in HGSOC sections **(D,E)**. Overview on a HGSOC section (x10) revealing clusters of brown (OATP5A1)-stained cells in the tumor **(E)**. Clusters of OATP5A1-positive cells at a higher magnification, x40 **(F)**.

and it was identified that *SLCO5A1* may be a potential positive prognostic factor for OS of HGSOC patients. Furthermore, the present findings suggested two networks of *SLCO* and ABC-transporter coding genes (*SLCO2B1/ABCC3* and *ABCB2/ABCB3/ABCC3/HER-2*) and demonstrated the expression of *SLCO1B7* in ovarian cancer samples.

Higher expression of all *SLCOs* in samples from serous ovarian cancer compared with benign ovarian tumor samples suggests the importance of this *SLCO*/OATP family for cancer progression. Many studies have revealed that transporters of the OATP family are functionally expressed in cancerous tissues, where they may be critical for determining the local concentration of endogenous metabolites such as steroid hormones, mediators in the inflammatory pathway and others as well as drugs. Thereby they can influence cancer biology and progression.

Particularly expression *of SLCO5A1* is of interest, because by using a combination of LASSO Cox regression and univariate Cox regression models, we showed that higher *SLCO5A1* expression in tissues of HGSOC patients had a significant positive impact on overall survival, a thus seems to have protective functions. The significant association of high *SLCO5A1* expression with the Yoshihara subclass 1 is in agreement with the positive effects on OS from or study (Pils et al., 2012). Further support of our findings is coming from data from the Human Protein Atlas where a trend for a better survival probability for ovarian cancer patients is associated with higher OATP5A1 mRNA expression levels (https://www.proteinatlas.org/ENSG00000137571-SLCO5A1/pathology).

These data clearly suggest that further studies in a larger collective of HGSOC patients should be performed to further explore the prognostic value of *SLCO5A1* in HGSOC. Furthermore, there is a general lack of studies on a potential prognostic effect of OATP5A1 for cancer patients; however, *SLCO5A1* expression has been reported in a number of tumors and the localization of the OATP5A1 protein has been shown in liver and breast tumors (Kindla et al., 2011; Wlcek et al., 2011).

The data also raise the question whether OATP5A1 functions as a transporter for known OATP substrates into cells (Hagenbuch and Gui, 2008; Stieger and Hagenbuch, 2014). Notably, a recent study in *SLCO5A1* transfected Sf9 insect cells indeed showed that OATP5A1 is capable of mediating the uptake of E2-glucuronide at an acidic pH (Patik et al., 2015). Because extensive lactate secretion from the anaerobic glycolysis leads to an acidification of the extracellular tumor environment (Kato et al., 2013), uptake processes for potential estrogen precursors driven by the proton gradient might also be important for the progression of hormone-dependent ovarian cancer cells. It is

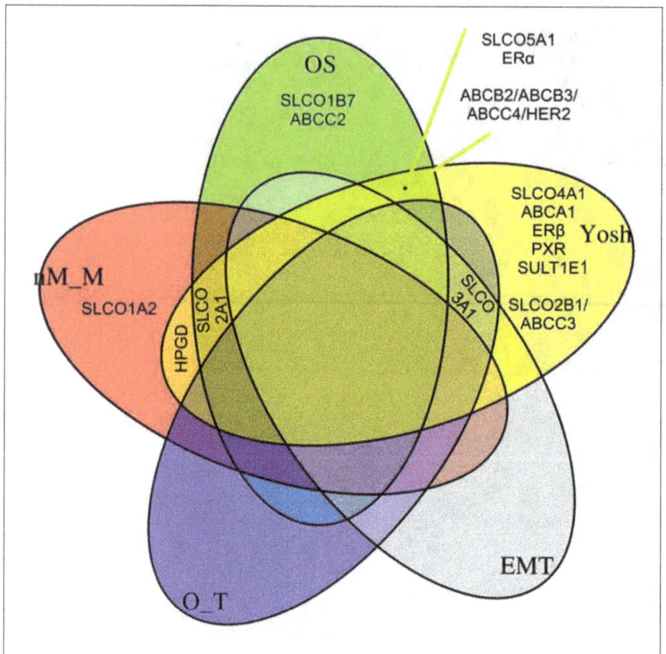

FIGURE 5 | Quintuple Venn plot. Overlapping genes/networks from the LASSO Cox regression model (*OS*, **Figure 2B**), a logistic regression model indicating a molecular subclassification system published by Yoshihara et al. (2009), and linear regression models (a gene signature indicating the epithelial-mesenchymal transition status (*EMT*), a gene signature indicating the putative origin of the tumors (Auer et al., 2017; Sukhbaatar et al., 2017), either ovarian surface epithelium or fallopian tube secretory epithelial cells (*O_T*), and to a signature indicating either miliary (M) or non-miliary (nM) tumor spread (*nM_M*) (Auer et al., 2015, 2016, 2017; Bachmayr-Heyda et al., 2016; Sukhbaatar et al., 2017). See also **Table 3**, where simple Spearman's rank correlation coefficients of all combinations given in Figure are shown.

worth to mentioning that pH-dependent transport of estrogen precursors was also described for the OATP2B1 in luminal A-like breast cancer (Matsumoto et al., 2015). Furthermore, the present results found that this OATP was upregulated in all HGSOC specimens investigated (see **Figure 1**).

The prominent cytosolic localization of OATP5A1 in ovarian cancer samples provides arguments against an important role of OATP5A1 in the transport of estrogen precursors or other substrates through the plasma membrane in HGSOC. For the uptake of compounds into the cells or extrusion of metabolites from cells to the extracellular space, plasma membrane localization would be required. However, OATP5A1 may still function as a transporter in intracellular organelles, which has been shown for a number of other transporters (Hediger et al., 2004). Also, intracellular sequestration of pharmacological agents may explain the increased resistance of HEK-293 cells to satraplatin after transfection with OATP5A1 (Olszewski-Hamilton et al., 2011). There is a strong possibility that OATP5A1 influences cancer progression by influencing cellular differentiation and migration directly. Studies in HeLa cells revealed that overexpression of OATP5A1 resulted in a reduction of cell proliferation and enhanced expression of genes that contribute to cell-cell adhesion, structural development and cell growth including desmocollin 3 and transglutaminase 2 (Sebastian et al., 2013).

However, a significant negative impact [a shift of HR to 3.74 (1.02–13.71; $p =$ 0.047)] on the OS was demonstrated for *SLCO4C1* as a single gene in the present study. *SLCO4C1* encodes the "kidney-specific" OATP4C1, a transporter for the excretion of uremic toxins to the urine (Toyohara et al., 2009). Because excretion of these toxins is impaired through kidney damage, upregulation of this transporter may reflect the damage to endothelium and other structures. With disease progression, other organs may be subjected to destruction by these toxins. As result, increased levels of uremic toxins can also damage the endothelium in extra-renal tissues, which may lead to an upregulation of OATP4C1 in tumors. This may explain the expression of *SLCO4C1* in a number of HGSOC samples and its absence in benign ovarian cysts in the present findings.

It is unclear which mechanism(s) may lead to the upregulation of *SLOC* genes in serous ovarian cancer. On the molecular levels, many mechanisms for epigenomic alterations are known that can change the gene expression pattern (Furihata et al., 2015). Both, (gene specific) hypermethylation and (global) hypomethylation of the DNA are commonly observed in various types of cancers incuding ovarian cancer (Kwon and Shin, 2011). Previous studies examined the expression of ct-OATO1B3 mRNA and indicated that DNA hypomethylation caused upregulation and that hypermethylation resulted in the suppression of ct-OATP1B3 mRNA expression in cancer cell lines (Imai et al., 2013; Sun et al., 2014).

Different transcription factors have been identified in the regulation of OATP expression. Importantly, the mRNA expression of a cancer-specific OATP1B3 variant is induced by the hypoxia-inducible factor (HIF-1α), which mediates cell survival under hypoxic conditions (Han et al., 2013). Apart from the *SLCO1B3* gene, binding sites for HIF-1α were also found in *SLCO4A1*, while binding sites for different transcription factors including HNF-α, NF-AT, c-Myc, NF-κB were found in different *SLCOs* using *in silico* structural analyses (http://www.genecards.org). For OATP5A1 expression, (http://www.genecards.org/cgi-bin/carddisp.pl?gene=SLCO5A1) a p53 binding site in the promoter of *SLCO5A1* was identified *in silico*. Because *TP53* is mutated in >95% of HGSOCs, missense mutations in the DNA-binding domain of *TP53* might be related to lower levels of *SLCO5A1* in HGSOC samples, Whether there is a correlation between *TP53* mutations, *SLCO5A1* levels and the prognosis for HGSOC patients. Further studies are required to elucidate this.

In the present study we identified two networks between genes coding for OATP transporters and ABC-efflux pumps. Although only a marginal impact of both networks was indicated according to the HR in univariate and multivariate COX analyses in our study, the network *ABCB2/ABCB3/ABCC4/HER-2* was indicated to be associated with the Yoshihara group 1 and a more favorable prognosis (Yoshihara et al., 2009; Pils et al., 2012).

The first identified co-expression network revealed *SLCO2B1* was connected with the *ABCC3* gene coding for the ABCC3 protein (MRP3). Notably, ABCC3 is implicated in drug resistance but also mediates the efflux of many glucuronidated metabolites formed from drugs. Therefore ABCC3 may be important for estrogen inactivation. Interestingly, a joint activity for OATP2B1 with another ABC-efflux pump, ABCG2 (BCRP), was described in a study on the human placenta, where the two transporters were thought to mediate uptake and excretion of sulfated estrogen precursors (Grube et al., 2007). However, considering that OATP2B1 may be an uptake transporter for estrogens, it has been suggested that a number of OATPs (OATP1A2, OATP1B1, OATP1B3, OATP1C1, OATP3A1, OATP4A1, and OATP5A1) (Stieger and Hagenbuch, 2014) and also LST-3TM12 and OATP6A1 (Patik et al., 2015; Malagnino et al., 2018) are capable of transporting estrogen precursors. Furthermore, the substrate specificity for E1S and DHEA-S differs widely between individual members and cells investigated. In serous ovarian cancer, *SLCO1B1, SLCO1C1,* and *SLCO6A1* were observed in a low number of samples only. This suggests that the contribution of individual OATPs for providing estrogen precursors to cancer cells may depend on the specific expression pattern in a certain tumor entity and its local environment.

The second identified co-expression network in serous ovarian cancer exists between ABC-transporters *(ABCB2, ABCB3,* and *ABCC4)* and *HER-2*. In this network, *ABCB3* and *ABCB2* are coding for the functional transporters TAP1 and TAP2 as part of the immune system. Endogenous peptides are transported by the TAP-complex from the cytosol to the endoplasmic reticulum and loaded onto MHC I for antigen processing. A down-regulation of the HLA class I antigen presentation machinery (APM) decreases recruitment of tumor-infiltrating lymphocytes, which leads to a reduction in the antitumor activity of the immune system (Aust et al., 2017). We previously showed that programmed death-ligand 1 (*PD-L1*) also known as CD274 on tumor cells is associated with reduced MHC I (APM) expression in HGSOC. This indicates two mutually exclusive immune-evasion mechanisms in ovarian cancer: down-regulation of T-cell mediated immunity by PD-L1 expression and silencing of self-antigen presentation by down-regulation of the MHC I complex (Aust et al., 2017). The correlation of the expression of this network with Yoshihara subclass 1 with a better prognosis also corresponds to the correlation of low MHC I expression with bad prognosis. Higher levels of ABCB2 and ABCB3 in ovarian tumors were previously shown to be associated with longer survival of patients (Auner et al., 2010). Upregulation of *ABCB2* and *ABCB3* in the antigen presentation pathway may therefore improve antigen-specific active immunotherapy and the outcome of an antibody-based therapy against HER-2. The forth component in the network is *ABCC4*, which codes for the ATP-efflux-pump ABCC4 (MRP4). ABCC4 substrates include cyclic nucleotides (cGMP, cAMP), anticancer drugs such as camptothecins, methotrexate and prostaglandins. By mediating nucleotide transport, ABCC4 influences various purinergic signaling pathways, which depending on the local conditions, either inhibits or stimulates cell survival, proliferation, invasion and metastasis in various types of cancer (Choi et al., 2003) and may lead to an altered expression of *HER-2* (Chen et al., 2016). Furthermore, ABCC4 is an important efflux transporter for the PGE_2 and may work with OATP2A1 and the PGE synthesizing/degrading enzymes *PTGS2,* and *PGDH* in the processing and degrading of PGE_2 synthesized in the arachidonic pathway. However, no direct co-expression for *ABCC4* with these enzymes or *SLCO2A1* was observed in our study, which was in contrast to previous data from a colon cancer study (Nomura et al., 2004).

An additional important finding of the present study was that *SLCO1B7,* which is a poorly characterized member of the *SLCO* family 1 member, was present in all samples in the cohort. A recent *in silico* analysis revealed that trans-splicing of *SLCO1B7* and *SLCO1B3* produced a novel OATP family 1 member, LST-3TM12. Furthermore, heterologous expression of *SLCO1B3* and *SLCO1B7* in HeLa cells leads to LST-3TM12 protein expression, resulting in an increased cellular accumulation of E2-glucuronide and DHEA-S (Malagnino et al., 2018). However, we did not observe significant co-expression of *SLCO1B7* with *SLCO1B3* in our cohort, but co-expression with the cancer-specific variant might be possible (Furihata et al., 2015; Thakkar et al., 2015). Therefore, future studies are warranted to elucidate the expression pattern of *SLCO1B7* with ct-*SLCO1B3* in cancer to elucidate whether a functional LST-3TM12 protein in HGSOC exits and to gain information to its relation to drug resistance and cancer progression.

Taken together, we indicated an analysis of a small but well-documented number of patients to elucidate the OATP mRNA expression pattern in HGSOC. However, the approach used in the present study did not address the complete biological heterogeneity nor did it identify all related genes.

In conclusion, we indicated upregulation of various *SLCO* transporters in HGSOC compared with benign cysts. Furthermore, we identified a network of *SLCO2B1* and *ABCC3* with relevance for estrogen turnover and a further network consisting of genes encoding 3ABC-efflux pumps and HER-2 with relevance for immune regulation. Additionally, an overlap with previously described signatures for a more favorable prognosis of patients with HGSOC was demonstrated for *SLCO5A1*.

AUTHOR CONTRIBUTIONS

TT, MS, RZ, and DC-T: Design and coordination of the study; MS, FM, DP, AG, and TT: Experimental part, analysis and interpretation of data; AG and DP: Bioinformatical and statistical analyses; TT, DP, MS, FM, with support of WJ, DM: Preparation of the manuscript; DC-T, RZ, IV, AV, JS, EB, and SM: Providing of sample and maintaining patient database. All authors read and approved the final manuscript.

ACKNOWLEDGMENTS

This work was supported by the 6th Framework Programme (FP6) Project of the European Union (EU) Ovarian Cancer: Diagnosis of a silent killer – OVCAD, no. 018698 (RZ, DC-T, TT, DP, and MS), the Austrian Science Fund (FWF; http://www.fwf.ac.at/): projects P23228-B19 (to DM) and I 3417-B31 (to WJ), and The Anniversary Fund of the Oesterreichische Nationalbank (OeNB): project Nr. 17278 (to DM).

SUPPLEMENTARY MATERIAL

Supplementary Figure 1 | Co-expressed gene networks. Genes used for GGM modeling are shown, which indicates the two networks that were revealed by the algorithm at the tuning parameter $K = 4$. The proportion of explained variation (PEV) values of the LASSO Cox regression models are shown for every tuning value between 1 and 8. As indicated, up to $K = 4$ a steady increase of the PEV was seen with no further increase beyond 4. Therefore, the model at $K = 4$ was used for all further analyses, which yielded two putative co-regulated networks: *SLCO2B1/ABCC3*, and *ABCB2(TAP1)/ABCB3(TAP2)/ABCC4/HER2*. These two networks were used for all analyses and represented by their first principal components (*cf.* **Supplementary Figure 2**).

Supplementary Figure 2 | Scatter plots showing the correlations of genes of both co-expressed networks with their first principal components (PC). Size coded values in the top-right square represent correlation coefficients and significance levels are indicated by $^{\circ}p < 0.1$, $^{***}p < 0.001$ (Spearman's correlations). Network 1: *SLCO2B1/ABCC3* **(A)**; Network 2: *ABCB2/ABCB3/ABCC4/HER-2* **(B)**.

Supplementary Table 1 | List of TaqMan® Gene Expression Assays for RT-qPCR. Assays were purchased from Applied Biosystems (Thermo Fisher, Waltham, MA) for RT-qPCR.

Supplementary Table 2 | Expression of *SLCOs* and genes coding for putative related ABC-transporters, enzymes, nuclear receptors, and HER-2 in 135 HGSOC samples.

REFERENCES

Alam, K., Farasyn, T., Ding, K., and Yue, W. (2018). Characterization of Liver- and Cancer-type-Organic Anion Transporting Polypeptide (OATP) 1B3 messenger RNA expression in normal and cancerous human tissues. *Drug Metab. Lett.* doi: 10.2174/1872312812666180326110146. [Epub ahead of print].

Auer, K., Bachmayr-Heyda, A., Aust, S., Grunt, T. W., and Pils, D. (2017). Comparative transcriptome analysis links distinct peritoneal tumor spread types, miliary and non-miliary, with putative origin, tubes and ovaries, in high grade serous ovarian cancer. *Cancer Lett.* 388, 158–166. doi: 10.1016/j.canlet.2016.11.034

Auer, K., Bachmayr-Heyda, A., Aust, S., Sukhbaatar, N., Reiner, A. T., and Grimm, C., (2015). Peritoneal tumor spread in serous ovarian cancer-epithelial mesenchymal status and outcome. *Oncotarget* 6, 17261–17275. doi: 10.18632/oncotarget.3746

Auer, K., Bachmayr-Heyda, A., Sukhbaatar, N., Aust, S., Schmetterer, K. G., and Meier, S. M., (2016). Role of the immune system in the peritoneal tumor spread of high grade serous ovarian cancer. *Oncotarget* 7, 61336–61354. doi: 10.18632/oncotarget.11038

Auner, V., Sehouli, J., Oskay-Oezcelik, G., Horvat, R., Speiser, P., and Zeillinger, R. (2010). ABC transporter gene expression in benign and malignant ovarian tissue. *Gynecol. Oncol.* 117, 198–201. doi: 10.1016/j.ygyno.2009.10.077

Aust, S., Felix, S., Auer, K., Bachmayr-Heyda, A., Kenner, L., Dekan, S., et al. (2017). Absence of PD-L1 on tumor cells is associated with reduced MHC I expression and PD-L1 expression increases in recurrent serous ovarian cancer. *Sci. Rep.* 7:42929. doi: 10.1038/srep42929

Bachmayr-Heyda, A., Auer, K., Sukhbaatar, N., Aust, S., Deycmar, S., Reiner, A., et al. (2016). Small RNAs and the competing endogenous RNA network in high grade serous ovarian cancer tumor spread. *Oncotarget* 7, 39640–39653. doi: 10.18632/oncotarget.9243

Bachmayr-Heyda, A., Aust, S., Auer, K., Meier, S. M., Schmetterer, K. G., and Pils, D. (2017). Integrative systemic and local metabolomics with impact on survival in high-grade serous ovarian cancer. *Clin. Cancer Res.* 23, 2081–2092. doi: 10.1158/1078-0432.CCR-16-1647

Banerjee, N., Allen, C., and Bendayan, R. (2012). Differential role of organic anion-transporting polypeptides in estrone-3-sulphate uptake by breast epithelial cells and breast cancer cells. *J. Pharmacol. Exp. Ther.* 342, 510–519. doi: 10.1124/jpet.112.192344

Bugde, P., Biswas, R., Merien, F., Lu, J., Liu, D. X., and Li, Y. (2017). The therapeutic potential of targeting ABC transporters to combat multi-drug resistance. *Expert Opin. Ther. Targets* 21, 511–530. doi: 10.1080/14728222.2017.1310841

Buxhofer-Ausch, V., Secky, L., Wlcek, K., Svoboda, M., Kounnis, V., Briasoulis, E., et al. (2013). Tumor-specific expression of organic anion-transporting polypeptides: transporters as novel targets for cancer therapy. *J. Drug Deliv.* 2013:863539. doi: 10.1155/2013/863539

Chekerov, R., Braicu, I., Castillo-Tong, D. C., Richter, R., Cadron, I., Mahner, L. et al. (2013). Outcome and clinical management of 275 patients with advanced ovarian cancer International Federation of Obstetrics and Gynecology II to IV inside the European Ovarian Cancer Translational Research Consortium-OVCAD. *Int. J. Gynecol. Cancer* 23, 268–275. doi: 10.1097/IGC.0b013e31827de6b9

Chen, Z., Shi, T., Zhang, L., Zhu, P., Deng, M., Huang, C., et al. (2016). Mammalian drug efflux transporters of the ATP binding cassette (ABC) family in multidrug resistance: a review of the past decade. *Cancer Lett.* 370, 153–164. doi: 10.1016/j.canlet.2015.10.010

Choi, K. C., Tai, C. J., Tzeng, C. R., Auersperg, N., and Leung, P. C. (2003). Adenosine triphosphate activates mitogen-activated protein kinase in pre-neoplastic and neoplastic ovarian surface epithelial cells. *Biol. Reprod.* 68, 309–315. doi: 10.1095/biolreprod.102.006551

Dong, Y., Wang, Z., Xie, G. F., Li, C., Zuo, W. W., Meng, G., et al. (2017). Pregnane X receptor is associated with unfavorable survival and induces chemotherapeutic resistance by transcriptional activating multidrug resistance-related protein 3 in colorectal cancer. *Mol. Cancer* 16:71. doi: 10.1186/s12943-017-0641-8

Dunkler, D., Michiels, S., and Schemper, M. (2007). Gene expression profiling: does it add predictive accuracy to clinical characteristics in cancer prognosis? *Eur. J. Cancer* 43, 745–751. doi: 10.1016/j.ejca.2006.11.018

Elsnerova, K., Mohelnikova-Duchonova, B., Cerovska, E., Ehrlichova, M., Gut, I., Rob, L., et al. (2016). Gene expression of membrane transporters: importance for prognosis and progression of ovarian carcinoma. *Oncol. Rep.* 35, 2159–2170. doi: 10.3892/or.2016.4599

Furihata, T., Sun, Y., and Chiba, K. (2015). Cancer-type organic anion transporting polypeptide 1B3: current knowledge of the gene structure, expression profile, functional implications and future perspectives. *Curr. Drug Metab.* 16, 474–485. doi: 10.2174/1389200216666150812142715

Giraud, C., Huet, S., and Verzelen, N. (2012). Graph selection with GGMselect. *Stat. Appl. Genet. Mol. Biol.* 11:3. doi: 10.1515/1544-6115.1625

Grube, M., Reuther, S. H., Meyer Zu Schwabedissen, Köck, K., Draber, K., Ritter, C., et al. (2007). Organic anion transporting polypeptide 2B1 and breast cancer resistance protein interact in the transepithelial transport of steroid sulfates in human placenta. *Drug Metab. Dispos.* 35, 30–35. doi: 10.1124/dmd.106.011411

Hagenbuch, B., and Gui, C. (2008). Xenobiotic transporters of the human organic anion transporting polypeptides (OATP) family. *Xenobiotica* 38, 778–801. doi: 10.1080/00498250801986951

Han, S., Kim, K., Thakkar, N., Kim, D., and Lee, W. (2013). Role of hypoxia inducible factor-1 α in the regulation of the cancer-specific variant of organic anion transporting polypeptide 1B3 (OATP1B3), in colon and pancreatic cancer. *Biochem. Pharmacol.* 86, 816–823. doi: 10.1016/j.bcp.2013.07.020

Hediger, M. A., Romero, M. F., Peng, J. B., Rolfs, A., Takanaga, H., and Bruford, E. A. (2004). The ABCs of solute carriers: physiological, pathological and therapeutic implications of human membrane transport proteinsIntroduction. *Pflugers Arch.* 447, 465–468. doi: 10.1007/s00424-003-1192-y

Holla, V. R., Backlund, M. G., Yang, P., Newman, R. A., and DuBois, R. N. (2008). Regulation of prostaglandin transporters in colorectal neoplasia. *Cancer Prev. Res.* 1, 93–99. doi: 10.1158/1940-6207.CAPR-07-0009

Imai, S., Kikuchi, R., Tsuruya,Y., Naoi, S., Nishida, S., Kusuhara, H., et al.(2013). Epigenetic regulation of organic anion transporting polypeptide 1B3 in cancer cell lines. *Pharm. Res.* 30, 2880–2890. doi: 10.1007/s11095-013-1117-1

Karam, A., Ledermann, J. A., Kim, J. W., Sehouli, J., Lu, K., and Ochiai, K. (2017). Fifth ovarian cancer consensus conference of the gynecologic cancer intergroup: first-line interventions. *Ann. Oncol.* 28, 711–717. doi: 10.1093/annonc/mdx011

Kato, Y., Ozawa, S., Miyamoto, C., Maehata, Y., Suzuki, A., Maeda, T., et al. (2013). Acidic extracellular microenvironment and cancer. *Cancer Cell Int.* 13:89. doi: 10.1186/1475-2867-13-89

Kindla, J., Rau, T. T., Jung, R., Fasching, P. A., Strick, R., and Stoehr, R. (2011). Expression and localization of the uptake transporters OATP2B1, OATP3A1 and OATP5A1 in non-malignant and malignant breast tissue. *Cancer Biol. Ther.* 11, 584–591. doi: 10.4161/cbt.11.6.14533

Kochel, T. J., and Fulton, A. M. (2015). Multiple drug resistance-associated protein 4 (MRP4), prostaglandin transporter (PGT), and 15-hydroxyprostaglandin dehydrogenase (15-PGDH) as determinants of PGE2 levels in cancer. *Prostaglandins Other Lipid Mediat.* 116–117, 99–103. doi: 10.1016/j.prostaglandins.2014.11.003

Kurman, R. J., and Shih Ie, M. (2016). The dualistic model of ovarian carcinogenesis: revisited, revised, and expanded. *Am. J. Pathol.* 186, 733–747. doi: 10.1016/j.ajpath.2015.11.011

Kwon, M. J., and Shin, Y. K. (2011). Epigenetic regulation of cancer-associated genes in ovarian cancer. *Int. J. Mol. Sci.* 12, 983–1008. doi: 10.3390/ijms12020983

Labidi-Galy, S. I., Papp, E., Hallberg, D., Niknafs, N., Adleff, V., and Noe, M. (2017). High grade serous ovarian carcinomas originate in the fallopian tube. *Nat. Commun.* 8:1093. doi: 10.1038/s41467-017-00962-1

Lusa, L., Miceli, R., and Mariani, L. (2007). Estimation of predictive accuracy in survival analysis using R and S-PLUS. *Comput. Methods Prog. Biomed.* 87, 132–137. doi: 10.1016/j.cmpb.2007.05.009

Malagnino, V., Hussner, J., Seibert, I., Stolzenburg, A., Sager, C. P., and Meyer Zu Schwabedissen, H. E. (2018). LST-3TM12 is a member of the OATP1B family and a functional transporter. *Biochem. Pharmacol.* 148, 75–87. doi: 10.1016/j.bcp.2017.12.012

Matsumoto, J., Ariyoshi, N., Sakakibara, M., Nakanishi, T., Okubo, Y., Shiina, N., et al. (2015). Organic anion transporting polypeptide 2B1 expression correlates with uptake of estrone-3-sulfate and cell proliferation in estrogen receptor-positive breast cancer cells. *Drug Metab. Pharmacokinet.* 30, 133–141. doi: 10.1016/j.dmpk.2014.10.005

Miow, Q. H., Tan, T. Z., Ye, J., Lau, J. A., Yokomizo, T., and Mori, S. (2015). Epithelial-mesenchymal status renders differential responses to cisplatin in ovarian cancer. *Oncogene* 34, 1899–1907. doi: 10.1038/onc.2014.136

Mueller, J. W., Gilligan, L. C., Idkowiak, J., Arlt, W., and Foster, P. A. (2015). The regulation of steroid action by sulfation and desulfation. *Endocr. Rev.* 36, 526–563. doi: 10.1210/er.2015-1036

Mungenast, F., Aust, S., Vergote, I., Vanderstichele, A., Sehouli, J., Braicu, E., et al. (2017). Clinical significance of the estrogen-modifying enzymes steroid sulfatase and estrogen sulfotransferase in epithelial ovarian cancer. *Oncol. Lett.* 13, 4047–4054. doi: 10.3892/ol.2017.5969

Nomura, T., Lu, R., Pucci, M. L., and Schuster, V. L. (2004). The two-step model of prostaglandin signal termination: *in vitro* reconstitution with the prostaglandin transporter and prostaglandin 15 dehydrogenase. *Mol. Pharmacol.* 65, 973–978. doi: 10.1124/mol.65.4.973

Nymoen, D. A., Hetland Falkenthal, T. E., Holth, A., Ow, G. S., Ivshina, A. V., and Davidson, B. (2015). Expression and clinical role of chemoresponse-associated genes in ovarian serous carcinoma. *Gynecol. Oncol.* 139, 30–39. doi: 10.1016/j.ygyno.2015.07.107

Obaidat, A., Roth, M., and Hagenbuch, B. (2012). The expression and function of organic anion transporting polypeptides in normal tissues and in cancer. *Annu. Rev. Pharmacol. Toxicol.* 52, 135–151. doi: 10.1146/annurev-pharmtox-010510-100556

Obermayr, E., Bednarz-Knoll, N., Orsetti, B., Weier, H. U., Lambrechts, S., and Brandt, B. (2017). Circulating tumor cells: potential markers of minimal residual disease in ovarian cancer? a study of the OVCAD consortium. *Oncotarget* 8, 106415–106428. doi: 10.18632/oncotarget.22468

Olszewski-Hamilton, U., Svoboda, M., Thalhammer, T., Buxhofer-Ausch, V., Geissler, K., and Hamilton, G. (2011). Organic anion transporting polypeptide 5A1 (OATP5A1) in Small Cell Lung Cancer (SCLC) cells: possible involvement in chemoresistance to satraplatin. *Biomark. Cancer* 3, 31–40. doi: 10.4137/BIC.S7151

Patik, I., Kovacsics, D., Német, O., Gera, M., Várady, G., Stieger, B., et al. (2015). Functional expression of the 11 human Organic Anion Transporting Polypeptides in insect cells reveals that sodium fluorescein is a general OATP substrate. *Biochem. Pharmacol.* 98, 649–658. doi: 10.1016/j.bcp.2015.09.015

Pils, D., Hager, G., Tong, D., Aust, S., Heinze, G., Kohl, M., et al. (2012). Validating the impact of a molecular subtype in ovarian cancer on outcomes: a study of the OVCAD Consortium. *Cancer Sci.* 103, 1334–1341. doi: 10.1111/j.1349-7006.2012.02306.x

Pradeep, S., Kim, S. W., Wu, S. Y., Nishimura, M., Chaluvally-Raghavan, P., and Sood, A. K. (2014). Hematogenous metastasis of ovarian cancer: rethinking mode of spread. *Cancer Cell* 26, 77–91. doi: 10.1016/j.ccr.2014.05.002

R Core Team (2018). *R: A language and environment for statistical computing.* Vienna: R Foundation for Statistical Computing. Available online at: https://www.R-project.org/

Rižner, T. L., Thalhammer, T., and Ozvegy-Laczka, C. (2017). The importance of steroid uptake and intracrine action in endometrial and ovarian cancers. *Front. Pharmacol.* 8:346. doi: 10.3389/fphar.2017.00346

Salomon-Perzynski, A., Salomon-Perzynska, M., Michalski, B., and Skrzypulec-Plinta, V. (2017). High-grade serous ovarian cancer: the clone wars. *Arch. Gynecol. Obstet.* 295, 569–576. doi: 10.1007/s00404-017-4292-1

Sebastian, K., Detro-Dassen, S., Rinis, N., Fahrenkamp, D., Muller-Newen, G., Merk, H., et al. (2013). Characterization of SLCO5A1/OATP5A1, a solute carrier transport protein with non-classical function. *PLoS ONE* 8:e83257. doi: 10.1371/journal.pone.0083257

Sissung, T. M., Ley, A. M., Strope, J. D., McCrea, E. M., Beedie, S., and Figg, W. D. (2017). Differential expression of OATP1B3 mediates unconjugated testosterone influx. *Mol. Cancer Res.* 15, 1096–1105. doi: 10.1158/1541-7786.MCR-16-0477

Stieger, B., and Hagenbuch, B. (2014). Organic anion-transporting polypeptides. *Curr. Top. Membr.* 73, 205–232. doi: 10.1016/B978-0-12-800223-0.00005-0

Sukhbaatar, N., Bachmayr-Heyda, A., Auer, K., Aust, S., Deycmar, S., Horvat, R., et al. (2017). Two different, mutually exclusively distributed, TP53 mutations in ovarian and peritoneal tumor tissues of a serous ovarian cancer patient: indicative for tumor origin? *Cold Spring Harb. Mol. Case Stud.* 3:a001461. doi: 10.1101/mcs.a001461

Sun, Y., Furihata, T., Ishii, S., Nagai, M., Harada, M., Shimozato, O., et al. (2014). Unique expression features of cancer-type organic anion transporting polypeptide 1B3 mRNA expression in human colon and lung cancers. *Clin. Transl. Med.* 3:37. doi: 10.1186/s40169-014-0037-y

Svoboda, M., Meshcheryakova, A., Heinze, G., Jaritz, M., Pils, D., Castillo-Tong, D., et al. (2016). AID/APOBEC-network reconstruction identifies pathways associated with survival in ovarian cancer. *BMC Genomics* 17:643. doi: 10.1186/s12864-016-3001-y

Svoboda, M., Wlcek, K., Taferner, B., Hering, S., Stieger, B., Tong, D., et al. (2011). Expression of organic anion-transporting polypeptides 1B1 and 1B3 in ovarian cancer cells: relevance for paclitaxel transport. *Biomed. Pharmacother.* 65, 417–426. doi: 10.1016/j.biopha.2011.04.031

Szakács, G., Paterson, J. K., Ludwig, J. A., Booth-Genthe, C., and Gottesman, M. M. (2006). Targeting multidrug resistance in cancer. *Nat. Rev. Drug Discov.* 5, 219–234. doi: 10.1038/nrd1984

Tamai, I., Nezu, J., Uchino, H., Sai, Y., Oku, A., Shimane, M., et al. (2000). Molecular identification and characterization of novel members of the human organic anion transporter (OATP) family. *Biochem. Biophys. Res. Commun.* 273, 251–260. doi: 10.1006/bbrc.2000.2922

Taylor, S., and Pollard, K. (2009). Hypothesis tests for point-mass mixture data with application to 'omics data with many zero values. *Stat. Appl. Genet. Mol. Biol.* 8.8. doi: 10.2202/1544 6115.1425

Thakkar, N., Kim, K., Jang, E. R., Han, S., Kim, D., and Lee, W. (2013). A cancer-specific variant of the SLCO1B3 gene encodes a novel human organic anion transporting polypeptide 1B3 (OATP1B3) localized mainly in the cytoplasm of colon and pancreatic cancer cells. *Mol. Pharm.* 10, 406–416. doi: 10.1021/mp3005353

Thakkar, N., Lockhart, A. C., and Lee, W. (2015). Role of Organic Anion-Transporting Polypeptides (OATPs) in Cancer Therapy. *AAPS J.* 17, 535–545. doi: 10.1208/s12248-015-9740-x

Torres, D., Kumar, A., Wallace, S. K., Bakkum-Gamez, J. N., Konecny, G. E., and Wang, C. (2017). Intraperitoneal disease dissemination patterns are associated with residual disease, extent of surgery, and molecular subtypes in advanced ovarian cancer. *Gynecol. Oncol.* 147, 503–508. doi: 10.1016/j.ygyno.2017.09.021

Toyohara, T., Suzuki, T., Morimoto, R., Akiyama, Y., Souma, T., Shiwaku, H., et al. (2009). SLCO4C1 transporter eliminates uremic toxins and attenuates hypertension and renal inflammation. *J. Am. Soc. Nephrol.* 20, 2546–2555. doi: 10.1681/ASN.2009070696

van de Steeg, E., van Esch, A., Wagenaar, E., Kenworthy, K. E., and Schinkel, A. H. (2013). Influence of human OATP1B1, OATP1B3, and OATP1A2 on the pharmacokinetics of methotrexate and paclitaxel in humanized transgenic mice. *Clin. Cancer Res.* 19, 821–832. doi: 10.1158/1078-0432.CCR-12-2080

Voutsadakis, I. A. (2016). Hormone receptors in serous ovarian carcinoma: prognosis, pathogenesis, and treatment considerations. *Clin. Med. Insights Oncol.* 10, 17–25. doi: 10.4137/CMO.S32813

Ween, M. P., Armstrong, M. A., Oehler, M. K., and Ricciardelli, C. (2015). The role of ABC transporters in ovarian cancer progression and chemoresistance. *Crit. Rev. Oncol. Hematol.* 96, 220–256. doi: 10.1016/j.critrevonc.2015.05.012

Wlcek, K., Svoboda, M., Riha, J., Zakaria, S., Olszewski, U., Dvorak, Z., et al. (2011). The analysis of organic anion transporting polypeptide (OATP) mRNA and protein patterns in primary and metastatic liver cancer. *Cancer Biol. Ther.* 11, 801–811. doi: 10.4161/cbt.11.9.15176

Yeung, T. L., Leung, C. S., Yip, K. P., Au Yeung, C. L., Wong, S. T., and Mok, S. C. (2015). Cellular and molecular processes in ovarian cancer metastasis. A review in the theme: cell and molecular processes in cancer metastasis. *Am. J. Physiol. Cell. Physiol.* 309, C444–C456. doi: 10.1152/ajpcell.00188.2015

Yoshihara, K., Tajima, A., Komata, D., Yamamoto, T., Kodama, S., Fujiwara, H., et al. (2009). Gene expression profiling of advanced-stage serous ovarian cancers distinguishes novel subclasses and implicates ZEB2 in tumor progression and prognosis. *Cancer Sci.* 100, 1421–1428. doi: 10.1111/j.1349-7006.2009.01204.x

Zeng, Y., and Breheny, P. (2016). Overlapping group logistic regression with applications to genetic pathway selection. *Cancer Inform.* 15, 179–187. doi: 10.4137/CIN.S40043

6

The Impacts of Genistein and Daidzein on Estrogen Conjugations in Human Breast Cancer Cells: A Targeted Metabolomics Approach

*Stefan Poschner[1], Alexandra Maier-Salamon[1], Martin Zehl[2], Judith Wackerlig[3], Daniel Dobusch[3], Bettina Pachmann[1], Konstantin L. Sterlini[1] and Walter Jäger[1,4]**

[1] Division of Clinical Pharmacy and Diagnostics, Department of Pharmaceutical Chemistry, University of Vienna, Vienna, Austria, [2] Department of Analytical Chemistry, Faculty of Chemistry, University of Vienna, Vienna, Austria, [3] Division of Drug Design and Medicinal Chemistry, Department of Pharmaceutical Chemistry, University of Vienna, Vienna, Austria, [4] Vienna Metabolomics Center (VIME), University of Vienna, Vienna, Austria

Correspondence:
Walter Jäger
walter.jaeger@univie.ac.at

The beneficial effect of dietary soy food intake, especially for women diagnosed with breast cancer, is controversial, as *in vitro* data has shown that the soy isoflavones genistein and daidzein may even stimulate the proliferation of estrogen-receptor alpha positive (ERα+) breast cancer cells at low concentrations. As genistein and daidzein are known to inhibit key enzymes in the steroid metabolism pathway, and thus may influence levels of active estrogens, we investigated the impacts of genistein and daidzein on the formation of estrogen metabolites, namely 17β-estradiol (E2), 17β-estradiol-3-(β-D-glucuronide) (E2-G), 17β-estradiol-3-sulfate (E2-S) and estrone-3-sulfate (E1-S) in estrogen-dependent ERα+ MCF-7 cells. We found that both isoflavones were potent inhibitors of E1 and E2 sulfation (85–95% inhibition at 10 μM), but impeded E2 glucuronidation to a lesser extent (55–60% inhibition at 10 μM). The stronger inhibition of E1 and E2 sulfation compared with E2 glucuronidation was more evident for genistein, as indicated by significantly lower inhibition constants for genistein [K_is: E2-S (0.32 μM) < E1-S (0.76 μM) < E2-G (6.01 μM)] when compared with those for daidzein [K_is: E2-S (0.48 μM) < E1-S (1.64 μM) < E2-G (7.31 μM)]. Concomitant with the suppression of E1 and E2 conjugation, we observed a minor but statistically significant increase in E2 concentration of approximately 20%. As the content of genistein and daidzein in soy food is relatively low, an increased risk of breast cancer development and progression in women may only be observed following consumption of high-dose isoflavone supplements. Further long-term human studies monitoring free estrogens and their conjugates are therefore highly warranted to evaluate the potential side effects of high-dose genistein and daidzein, especially in patients diagnosed with ERα+ breast cancer.

Keywords: soy, genistein, daidzein, breast cancer, estrogens, metabolomics

Abbreviations: CYP, cytochrome P450 enzyme; DMEM, Dulbecco's modified Eagle's medium; DMSO, dimethyl sulfoxide; DPBS, Dulbecco's phosphate-buffered saline; E1, estrone; E1-S, estrone-3-sulfate; E2, 17β-estradiol; E2-G, 17β-estradiol-3-(β-D-glucuronide); E2-S, 17β-estradiol-3-sulfate; E3, estriol (16α-OH-17β-estradiol); EIC, extracted ion chromatogram; ERα, estrogen receptor alpha; ERβ, estrogen receptor beta; ESI, electro-spray ionization; 17β-HSD, 17β-hydroxysteroid dehydrogenase; K_i, inhibition constant; K_m, Michaelis constant; LC-HRMS, liquid chromatography-high resolution mass spectrometry; LLOQ, lower limit of quantification; SD, standard deviation; SPE, solid phase extraction; SULT, sulfotransferase; UGT, UDP-glucuronosyl transferase; V_{max}, maximum reaction velocity.

INTRODUCTION

Breast cancer is the most prevalent cancer in women and the second leading cause of cancer-related deaths among females worldwide (Ferlay et al., 2015). Chemoprevention in combination with anticancer treatment is therefore crucial to reduce rates of morbidity and mortality. Evidence from epidemiological and experimental studies indicates that several natural products may act as chemopreventive agents and inhibit mammary carcinogenesis (Pan et al., 2015). Among these products is soy, which contains variable amounts of genistein and daidzein as the major isoflavones (approximately 47 and 44%, respectively) and minor amounts of glycitein (approximately 9% of the total isoflavones in soybeans). The genistein and daidzein content is therefore also predominant in soy-derived foods and dietary supplements (Wiseman et al., 2002; Clarke et al., 2008).

Epidemiological studies have indicated that soy intake post-diagnosis not only improves prognosis but is also associated with statistically significant reductions in breast cancer recurrence (Kang et al., 2010; Chi et al., 2013). However, based on the weak estrogen-like effects of the isoflavones genistein and daidzein, some researchers and clinicians are concerned that a high soy intake may increase the cancer risk. Indeed, *in vitro* studies have shown that both genistein and daidzein stimulate the proliferation of MCF-7 human estrogen-receptor alpha positive (ERα+) breast cancer cells at low concentrations, but inhibit tumor growth at higher doses. In ER alpha negative (ERα−) cells (MDA-MB-231), this biphasic effect is not observed; both phytoestrogens exhibit an anti-proliferative effect only. This indicates that the proliferative effect of genistein and daidzein, as observed at low doses, is ERα-mediated, while ERβ, which is expressed at low levels in both MCF-7 and MDA-MB-231 cells, seems to oppose ERα actions and exhibits anti-migratory and anti-invasive properties (Vladusic et al., 2000; Al-Bader et al., 2011; Wang et al., 2012; Uifălean et al., 2016).

Besides an ERα-mediated interaction, low concentrations of both isoflavones can also induce cell proliferation via G protein coupled estrogen receptor 1 (GPER1) by stimulating cAMP production, intracellular Ca^{2+} mobilization and cSrc activation. Subsequently, the transactivation of the epidermal growth factor receptor (EGFR) is triggered, leading to an activation of downstream signaling pathways such as PI3K/Akt and MAPK/ERK (Uifălean et al., 2016).

In addition to ERα interaction and activation of signaling pathways, the stimulatory effect of genistein and daidzein on ERα+ breast cancer cells might also be linked to increased steroid hormone levels, which drive cellular proliferation and thus are an important factor for carcinogenesis (Folkerd and Dowsett, 2013). Mechanism for altered steroid levels between ERα+ and ERα− breast cancer cells include differences in estrogen metabolism. Indeed, incubation of human ERα+ MCF-7 breast cancer cells with E1 for 24 h resulted in a more than sevenfold higher formation of estrogen sulfates compared to ERα− MDA-MB-231 cells, as cellular SULT expression is significantly higher in MCF-7 cells (Pasqualini, 2009). However, estrogen conjugates do not promote ER-mediated activity but represent a local reservoir of native E1 and E2 after hydrolysis by sulfatases (Samavat and Kurzer, 2015). Interestingly, a previous human trial demonstrated that participants who consumed a high-soy diet for 13 months showed a non-significant increase of urinary E2 levels of 18% (Maskarinec et al., 2012), suggesting a possible role of E2 in the observed increased cellular growth of ERα+ breast tumors by genistein and daidzein.

This prompted us to hypothesize that genistein and daidzein might dose-dependently alter steroid hormone levels by inhibiting the conjugation of estrogens and their precursors. Our hypothesis was supported by *in vitro* studies showing that soy isoflavonoids are able to inhibit various enzymes involved in the metabolism of estrogens, including cytochrome P450 3A4 (CYP3A4), 17β-HSD, SULTs, and UGTs (Mesía-Vela and Kauffman, 2003; Mohamed and Frye, 2011; Ronis, 2016; Cassetta et al., 2017).

Whether soy components influences the estrogen metabolism is not yet known. Therefore, the aim of the present study was to investigate the impacts of genistein and daidzein on estrogen metabolism in human ERα+ MCF-7 breast cancer cells. For this purpose, a newly established specific and sensitive analytical LC-HRMS assay was conducted to simultaneously quantify the main steroids of the estrogenic pathway namely E1, E2, estriol (16α-OH-17β-estradiol, E3), E1-S, E2-G and E2-S (Rižner, 2013; Mueller et al., 2015). The outcomes of metabolism were subsequently correlated with cell growth in order to better understand the effects of soy isoflavones in ERα+ breast cancer.

MATERIALS AND METHODS

Materials

16α-hydroxy-17β-estradiol (E3), E2, 17β-estradiol-3-(β-D-glucuronide) sodium salt (E2-G) and E1, as well as acetic acid, acetonitrile, ammonium acetate, DMSO, genistein and daidzein, were purchased from Sigma–Aldrich Chemical Co. (Munich, Germany). 17β-estradiol-3-sulfate sodium salt (E2-S) and estrone-3-sulfate sodium salt (E1-S) were obtained from Steraloids, Inc. (Newport, RI, United States). 16α-hydroxy-17β-estradiol-2,4,17-d_3 (E3-d_3), 17β-estradiol-2,4,16,16-d_4 (E2-d_4), 17β-estradiol-16,16,17-d_3-3-(β-D-glucuronide) sodium salt (E2-G-d_3), 17β-estradiol-2,4,16,16-d_4-3-sulfate sodium salt (E2-S-d_4), estrone-2,4,16,16-d_4 (E1-d_4) and estrone-2,4,16,16-d_4-3-sulfate sodium salt (E1-S-d_4) were purchased from C/D/N Isotopes, Inc. (Pointe-Claire, QC, Canada). Purified water was obtained using an arium® pro ultrapure water system (Sartorius AG, Göttingen, Germany).

Cell Proliferation Studies

MCF-7 breast cancer cells were purchased from the American Type Culture Collection (ATCC; Rockville, MD, United States). All experiments were performed during the exponential growth phase of the cell line. MCF-7 cells were routinely cultivated at 37°C (95% humidity and 5% CO_2) in phenol red-free Dulbecco's Modified Eagle Medium F-12 (DMEM/F-12; Invitrogen, Karlsruhe, Germany), fortified with 1% PenStrep®-solution and 10% fetal bovine serum (Invitrogen). For experimental conditions, cells were seeded at a density of 1.0×10^6 cells per well and allowed to attach for 24 h. Prior to the application of genistein and daidzein, cells were washed twice with DPBS (Invitrogen), and DMEM/F-12, containing 10% HyClone® heat-inactivated charcoal-stripped fetal bovine serum (THP Medical Products, Vienna, Austria), was subsequently added to exclude external hormones. To evaluate the potential influence of genistein and daidzein on MCF-7 cell proliferation, cells were incubated for 48 h with E1 (100 nM) as an estrogen precursor in the presence of 1, 5, and 10 μM genistein or daidzein, respectively. Genistein, daidzein and E1 were dissolved in DMSO prior to their addition to the cell medium to give a final DMSO concentration of 0.05%. Prior to cell counting with a Coulter® Z1 cell counter (Beckman Coulter GmbH, Krefeld, Germany), supernatant medium was removed and cells were detached using 400 μl TrypLe® solution (Invitrogen). The effect of E1 (10, 25, 50, 75, and 100 nM) on the growth of MCF-7 cells was also determined using the same protocol as for genistein and daidzein. All experiments were performed in triplicate and the data are reported as means ± SD of all values.

Inhibition Studies

MCF-7 breast cancer cells were cultivated in the presence of HyClone® heat-inactivated charcoal-stripped fetal bovine serum as described above, and then treated with increasing concentrations of E1 (10, 25, 50, 75, and 100 nM) in the presence of 1, 5, and 10 μM genistein or daidzein, respectively. After 24 and 48 h, 2000 μl media aliquots were mixed with 20 μl deuterated internal standard solution and pre-cleaned by SPE on Oasis HLB 1 cc SPE cartridges (30 mg; Waters Corporation, Milford, MA, United States), as described previously (Poschner et al., 2017). Briefly, reconditioning of the cartridges was achieved using 2 × 1.0 ml acetonitrile and 3 × 1.0 ml ammonium acetate buffer (10 mM, pH = 5.0). Subsequently, samples were loaded onto the SPE cartridges and washed with 1 × 1.0 ml ammonium acetate buffer (10 mM, pH = 5.0) and 2 × 1.0 ml acetonitrile/ammonium acetate buffer (10 mM, pH 5.0) 10:90 (v/v). Analytes were then eluted using 2 × 650 μl acetonitrile/ammonium acetate buffer (10 mM, pH = 5.0) 95:5 (v/v), evaporated to dryness, and reconstituted in 270 μl acetonitrile/ammonium acetate buffer (10 mM, pH = 5.0) 25:75 (v/v). After media collection, cells were washed five times with 2.0 ml DPBS, detached using 200 μl TrypLE® solution (37°C, 15 min), mixed with 800 μl DPBS and transferred into plastic vials. Aliquots of these suspensions (100 μl each) were used to determine the exact number of cells per sample well. For this, the aliquots were diluted 100-fold and counted using a Coulter® Z1 cell counter. To additionally quantify cytosolic steroid levels, the remaining cell suspensions (900 μl each) were gently centrifuged (1000 rpm, 8 min) and the supernatants were discarded. The cell pellets were subsequently resuspended in 100 μl aqueous ammonium acetate buffer (10 mM, pH = 5.0) and lysed by five freeze-thaw-cycles in liquid nitrogen (3 min each), followed by thawing at ambient temperature. Ammonium acetate buffer (1000 μl) was then added and the suspensions were centrifuged (14000 rpm, 5 min), and the clear supernatants were concentrated using the SPE protocol described above. All processed samples were then stored at −80°C until further LC-HRMS analysis. Four biologically independent experiments were performed, and reported values represent the overall means ± SD of all determinations.

LC-HRMS Assay

E1, E1-S, E2, E2-S, E2-G, and E3 were quantified using an LC-HRMS assay, validated according to the ICH Q2(R1) guidelines as described previously (Poschner et al., 2017). LC was performed using an UltiMate 3000 RSLC-series system (Dionex; Thermo Fisher Scientific, Inc., Germering, Germany) coupled to a maXis HD ESI-Qq-TOF mass spectrometer (Bruker Corporation, Bremen, Germany). Solvent A was aqueous ammonium acetate buffer (10 mM, pH = 5.0) and solvent B was acetonitrile. A Phenomenex Luna® 3 μm C18(2) 100 Å LC column (250 mm × 4.6 mm I.D.; Phenomenex, Inc., Torrance, CA, United States), preceded by a Hypersil® BDS-C18 guard column (5 μm, 10 mm × 4.6 mm I.D.; Thermo Fisher Scientific, Inc.) and maintained constantly at 43°C, was used for steroid separation at a flow rate of 1 ml/min. The injection volume was 100 μl for each sample. The gradient used was as follows: 25% solvent B at 0 min, 56.3% solvent B at 19 min, a washing step at 90% solvent B from 19.5 to 24.0 min and column re-equilibration with 25% solvent B from 24.5 to 30.5 min. The ESI ion source settings were as follows: Capillary voltage, −4.5 kV; nebulizer, 1.0 bar N_2; dry gas flow rate, 8.0 l/min N_2; and dry temperature, 200°C. The ion transfer parameters were set to 400 Vpp funnel RF and 300 Vpp multipole RF, the quadrupole ion energy was 8.0 eV and the collision cell parameters were as follows: Collision energy, 10.0 eV; collision RF, 1100 Vpp; transfer time, 38 μs; and pre-pulse storage, 18 μs. Full-scan mass spectra were recorded in the range of *m/z* 150–500. Control samples consisting of unspiked cell culture medium showed no detectable background traces of the analyzed hormones. To ensure accurate quantification results, quality control samples, containing each analyte at a concentration of 6-fold or 600-fold of the respective lower limits of quantification (LLOQs), were analyzed in triplicate with each LC batch. The LLOQs were determined as follows: E1, 19.0 pg/ml; E1-S, 4.0 pg/ml; E2, 140.9 pg/ml; E2-S, 3.4 pg/ml; E2-G, 12.0 pg/ml; E3, 28.4 pg/ml cell medium.

Data Analysis

Liquid chromatography-high resolution mass spectrometry data were analyzed using Compass DataAnalysis 4.2 and QuantAnalysis 2.2 software (Bruker Corporation). EICs were created for each analyte and internal standard pair, from which the respective peak areas were determined to calculate the analyte/internal standard ratios for quantification. Kinetic analysis of estrogen metabolite formation in the presence and absence of genistein or daidzein using E1 as an estrogen precursor (10–100 nM for 48 h) was performed. All data best fitted to the Michaelis–Menten model: $V = V_{max} \times [S] / (K_m + [S])$, where V is the rate of the reaction, V_{max} is the maximum reaction velocity, K_m is the Michaelis constant and $[S]$ is the substrate concentration. Kinetic parameters were calculated

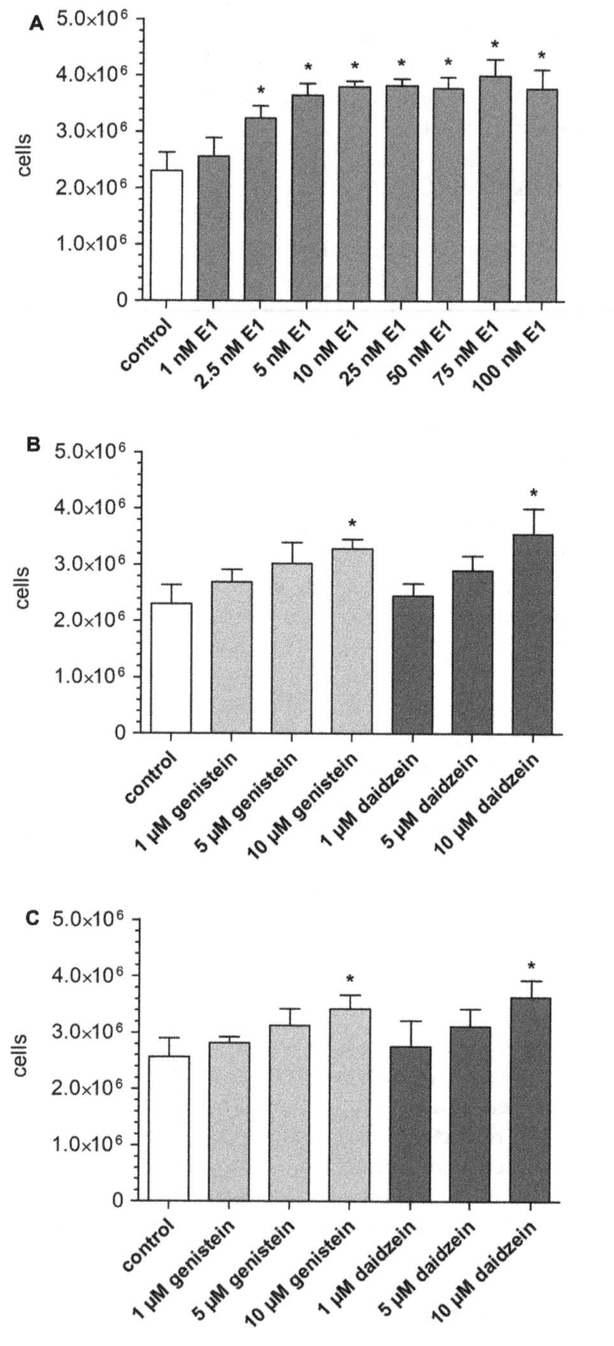

FIGURE 1 | Influence of E1 and soy isoflavones on MCF-7 breast cancer cell proliferation. Cells were incubated for 48 h with **(A)** increasing concentrations of E1 (1–100 nM; control: DMSO), **(B)** increasing concentrations of genistein and daidzein (1–10 µM; control: DMSO) and **(C)** increasing concentrations of genistein and daidzein (1–10 µM) in the presence of 1 nM E1 (control: 1 nM E1 in DMSO). All data represent the means ± SD of three independent biological replicates. Asterisks (*) indicate significantly different mean values in comparison to the controls ($P < 0.05$).

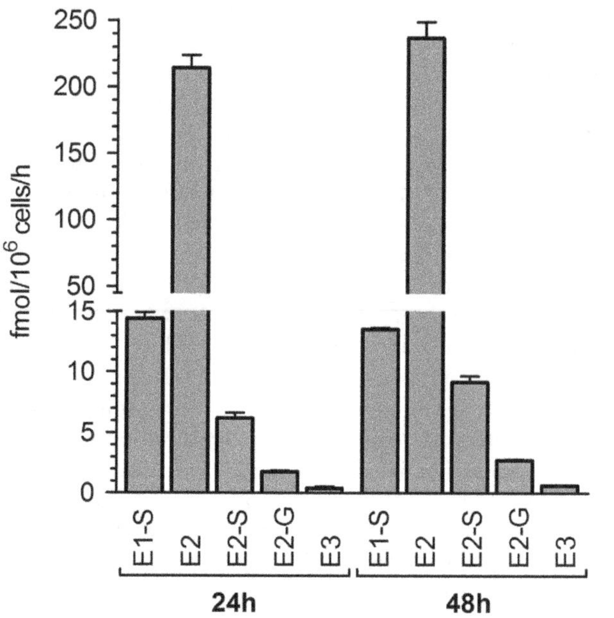

FIGURE 2 | Pattern of estrogen metabolite formation rates by MCF-7 cells. Cells were incubated with 100 nM E1 as a hormone precursor, and medium aliquots were analyzed for estrogen metabolites at 24 and 48 h. Data represent the means ± SD of three independent biological replicates.

using GraphPad Prism 6.0 software (GraphPad Software Inc., La Jolla, CA, United States). Inhibition modes were determined from Lineweaver–Burk plots, and corresponding K_i were calculated by plotting the slopes of the primary Lineweaver–Burk plots against the respective inhibitor concentrations using GraphPad Prism 6.0. The same software package was used for statistical analyses. All values were expressed as means ± SD and the Student's *t*-test and ANOVA with Tukey's post-test were used to compare differences between control samples and treatment groups. The statistical significance level was set to $P < 0.05$.

RESULTS

Influence of Estrone and Soy Isoflavones on MCF-7 Cell Proliferation

To assess the influence of E1 on MCF-7 cancer cell growth, cells were incubated with increasing concentrations of E1 for 48 h, detached by application of TrypLe® solution and counted using a Coulter® Z1 cell counter. Compared with control samples (containing DMSO only), the number of viable MCF-7 cells was significantly increased in the presence of E1 ($2.31 \pm 0.33 \times 10^6$ vs. $3.99 \pm 0.31 \times 10^6$ cells) (**Figure 1A**), confirming the hormone-dependency of the MCF-7 cell line. The observed proliferative effect of E1 on the breast cancer cells was concentration-dependent with a mean maximum cell growth increase of 73% at 75 nM E1. Additionally, we evaluated the effect of E1 in combination with the soy isoflavones genistein or daidzein on MCF-7 cell growth. For this purpose, cells were co-incubated with 0, 1, 2.5, and 100 nM E1 as a hormone precursor in the presence of increasing concentrations of genistein or daidzein (1–10 µM). These concentrations were chosen as they represent plasma levels measured after the administration of isoflavone supplements. As shown in **Figure 1B**, the presence of both isoflavones in the absence of E1 had a significant effect on cell proliferation (+42% for genistein and +54% for daidzein). Co-incubation with the isoflavones and 1 nM E1 led to similar results with a mean cell number increase of +34% for genistein and +42% for daidzein (**Figure 1C**). When the E1 concentration was further increased to 2.5 nM, we observed only a slightly higher cell growth (+16 and +15%, respectively) compared to the incubation with E1 alone. In the presence of 100 nM E1, genistein and daidzein did not show any further increase of cellular growth because of the already high cell number stimulated by E1.

Formation of Estrogen Metabolites by MCF-7 Cells

In preliminary experiments, MCF-7 breast cancer cells were treated with 100 nM E1 as a hormone precursor and cell media aliquots were analyzed for E1 and its metabolites after 24 and 48 h. By using a highly specific and sensitive LC-HRMS assay, five biotransformation products could be quantified besides the precursor E1 in the cellular medium (**Figure 2**). As metabolite formation showed a linear trend with time up to 48 h, incubations in all further experiments were finalized after this time-span as it ensured the most precise quantification of the biotransformation products.

E2 represented the main metabolite in the cellular supernatant, with a mean formation rate of 233.1 ± 6.9 fmol/10^6 cells/h after 48 h (**Figure 2** and **Table 1**). It was further sulfated and glucuronidated to E2-S and E2-G, with a markedly favoritism for the sulfated product (9.15 ± 1.21 vs. 2.76 ± 0.37 fmol/10^6 cells/h). In addition to the conjugation reactions, E2 was also hydroxylated to E3, though this was a minor metabolite in MCF-7 cells with a formation rate of only 0.65 ± 0.05 fmol/10^6 cells/h. Alongside the two E2 conjugates, we also observed the sulfation of the precursor E1 to E1-S (13.5 ± 2.1 fmol/10^6 cells/h). Concomitant with the formation of these five metabolites, the E1 concentration in the medium decreased by 29% from 100 nM to 71.0 ± 0.9 nM after 48 h. The total molar proportion of all five metabolites was 28.9% indicating that these five biotransformation products represent almost 100% of all metabolites formed from the precursor E1 by the MCF-7 cells (un-metabolized E1 + total detected metabolites: 99.9%). Interestingly, intracellular metabolite concentrations in all samples were below the respective detection limits (data not shown).

Kinetic profiles for the formation of estrogen metabolites by MCF-7 cells were then evaluated over an E1 concentration range of 10–100 nM for 48 h. 17β-HSD-mediated formation of the main metabolite E2 best fitted to the Michaelis–Menten model, with a mean V_{max} value of 464.5 ± 39.2 fmol/10^6 cells/h and a mean K_m value of 95.4 ± 14.0 nM (**Table 2**). E2-S and E2-G formation also exhibited Michaelis–Menten kinetics with similar K_m values (95.9 ± 5.4 and 92.7 ± 9.0 nM, respectively), though the V_{max} value for sulfation was 3.3-fold higher than that for glucuronidation (18.3 ± 0.7 vs. 5.52 ± 0.37 fmol/10^6 cells/h), confirming the preference for E2 sulfation by MCF-7 cells. Kinetic parameters calculated for the sulfation of the precursor E1 (V_{max} = 26.8 ± 2.3 fmol/10^6 cells/h, K_m = 88.3 ± 11.3 nM) were comparable to those for E2 sulfation, probably because both are substrates of the same enzyme isoforms SULT1A1 and SULT1E1 (Harris et al., 2004). Evaluation of the kinetic profile for E3 formation was not possible, as only the highest E1 concentration (100 nM) but not the lower ones, resulted in E3 concentrations above the LLOQ of the presented assay.

Inhibition of Estrogen Conjugations by Genistein

To assess the possible inhibitory effect of genistein on estrogen metabolism, MCF-7 cells were first treated with E1 (100 nM) for 48 h in the presence and absence of increasing genistein concentrations (1, 5, and 10 μM). As shown in **Table 1**, a marked inhibition of E1 and E2 conjugation by this isoflavone was observed (Supplementary Figure S1A). Even in the presence of 1 μM genistein, the formation rates of E1-S, E2-S and E2-G decreased by approximately 25–35% compared to control. At 10 μM genistein, the inhibition was more obvious, and more pronounced for sulfation than for glucuronidation. The formation rates of E1-S and E2-S were reduced by approximately 90–95%, respectively, compared with the control (E1-S, 1.27 ± 0.22 vs. 13.5 ± 2.1 fmol/10^6 cells/h; E2-S, 0.54 ± 0.05 vs.

TABLE 1 | Estrogen metabolism by MCF-7 cells in the presence of genistein and daidzein.

Inhibitor	E2 (fmol/10^6 cells/h)	E1-S (fmol/10^6 cells/h)	E2-S (fmol/10^6 cells/h)	E2-G (fmol/10^6 cells/h)
Control	233.1 ± 6.9	13.5 ± 2.1	9.15 ± 1.21	2.76 ± 0.37
1 μM genistein	242.1 ± 16.7	10.2 ± 1.8	**5.90 ± 0.76***	**2.12 ± 0.34***
5 μM genistein	**264.0 ± 8.8***	**2.26 ± 0.27***	**1.12 ± 0.37***	**1.41 ± 0.33***
10 μM genistein	**277.2 ± 18.2***	**1.27 ± 0.22***	**0.54 ± 0.05***	**1.06 ± 0.10***
1 μM daidzein	244.2 ± 9.0	**8.15 ± 1.26***	**5.91 ± 1.27***	2.39 ± 0.27
5 μM daidzein	**260.7 ± 19.2***	**3.11 ± 0.34***	**1.27 ± 0.34***	**1.94 ± 0.30***
10 μM daidzein	**275.4 ± 5.9***	**2.00 ± 0.30***	**0.69 ± 0.16***	**1.26 ± 0.15***

Cells were incubated with increasing concentrations of the soy isoflavones genistein and daidzein and 100 nM E1 as hormone precursor for 48 h. All data represent the means ± SD of four independent biological replicates. Values in bold and marked with an asterisk (*) are significantly different in comparison to the control values ($P < 0.05$).

TABLE 2 | Kinetic parameters of estrogen metabolism by MCF-7 cells in the presence of genistein and daidzein.

Inhibitor	E2		E1-S		E2-S		E2-G	
	V_{max} (fmol/10^6 cells/h)	K_m (nM)	V_{max} (fmol/10^6 cells/h)	K_m (nM)	V_{max} (fmol/10^6 cells/h)	K_m (nM)	V_{max} (fmol/10^6 cells/h)	K_m (nM)
Control	464.5 ± 39.2	95.4 ± 14.0	26.8 ± 2.3	88.3 ± 11.3	18.3 ± 0.7	95.9 ± 5.4	5.52 ± 0.37	92.7 ± 9.0
1 μM genistein	463.3 ± 39.7	87.1 ± 13.4	**19.1 ± 2.0***	84.1 ± 12.9	**13.5 ± 0.6***	98.2 ± 4.5	**4.13 ± 0.34***	91.3 ± 10.9
5 μM genistein	520.7 ± 32.9	95.2 ± 10.5	**4.28 ± 0.42***	91.6 ± 12.9	**2.19 ± 0.07***	96.8 ± 4.5	**2.84 ± 0.20***	106.4 ± 10.3
10 μM genistein	**543.9 ± 31.6***	93.8 ± 9.51	**2.58 ± 0.25***	93.9 ± 13.3	**1.04 ± 0.07***	97.8 ± 9.8	**2.16 ± 0.06***	106.3 ± 9.1
1 μM daidzein	488.2 ± 36.4	96.4 ± 12.4	**17.1 ± 1.4***	102.6 ± 11.5	**11.9 ± 0.9***	101.2 ± 10.8	**4.83 ± 0.27***	98.0 ± 7.8
5 μM daidzein	508.7 ± 22.7	95.6 ± 7.39	**6.43 ± 0.28***	104.4 ± 14.3	**2.64 ± 0.22***	102.8 ± 11.9	**3.99 ± 0.18***	100.4 ± 6.6
10 μM daidzein	**543.5 ± 32.9***	96.8 ± 10.1	**4.20 ± 0.47***	105.7 ± 16.5	**1.35 ± 0.11***	98.6 ± 11.9	**2.63 ± 0.32***	105.6 ± 18.3

Cells were incubated with increasing concentrations of the soy isoflavones genistein and daidzein and 10 to 100 nM E1 as hormone precursor for 48 h. All data represent the means ± SD of four independent biological replicates. Values in bold and marked with an asterisk (*) are significantly different in comparison to the control values ($P < 0.05$).

9.15 ± 1.21 fmol/10^6 cells/h), whereas E2-G formation was only reduced by approximately 60% (1.06 ± 0.10 vs. 2.76 ± 0.37 fmol/10^6 cells/h). Genistein also showed a pronounced inhibition on E3 formation (data not shown); based on its low concentration in the cellular medium, the corresponding K_i could not be calculated.

In order to determine the kinetic parameters for the observed inhibition processes, cells were treated with 10–100 nM E1 as hormone precursor and increasing concentrations of genistein (1–10 μM). As shown in **Figure 3**, the presence of genistein did not alter the kinetic profiles for E1 or E2 conjugations; the data still best-fitted to the Michaelis–Menten kinetic model. However, the mean V_{max} values for the formation of the conjugates were significantly decreased by increasing genistein concentrations, while the corresponding K_m values were almost unaffected (**Table 2**). In order to gain further insight into the inhibition process, we determined the mode of inhibition by genistein on E1 and E2 metabolism and calculated the corresponding K_i by plotting the slopes of the primary Lineweaver–Burk plots against the respective inhibitor concentrations (**Figure 3**). As reported in **Table 3**, non-competitive inhibition by genistein was confirmed for all E1 and E2 conjugates, as initially indicated by the altered V_{max} values and the almost unchanged K_m values (**Table 2**). The more pronounced inhibition of E1 and E2 sulfation over E2 glucuronidation by genistein (**Figure 3**) was also reflected by significantly lower K_i values for sulfation (E2-S, 0.32 μM and E1-S, 0.76 μM vs. E2-G, 6.01 μM), indicating decreased rates of sulfate formation even at very low genistein concentrations.

Inhibition of Estrogen Conjugations by Daidzein

Analogous to the cell experiments conducted with genistein, we first investigated the possible inhibition of E1 and E2 metabolism by daidzein. Again, the formation rates of E1-S, E2-S and E2-G were significantly decreased by approximately 15–40% compared to control, even at 1 μM daidzein (**Table 1** and Supplementary Figure S1B). The increase in daidzein concentration to 10 μM led to more pronounced suppression of E1 and E2 sulfation by approximately 85 and 90% compared to control (E1-S, 2.00 ± 0.30 vs. 13.5 ± 2.1 fmol/10^6 cells/h; E2-S, 0.69 ± 0.16 vs. 9.15 ± 1.21 fmol/10^6 cells/h), while E2 glucuronidation was only reduced by approximately 55% (1.26 ± 0.15 vs. 2.76 ± 0.37 fmol/10^6 cells/h). Like genistein, also daidzein showed a pronounced inhibition of the very minor metabolite E3 (data not shown). However, based on its low concentration in the cellular medium, we were not able to calculate the kinetics for its inhibition.

Figure 4 and **Table 2** show the Michaelis–Menten parameters for the formation of E1-S, E2-S, and E2-G by MCF-7 cells in the presence of increasing daidzein concentrations (1–10 μM). The V_{max} and K_m values were comparable to those calculated for the inhibition by genistein. The observed decrease in V_{max} values and unaltered K_m values, together with the corresponding Lineweaver–Burk plots, again indicated that a non-competitive mechanism was the most likely mode of inhibition by daidzein. As shown in **Table 3**, the K_i values were also significantly

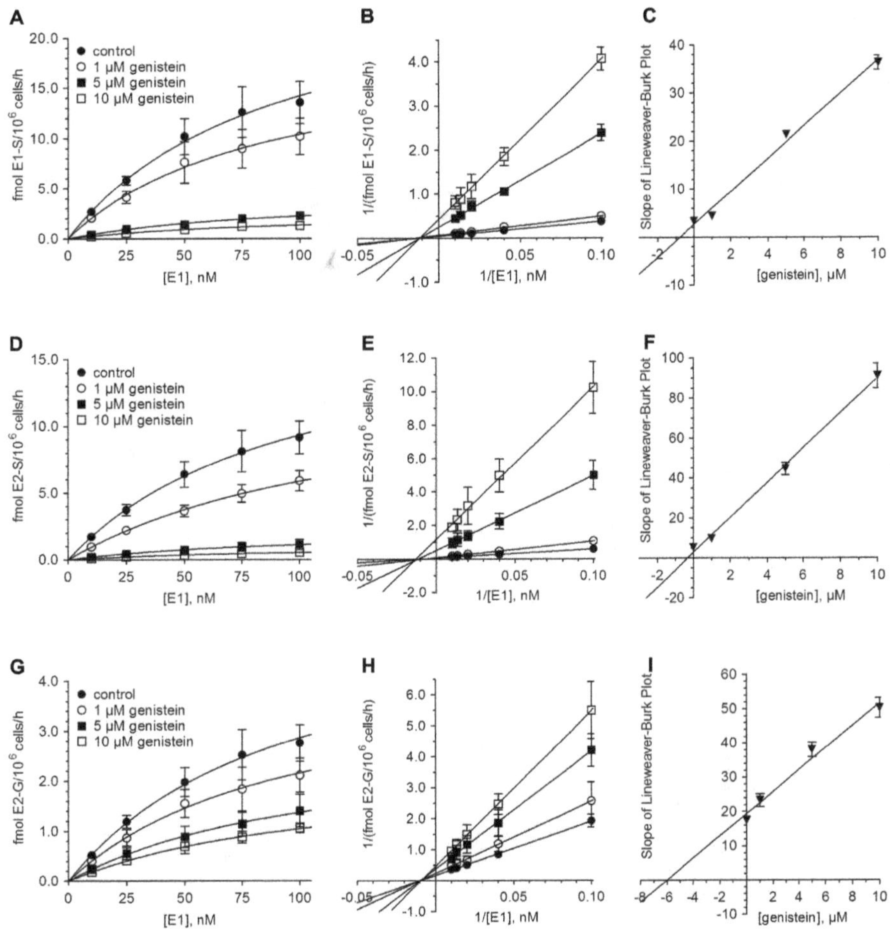

FIGURE 3 | Inhibition of estrogen conjugation by genistein. The kinetics of **(A–C)** E1 sulfation, **(D–F)** E2 sulfation and **(G–I)** E2 glucuronidation were calculated following incubation of MCF-7 cells with 10 to 100 nM E1 for 48 h in the presence (1–10 μM) and absence of genistein. Data is displayed in Michaelis–Menten, Lineweaver–Burk and K_i value plots. All data represent the means ± SD of four independent biological replicates.

lower for sulfation compared with glucuronidation [E2-S (0.48 μM) < E1-S (1.64 μM) < E2-G (7.31 μM)].

Effect of Genistein and Daidzein on E2 Formation

Concomitant with the observed suppression of SULT- and UGT-mediated conjugation of E1 and E2, we observed a minor but statistically significant increase in E2 formation (**Figure 5**). When MCF-7 cells were exposed to 100 nM E1 in the presence of 1 μM isoflavone, E2 levels were elevated by approximately 4–5% (242.1 ± 16.7 fmol/10^6 cells/h for genistein and 244.2 ± 9.0 fmol/10^6 cells/h for daidzein) compared to control (233.1 ± 6.9 fmol/10^6 cells/h). Inhibition of E1 and E2 conjugation with 10 μM genistein or daidzein further increased E2 formation by ~20% compared to control (277.2 ± 18.2 fmol/10^6 cells/h for genistein and 275.4 ± 5.9 fmol/10^6 cells/h for daidzein) (**Table 1**).

In parallel, V_{max} values increased from 464.5 ± 39.2 fmol/10^6 cells/h to 543.9 ± 31.6 or 543.5 ± 32.9 fmol/10^6 cells/h, when cells were treated with 10 μM genistein or daidzein, respectively.

TABLE 3 | Inhibition constants (K_i) and modes of inhibition.

Isoflavone	Metabolic activity	K_i (μM)	Mode of inhibition
Genistein	E1 sulfation	0.76	Non-competitive
	E2 sulfation	0.32	Non-competitive
	E2 glucuronidation	6.01	Non-competitive
Daidzein	E1 sulfation	1.64	Non-competitive
	E2 sulfation	0.48	Non-competitive
	E2 glucuronidation	7.31	Non-competitive

K_i values were obtained by plotting the slopes of the respective Lineweaver–Burk plots against isoflavone concentration. All data represent the means ± SD of four independent biological replicates.

As already shown for E1 and E2 conjugates, K_m values were not affected by either isoflavone.

DISCUSSION

To the best of our knowledge, the present study was the first to investigate the concentration-dependent impacts of the

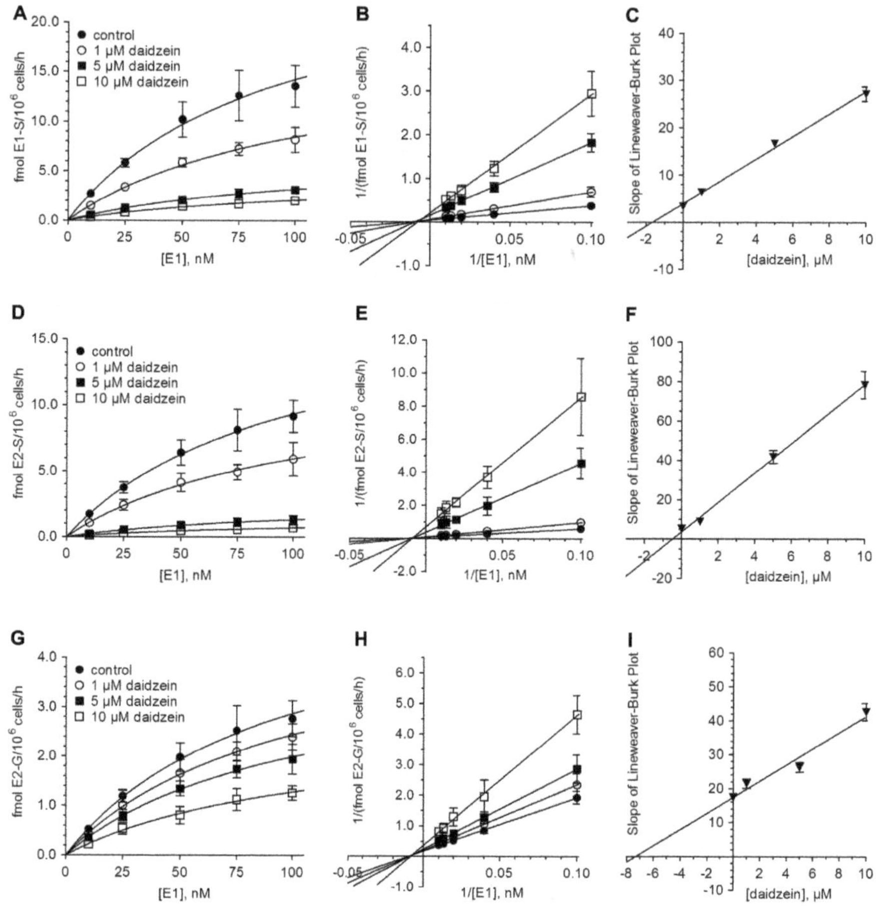

FIGURE 4 | Inhibition of estrogen conjugation by daidzein. The kinetics of **(A–C)** E1 sulfation, **(D–F)** E2 sulfation and **(G–I)** E2 glucuronidation were calculated following incubation of MCF-7 cells with 10 to 100 nM E1 for 48 h in the presence (1–10 µM) and absence of daidzein. Data is displayed in Michaelis–Menten, Lineweaver–Burk and K_i value plots. All data represent the means ± SD of four independent biological replicates.

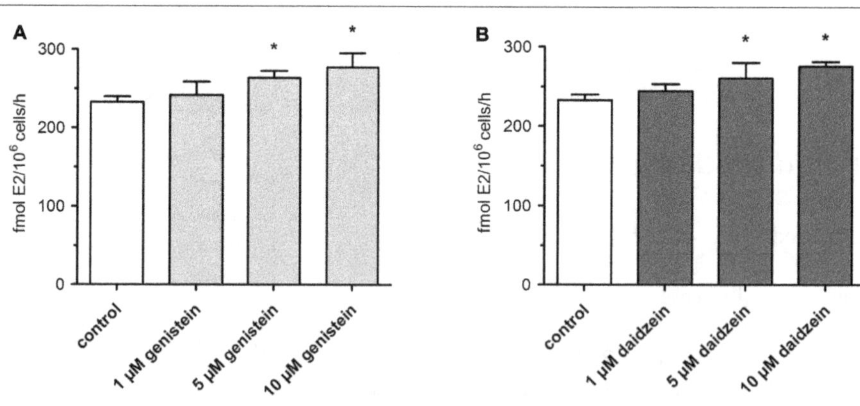

FIGURE 5 | Formation of active E2 by MCF-7 breast cancer cells. Cells were incubated with 100 nM E1 in the presence of **(A)** genistein or **(B)** daidzein. All data represent the means ± SD of four independent biological replicates. Asterisks (*) indicate significantly different mean values in comparison to the controls ($P < 0.05$).

soy isoflavones genistein and daidzein on the formation of estrogen conjugates in human ERα+ breast cancer cells (MCF-7). When cells were exposed solely to the hormone precursor E1, proliferation increased up to 1.6-fold. A stimulatory effect on cell proliferation was also observed when cells were incubated with genistein or daidzein (1–10 µM) in the absence or in the presence of low E1 concentrations (1 and 2.5 nM). Our findings are in line with previous studies that have also reported a stimulatory effect

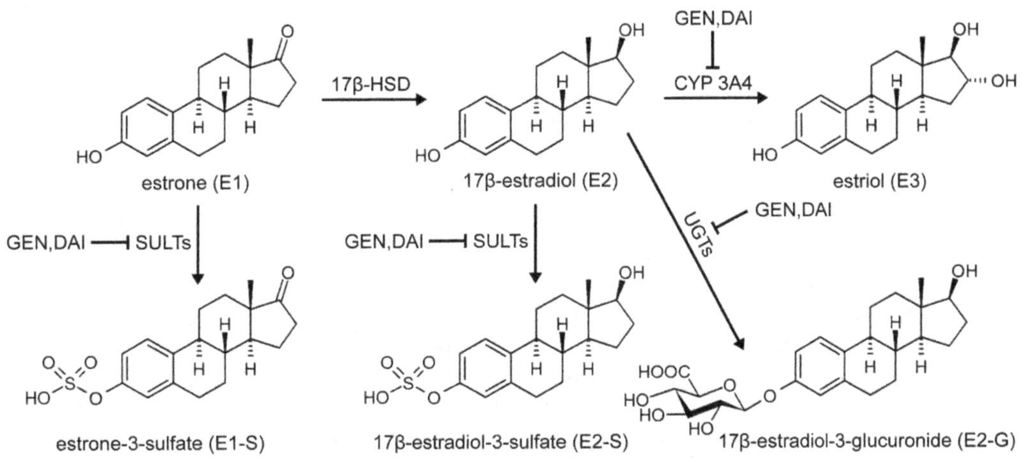

FIGURE 6 | Effect of soy isoflavones on estrogen metabolism in MCF-7 cells. Genistein (GEN) and daidzein (DAI) inhibit the formation of E1-S, E2-S, E2-G and E3, thereby increasing active E2 levels.

of these isoflavone concentrations on MCF-7 cell growth (Chen et al., 2015; Wei et al., 2015). Our data also correlate with the *in vitro* study by Kuiper et al. (1998), which shows that genistein presents a 20- to 30-fold higher binding affinity for ERβ than for ERα while daidzein has only a fivefold increased affinity for ERβ, explaining the observed slightly increased proliferative effect of daidzein on ERα+ MCF-7 cell growth (**Figure 1**).

After an incubation-period of 48 h, we were able to observe the formation of five metabolites, namely E1-S, E2, E2-S, E2-G and E3. Based on Michaelis–Menten parameters, the predominant metabolite was E2 (V_{max}, 464.5 ± 39.2 fmol/10^6 cells/h), while the conjugates E1-S, E2-S and E2-G exhibited significantly lower V_{max} values. Estimations of K_m values for E1-S, E2, E2-S and E2-G gave comparable results, indicating similar affinities to 17β-HSD, SULTs and UGTs. The CYP3A4-mediated hydroxylation of E2 to E3, however, represented only a very minor metabolic pathway by MCF-7 cells, as the formation of E3 could not be quantified at E1 concentrations of <100 nM.

Sulfation is therefore the main conjugation pathway of estrogens in MCF-7 cells as it accounted for 8.64% of total metabolites rate compared to only 1.05% for glucuronidation. The CYP3A4-mediated formation of E3 is negligible with a proportion of only 0.25% of the total E1 metabolism. These data are in line with previous *in vitro* investigations, which revealed a more than sevenfold higher formation of estrogen sulfates in human ERα+ MCF-7 breast cancer cells than ERα− MDA-MB-231 cells after incubation with E1 for 24 h, based on significantly higher SULT expression (Pasqualini, 2009). Higher SULT expression in ERα+ breast tumors compared to ERα− breast cancer tissues was also found in human primary tumor tissue samples (Adams et al., 1979).

When the cells were incubated with E1 in the presence of soy isoflavones (up to 10 μM), estrogen conjugations were markedly decreased. Genistein inhibited E1-S and E2-S formation by 90 and 95% compared to control, while E2 glucuronidation was less affected and only decreased by 60%. Interestingly, daidzein, which differs from genistein only by the absence of a hydroxyl group in position 5, showed slightly weaker inhibitory effects (E1-S, 85%; E2-S, 90%; E2-G, 55%). These findings are in accordance with previous data, which also reported a stronger inhibition of E1 and E2 sulfation by genistein than by daidzein, potentially due to a higher potency of this isoflavone against SULT1A1 (Mesía-Vela and Kauffman, 2003). Kinetic analysis in combination with corresponding Lineweaver–Burk plots showed that both isoflavones non-competitively inhibited estrogen conjugations by MCF-7 cells, with very low K_i values for E1 sulfation (genistein, 0.76 μM; daidzein, 1.64 μM). E2 sulfation was affected to an even greater extent by either isoflavone (genistein, 0.32 μM; daidzein, 0.48 μM). By contrast, the calculated K_i values for E2 glucuronidation were markedly higher (genistein, 6.01 μM; daidzein, 7.31 μM), confirming the stronger impact of isoflavone treatment on sulfation compared with glucuronidation. Non-competitive inhibition of E1 and E2 metabolite formation by both isoflavones is of clinical importance, as it suggests that the extent of inhibition depends only on the inhibitor concentration (indicated by marked decreases in V_{max}) and not on the binding of E1 and E2 to the respective enzymes (indicated by largely unaltered K_m values).

Whether dietary soy intake or high-dose isoflavone supplements may cause or exacerbate breast cancer in post-menopausal women remains controversial. Although soy food and its isoflavones have been widely investigated in the past few decades as cancer chemopreventives, conflicting data regarding their efficacy and safety have been reported. Population-based studies (Nechuta et al., 2012; Zhang et al., 2017) have indicated beneficial effects of dietary soy food consumption for women diagnosed with ERα− breast cancer, such as reduced risk of mortality and improved treatment outcomes; however, these effects have not been observed in patients expressing ERα. Clinical trials have also raised concerns that isoflavone intake may drive cancer cell proliferation (Shike et al., 2014) and significantly increase the Ki-67 labeling index in premenopausal women (Khan et al., 2012). Therefore, understanding of the metabolic interplay between genistein, daidzein and the concentration of active E2, which is associated with breast cancer risk and progression (Folkerd and Dowsett, 2013), is crucial for risk assessments.

Concomitant with the observed inhibition of E1 and E2 conjugation, genistein and daidzein caused a minor, but statistically significant increase of approximately 20% in the active E2 levels (**Figure 5**). Based on increased E2 formation in the presence of genistein and daidzein, inhibition of 17β-HSD can be excluded. Our data are in contrast to a very recent study showing an inhibition of this enzyme by genistein (Cassetta et al., 2017). This discrepancy might be explained by the fact that the authors used purified recombinant 17β-HSD from the filantous fungus *Cochliobolus lunatus* and not a human enzyme which might differ in activity. Both isoflavones, however, significantly inhibited the activity of cellular SULTs responsible for the formation of E1-S thereby increasing the E1 pool and consequently leading to a higher E2-formation by 17β-HSD. Furthermore, genistein and daidzein also demonstrated a pronounced inhibition of E2-S, E2-G and E3 formation thereby contributing to the observed increased E2 level (**Figure 6**).

The observed increase in E2 in our *in vitro* model was also found in a previous human trial which examined the effect of soy foods on urinary estrogens in premenopausal women (Maskarinec et al., 2012). Participants who consumed a high-soy diet for 13 months showed a non-significant increase of urinary E2 levels of 18%. These findings were confirmed by a meta-analysis (Hooper et al., 2009), in which the authors also reported a small, non-significant increase in total estradiol concentrations of 14% in post-menopausal women following soy isoflavone consumption. Although both studies observed a minor, non-significant increase in urinary E2 levels, soy food consumption should be considered safe, as even the daily intake of two dietary servings of soy powder (25 g each) for up to 30 days lead to mean total plasma levels (parent compound, glucuronides and sulfates) of only 11.6 ng/ml (0.042 μM) for genistein and 6.7 ng/ml (0.026 μM) for daidzein (Shike et al., 2014). These concentrations are far below our calculated K_i values (0.3–1.6 μM for E1 and E2 sulfates, and 6.0–7.3 μM for E2 glucuronide) therefore suggesting no significant effect of dietary soy intake on estrogen metabolism.

On the other hand, daily high-dose supplementation with genistein (600 mg) and daidzein (300 mg) for 84 days has been found to increase the trough plasma levels up to a concentration of 15 μg/ml (55 μM) total isoflavones (Pop et al., 2008). Taking into account that the majority of isoflavones are extensively metabolized *in vivo* (up to 98%), the remaining free genistein and daidzein plasma concentrations would reach approximately 1 μM, which is still high enough to inhibit E1 and E2 sulfation, while leaving E2 glucuronidation unaffected. Whether genistein or daidzein glucuronides and sulfates also exhibit an inhibitory activity toward E1 and E2 conjugation is not known yet. However, any additive inhibitory effects would further increase the plasma concentration of free E2 following isoflavone supplementation.

CONCLUSION

The present work identified a non-competitive inhibition of E1 and E2 conjugation by low micromolar concentrations of soy isoflavones in the human breast cancer cell line MCF-7, which leads to a minor but statistically significant increase in unconjugated E2 of approximately 20%. As the content of genistein and daidzein in soy food is relatively low, an increased risk of breast cancer development and progression in women might only be observed after the continuous consumption of high-dose isoflavone supplements. Further long-term human studies monitoring free estrogens and their conjugates are therefore highly warranted to evaluate the efficacy and safety of high-dose genistein and daidzein supplementation, especially in patients diagnosed with ERα+ breast cancer.

AUTHOR CONTRIBUTIONS

SP performed all the cell culture experiments, the LC-HRMS analysis and the data analysis, and contributed to the manuscript. AM-S analyzed the data and contributed to the manuscript. MZ, JW, and DD performed the LC-HRMS analysis. BP and KS cultivated the MCF-7 cells and performed inhibition experiments; and WJ planned the experiments, analyzed the data and wrote the final version of the manuscript.

ACKNOWLEDGMENTS

This research was supported by a grant from the Austrian Science Fund (FWF) [I 3417-B31] awarded to WJ.

REFERENCES

Adams, J. B., Pewnim, T., Chandra, D. P., Archibald, L., and Foo, M. S. (1979). A correlation between estrogen sulfotransferase levels and estrogen receptor status in human primary breast carcinoma. *Cancer Res.* 39, 5124–5126.

Al-Bader, M., Ford, C., Al-Ayadhy, B., and Francis, I. (2011). Analysis of estrogen receptor isoforms and variants in breast cancer cell lines. *Exp. Ther. Med.* 2, 537–544. doi: 10.3892/etm.2011.226

Cassetta, A., Stojan, J., Krastanova, I., Kristan, K., Brunskole Švegelj, M., Lamba, D., et al. (2017). Structural basis for inhibition of 17β-hydroxysteroid dehydrogenases by phytoestrogens: the case of fungal 17β-HSDcl. *J. Steroid Biochem. Mol. Biol.* 171, 80–93. doi: 10.1016/j.jsbmb.2017.02.020

Chen, J., Duan, Y., Zhang, X., Ye, Y., Ge, B., and Chen, J. (2015). Genistein induces apoptosis by the inactivation of the IGF-1R/p-Akt signaling pathway in MCF-7 human breast cancer cells. *Food Funct.* 6, 995–1000. doi: 10.1039/c4fo01141d

Chi, F., Wu, R., Zeng, Y. C., Xing, R., Liu, Y., and Xu, Z. G. (2013). Post-diagnosis soy food intake and breast cancer survival: a meta-analysis of cohort studies. *Asian Pac. J. Cancer Prev.* 14, 2407–2412.

Clarke, D. B., Bailey, V., and Lloyd, A. S. (2008). Determination of phytoestrogens in dietary supplements by LC-MS/MS. *Food Addit. Contam. Part A Chem. Anal. Control Expo. Risk Asses.* 25, 534–547. doi: 10.1080/02652030701658340

Ferlay, J., Soerjomataram, I., Dikshit, R., Eser, S., Mathers, C., Rebelo, M., et al. (2015). Cancer incidence and mortality worldwide: sources, methods and major patterns in GLOBOCAN 2012. *Int. J. Cancer.* 136, E359–E386. doi: 10.1002/ijc.29210

Folkerd, E., and Dowsett, M. (2013). Sex hormones and breast cancer risk and prognosis. *Breast* 22(Suppl. 2), 38–43. doi: 10.1016/j.breast.2013.07.007

Harris, R. M., Wood, D. M., Bottomley, L., Blagg, S., Owen, K., Hughes, P. J., et al. (2004). Phytoestrogens are potent inhibitors of estrogen sulfation: implications for breast cancer risk and treatment. *J. Clin. Endocrinol. Metab.* 89, 1779–1787.

Hooper, L., Ryder, J. J., Kurzer, M. S., Lampe, J. W., Messina, M. J., Phipps, W. R., et al. (2009). Effects of soy protein and isoflavones on circulating hormone concentrations in pre- and post-menopausal women: a systematic review and meta-analysis. *Hum. Reprod. Update* 15, 423–440. doi: 10.1093/humupd/dmp010

Kang, X., Zhang, Q., Wang, S., Huang, X., and Jin, S. (2010). Effect of soy isoflavones on breast cancer recurrence and death for patients receiving adjuvant endocrine therapy. *CMAJ* 182, 1857–1862. doi: 10.1503/cmaj.091298

Khan, S. A., Chatterton, R. T., Michel, N., Bryk, M., Lee, O., Ivancic, D., et al. (2012). Soy isoflavone supplementation for breast cancer risk reduction: a randomized phase II trial. *Cancer Prev. Res.* 5, 309–319. doi: 10.1158/1940-6207.CAPR-11-0251

Kuiper, G. G., Lemmen, J. G., Carlsson, B., Corton, J. C., Safe, S. H., van der Saag, P. T., et al. (1998). Interaction of estrogenic chemicals and phytoestrogens with estrogen receptor beta. *Endocrinology* 139, 4252–4263.

Maskarinec, G., Morimoto, Y., Heak, S., Isaki, M., Steinbrecher, A., Custer, L., et al. (2012). Urinary estrogen metabolites in two soy trials with premenopausal women. *Eur. J. Clin. Nutr.* 66, 1044–1049. doi: 10.1038/ejcn.2012.71

Mesía-Vela, S., and Kauffman, F. C. (2003). Inhibition of rat liver sulfotransferases SULT1A1 and SULT2A1 and glucuronosyltransferase by dietary flavonoids. *Xenobiotica* 33, 1211–1220.

Mohamed, M. E., and Frye, R. F. (2011). Effects of herbal supplements on drug glucuronidation. Review of clinical, animal, and in vitro studies. *Planta Med.* 77, 311–321. doi: 10.1055/s-0030-1250457

Mueller, J. W., Gilligan, L. C., Idkowiak, J., Arlt, W., and Foster, P. A. (2015). The regulation of steroid action by sulfation and desulfation. *Endocr. Rev.* 36, 526–563. doi: 10.1210/er.2015-1036

Nechuta, S. J., Caan, B. J., Chen, W. Y., Lu, W., Chen, Z., Kwan, M. L., et al. (2012). Soy food intake after diagnosis of breast cancer and survival: an in-depth analysis of combined evidence from cohort studies of US and Chinese women. *Am. J. Clin. Nutr.* 96, 123–132. doi: 10.3945/ajcn.112.035972

Pan, M. H., Chiou, Y. S., Chen, L. H., and Ho, C. T. (2015). Breast cancer chemoprevention by dietary natural phenolic compounds: specific epigenetic related molecular targets. *Mol. Nutr. Food Res.* 59, 21–35. doi: 10.1002/mnfr.201400515

Pasqualini, J. R. (2009). Estrogen sulfotransferases in breast and endometrial cancers. *Ann. N. Y. Acad. Sci.* 1155, 88–98. doi: 10.1111/j.1749-6632.2009.04113.x

Pop, E. A., Fischer, L. M., Coan, A. D., Gitzinger, M., Nakamura, J., and Zeisel, S. H. (2008). Effects of a high daily dose of soy isoflavones on DNA damage, apoptosis and estrogenic outcomes in healthy, postmenopausal women – a phase I clinical trial. *Menopause* 15, 684–692. doi: 10.1097/gme.0b013e318167b8f2

Poschner, S., Zehl, M., Maier-Salamon, A., and Jäger, W. (2017). Simultaneous quantification of estrogens, their precursors and conjugated metabolites in human breast cancer cells by LC-HRMS without derivatization. *J. Pharm. Biomed. Anal.* 138, 344–350. doi: 10.1016/j.jpba.2017.02.033

Rižner, T. L. (2013). Estrogen biosynthesis, phase I and phase II metabolism, and action in endometrial cancer. *Mol. Cell. Endocrinol.* 381, 124–139. doi: 10.1016/j.mce.2013.07.026

Ronis, M. J. (2016). Effects of soy containing diet and isoflavones on cytochrome P450 enzyme expression and activity. *Drug Metab. Rev.* 48, 331–341. doi: 10.1080/03602532.2016.1206562

Samavat, H., and Kurzer, M. S. (2015). Estrogen metabolism and breast cancer. *Cancer Lett.* 356, 231–243. doi: 10.1016/j.canlet.2014.04.018

Shike, M., Doane, A. S., Russo, L., Cabal, R., Reis-Filho, J. S., Gerald, W., et al. (2014). The effects of soy supplementation on gene expression in breast cancer: a randomized placebo-controlled study. *J. Natl. Cancer Inst.* 106:dju189. doi: 10.1093/jnci/dju189

Uifălean, A., Schneider, S., Gierok, P., Ionescu, C., Iuga, C. A., and Lalk, M. (2016). The impact of soy isoflavones on MCF-7 and MDA-MB-231 breast cancer cells using a global metabolomic approach. *Int. J. Mol. Sci.* 17:E1443. doi: 10.3390/ijms17091443

Vladusic, E., Hornby, A., Guerra-Vladusic, F., Lakins, J., and Lupu, R. (2000). Expression and regulation of estrogen receptor beta in human breast tumors and cell lines. *Oncol. Rep.* 7, 157–224. doi: 10.3892/or.7.1.157

Wang, D., Huang, P., Zhu, B., Sun, L., Huang, Q., and Wang, J. (2012). Induction of estrogen receptor (-36 expression by bon morphogenetic protein 2 in breast cancer cell lines. *Mol. Med. Rep.* 6, 591–596. doi: 10.3892/mmr.2012.945

Wei, Y. K., Gamra, I., Davenport, A., Lester, R., Zhao, L., and Wei, Y. (2015). Genistein induces cytochrome P450 1B1 gene expression and cell proliferation in human breast cancer MCF-7 cells. *J. Environ. Pathol. Toxicol. Oncol.* 34, 153–159.

Wiseman, H., Casey, K., Clarke, D. B., Barnes, K. A., and Bowey, E. (2002). Isoflavone aglycon and glucoconjugate content of high- and low-soy U.K. foods used in nutritional studies. *J. Agric. Food Chem.* 50, 1404–1410.

Zhang, F. F., Haslam, D. E., Terry, M. B., Knight, J. A., Andrulis, I. L., Daly, M. B., et al. (2017). Dietary isoflavone intake and all-cause mortality in breast cancer survivors: the breast cancer family registry. *Cancer* 123, 2070–2079. doi: 10.1002/cncr.30615

Physiology and Pathophysiology of Steroid Biosynthesis, Transport and Metabolism in the Human Placenta

*Waranya Chatuphonprasert[1,2], Kanokwan Jarukamjorn[3] and Isabella Ellinger[1]**

[1] *Pathophysiology of the Placenta, Department of Pathophysiology and Allergy Research, Center for Pathophysiology, Infectiology and Immunology, Medical University of Vienna, Vienna, Austria,* [2] *Faculty of Medicine, Mahasarakham University, Maha Sarakham, Thailand,* [3] *Research Group for Pharmaceutical Activities of Natural Products Using Pharmaceutical Biotechnology (PANPB), Faculty of Pharmaceutical Sciences, Khon Kaen University, Khon Kaen, Thailand*

Correspondence:
Isabella Ellinger
Isabella.ellinger@meduniwien.ac.at

The steroid hormones progestagens, estrogens, androgens, and glucocorticoids as well as their precursor cholesterol are required for successful establishment and maintenance of pregnancy and proper development of the fetus. The human placenta forms at the interface of maternal and fetal circulation. It participates in biosynthesis and metabolism of steroids as well as their regulated exchange between maternal and fetal compartment. This review outlines the mechanisms of human placental handling of steroid compounds. Cholesterol is transported from mother to offspring involving lipoprotein receptors such as low-density lipoprotein receptor (LDLR) and scavenger receptor class B type I (SRB1) as well as ATP-binding cassette (ABC)-transporters, ABCA1 and ABCG1. Additionally, cholesterol is also a precursor for placental progesterone and estrogen synthesis. Hormone synthesis is predominantly performed by members of the cytochrome P-450 (CYP) enzyme family including CYP11A1 or CYP19A1 and hydroxysteroid dehydrogenases (HSDs) such as 3β-HSD and 17β-HSD. Placental estrogen synthesis requires delivery of sulfate-conjugated precursor molecules from fetal and maternal serum. Placental uptake of these precursors is mediated by members of the solute carrier (SLC) family including sodium-dependent organic anion transporter (SOAT), organic anion transporter 4 (OAT4), and organic anion transporting polypeptide 2B1 (OATP2B1). Maternal–fetal glucocorticoid transport has to be tightly regulated in order to ensure healthy fetal growth and development. For that purpose, the placenta expresses the enzymes 11β-HSD 1 and 2 as well as the transporter ABCB1. This article also summarizes the impact of diverse compounds and diseases on the expression level and activity of the involved transporters, receptors, and metabolizing enzymes and concludes that the regulatory mechanisms changing the physiological to a pathophysiological state are barely explored. The structure and the cellular composition of the human placental barrier are introduced. While steroid production, metabolism and transport in the placental syncytiotrophoblast have been explored for decades, few information is available for the role of placental-fetal endothelial cells in these processes. With regard to placental structure and function, significant differences exist between species. To further decipher physiologic pathways and their pathologic alterations in placental steroid handling, proper model systems are mandatory.

Keywords: cholesterol, progestagens, estrogens, glucocorticoids, gestational diabetes mellitus, preeclampsia, intrauterine growth retardation, oxysterols

INTRODUCTION

The placenta is a multifunctional organ enabling optimal fetal growth. Structure and function can adapt to diverse external stressors. In case of failure of adaptation or inadequate placental development, fetal survival or fetal growth and development are endangered and developmental programming of adult diseases may occur (Barker and Thornburg, 2013; Burton et al., 2016; Arabin and Baschat, 2017). Moreover, the placenta contributes to maternal diseases such as preeclampsia, which predispose the mother to lifelong illness (Bokslag et al., 2016).

Essential placental functions are biosynthesis, metabolism, and transport of cholesterol, sex hormones and glucocorticoids. This article summarizes placental handling of these steroids under physiologic conditions and gives an overview on changes observed due to maternal diseases and exogenous influences. Whenever possible, data obtained in human placenta or human *in vitro* systems are referenced. We also draw attention to open research questions.

THE HUMAN PLACENTAL BARRIER AND PLACENTAL MODEL SYSTEMS

The hemochorial human placenta results from a deep invasion of embryonic cells during implantation. The mature human placenta is a disk delimited by chorionic and basal plate (**Figure 1A**), which enclose the intervillous space filled with maternal blood. The basal plate contacts the uterine wall. From the chorionic plate, both umbilical cord and the branched chorionic villi originate. The cells of the chorionic villi form the "placental barrier," which prevents direct contact of maternal and fetal blood. Biosynthesis, metabolism, and transport of steroids occur in the chorionic villi (Benirschke et al., 2012).

Chorionic villi are composed of several cell types (Jones and Fox, 1991; Benirschke et al., 2012). The STB, an epithelial multinucleated syncytium, covers the surface of the chorionic villi. The microvillous apical membrane of the STB contacts maternal blood, while the basal plasma membrane of the STB is directed toward the stromal core of the villi. Apical and basal plasma membranes of the STB are often regarded as the most important membrane barriers in the materno-fetal transport processes. Nutrients, hormones, or fetal waste products traverse the STB by different transport mechanisms (Desforges and Sibley, 2010; Brett et al., 2014). Mononuclear CTB are located below the STB. They proliferate and fuse into the STB, thus supporting growth and regeneration of this layer. Early in pregnancy, CTBs form a continuous layer beneath the STB (**Figure 1B**). With progressing pregnancy, CTBs transform from a cuboidal into a flat phenotype. The CTB layer becomes incomplete, but maintains a functional network due to multiple interconnecting cell processes (Jones et al., 2008; **Figure 1C**).

The stromal core of the chorionic villi contains fetal blood vessels delineated by pFECs (Burton et al., 2009), macrophages (Reyes et al., 2017) and additional stromal cells (Sati et al., 2007), which are all embedded in a non-cellular matrix. pFECs are non-fenestrated endothelial cells. Early placental pFECs are probably more permeable than term pFECs. Recent years of research have demonstrated the importance of pFEC function for the fetal development (Wadsack et al., 2012). Heterogeneity of pFECs in the macro-circulation (umbilical cord) and microcirculation (chorionic villi) was shown *in situ* (Lang et al., 1993) and *in vitro* (Lang et al., 2003). Moreover, venous and arterial pFECs, which differ in their phenotypic, genotypic, and functional characteristics, have been described (Lang et al., 2008). The term placenta has a high degree of vascularity (Zhang et al., 2002). The capillaries closely approximate the villous covering, thereby forming "vasculosyncytial membranes" that are important for materno-fetal exchange processes (Burton et al., 2009). Thus, the term maternal–fetal interface or placental barrier consists of a thin cytoplasmic layer of STB apposed to a capillary (**Figure 1C**). Between the STB and pFEC the extracellular matrix is reduced to their fused basal laminae. STB and pFEC actively regulate uptake, metabolism, and transfer/exchange of molecules, while the non-cellular structures probably act as filters and provide transient storage capability (Benirschke et al., 2012).

The placenta undergoes significant anatomical changes in the course of pregnancy (Kingdom et al., 2000), which are relevant to maintain appropriate placental function as pregnancy progresses. Hormones in the fetal and maternal circulations have an important role in determining the placental phenotype (Fowden et al., 2015). As a developing organ that constantly adapts to the maternal environment, not only the structure, but also the transcriptome changes over time (Cox et al., 2015). In line with this, expression of various placental genes involved in biosynthesis, transfer or metabolism of steroids changes during pregnancy (see below).

Abbreviations: 7-DHC, 7-dehydrocholesterol; ABC, ATP-binding cassette; ACAT, Acyl-coenzyme A:cholesterol acyltransferase; ACTH, adrenocorticotropic hormone; A-dione, androstenedione; Apo, Apolipoprotein; ART, assisted reproductive technologies; BCRP, breast cancer resistance protein; CEH, cholesteryl ester hydrolase; CRH, corticotropin-releasing hormone; CTB, cytotrophoblasts; CYP, cytochrome P450; DHCR7, 7-dehydrocholesterol reductase; DHEA, dehydroepiandrosterone; DHEA-S, dehydroepiandrosterone sulfate; E1, estrone; E2, estradiol; E3, estriol; ER, endoplasmic reticulum; GDM, gestational diabetes mellitus; GR, glucocorticoid receptor; hCG, human chorionic gonadotropin; HDL, high-density lipoprotein; HMG-CoA, 3-hydroxy-3-methylglutaryl-coenzyme A; HMGR, HMG-CoA reductase; HPA axis, hypothalamic–pituitary–adrenal axis; HPEC, (isolated) human placental epithelial cells; HSD, hydroxysteroid dehydrogenase; HSP, heat shock protein; HUVEC, human umbilical vein endothelial cells; INSIG, insulin induced gene; IUGR, intrauterine growth retardation; LDL, low-density lipoprotein; LDLR, LDL receptor; LRP, LDLR-related protein; LXR, liver X receptor; MTP, microsomal triglyceride transfer protein; NPC, Niemann-Pick C; OAT, organic anion transporter; OATP, organic anion transporting polypeptide; OHC, hydroxycholesterol; OHP, hydroxyprogesterone; ORP, OSB-related protein; OSBP, oxysterol binding proteins; oxLDL, oxidized LDL; PCOS, polycystic ovary syndrome; PDI, protein disulfide-isomerase; pFEC, placental-fetal endothelial cells; PKA, protein kinase A; PM, particulate matter; RCT, reverse cholesterol transport; ROR, RAR-related orphan receptors; ROS, reactive oxygen species; RXR, retinoid X receptor; -S, -sulfate; SCAP, SREBP cleavage-activating protein; SCP, sterol carrier protein; SF, steroidogenic factor; sFlt1, soluble fms-like tyrosine kinase 1; SLC, solute carrier; SLCO, SLC transporter, SOAT, sodium-dependent organic anion transporter; SLOS, Smith-Lemli-Opitz syndrome; Sp1, Specific protein 1; SRB1, scavenger receptor class B type I; SRE, sterol regulatory element; SREBP, SRE-binding protein; StAR/STARD1, steroidogenic acute regulatory protein; START, StAR-related lipid transfer; STB, syncytiotrophoblast; STS, steroid sulfatase; SULT, sulfotransferase; TLR, Toll-like receptor; VLDL, very low-density lipoprotein; VLDLR, VLDL receptor.

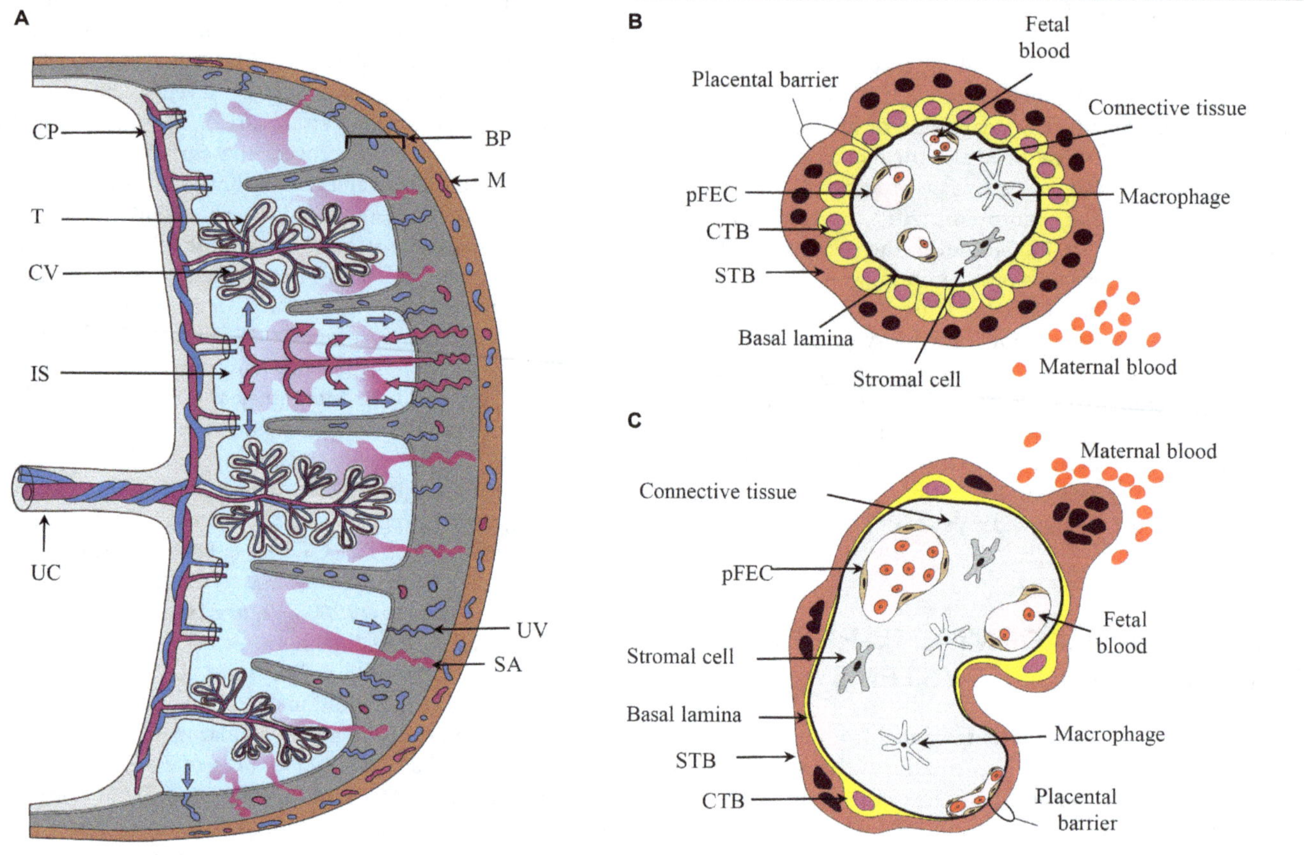

FIGURE 1 | The placental barrier. **(A)** Schematic depiction of the main structural elements of the human placenta. From the chorionic plate (CP), the umbilical cord (UC), and the chorionic villi (CV) originate. The umbilical vein carries oxygen- and nutrient-rich blood from the placenta to the fetus, while two arteries transport deoxygenated blood and waste products from the fetus to the placenta. The intervillous space (IS) is filled with maternal blood that enters this cavity via remodeled and opened maternal spiral arteries (SA) and leaves via uterine veins (UV). Cells in direct contact with maternal blood are the villous trophoblasts (T). The basal plate (BP) contains extravillous trophoblasts and decidual cells. **(B,C)** Schematic representation of first trimester **(B)** and term trimester chorionic villi **(C)** depicting the major cell types and the placental barrier. CTB , cytotrophoblast; M, myometrium of the maternal uterus, pFECs, placental-fetal endothelial cells; STB, syncytiotrophoblast.

The structure of the placenta is species-specific. Thus, no perfect animal model for the human placenta exists and special care must be taken with extrapolation of data from one species to another. Higher order primates including old world monkeys such as baboons are most closely aligned to humans with respect to structure as well as regulation of steroidogenesis (Pepe and Albrecht, 1995; Grigsby, 2016). Species-specific placental anatomy, endocrine function or advantages and limitations of relevant animal models to study the function of the human placenta in health and disease are detailed in various review articles (Malassine et al., 2003; Carter, 2007; Fowden et al., 2015; Carter and Enders, 2016; Grigsby, 2016; Hafez, 2017).

Placental functions can also be studied in human *ex vivo* models such as the isolated perfused placenta and placental villous tissue explants. Commonly used *in vitro* models are (1) isolated and *in vitro* cultured placental primary cells including trophoblasts as well as primary arterial and venous pFECs; (2) diverse, mainly trophoblastic cell lines derived by either transfection or spontaneous mutation including the choriocarcinoma cell lines BeWo, JEG-3, and Jar; and (3) isolated membrane vesicles (Lang et al., 2008; Prouillac and Lecoeur, 2010; Orendi et al., 2011; Cvitic et al., 2013; Myllynen and Vahakangas, 2013; Gohner et al., 2014; Steinberg and Robins, 2016). Choriocarcinoma cell lines are the most extensively used cell models. Their disadvantage is their origin from tumors. GeneChip analysis has revealed considerable differences between the gene expression patterns of choriocarcinoma cell lines and primary placental cells (Bilban et al., 2010). Thus, results obtained in cell lines should always be interpreted carefully and best be confirmed in other *in vitro* or *ex vivo* models. Over the last years co-cultures of trophoblast cells with endothelial cells have been established in order to mimic the entire placental barrier (Levkovitz et al., 2013a,b; Blundell et al., 2016, 2018). In the future, they may become attractive models to study transplacental transport processes and functional interdependence of cells.

CHOLESTEROL

Cholesterol (**Figure 2B**) is an essential component of cell membranes influencing their integrity, fluidity, and permeability,

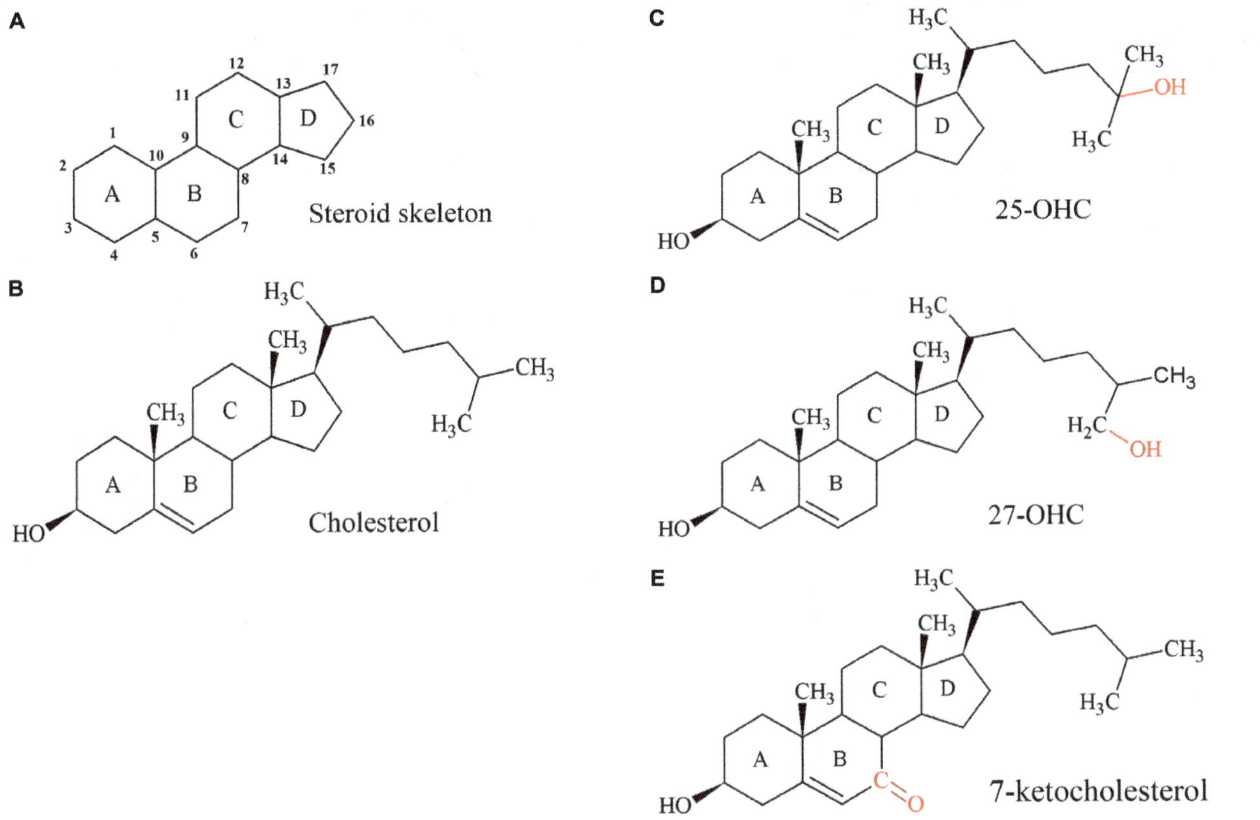

FIGURE 2 | Structures of the steroid skeleton, cholesterol, and common oxysterols. **(A)** All steroids have the same basic perhydro-1,2-cyclopentenophenanthrene skeleton. Letters designate each ring, the carbon atoms are numbered. A slight variation in this skeleton or the introduction of functional groups result in various classes of steroids. **(B)** Unesterified cholesterol contains this skeleton with a hydroxyl group, two methyl groups, and a hydrogen tail. In the esterified form, a fatty acid would be bound to the hydroxyl group by an ester bond. **(C)** 25-hydroxycholesterol (25-OHC), the most extensively studied oxysterol. **(D)** Oxysterol 27-hydroxycholesterol (27-OHC). **(E)** Oxysterol 7-ketocholesterol. Red molecules indicate the positions of hydroxylation **(C,D)** or oxidation **(E)** of cholesterol to 25- or 27-OHC, or 7-ketocholesterol, respectively. Oxysterols are intermediates of cholesterol catabolism and act as signaling molecules with regulatory impact on various cellular processes including lipid metabolism.

equally important for the growing placenta and fetus. The human placenta needs more than 1 g of cholesterol for tissue growth (Pratt et al., 1946) and the term human placenta manufactures approximately 400 mg of sex steroids from the precursor cholesterol per day (Knopp et al., 1981). Cholesterol is essential for myelination (Snipes and Suter, 1997) and as an activator and propagator of the sonic hedgehog-signaling pathway (Blassberg and Jacob, 2017). Thus, cholesterol is indispensable for patterning and development of the fetal nervous system.

Oxysterols are structurally closely related to cholesterol (**Figures 2C–E**) and have regulatory functions in cholesterol metabolism (Schroepfer, 2000; Mutemberezi et al., 2016; Sun et al., 2018). They are not only generated by enzymes, but also formed by autoxidation and thus accumulate under increased oxidative stress (Zarrouk et al., 2014).

According to the WHO, in 2008 the global prevalence of raised total cholesterol among female adults ($\geq$5.0 mmol/l) was 40%; thus, hypercholesterolemia became a major health care problem. Various studies have indicated that maternal hypercholesterolemia (Napoli et al., 1997, 1999; Marceau et al., 2005; Catov et al., 2007; Zhang et al., 2017), but also maternal hypocholesterolemia (Sattar et al., 1999; Edison et al., 2007) negatively impact pregnancy outcome. Among the observed consequences are preterm delivery (Marceau et al., 2005; Catov et al., 2007; Edison et al., 2007), low birth weight (Marceau et al., 2005), IUGR (Sattar et al., 1999), and changes in the fetal aorta that determine the long-term susceptibility of children to fatty-streak formation and subsequent atherosclerosis (Napoli et al., 1997, 1999). Furthermore, altered mRNA expression levels of placental lipoprotein receptors involved in cholesterol uptake were observed (Ethier-Chiasson et al., 2007; Zhang et al., 2017).

As described below, also diseases of pregnancy and various endogenous and exogenous compounds can affect the placental proteins involved in cholesterol biosynthesis, metabolism, and transport. The long-term consequences for the fetus are hardly known. Thus, we need to further explore the regulation of cholesterol-associated pathways in placentas in healthy and diseased pregnancies in order to understand the correlation between observed changes *in utero* and diseases developing during later lives.

Cholesterol Biosynthesis and Homeostasis

Cellular cholesterol homeostasis includes tightly regulated processes, which are summarized in **Figure 3** (Ikonen, 2006; Cerqueira et al., 2016; Soffientini and Graham, 2016). Intracellular cholesterol synthesis starts from acetyl-coenzyme A (acetyl-CoA). Lanosterol, the first sterol, feeds into two pathways, the Bloch (Bloch, 1965) and the Kandutsch–Russell (Kandutsch and Russell, 1960) pathway that both result in cholesterol production. The rate-limiting and committed step is the conversion of HMG-CoA to mevalonate mediated by HMGR. HMGR is regulated by endogenous molecules including transcription factor SREBP2 (Shimano and Sato, 2017) as well as the statin drugs (Lamon-Fava, 2013). Excess cellular cholesterol gets fatty-acylated by the action of ACAT, to form cholesteryl esters for storage in cytoplasmic lipid droplets; the inverse reaction is controlled by, e.g., CEH (Miller and Bose, 2011; Korber et al., 2017).

Cholesterol synthesis and HMGR activity in human (Hellig et al., 1970; Telegdy et al., 1970; Boguslawski and Sokolowski, 1984) as well as baboon placenta (Khamsi et al., 1972; Shi et al., 1999) decrease as pregnancy progresses. There are estimates

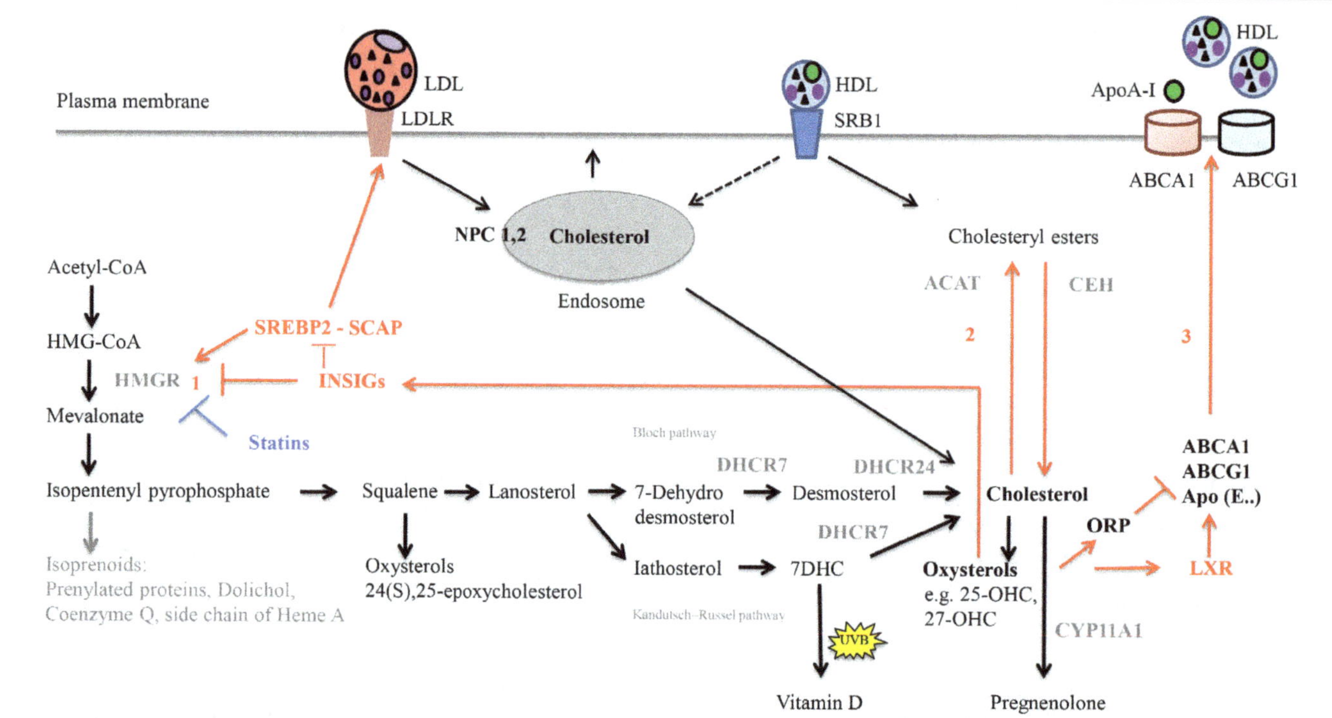

FIGURE 3 | Important steps in cholesterol synthesis and homeostasis. Cholesterol synthesis occurs via the mevalonate pathway and involves over 20 enzymes. It starts from acetyl-CoA in the cytosol, but all steps downstream of 3-hydroxy-3-methylglutaryl-coenzyme A (HMG-CoA) occur in the smooth endoplasmic reticulum. Lanosterol, the first sterol, feeds either into the Bloch pathway or the Kandutsch–Russell pathway. In these pathways, cholesterol is produced from either desmosterol or 7-dehydrocholesterol (7-DHC), by the enzymes 24-dehydrocholesterol reductase (DHCR24) and 7-dehydrocholesterol reductase (DHCR7), respectively. Gene mutations of the enzyme DHCR7 result in Smith-Lemli-Opitz syndrome, SLOS, with increased levels of cholesterol precursors and reduced levels of cholesterol. In the skin, 7-DHC can be converted to vitamin D by UVB light. Diverse oxysterols are produced enzymatically from cholesterol, its precursors but also during subsequent steroid hormone synthesis. The rate limiting step in cholesterol synthesis is catalyzed by 3 HMG-CoA reductase (HMGR). Cellular homeostasis of cholesterol is maintained by three distinct mechanisms (red arrows). (1) Regulation of HMGR activity and levels to control cholesterol biosynthesis occurs by feed-back inhibition, control of gene expression, rate of enzyme degradation, and phosphorylation–dephosphorylation. For example, the transcription factor sterol regulatory element-binding protein 2 (SREBP2) positively regulates the gene expression of HMGR. Rising cholesterol and oxysterol levels reduce the rate of cholesterol biosynthesis by modulating the activities of insulin-induced gene (INSIG) proteins. When activated, INSIG both promotes the ubiquitination and consequent destabilization of HMGR and inhibits the transcriptional activity of SREBP2 by retaining it in complex with SREBP cleavage-activating protein (SCAP) in the endoplasmic reticulum. (2) Rising cholesterol levels also activate acyl-coenzyme A:cholesterol acyltransferase (ACAT), which esterifies cholesterol leading to its sequestration in cytosolic lipid droplets. Through hydrolysis via the cholesteryl ester hydrolase (CEH) enzyme system, the cholesteryl esters can be reused later. (3) Regulation of cholesterol uptake and export via low-density lipoprotein (LDL)-receptor-mediated uptake and high-density lipoprotein HDL-mediated reverse transport, respectively. Oxysterols activate liver-X receptor (LXR) transcription factors, which positively regulate the transcription of proteins that drive cholesterol efflux from the cell (ABC transporter, ABCA1 and ABCG1), and sequester it in lipoprotein particles containing Apolipoprotein E (ApoE) in the circulatory system. Activation of oxysterol binding protein-related proteins (ORP) by oxysterols negatively regulates cholesterol efflux by promoting ABCA1 ubiquitination and degradation. Following binding of lipoprotein particles (LDL and HDL) to their respective receptors [LDLR, Scavenger receptor class B type 1 (SRB1)], they are internalized into endosomes. Alternatively, HDL particles can transfer cholesteryl esters to the plasma membrane (selective lipid uptake) without requirement for endocytosis. Within endosomes, Niemann-Pick C1 (NPC1) and NPC2 are critical for the egress of internalized cholesterol from endosomes; they act together to redistribute cholesterol to the ER. Statins are HMGR inhibitors. The net result of statin treatment is an increased cellular uptake of LDLs, since the intracellular synthesis of cholesterol is inhibited and cells are therefore dependent on extracellular sources of cholesterol.

that *de novo* cholesterol synthesis in the term human placenta provides only 1–2% of the cholesterol required for progesterone biosynthesis (Simpson et al., 1978). But the extent of cholesterol synthesis is species-specific; rabbit placentas near term exhibit a high level of HMGR expression and activity (Montoudis et al., 2003; Marseille-Tremblay et al., 2007).

Human pregnancy is characterized by maternal hyperlipidemia especially during the last trimester (Herrera et al., 2006). High maternal estrogen concentrations and maternal insulin-resistance stimulate hepatic VLDL production. Triglyceride and cholesterol concentrations in LDL and HDL particles rise, providing ample cholesterol fuel for the STB (Winkler et al., 2000; Herrera, 2002; Weissgerber and Wolfe, 2006). In contrast, maternal serum cholesterol levels in pregnant rabbits drop significantly compared to the non-pregnant state (Marseille-Tremblay et al., 2007).

With advancing gestational age, maternal serum-derived cholesterol replaces endogenously produced cholesterol as the major substrate of placental progesterone production in humans and baboons (Baird et al., 1973; Babischkin et al., 1997a,b; Henson, 1998; Shi et al., 1999). Addition of LDL to primary trophoblast cultures drastically suppresses *de novo* cholesterol synthesis, stimulates progesterone production and inhibits cholesteryl ester-forming ACAT (Winkel et al., 1980a,b, 1981). Likewise, addition of HDL_2 stimulates progesterone secretion *in vitro* (Lasuncion et al., 1991). Trophoblasts isolated from healthy early, mid, and late baboon gestation show an upregulation of LDLR in mid and late gestation, while HMGR activity is reduced (Henson et al., 1997). Nevertheless, when external LDL supply is reduced *in vivo* or *in vitro*, human and baboon trophoblasts continue to produce sufficient progesterone due to endogenous cholesterol production (Simpson et al., 1978; Moise et al., 1986; Parker et al., 1986; Henson et al., 1991). In choriocarcinoma cells, an inverse relationship between the lipoproteins in the culture medium and the HMGR activity was demonstrated (Simpson et al., 1978). Together, these data suggest feedback inhibition of maternal-derived cholesterol on endogenous cholesterol synthesis and cholesteryl ester formation in human and baboon STB.

Impact of Exogenous and Endogenous Factors on Placental Cholesterol Biosynthesis

Inconsistent with feedback inhibition by cholesterol, maternal hypercholesterolemia does neither change placental HMGR protein levels nor change placental cholesterol or cholesteryl ester content (Marseille-Tremblay et al., 2008).

From other tissues, age- and gender-related dysregulation of cholesterol metabolism, and specifically of HMGR regulation are known (Trapani and Pallottini, 2010). A hint for placenta-specific regulation of cholesterol biosynthesis is the observation that maternal hypercholesterolemia causes an increase in the placental expression of the transcription factor SREBP-2 (Marseille-Tremblay et al., 2008). Scarce information is available on regulation of the placental SREBP – SCAP – INSIG system (**Figure 3**). In the Golden Syrian hamster, suppression of sterol synthesis by exogenous sterol is blunted in placenta and other developing tissues when compared to parental tissues. This lack of response appears to be mediated at least partly through the SCAP:INSIGs ratio, which is 1.8-fold greater in the placenta as compared to the adult liver (Yao et al., 2007). Neither in human nor baboon placenta regulation of these molecules has been investigated so far, but this topic might be of relevance in the context of ART, which are increasingly applied today. Among the observed adverse neonatal outcomes in pregnancies conceived through *in vitro* fertilization and intracytoplasmic sperm injection are low birth weight and small size for gestational age. Interestingly, a recent study performed in humans (Lou et al., 2014) found that placenta and fetus from ART pregnancies showed altered transcript levels of *INSIG1* and *SREBF1*. The enhanced gene expression correlated with lower methylation rates of INSIG1 and SREBF1. The authors hypothesized an impact of ART on the placental/fetal cholesterol metabolism with consequences for the future life of the offspring (Collier et al., 2009). More research is required to confirm this theory.

Estrogen production is significantly (3–8 times at term) increased during pregnancy. The elevated estrogen levels were suggested to stimulate cholesterol uptake via increased LDLR expression as well as progesterone production via increased P450scc enzyme activity in cultured primary trophoblasts (Pepe and Albrecht, 1995; Grimes et al., 1996). In contrast, activities of the placental enzymes HMGR, ACAT, or CEH were found unaffected by estrogen (Babischkin et al., 1997a). This contrasts with estrogen-influenced HMGR regulation in other species and tissues (Trapani et al., 2010).

Recently, an impact of GDM on cholesterol synthesis and esterification in isolated and cultured human placental endothelial cells (HPECs) has been observed. The authors of the study suspected that higher intracellular ROS levels in GDM upregulated HMGR, increased *de novo* cholesterol biosynthesis and ACAT1 expression, but the underlying mechanisms remain to be identified (Sun et al., 2018).

Statins, inhibitors of HMGR, are increasingly prescribed to women of reproductive age (Forbes et al., 2015), but in experiments with first trimester placental explants or isolated first trimester trophoblasts, statins revealed detrimental effects on trophoblast growth (Forbes et al., 2008). Statins not only significantly decreased progesterone secretion (Kenis et al., 2005). They also inhibited proliferation (Forbes et al., 2015) and migration (Tartakover-Matalon et al., 2007) of trophoblasts. Isoprenylation, which also depends on HMGR activity (**Figure 3**), is required for cell proliferation, migration, metabolism, and protein glycosylation and thus, proper development of embryo and placenta. The existing data suggest that statins should be avoided during the first trimester of pregnancy (Ermini et al., 2017). On the other hand, there is evidence that statins, due to their anti-proliferative, anti-invasive, anti-inflammatory, and anti-angiogenic effects might be useful in treatment of various obstetric and gynecologic conditions including endometriosis, PCOS, ovarian cancer, preeclampsia, and antiphospholipid syndrome (Esteve-Valverde et al., 2018; Zeybek et al., 2018). Further studies are required to understand the mechanisms of action of statins during gestation. Moreover, clinical trials to investigate the efficacy, safety, and appropriate dosage of different statins during pregnancy are needed.

In summary, the regulation of placental cholesterol synthesis requires further characterization, but species-specific placental structure and function should be considered. Many of the involved enzymes are regulated at multiple levels (Shi et al., 1999). Besides total mRNA and protein levels, DNA- and protein modifications and protein activities should be analyzed to obtain conclusive information about the mechanism of regulation. Since placental tissue is a mixture of different cell types, analysis of purified cell populations should be preferred over total tissue analysis to decipher cell type-specific regulation of protein expression (Shi et al., 1999).

Maternal Lipoprotein Particle Uptake by the STB

Fetuses produce a significant fraction of the required cholesterol via endogenous synthesis. In humans, genetic defects in *de novo* cholesterol synthesis result in severe congenital birth defects. SLOS is caused by a deficiency of DHCR7 (**Figure 3**), which catalyzes the conversion of 7-DHC to cholesterol (Jira, 2013; Kanungo et al., 2013). SLOS fetuses with null mutations in DHCR7 exhibit no endogenous cholesterol synthesis, but they have some cholesterol in tissues and blood at birth indicating placental cholesterol transfer (Tint et al., 1995).

Amount and period of materno-fetal cholesterol transport remain under debate. Extrapolation of data from non-human species is difficult as the quantity of cholesterol derived from the maternal circulation differs (Connor and Lin, 1967; Pitkin et al., 1972; Cavender et al., 1995; Woollett, 1996, 2005; Jurevics et al., 1997; Woollett and Heubi, 2000; Herrera, 2002) ranging from very low levels in rat (Belknap and Dietschy, 1988; Jurevics et al., 1997) to more than 40% in the rhesus monkey (Pitkin et al., 1972). Studies in humans revealed that materno-fetal cholesterol transfer occurred throughout pregnancy (Plotz et al., 1968; Hellig et al., 1970; Lin et al., 1977). However, mainly during early development maternal cholesterol serves as the primary source of fetal cholesterol (Napoli et al., 1997; Baardman et al., 2012).

Subsequently, we summarize the mechanisms of placental cholesterol uptake and transport (**Figure 4**). Cholesterol transport across the secondary yolk sac that may participate in nutrition of the human fetus during the first trimester (Burton et al., 2001) was reviewed elsewhere (Baardman et al., 2013).

In plasma, cholesterol is associated with different types of lipoprotein particles. Among them, LDLs carry 65–70% of circulating plasma cholesterol. Lipoprotein particles can interact with the plasma membrane of target cells via members of the LDLR family including LDLR, VLDLR, LRP1, LRP2 (megalin), or LRP8 (apoE receptor 2) (Go and Mani, 2012).

The presence of LDL-specific binding sites was shown throughout pregnancy in preparations of microvillous placental membranes, representing enriched apical STB plasma membranes (Alsat et al., 1982, 1984; Rebourcet et al., 1986; Naoum et al., 1987). Expression of LDLR mRNA in baboon STB increases with advancing pregnancy (Albrecht et al., 1995). Estrogen, but also depletion of cholesterol upregulate LDLR expression (Henson et al., 1991, 1997; Pepe and Albrecht, 1995; Grimes et al., 1996; Babischkin et al., 1997a,b). But conflicting data concerning the regulation of LDLR mRNA levels in total placental tissue in the course of human pregnancy exist (Furuhashi et al., 1989; Albrecht et al., 1995; Murata et al., 1996; Plosch et al., 2010). Additional expression of LDLR in stromal cells in the chorionic villi (Kamper et al., 2017) and cell-type specific receptor regulation may account for that discrepancy.

The transfer of lipids between HDL and target cells is incompletely understood. A number of proteins and receptors have been described to bind HDL. After receptor binding, HDL associated lipids are transferred to cells predominantly without catabolism of the particle. Transfer of cholesteryl esters to the accepting plasma membrane is known as "selective uptake" (Linton et al., 2017). An alternative pathway comprising endocytosis of whole HDL particles followed by resecretion exists. Neither the connection between HDL endocytosis and selective lipid uptake nor the physiological relevance of HDL uptake is fully clarified. SRB1 (in humans also termed CLA-1) is a multiple ligand receptor able to facilitate uptake of cholesteryl esters from HDL. SRB1 can also mediate whole HDL particle endocytosis (Rohrl and Stangl, 2013).

HDL binding-sites as well as SRB1 were found on isolated placental microvillous and basal plasma membranes of the STB (Alsat and Malassine, 1991; Lafond et al., 1999). *In situ*, SRB1 localizes to first and third trimester trophoblasts as well as term pFECs (Landers et al., 2018). Cultured first trimester trophoblasts expressed SRB1, exhibited selective cholesteryl ester-uptake from HDL_3, but also displayed considerable HDL endocytosis and degradation. In term cultured trophoblasts, SRB1 expression was lower. Likewise, selective uptake as well as HDL degradation were decreased compared to first trimester cells, but were still elevated compared to other tissues (Wadsack et al., 2003). *In vitro*, SRB1 involvement in selective cholesteryl ester-uptake from HDL_3 was demonstrated (Wadsack et al., 2003). In total placental tissue highest SRB1 expression levels were observed in term placenta (Plosch et al., 2010), which might be explained by the expression of SRB1 in pFECs (Stefulj et al., 2009) and the increase of the proportion of vessels from 37% in first trimester to 63% at term (Zhang et al., 2002). In pregnant women with high serum cholesterol levels, LDLR expression, but not SRB1 protein expression is down-regulated (Ethier-Chiasson et al., 2007). Cell-type specific, *SRB1* gene transcription can be regulated by hormones, including hCG and estrogen (Landschulz et al., 1996; Fukata et al., 2014). Whether and how SRB1 expression in human STB and pFECs is influenced by these hormones, remains to be determined.

VLDL binds to term placental microvillous membranes (Naoum et al., 1987) and the triglyceride-enriched VLDL is an important fatty acid supplier for the fetus. Hydrolysis of VLDL-associated triglycerides is mediated by lipases such as lipoprotein lipase, which are expressed at the apical membrane of the STB (Bonet et al., 1992; Lindegaard et al., 2005). While the placenta also expresses several receptors for apolipoprotein (Apo)E-enriched particles, including VLDLR (Gafvels et al., 1993; Wittmaack et al., 1995; Murata et al., 1996), LRP1 (Gafvels

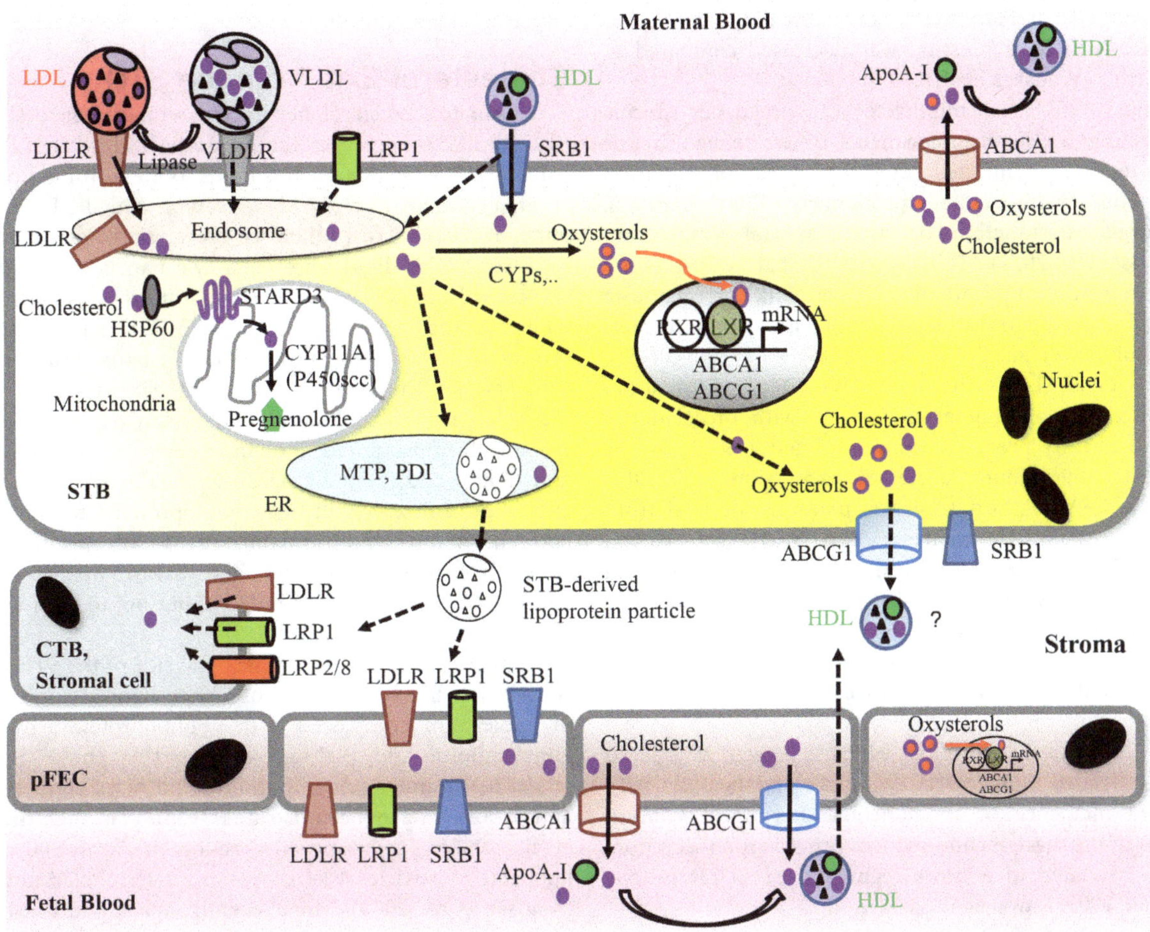

FIGURE 4 | Proposed model for placental uptake of cholesterol from maternal lipoproteins, cholesterol metabolism, and materno-fetal transport of cholesterol. For detailed information, see text. Solid arrows indicate pathways that have been demonstrated *in vitro*. Dashed arrows indicate hypothetic routes. Apo, Apolipoprotein; ABC transporters, ATP-binding cassette transporters; CYPs, cytochrome P-450 enzymes; CTB, cytotrophoblast; pFECs, placental-fetal endothelial cells; HDL, high-density lipoprotein; HSP, heat shock protein; LDL, low-density lipoprotein; LDLR, low-density lipoprotein receptor; LRP, lipoprotein receptor-related proteins; LXR, liver X receptor; PDI, protein disulfide isomerase; MTP, microsomal triglyceride transfer protein; RXR, retinoid X receptor; SRB1, scavenger receptor class B type 1; STARD3, StAR-related lipid transfer domain protein 3; STB, syncytiotrophoblast; VLDL, very low-density lipoprotein; VLDLR, very low-density lipoprotein receptor.

et al., 1992; Cao et al., 2014; Kamper et al., 2017), LRP2 (Burke et al., 2013; Kamper et al., 2017), and LRP8 (Kim et al., 1996; Ulrich et al., 2016), their involvement in cholesterol uptake by the STB has never been demonstrated. A mutation in human LRP2 gives rise to severe congenital anomalies in the offspring (Kantarci et al., 2007). This may indicate an important role of LRP2 in placental cholesterol transport, but LRP2 is a multiligand receptor and thus, may serve different roles in trophoblast biology (Coukos et al., 1994; Go and Mani, 2012).

Impact of Diseases and Exogenous Compounds on Placental Lipoprotein Receptor Expression

GDM is a glucose intolerance, which is first recognized during pregnancy, but usually resolves after birth. In Europe, it has a prevalence of 5.4% (Eades et al., 2017). The most common adverse outcome is high fetal birth weight (macrosomia). Placental abnormalities include increased incidence of villous immaturity, increased measures of angiogenesis, and higher placental weight. GDM is also associated with a higher risk of maternal and fetal complications including development of type 2 diabetes in later life (Huynh et al., 2015; Gallo et al., 2016; Rani and Begum, 2016). In GDM, altered maternal and neonatal lipid profiles were observed. Moreover, expression of LDLR and SRB1 was induced (Dube et al., 2013).

IUGR is observed in 5–10% of pregnancies. Due to a compromised placental function, the fetus does not reach its intrauterine potential for growth and development. As the second leading cause of perinatal mortality IUGR is responsible for 30% of stillborn infants. Long-term health defects include impaired neurological and cognitive development and cardiovascular or endocrine diseases in adulthood (Nardozza et al., 2017). IUGR is associated with a decreased supply of nutrients and/or oxygen to the growing fetus. Placental LDLR expression was found increased, while SRB1 expression was decreased compared to healthy controls (Wadsack et al., 2007).

Preeclampsia is a multifactorial pregnancy-specific disease affecting 3–5% of pregnancies. It is defined by *de novo* hypertension manifested after 20 weeks of gestation in combination with either proteinuria (300 mg/day), maternal organ dysfunction or uteroplacental dysfunction (Tranquilli et al., 2014). IUGR and premature birth are clinically relevant complications. In addition, preeclampsia affects the long-term outcome of both mothers and their offspring (Bokslag et al., 2016). Serum levels of triglycerides, LDLs, small dense LDLs that are susceptible to oxidation, as well as oxLDLs are higher in women with preeclampsia compared to healthy pregnant women (Chigusa et al., 2013). Murata et al. (1996) found decreased expression of VLDLR and LDLR mRNA in third trimester placentas derived from preeclamptic women. Hentschke et al. (2013) reported no differences in LDLR, LRP1, SRB1 mRNA levels when comparing placentas of healthy and preeclamptic women. But they observed reduced LRP1 mRNA expression in placentas of preeclamptic mothers delivering small-for-gestational-age babies compared to healthy controls (Hentschke et al., 2013).

Maternal exposure to cadmium, which is present in tobacco smoke, is associated with low birth weight and possibly with an increased incidence of spontaneous abortion. Cadmium accumulates in the placenta and reduces progesterone secretion. Partly, this is related to a down-regulation of LDLR mRNA (Jolibois et al., 1999; Kawai et al., 2002).

In summary, the human placenta expresses several receptors for lipoprotein particles. For most receptors, their involvement in and individual contribution to placental cholesterol uptake remains unexplored. Moreover, regulation of receptor expression under physiologic and pathologic conditions of pregnancy has been barely investigated.

Intracellular Cholesterol Transport in the STB

After internalization into acidic endosomal compartments, dissociation of receptor-ligand complexes occurs. The receptors return to the plasma membrane, while lipoprotein particles enter the lysosomal route for degradation. Cholesterol incorporates into the endosomal/lysosomal membranes by coordinated actions of NPC1 and NPC2. Cholesterol transport to mitochondria for steroidogenesis is achieved by lipid transfer proteins including StAR/STARD1 and other members of the START domain protein family (Elustondo et al., 2017). Cholesterol transport to other cellular targets, e.g., the plasma membrane occurs by vesicular and non-vesicular means, the latter involving cholesterol binding to various proteins (Miller and Auchus, 2011; Luo et al., 2017). Although expression of some intracellular cholesterol transporting proteins including NPCs, NPC1-Like1, ABC-transporters ABCA2, SCP-x, STARD3, and HSP60 has been demonstrated in human term placenta (Tuckey et al., 2004; Burke et al., 2009; Monreal-Flores et al., 2017), the mechanism of intracellular cholesterol transport in STB remains largely uncharacterized.

Cholesterol Exit From the STB

To eliminate cholesterol, hepatocytes secrete lipoprotein particles (Sacks, 2015). Secretion requires ApoB and the ER-localized cofactor MTP. MTP transfers lipids to the forming lipoproteins. It is a dimer of a 97-kDa protein and PDI (Walsh and Hussain, 2017). Most other cell types release excess cholesterol to extracellular lipid acceptors. Mechanisms accounting for cholesterol efflux include passive diffusion as well as active pathways mediated by ABCA1, ABCG1, and SRB1. Several factors including cellular cholesterol status, lipid transporter activity, and the nature of extracellular acceptors, influence the efficiency of cholesterol efflux. ABCA1 and ABCG1 are specifically important for the elimination of cholesterol from cells and tissues and for the biogenesis of HDL. ABCA1 stimulates cholesterol efflux to lipid-free apolipoproteins, predominantly to apoA-I, but also ApoE. In contrast, ABCG1 promotes efflux of cholesterol and oxysterols to HDL. SRB1 can mediate cholesterol efflux from peripheral cells to HDL, but not to lipid-free apoA-I (Phillips, 2014; Favari et al., 2015).

Efflux of cholesterol from the basal side of the STB is unclear. It may occur via secretion of either lipoprotein particles or of cholesterol complexed with apolipoproteins. ApoB, MTP large subunit and PDI are expressed in the STB (Kamper et al., 2017) and unique lipoprotein particles containing ApoB and ApoA-I have been isolated from placental tissue (Park et al., 1988). Furthermore, secretion of ApoB-100-containing lipoprotein particles was shown from term placental biopsies (Madsen et al., 2004). More recently, apical and basal secretion of ApoB in polarized grown BeWo cells was demonstrated (Kamper et al., 2017). Cholesterol complexed with ApoB or lipoprotein particles and secreted from the basal membranes of the STB could provide cholesterol and other lipids not only to pFECs and consequently to the fetus, but also to CTBs as well as stromal cells of the chorionic villi given that these cells express the relevant apolipoprotein receptors. Indeed, *in situ* expression of lipoprotein receptors such as LDLR or LRP1 on placental cells including pFECs or LRP2 on the CTB was shown (Kamper et al., 2017). This would enable uptake of STB-derived lipoprotein-associated cholesterol. In support of the idea that intact lipoproteins reach stromal cells of the villi, a capability to hydrolyze VLDL-triglycerides has been demonstrated on isolated placental macrophages (Bonet et al., 1992). However, how placental macrophages or other stromal cells cover their cholesterol requirements is currently unknown.

Apical secretion of ApoE from the STB was suggested to facilitate uptake of maternal non-LDL lipoprotein particles (Rindler et al., 1991); likewise, apical secretion of ApoB, which was observed in BeWo cells (Kamper et al., 2017), could be of relevance for regulation or induction of cholesterol uptake by trophoblasts. Moreover, apical secretion of apolipoproteins may enable RCT from the STB via apically expressed ABCA1 or SRB1 (see below). However, these speculations require further investigation.

Alternatively, cholesterol can exit the STB via ABCA1 and ABCG1, which stimulate efflux of cholesterol and oxysterols (Aye et al., 2009). Both transporters exhibit high expression in the placenta (Albrecht et al., 2007; Stefulj et al., 2009; Aye et al., 2010; Bhattacharjee et al., 2010; Nikitina et al., 2011; Bloise et al., 2016). They localize to apical (ABCA1) and basal membrane (ABCG1) of the STB and to the luminal surface of the pFEC (Albrecht et al., 2007; Stefulj et al., 2009; Aye et al., 2010; Baumann et al., 2013), but contradictory localization data also exist (Bhattacharjee et al., 2010; Nikitina et al., 2011). In cultured trophoblasts, up- or down-regulation of ABCA1 and ABCG1 stimulated or reduced, respectively, cellular cholesterol efflux (Aye et al., 2010). The presence of SRB1 at the apical and basal membrane of the STB (Lafond et al., 1999) would allow for bidirectional transport of liposoluble molecules to and from lipoprotein particles (Cao et al., 1997). In polarized grown BeWo cells, basal efflux of cholesterol was highest to HDL, and was suggested to occur via either SRB1 (Schmid et al., 2003), or ABCG1 (Woollett, 2011). However, expression and subcellular localization of SRB1, ABCA1, and ABCG1 seem to differ between BeWo cells and primary trophoblasts (Woollett, 2011). In any way, an efflux of cholesterol from the basal membrane of the STB via ABCG1 or SRB1 requires appropriate cholesterol acceptor molecules within the stroma of the villi. This has not been described.

Cholesterol Transport by pFECs

Uptake of cholesterol by pFECs remains unknown. Efflux of cholesterol via ABCA1 and ABCG1 to apolipoproteins or HDL particles, respectively, has been confirmed in isolated term HPECs, while SRB1 does not contribute to HDL-mediated cholesterol release (Stefulj et al., 2009; Sun et al., 2018). Appropriate cholesterol acceptor molecules (HDL and ApoE) are available in the fetal circulation (Bansal et al., 2005).

Regulation of ABC-Transporters via LXR in Health and Diseases

LXRs are "sterol sensors" responsible for protecting cells from cholesterol overload. LXR-activation by oxysterols (see below), but not cholesterol, induces transcriptional activity of the LXR/RXR heterodimer. This results in reduced intracellular cholesterol synthesis as well as cholesterol uptake, but induced expression of molecules implicated in RCT including ABCA1, ABCG1, and ApoE (Zhao and Dahlman-Wright, 2010; Soffientini and Graham, 2016; see **Figure 3**). Although oxysterols are generally perceived as endogenous agonists of LXR, some can act as antagonists (Mutemberezi et al., 2016). Due to their role in lipid metabolism, LXRs are considered as relevant drug targets. The synthetic ligands T0901317 and GW3965 are important tools in biomedical research. Unfortunately, they have poor LXR subtype selectivity and T0901317 is not only an LXR ligand, but also displays agonistic effects on farnesoid X receptor and pregnane X receptor (Zhao and Dahlman-Wright, 2010).

LXR-α and LXR-β as well as RXR can be detected throughout gestation, with increased expression of LXRs in preterm and term placentas (Marceau et al., 2005; Plosch et al., 2010). Preeclampsia or GDM were found to influence expression of LXRs in some (Weedon-Fekjaer et al., 2010b), but not all studies (Plosch et al., 2010).

LXR controls expression of ABCA1 and ABCG1 in cultured trophoblasts (Aye et al., 2010) and HPECs (Stefulj et al., 2009; Sun et al., 2018). Oxysterols or T0901317 increase cholesterol efflux, while LXR-inhibitors or siRNA-mediated LXR knock down decrease cholesterol efflux. As key regulators of the lipid metabolism, LXRs also play a regulatory role in fatty acid metabolism in trophoblast cells (Weedon-Fekjaer et al., 2010a).

Recently, upregulation of ABCA1 and ABCG1 in HPECs derived from GDM placentas compared to control placentas was shown. Upregulation was the consequence of GDM-induced increased ROS-formation, increased ROS-derived oxysterol levels and subsequent LXR activation. The resulting enhanced cholesterol efflux protected the cells from cholesterol overload due to GDM-induced increased cholesterol biosynthesis. Thus, the LXR-mediated upregulation of ABC-transporters in GDM appeared to restore cholesterol homeostasis (Sun et al., 2018). Alterations of expression levels of ABCA1 and ABCG1 in total placental tissue in case of pregnancy diseases such as GDM, preeclampsia, hypoxia, or antiphospholipid-syndrome were reported, but the results are partly inconsistent (Albrecht et al., 2007; Plosch et al., 2007, 2010; Korner et al., 2012; Baumann et al., 2013; Chigusa et al., 2013; Dube et al., 2013; Liu et al., 2014; Huang et al., 2018).

ABCA1 and ABCG1 also efflux oxysterols (Stefulj et al., 2009; Aye et al., 2010; Sun et al., 2018). In cultured trophoblasts, both transporters were shown to prevent accumulation of the oxysterols 25-hydroxycholesterol (25-OHC) and 7-ketocholesterol (**Figures 2C,E**), which exhibit cytotoxic potential at higher concentrations (Aye et al., 2010). ABCA1 expression increases during trophoblast syncytialization *in vitro* (Keelan et al., 2011). ABCA1 localization at the apical STB membrane *in situ* (**Figure 4**) may ensure efflux and thus placental elimination of oxysterols into maternal blood.

Oxysterols and Pregnancy

Many different oxysterols have been identified; they are formed by either free radical oxidation or by enzyme-mediated mechanisms (Mutemberezi et al., 2016). Oxysterols exhibit multifaceted functions. Some oxysterols are important regulators of cholesterol homeostasis (**Figures 3, 4**). 27-OHC (**Figure 2D**), produced from cholesterol by the enzyme CYP27A1, is the most prominent oxysterol in the bloodstream of human adults (Bjorkhem, 2002). *In vitro*, 27-OHC inhibits cholesterol synthesis by negative feedback regulation of HMGR. 27-OHC is an agonist of LXR stimulating cholesterol efflux from cells. Increased CYP27A1 and/or 27-OHC levels might reflect the attempt to remove excess cholesterol from cells and to limit lipid peroxidation. Some studies show that diseases of pregnancy such as preeclampsia are associated with altered expression of placental CYP27A1 protein and altered levels of 27-OHC in placenta, maternal, and/or fetal serum. But these studies are partly contradictory and the mechanism behind the alteration and the impact of these changes on placental cholesterol metabolism remains to be determined (Moon et al., 2014; Mistry et al., 2017; Winkler et al., 2017).

Oxysterols are major components of oxLDL. They contribute to the pathophysiology of atherosclerosis, and are found at increased levels in atherosclerotic lesions (Vejux et al., 2008; Levitan et al., 2010). OxLDL serum levels rise even during normal gestation (Belo et al., 2004; Makedou et al., 2011). Elevated levels of oxLDL and oxysterols have been identified in maternal serum in preeclampsia, pregnancy-induced hypertension, GDM, and diabetes mellitus type I as well as in the cord blood of neonates with IUGR or GDM (Bodzek et al., 2002a,b; Uzun et al., 2005; Qiu et al., 2006; Kim et al., 2007; Leduc et al., 2011; Moon et al., 2014; Sun et al., 2018). Overall, the cytotoxic and pro-inflammatory activities of oxysterols contribute to the development of many diseases associated with oxidative stress (Vejux et al., 2008; Zarrouk et al., 2014).

Oxysterols can influence various aspects of trophoblast function. The oxysterols 25-OHC and 7-keto-cholesterol (**Figures 2C,E**), which are present in oxLDLs, reduce trophoblast invasion via activation of LXR (Pavan et al., 2004; Fournier et al., 2008). Moreover, 25-OHC inhibits syncytialization of CTB (Aye et al., 2011). Oxysterols increase the release of soluble endoglin, a molecule present at elevated concentrations in the maternal circulation in women with preeclampsia, via increased expression of matrix metalloproteinase 14 in the placenta (Valbuena-Diez et al., 2012; Brownfoot et al., 2014). Oxysterols promote the production of pro-inflammatory cytokines in placental trophoblasts, via activation of TLR 4 thus providing a mechanistic link between oxidative stress in pregnancy and placental inflammation. This pro-inflammatory action of oxysterols predominated over simultaneously observed anti-inflammatory effects mediated by oxysterols via LXR activation (Aye et al., 2012). It has been speculated that LXR activation indirectly supports the repression of TLR target genes activation. LXR activation results in increased placental expression of ABCA1 and ABCG1 (Stefulj et al., 2009; Aye et al., 2010; Sun et al., 2018). This may change cellular oxysterol levels as well as alter the cholesterol content of the membrane microdomains required for TLR signaling by promoting cholesterol efflux.

The dual (pro-inflammatory/anti-inflammatory) role of oxysterols observed in trophoblast cells (Aye et al., 2012) already indicates the complexity associated with these molecules. In addition, a study by Larkin et al. (2014) revealed that the effects of oxysterols on trophoblasts are concentration dependent. 25-OHC applied at higher (100 μM) concentrations was found to be cytotoxic, to inhibit differentiation as well as progesterone secretion of trophoblast cells. In contrast, low (10 μM) concentrations stimulated differentiation, progesterone secretion and ABCA1 expression, and reduced SRBP2, LDLR and HMGR expression (Larkin et al., 2014). To add to the complexity, not all of these cellular effects are mediated via LXR (Larkin et al., 2014). Oxysterols are known to interact with many proteins. RORα and RORγ are other nuclear receptors binding oxysterols. RORs are transcription activators and RORγ was shown to regulate hepatic lipid metabolism. Loss of RORγ reduces the expression of a number of lipid metabolic genes, which in turn reduces the levels of triglycerides, cholesterol, and bile acids in liver and blood. 25-OHC is an agonist of RORγ, while other oxysterols may function as inverse agonists (Mutemberezi et al., 2016; Jetten et al., 2018). Oxysterols including 25-OHC are able to bind INSIGs, which induces interaction of INSIGs and SCAP and consequently inhibits SREBP activation. 25-OHC can regulate cholesterol synthesis by interaction with NPC1 and 2. Finally, 25-OHC can bind to OSBP and ORPs and modify their function (**Figure 3**). ORP8 can modulate ABCA1 expression and thereby influence cholesterol efflux (Mutemberezi et al., 2016).

To conclude, oxysterols can compromise placental formation, regeneration, and function, but also are important regulators of placental cholesterol metabolism and probably other physiological processes. Their effect may depend on the identity and concentration of the local oxysterol compound and the available intracellular binding partners. ABCA1 and ABCG1 were shown to prevent the toxic effects of oxysterols on placental and fetal development and function, and reduce the risks associated with diseases of pregnancy such as GDM. But altered regulation of these receptors or oxysterol binding partners in the case of pregnancy-associated diseases in combination with increased levels of oxysterols might (further) compromise placental function.

Our knowledge of function and regulation of oxysterols in the context of pregnancy and regulation of cholesterol metabolism remains limited. We need to explore the types of oxysterols induced during healthy and diseased pregnancy, and learn whether they are generated mainly by enzymes or by autoxidation. It remains to be determined whether they act primarily early (around implantation) or late in pregnancy. Published data are often contradictory. This might be related to problems associated with reliable measurements of oxysterols that are quite susceptible to autoxidation and the fact that oxysterol production is influenced by several factors including cell type, mode of experimentation or circadian variations (Schroepfer, 2000; Mutemberezi et al., 2016).

STEROID HORMONES

Steroid hormones comprise sex steroids and corticosteroids. In adults, the sex steroids – progestagens, estrogens, and androgens – are produced in ovaries and testes, while the corticosteroids – glucocorticoids and mineralocorticoids – are released from the adrenal cortex (Miller and Auchus, 2011; Miller, 2017). During pregnancy, the placental STB becomes a major source of progesterone (at term around 250 mg/day) and estrogens (at term around 100–120 mg/day). Fetal organs (adrenal cortex and liver), in contrast, synthesize corticosteroids and the androgens DHEA, DHEA-S, 16α-hydroxy-DHEA, and 16α-hydroxy-DHEA-S (Evain-Brion and Malassine, 2003; Costa, 2016; Pasqualini and Chetrite, 2016). These hormones are transfered between placental and fetal compartment and are subjected to transformation. Partly, fetus and placenta have complementary enzyme activities and thus are interdependent. Moreover, the hormones also reach the maternal compartment. For more information about steroid hormone exchange between fetus, placenta and mother the reader is referred to Pasqualini and Chetrite (2016). Proper function and interaction of the steroid producing tissues and the involved enzymes and transporters is crucial since the intrauterine exposure of the offspring to abnormal levels of glucocorticoids (Miranda and Sousa, 2018) or sex steroids (Cardoso et al., 2015; Pluchino et al., 2016) can negatively impact fetal development. Furthermore, abnormal concentrations of steroid hormones during pregnancy can increase the maternal risk for malignant diseases (Schock et al., 2014). The following chapters summarize the mechanisms of uptake, synthesis, and transformation of steroid hormones at the human placental barrier and highlight circumstances that cause alterations.

Steroid hormones are derived from cholesterol and thus have closely related structures based on the common steroid skeleton (**Figure 2A**). The major classes of enzymes required for the production of steroid hormones are the CYP heme-containing proteins (P450 and CYPs) and the HSDs. CYPs important for steroid hormone synthesis are CYP11A1, which is a mitochondrial protein, as well as CYP17A1, CYP19A1, and CYP21A2, all located in the ER. CYPs catalyze the hydroxylation and cleavage of steroid substrates, while reduction and oxidation of steroid hormones are effected by isoforms of 3βHSDs and 17βHSDs. Cell-type specific, HSDs localize to the membranes of either mitochondria or ER (Payne and Hales, 2004; Miller and Auchus, 2011). The major placental transporter families are SLCs and the ABC-transporters. SLCOs usually mediate influx of their substrates. They participate in uptake of hydrophilic or charged molecules such as sulfated steroids. In contrast, ABC-transporters mediate the efflux of substrates (Joshi et al., 2016; Walker et al., 2017).

Sex Steroids and the Placenta

Progesterone

Progesterone (P4) is the major and most relevant progestagen. In humans, the ovarian corpus luteum secretes progesterone until week 8 of gestation, thereafter, the placenta completely takes over the production (Malassine et al., 2003).

Progesterone exerts many functions. Briefly, it is an intermediate in the production of other steroid hormones (**Figures 5, 6**) and a neurosteroid involved in brain function. Progesterone is crucial for a successful pregnancy as it supports blastocyst implantation, maintains pregnancy, and prepares the mammary glands for lactation (Miller and Auchus, 2011; Halasz and Szekeres-Bartho, 2013; Costa, 2016; Di Renzo et al., 2016). Progesterone and synthetic progestins are successfully used for the prevention of preterm birth and for treatment of various gynecological disorders (Di Renzo et al., 2012, 2016).

The action of progesterone on target tissues is mediated by two progesterone receptor isoforms (A and B) that function as ligand-activated transcription factors. Under physiological conditions, the withdrawal of progesterone receptor-mediated signaling triggers menstruation and parturition (Wetendorf and DeMayo, 2012, 2014; Patel et al., 2015). Likewise, pathologic deregulation of the progesterone-receptor signaling pathway is associated with preterm delivery (Patel et al., 2015; Tiwari et al., 2016). For example, poor pregnancy outcome due to hepatitis E virus infection is related to low expression of functional progesterone receptors and high expression of receptor haplotypes exhibiting reduced response to progesterone (Romano et al., 2007; Bose et al., 2011).

Physiology and Pathophysiology of Progesterone Synthesis

Synthesis of progesterone starts within mitochondria (**Figures 4, 6**). Cholesterol has to be loaded into the outer mitochondrial membrane in a process that is not entirely understood (Miller and Auchus, 2011; Miller, 2017). In most steroidogenic tissues, the transport of cholesterol from the outer to the inner mitochondrial membrane is mediated by StAR, which can be acutely stimulated by tissue-specific trophic hormones (Miller, 2013); however, StAR is not expressed in human placenta (Sugawara et al., 1995). Instead, StAR-like protein, STARD3 (or MLN64) (Bose et al., 2000; Tuckey et al., 2004) as well as HSP60 are involved in mitochondrial cholesterol import in the placenta (Tuckey, 2005; Olvera-Sanchez et al., 2011; Esparza-Perusquia et al., 2015; Monreal-Flores et al., 2017). In JEG-3 cells, HSP60 additionally participates in delivery of cholesterol to the metabolizing enzyme CYP11A1 (Monreal-Flores et al., 2017). STARD3 action requires a complex multicomponent molecular machine on the outer mitochondrial membrane, which includes, among other factors, the translocator protein TSPO. In obese women (BMI 38.8 ± 6.4 kg/m^2), who exhibit altered insulin sensitivity and leptin level, the serum levels of progesterone as well as estradiol were significantly reduced. While expression of key enzymes of placental progesterone and estrogen synthesis (CYP11A1, 3β-HSD1, and 17β-HSD1) was not altered, the expression levels of TSPO as well as the cholesterol content in placental mitochondria were decreased. *In vitro*, long chain fatty acids and LPS could reduce TSPO expression (Lassance et al., 2015).

After mitochondrial import, cholesterol is hydroxylated at two positions (C-20 and C-22) and the cholesterol side chain is cleaved off by P450 side-chain cleaving enzyme (P450scc or CYP11A1; **Figures 5, 6**; Hochberg et al., 1974; Slominski et al., 2015b). CYP11A1 is a rate-limiting enzyme of steroidogenesis and converts cholesterol to pregnenolone, the precursor of all other steroid hormones (Hanukoglu, 1992; Miller and Auchus, 2011; Miller, 2013). Moreover, CYP11A1 is also a metabolizing enzyme for other sterols. It mediates conversion of 7-DHC to 7-dehydropregnenolone and hydroxylates the side chain of vitamin D (Slominski et al., 2005, 2006, 2009, 2012, 2015a,b).

CYP11A1 localizes exclusively to the STB (Li et al., 2005; He et al., 2013). The placental CYP11A1 protein expression level remain constant from first to term trimester (Henderson et al., 2008; He et al., 2013). The major regulatory factor for *CYP11A1* gene expression in other steroidogenic tissues, SF-1, is absent in the human placenta. Instead, human placental *CYP11A1* gene expression is tightly regulated by one activator (LBP-1b) and two repressor proteins (LBP-9 and LBP-32). In analogy to CYP11A1, these proteins are expressed already very early in pregnancy and localize to the STB (Henderson et al., 2008).

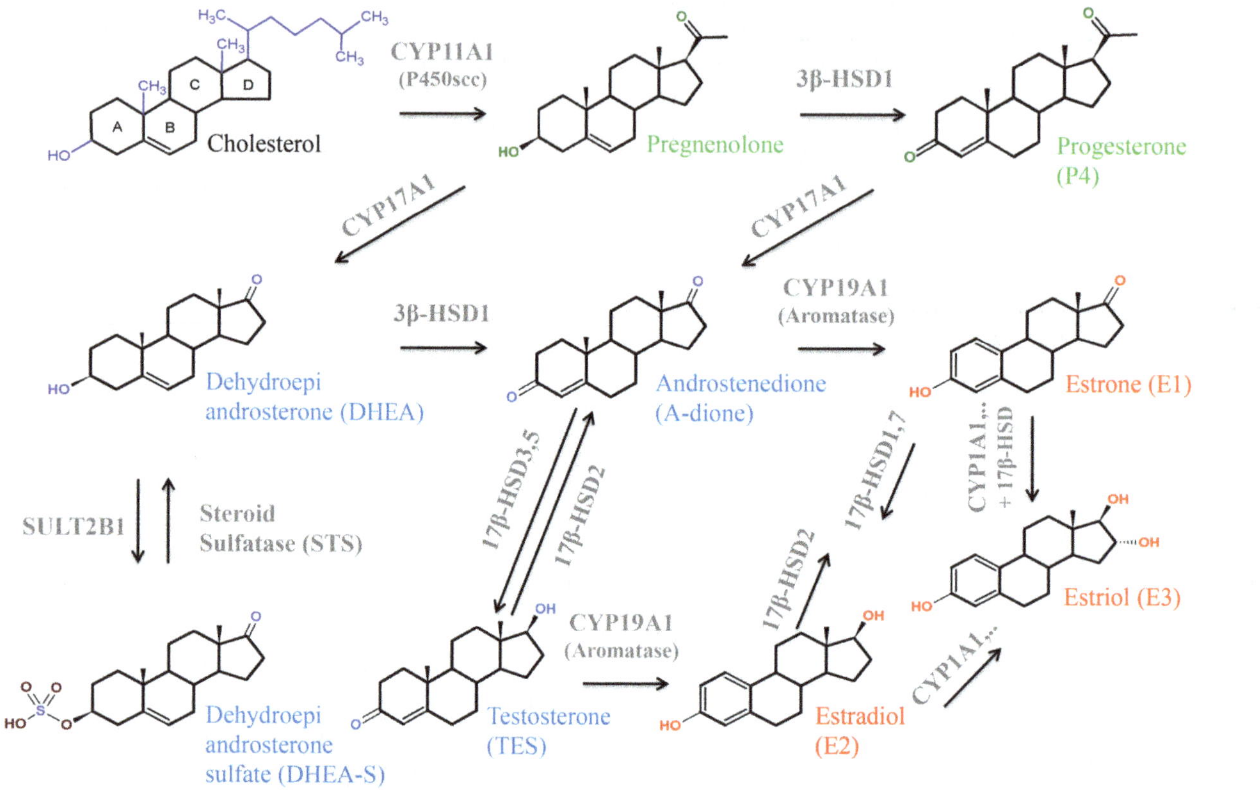

FIGURE 5 | Structures and interconversion of the sex-steroids progestagens (green), estrogens (red), and androgens (blue) starting from cholesterol. For detailed information, see text. Arrows indicate metabolizing processes by respective enzymes (gray). CYPs, cytochrome P-450 enzymes; HSD, hydroxysteroid dehydrogenase; SULT, sulfotransferase.

CYP11A1 is upregulated at both mRNA and protein level in placentas of women with severe preeclampsia. Overexpression of CYP11A1 reduces trophoblastic cell proliferation and induces apoptosis in the HTR8/SVneo extravillous trophoblast cell line through activation of caspase-3 expression (Enquobahrie et al., 2008; He et al., 2013). In line with increased expression of CYP11A1 during preeclampsia, the level of pregnenolone (and progesterone) is increased in preeclamptic women (Moon et al., 2014). CYP11A1 is also involved in lipid peroxidation. Based on results obtained in isolated placental mitochondria and JEG-3 cells, it has been speculated that not only excess progesterone synthesis but also production of lipid peroxides by increased expression of placental CYP11A1 may contribute to the pathogenesis of preeclampsia (Zabul et al., 2015).

In contrast, life style factors like smoking or cocaine may inhibit progesterone synthesis. Cadmium, which is found in cigarette smoke, reduces CYP11A1 mRNA expression as well as progesterone synthesis in human cultured trophoblasts (Kawai et al., 2002). A study in pregnant rats treated with cocaine demonstrated significantly reduced maternal serum levels of pregnenolone and progesterone as well as reduced mRNA and protein expression of CYP11A1 and STARD3 (Wu et al., 2012).

Pregnenolone is converted to progesterone by 3β-HSD1 in the ER (**Figures 5, 6**; Miller and Auchus, 2011; Liu et al., 2016). 3β-HSD1 is exclusively expressed in the placental STB (Ian Mason, 1993; Li et al., 2005), while 3β-HSD2 is predominantly expressed in the adrenal gland and gonads (Labrie et al., 1992; Ian Mason, 1993). Besides pregnenolone, human 3β-HSD1 can also use 17α-hydroxypregnenolone and DHEA as substrates (Hanukoglu, 1992). Various endogenous hormones including estradiol, insulin, insulin-like growth factor, calcitriol, leptin, and CRH can modulate progesterone synthesis (Costa, 2016). Unfortunately, also environmental toxins influence activity of 3β-HSD1 and thus progesterone synthesis. Evidence for this was obtained in the choriocarcinoma cell line JEG-3. Fine PM (<2.5 μm, PM2.5) is a leading air pollutant and exposure to PM2.5 during the prenatal period increases the risk of adverse pregnancy outcome. Exposure of cells to PM2.5 causes reduced progesterone secretion as well as reduced expression of 3β-HSD1 and CYP11A1 mRNA and protein (Wang et al., 2017). The fungicide tributyltin lowers progesterone production and acts as a moderate inhibitor of 3β-HSD1 (Cao et al., 2017). Likewise, the insecticides methoxychlor and its metabolite hydroxychloroquine inhibit progesterone as well as estradiol production; these substances are potent 3β-HSD1 inhibitors (Liu et al., 2016). In contrast, ochratoxin A, a common food-borne mycotoxin, induces the expression of 3β-HSD1, leading to a significant increase of progesterone production (Woo et al., 2013).

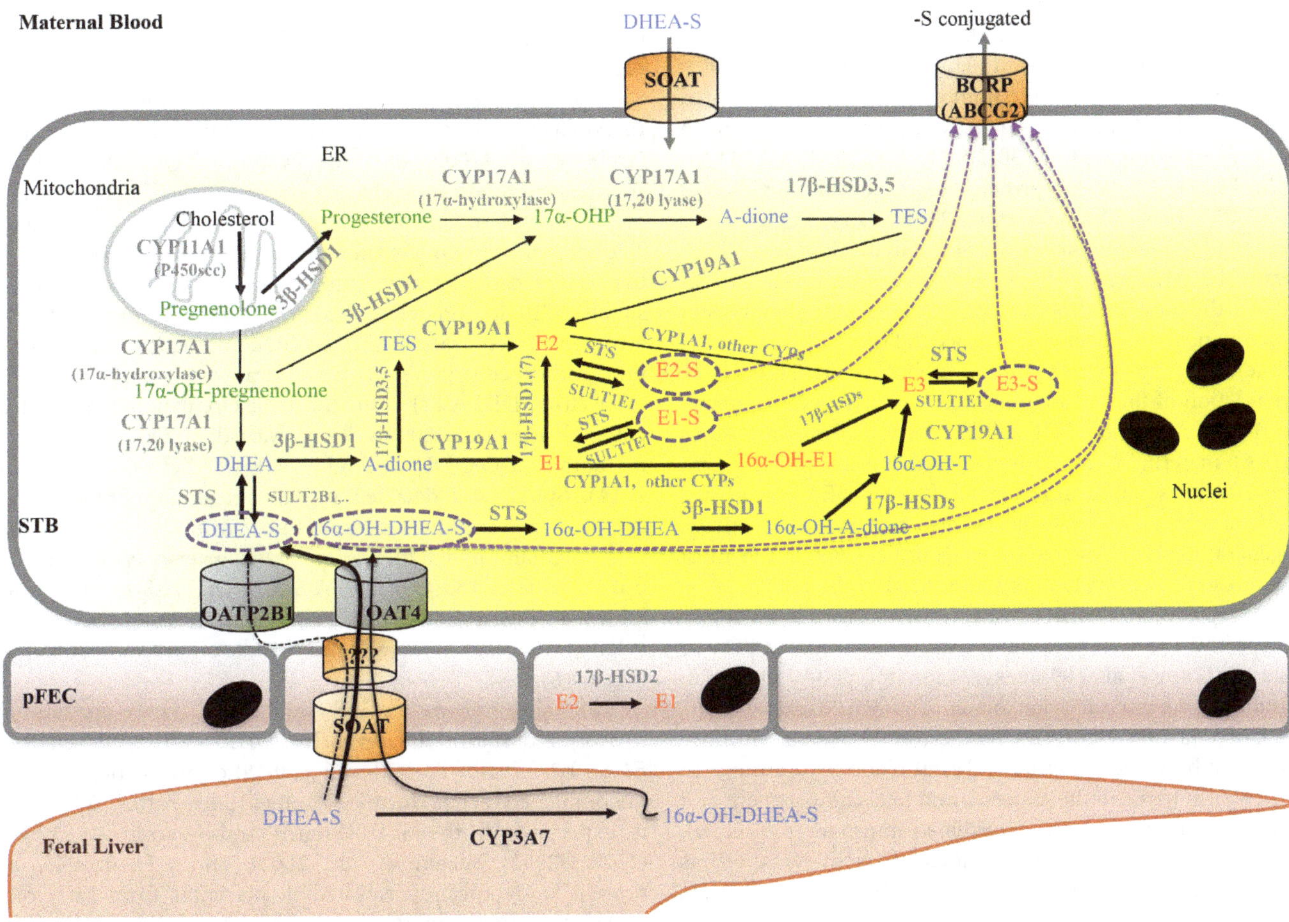

FIGURE 6 | Proposed model for placental progesterone and estrogen synthesis. For detailed description, see text. Progestagens are shown in green, estrogens in red, and androgens in blue color. Solid arrows indicate enzymatic steps that have been demonstrated in human placenta; respective enzymes are shown in gray. Dashed arrows indicate hypothetic routes of transport of sulfate-conjugated compounds. Dashed purple circles highlight sulfate-conjugated compounds that require transporters for uptake into (SOAT, OAT4, and OATP2B1) and export (ABCG2) from cells. A-dione, androstenedione; ABC transporters, ATP-binding cassette transporters; BCRP, breast cancer resistance protein; DHEA, dehydroepiandrosterone; DHEA-S, dehydroepiandrosterone sulfate; CYPs, cytochrome P-450 enzymes; E1, estrone; E1-S, estrone sulfate; E2, Estradiol; E2-S, estradiol sulfate; E3, estriol; E3-S, estriol sulfate; ER, endoplasmatic reticulum; pFEC, placental-fetal endothelial cell; -OH-, -Hydroxy-; 17α-OHP, 17α-hydroxyprogesterone; HSD, hydroxysteroid dehydrogenase; OAT4, organic anion transporter 4; OATP2B1, organic anion transporting polypeptide 2B1; SOAT, sodium-dependent organic anion transporter; STS, steroid sulfatase; SULT, sulfotransferase; STB, syncytiotrophoblast; TES, testosterone.

Estrogens

The group of estrogen steroids comprises estrone (E1), estradiol, (E2), estriol (E3), and estetrol (E4). Among these, estradiol is the most abundant estrogen. Estrogen's multiple functions have been summarized on several occasions and include stimulation of utero-placental blood flow, endometrial growth and differentiation, contraction of the myometrium and proliferation of the mammary epithelium (Mesiano, 2001; Costa, 2016). As detailed in the chapter on cholesterol, estrogens also regulate expression of genes required for placental cholesterol supply. They exert their effect via different types of receptors, the nuclear estrogen receptors α and β as well as membrane-associated receptors. The synthesis of estrogens is controlled by diverse endogenous hormones such as estradiol, cortisol, calcitriol, CRH, hCG, insulin, and leptin (Costa, 2016).

Physiology and Pathophysiology of Estrogen Synthesis

Synthesis of estrogens involves several enzymes and transporters (**Figures 5, 6**). CYP17A1 (or P450c17) is a bifunctional enzyme with 17α-hydroxylase and 17,20-lyase activities that converts pregnenolone to 17α-hydroxypregnenolone and subsequently to DHEA. Alternatively, progesterone can be converted to 17α-hydroxyprogesterone (17α-OHP) and then to A-dione (Escobar and Carr, 2011; Thomas and Potter, 2013). Early studies in human placentas and choriocarcinoma cell lines could not demonstrate placental CYP17A1 activity or mRNA expression (Siiteri and MacDonald, 1966; Bahn et al., 1981; Voutilainen and Miller, 1986). The concept emerged that the placenta was unable to convert pregnenolone and progesterone to the androgen products. Thus, compulsive import of sulfated fetal C19-androgens, 16α-hydroxylated DHEA-S and DHEA-S, which are further processed into estrogens by placental STS, 3βHSD1, CYP19A1 (aromatase), and 17βHSD isoenzymes, was assumed. However, more recent studies (Pezzi et al., 2003; Escobar et al., 2011; Noyola-Martinez et al., 2017) demonstrated placental CYP17A1 mRNA expression, although at a much lower level as compared to 3β-HSD1, CYP19A1, CYP11A1, and 17β-HSD3. CYP17A1 protein was detected in placental STB and JEG-3 cells (Escobar et al., 2011). 17α-OHP synthesis by CYP17A1 in trophoblasts is regulated by the cAMP/PKA pathway (Escobar and Carr, 2011). The authors estimated that 20–30% of the estrogen produced during pregnancy could result from pregnenolone conversion by placental CYP17A1.

While endogenous production of DHEA in the STB occurs, a large fraction of the sulfo-conjugated C19-estrogen precursors 16α-OH-DHEA-S and DHEA-S is derived from the fetus (**Figure 6**); maternal DHEA-S is also used, but to a minor extent (Kallen, 2004; Pasqualini and Chetrite, 2016). DHEA is produced in the fetal adrenal gland, which is also rich in SULT activity, thus generating DHEA-S. 16α-OH-DHEA-S, that is the most abundant estrogen precursor, is synthesized in the fetal liver by 16α-hydroxylation of DHEA-S via CYP3A7 (Leeder et al., 2005). Fetal hepatic CYP3A7 expression is detected around day 50 to 60 of gestation (Yang et al., 1994); expression of CYP3A7 in human placenta remains unclear (Hakkola et al., 1996; Maezawa et al., 2010). Unconjugated estrogens, synthesized by the placenta, are released into both the maternal and fetal blood by diffusion. In part, they get sulfated in the maternal and fetal compartment and re-enter the placenta by carrier-mediated transport (see below). Moreover, the human placenta exhibits STS activity as well as SULT activities (e.g., SULT1E1 and SULT2B1) (Stanley et al., 2001; Miki et al., 2002; He et al., 2004) and thus can convert unconjugated estrogens (or other substrates) into sulfated forms and *vice versa*, respectively. For more information on the function of sulfated steroid hormones in reproduction, the reader is referred to Geyer et al. (2017).

Uptake of conjugated fetal and maternal steroids requires placental expression of appropriate transport systems (Geyer et al., 2017). The human SLC family 22 member 11 (SLC22A11) also known as OAT4, is predominantly expressed in placenta and kidney (Cha et al., 2000). In placenta, OAT4 was detected at the basal plasma membrane of the STB as well as on the CTB in first- and third-trimester placentas (Ugele et al., 2003; Noguchi et al., 2015; Tomi et al., 2015). Studies using isolated basal membrane fractions of placental STB, primary trophoblasts, JEG-3 cells as well as OAT4-transfected cell lines demonstrated uptake of sulfated steroids, including DHEA-S, 16α-OH-DHEA-S and sulfated estrogens via OAT4 (Cha et al., 2000; Ugele et al., 2008; Schweigmann et al., 2014; Tomi et al., 2015). PKA regulates OAT4-mediated transport of sulfated steroids (Tomi et al., 2014). The SLC OAT family member 2B1 (SLCO2B1, OATP2B1, and OATP-B) is also expressed at the basal surface of the STB and on the CTB (St-Pierre et al., 2002). However, 16α-OH-DHEA-S is not a substrate of SLCO2B1. SLCO2B1 can transport sulfated estrogens, while conflicting data exist about whether DHEA-S is a substrate of this transporter (Grube et al., 2007; Ugele et al., 2008; Schweigmann et al., 2014). SLCO2B1 activity is regulated by unconjugated steroid hormones (Grube et al., 2006). The BCRP (ABCG2) is found on the apical surface of placental STB (Nakamura et al., 1997). Placental ABCG2 appears regulated by several endogenous factors (including hormones) as well as exogenous factors (Hahnova-Cygalova et al., 2011). In ABCG2/OATP2B1-overexpressing epithelial MDCKII cells, Grube et al. (2007) obtained evidence that OATP2B1 and ABCG2 together mediate basolateral-to-apical directed transport of the steroid sulfates E3-S and DHEA-S (Grube et al., 2007). Thus the current concept for uptake of fetal sulfated steroid is that OAT4 can transport sulfo-conjugated estrogens as well as sulfated C19-steroid precursors for placental *de novo* synthesis of estrogens. In contrast, OATP2B1 (in combination with ABCG2) may rather contribute to the clearance of estrogen sulfates (as well as DHEA-S?) from the fetal circulation (Ugele et al., 2003; Grube et al., 2007). SOAT was identified as transporter for both 16α-OH-DHEA-S and DHEA-S (Schweigmann et al., 2014). SOAT was detected in the apical membrane of STB as well as on pFECs in the third trimester of pregnancy (Schweigmann et al., 2014). This transporter may thus mediate uptake of fetal 16α-OH-DHEA-S and DHEA-S by pFECs and maternal DHEA-S by the STB. A mechanism for exit of sulfated steroids at the abluminal side of pFECs is unknown (**Figure 6**).

STS, also known as aryl sulfatase C is responsible for hydrolysis of steroid sulfates such as DHEA-S, 16α-OH-DHEA-S, E1-S, E2-S, and E3-S, leading to the production of their unconjugated active forms (Thomas and Potter, 2013). STS is expressed in the STB (French and Warren, 1965; Miki et al., 2002; Suzuki et al., 2003) and STS mRNA and protein is significantly elevated in placentas from early onset preeclamptic women (Gratton et al., 2016). In preeclampsia, anti-angiogenic factors such as soluble fms-like tyrosine kinase (sFlt)1 disrupt the maternal endothelium by binding circulating angiogenic factors, which causes the symptomatic second stage of preeclampsia including dysregulated placental perfusion and ischemia (Maynard et al., 2003). Silencing of STS in primary placental trophoblasts resulted in a significant decrease in sFlt1 secretion and a significant reduction in sFlt1 transcription (Gratton et al., 2016). Thus, it was speculated that high STS expression could contribute to preeclampsia via altered sFlt1 regulation (Gratton et al., 2016).

3β-HSD1 catalyzes the conversion of DHEA into A-dione, which is further transformed to estrone by the P450 aromatase (CYP19A1). CYP19A1 could also convert testosterone into estradiol (Hanukoglu, 1992; Thomas and Potter, 2013), but affinity of CYP19A1 for A-dione is much higher (Yoshida and Osawa, 1991). Placental CYP19A1 expression and function are diminished in pregnancies complicated by preeclampsia compared to controls (Perez-Sepulveda et al., 2015). PCOS is a common endocrinal metabolic disorder, affecting approximately 5–10% of women at reproductive age. It is characterized by ovulatory/menstrual irregularity, polycystic ovaries, and hyperandrogenism, including progesterone resistance (Goodarzi et al., 2011; Piltonen et al., 2015). In placental tissue from women with PCOS, reduced activities of CYP19A1 and increased activities of 3β-HSD1 were observed when compared to control women. Moreover, women with PCOS showed higher A-dione and testosterone concentrations compared to normal pregnant women (Maliqueo et al., 2013).

17β-HSDs are also known as 17-ketosteroid reductases. They catalyze the reversible conversion of 17-keto and 17β-hydroxy groups in androgens and estrogens, including A-dione, DHEA, and estradiol. The direction of the reaction depends on the substrate (Hanukoglu, 1992; Thomas and Potter, 2013). 17β-HSD1 predominantly catalyzes the NADPH-promoted stereospecific reduction of estrone to the more active estradiol (Thomas and Potter, 2013; Herman et al., 2016). 17β-HSD2 shows oxidative activity and is capable of catalyzing the conversion of estradiol, testosterone, and dihydrotestosterone to their less-active 17-keto forms, estrone, A-dione, and 5α-androstanedione, respectively (Rantakari et al., 2008). These two enzymes were found to have different locations in the placenta. While 17β-HSD1 was detected in the STB already at week 4 of gestation, 17β-HSD2 was expressed in the pFEC and detected only after week 12 of gestation. 17β-HSD2 was suggested to prevent the excessive passage of active estrogens into the fetal circulation by catalyzing the inactivation of estradiol to estrone within the pFECs (Takeyama et al., 1998; Bonenfant et al., 2000; Drolet et al., 2007). Placental expression of 17β-HSD3, which is involved in testosterone formation, is increased in preeclamptic women (Shao et al., 2017). 17β-HSD5 protein (Phillips et al., 2014) and 17β-HSD7 mRNA (Krazeisen et al., 1999) expression were shown in human placenta.

Estriol is mainly synthesized from 16α-OH-DHEA-S, but, alternatively, can be converted from estrone or estradiol. This requires expression of enzymes with 16α-hydroxylase activity such as CYP1A1 (Duttaroy and Basak, 2015; **Figure 6**).

Overall, in preeclampsia, and specifically early onset preeclampsia, several of the placental enzymes involved in progesterone and estrogen formation and transformation show altered expression. Moreover, the placental expression levels of steroid receptors (estrogen receptor α and β, progesterone receptor) can change in preeclampsia (Park et al., 2018). Whether the alterations are a consequence of preeclampsia or precede the disease is not known. Maternal serum progesterone and estrogen levels are found reduced, while androgen levels are increased in preeclampsia (Ghorashi and Sheikhvatan, 2008; Hertig et al., 2010; Bussen and Bussen, 2011; Sharifzadeh et al., 2012; Acikgoz et al., 2013; Moon et al., 2014; Perez-Sepulveda et al., 2015; Shao et al., 2017; Shin et al., 2018; Wan et al., 2018). But data remain partly conflicting, which might be due to diverging characteristics of the patients selected.

Most of the reports are mainly descriptive without any analysis of mechanisms causing the underlying changes. One exception is a recent study describing a significant up-regulation of microRNA (miR-22) in placentas derived from preeclamptic women (Shao et al., 2017). MicroRNAs (miRNAs) are small non-coding RNAs of about 22 nucleotides in length that play a critical role in post-transcriptional gene regulation (Bartel, 2009). The authors demonstrated significantly increased testosterone and reduced estradiol levels in plasma samples as well as increased placental expression levels of 17β-HSD3 and reduced placental aromatase expression in women with early onset preeclampsia. Furthermore, increased levels of the miR-22 were detected mainly in placental villous and extravillous trophoblasts. JEG-3 cells were then used to explore the mechanism behind the changes. Increasing testosterone concentrations repressed the expression of aromatase and estrogen receptor α and the production of E2. Testosterone caused increased miR-22 expression, which directly inhibited estrogen receptor α expression. The altered estrogen receptor α signaling decreased aromatase expression and estradiol production. Unfortunately, the question how 17β-HSD3 is induced by preeclampsia remains open. 17β-HSD1 also appears dysregulated – albeit significantly reduced – in preeclamptic placentas, most likely due to upregulation of miR-210 and miR-518c, which were confirmed to target 17β-HSD1 (Ishibashi et al., 2012). Dysregulation of miRNAs in preeclamptic placentas has also been reported by Hu et al. (2009) and Zhu et al. (2009).

The adrenocortical carcinoma cell line NCI-H295R is an established cellular model to study adverse effects on steroidogenesis of numerous substances including heavy metals such as cadmium (Knazicka et al., 2015) or industry-derived environmental toxins such as perfluoroalkyl acids (Kang et al., 2016). Various substances have already been found to change steroid production and thus it might be expected that these molecules could also impact placental steroidogenesis. For cadmium, this has already been demonstrated (Kawai et al., 2002), but further functional studies are required. In this context the recently established co-culture models of choriocarcinoma cells (JEG-3 or BeWo) with H295R cells should be considered for future analysis. The H295R/BeWo co-culture model offers the opportunity to evaluate the effects of chemical exposures on androgen and estrogen biosynthesis, as well as on various other aspects of feto–placental communication (Hudon Thibeault et al., 2017; Drwal et al., 2018; Thibeault et al., 2018).

Glucocorticoids and the Placenta

Glucocorticoids or glucocorticosteroids are produced by the adrenal cortex in response to cues such as stress or illness under the control of the HPA-axis. The name glucocorticoid is derived from their ability to promote gluconeogenesis in the liver and their synthesis in the adrenal cortex (Castro et al., 2011). The natural human glucocorticoid is cortisol (**Figure 7**). In the adult, these signals stimulate the hypothalamus to release CRH, which in turn cause the release of ACTH from the anterior pituitary. ACTH induces synthesis of glucocorticoids from cholesterol in the adrenal glands, which exerts a negative feedback on the release of CRH and ACTH (**Figure 8**).

Glucocorticoids coordinate many functions such as inflammatory and immune responses, metabolic homeostasis, cognitive function, reproduction, and development. At the cellular level, glucocorticoids exert their effects by binding to the GR that is almost ubiquitously expressed and induces target gene transcription. The classical model of GR transactivation involves GR dimerization and binding at glucocorticoid response elements (GREs) leading to co-activator recruitment and activation of transcription from proximate promoters (Pavek and Smutny, 2014; Whirledge and DeFranco, 2018). GR is

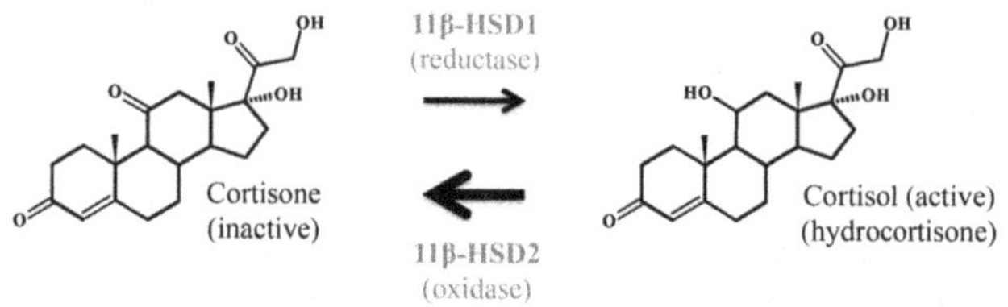

FIGURE 7 | Interconversion of cortisol and the inactive metabolite cortisone by 11β-hydroxysteroid dehydrogenases type 1 and 2. 11β-HSD1 exerts mainly reductase activity *in vivo*, while 11β-HSD2 metabolizes the conversion of cortisol to cortisone. In human placenta, conversion from cortisol to cortisone predominates at all gestational ages, but increasing conversion of cortisone to cortisol in homogenized human placental tissue toward term indicates a predominant reductase activity of 11β-HSD1.

expressed in STB and CTB as well as in JEG-3 and BeWo cell lines (Pavek and Smutny, 2014). Cortisol stimulates productions of placental hormones such as CRH and hCG (Robinson et al., 1988; Ni et al., 2009). Increased cortisol levels in the placenta are linked to the induction of estrogen synthesis, which precedes the onset of parturition in human. Induction of CYP19A1 in trophoblast cultures in response to cortisol was shown to occur via activation of the cAMP/PKA pathway by CRH and hCG and the subsequent induction of transcription factor Sp1 (Wang et al., 2012, 2014; **Figure 8**).

Placental CRH Synthesis and Function

CRH is the major mediator of adaptive response to stressors and is synthesized by several organs (Koutmani et al., 2013; Slominski et al., 2013). During pregnancy, the CRH concentration in maternal plasma increases substantially and reaches levels that are 1,000–10,000 times that of non-pregnant women. The major CRH source during pregnancy is the placenta that can also produce ACTH (Bicknell, 2008; Gangestad et al., 2012; Thomson, 2013). CRH is synthesized in the STB from first to third trimester (Riley et al., 1991; Warren and Silverman, 1995). In humans and great apes CRH levels rise exponentially throughout pregnancy to peak at labor. Rodents, in contrast, do not exhibit placental CRH production (Heussner et al., 2016). Placental CRH production may have evolved in primates to stimulate fetal ACTH release and adrenal steroidogenesis, in order to guarantee sufficient synthesis of DHEA, a precursor for placental sex hormone synthesis. Concomitant stimulation of fetal cortisol and DHEA by placental CRH would couple the glucocorticoid effects on fetal organ maturation with the timing of parturition. While glucocorticoids inhibit hypothalamic CRH synthesis and secretion (Frim et al., 1990), they paradoxically stimulate placental CRH expression (Robinson et al., 1988; Jones et al., 1989; Wang et al., 2014).

CRH operates via activation of two receptors, CRH-receptor type 1 and type 2 (Grammatopoulos and Ourailidou, 2017), which are expressed in the human placenta (Florio et al., 2000). Placental CRH exhibits many functions in pregnancy and parturition. To name a few, CRH modulates placental glucose transporter expression (Gao et al., 2012) and stimulates estradiol production by induction of STS, CYP19A1, and 17β-HSD1 expression in trophoblasts (You et al., 2006). CRH impacts on the expression levels of several other placental hormones including ACTH (Challis et al., 1995) and prostaglandin (Gao et al., 2008). Progesterone is an inhibitor of CRH production (Karalis et al., 1996; Ni et al., 2004; Sfakianaki and Norwitz, 2006) and also a competitive antagonist of cortisol binding to GR (Majzoub and Karalis, 1999). On the other hand, CRH inhibits progesterone production by suppression of CYP11A1 and 3β-HSD1 (Jeschke et al., 2005; Yang et al., 2006). CRH is involved in the timing of birth by regulation of estrogen and progesterone levels as they control the contractile properties of the myometrium (Majzoub and Karalis, 1999; Gangestad et al., 2012; Thomson, 2013).

Placental Cortisol Metabolism and Transport in Health and Disease

Glucocorticoids are important during pregnancy and for fetal development. Fetal glucocorticoid synthesis is only partially influenced by the HPA axis, but instead is primarily regulated by differential expression of the enzymes required for glucocorticoid synthesis. Moreover, maternal glucocorticoids can potentially cross the placenta. To enable pregnancy and ensure proper fetal development, glucocorticoid signaling occurs during three period of gestation: early in pregnancy to enable implantation, between week 7 and 14 to enable fetal-adrenal development, repress DHEA synthesis and enable female genital development and finally during the third trimester. Fetal serum glucocorticoid levels must increase significantly before birth in order to ensure proper development of the lungs and several other organs (Busada and Cidlowski, 2017). On the other hand, the fetus should not be exposed to excessive levels of glucocorticoids; this can suppress fetal growth and program the fetus for life-long diseases such as hypertension, glucose intolerance, diabetes, and strokes (Moisiadis and Matthews, 2014a,b; Konstantakou et al., 2017).

In the adrenal gland, cortisol synthesis is initiated by 21-hydroxylase (CYP21A2) (Hanukoglu, 1992). CYP21A2 converts progesterone as well as 17α-OH-progesterone, through a hydroxylation at position C21, into 11-deoxycorticosterone and 11-deoxycortisol, respectively. After catalyzation by CYP21A2, 11β-hydroxylase (CYP11B1), and 11β-HSD are the key molecules mediating and regulating tissue-specific glucocorticoid actions. CYP11B1 catalyzes 11-deoxycorticosterone and 11-deoxycortisol to corticosterone and cortisol, respectively. There has been no evidence so far of CYP21A2 or CYP11B1 expression in human placenta. However, 11β-HSD type 1 and 2 isozymes are expressed in the placenta and the fetal membranes (Heussner et al., 2016; Yang et al., 2016; Konstantakou et al., 2017). 11β-HSD2 is an oxidase converting cortisol to the inactive 11-keto metabolite, cortisone. 11β-HSD1, in contrast, preferentially acts as a reductase *in vivo*, mediating the NADPH-dependent conversion of cortisone to cortisol (**Figure 7**). In line with this, Giannopoulos et al. (1982) reported increasing conversion of cortisone to cortisol in homogenized human placental tissue toward term, although conversion from cortisol to inactive cortisone predominated at all gestational ages.

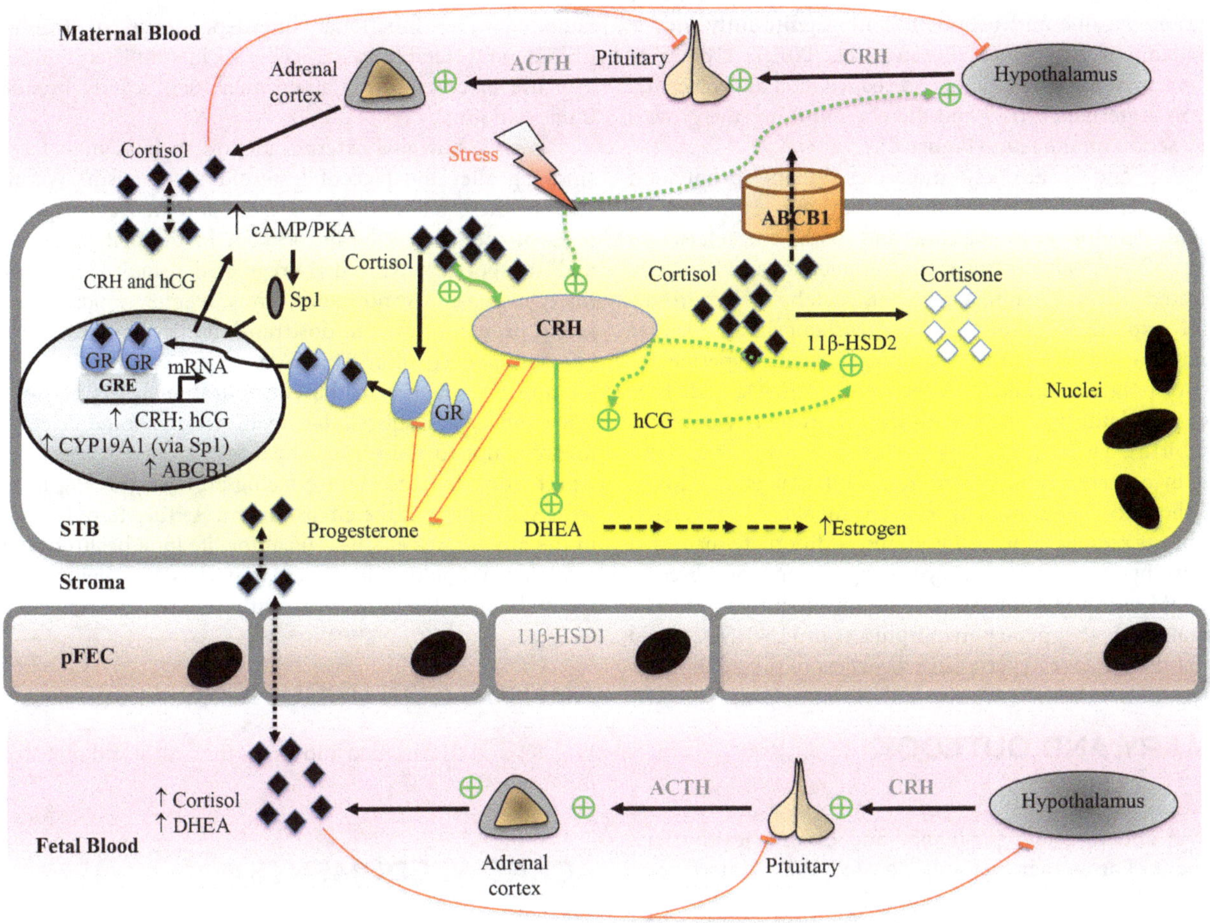

FIGURE 8 | Proposed model for placental glucocorticoid (cortisol) function and metabolism. For detailed description, see text. Cortisol can diffuse across cell membranes and regulate target protein expression directly via glucocorticoid receptor (GR) or indirectly via other transcription factors (e.g., Sp1). Placental corticotropin-releasing hormone (CRH) is the major mediator of adaptive response to stressors during pregnancy. Cortisol stimulates placental CRH expression, which regulates placental hormone levels (e.g., hCG, estrogen, progesterone, and 11β-HSD2). Red arrows indicate inhibiting/negative feedback pathways, while green arrows indicate stimulating pathways. ABC transporters, ATP-binding cassette transporters; ACTH, adrenocorticotropic hormone; CRH, corticotropin-releasing hormone; DHEA, dehydroepiandrosterone; GRE, glucocorticoid response element; HSD, hydroxysteroid dehydrogenase; hCG, human chorionic gonadotropin; pFEC, placental-fetal endothelial cell; PKA, protein kinase A; Sp1, specificity protein 1 transcription factor; STB, syncytiotrophoblast.

Cortisol is required during early pregnancy for the establishment of gestation (Michael and Papageorghiou, 2008). 11β-HSD1 and GR are localized widely in the decidual stroma and epithelium, while the distribution of 11β-HSD2 is mainly confined to the decidual epithelium and scarcely observed in the decidual stroma. Furthermore, 11β-HSD1 is localized only in the fetal blood vessels in the interstitial core of the villous tissue but not in the extravillous trophoblast, CTB and STB. 11β-HSD2 expression is mainly restricted to the STB. The distribution pattern of 11β-HSD1 suggests that higher concentrations of cortisol are required on the maternal side than on the fetal side in early pregnancy (Yang et al., 2016).

Cortisol levels in the maternal circulation rise toward term (Goldkrand et al., 1976). As steroid hormones use free diffusion to enter target cells, maternal cortisol reaches placental cells. Overexposure of the fetus to glucocorticoids during pregnancy reduces birth weight and can be detrimental to fetal development. In the human placenta, 11β-HSD2 acts as a major "barrier" to materno-fetal cortisol transfer as shown in the isolated perfused placenta (Stirrat et al., 2018). 11β-HSD2 is localized abundantly in the STB (Yang et al., 2016) and generates a cortisone-to-cortisol-ratio >1 (Heussner et al., 2016). CRH and cortisol induce the expression of 11β-HSD2 in isolated trophoblasts (van Beek et al., 2004; Fahlbusch et al., 2012). Furthermore, cortisol stimulates hCG production in trophoblasts (Wang et al., 2014) and the upregulation of 11β-HSD2 expression in trophoblasts by cortisol may be mediated in part by hCG (Ni et al., 2009). Nevertheless, the conversion of cortisol is incomplete and a fraction of cortisol remains unmetabolized (Sun et al., 1999). The energy-dependent drug-efflux pump ABCB1 may mediate export of glucocorticoids from cells (Uhr et al., 2002). Studies in BeWo cells suggested that this transporter could contribute to the placental glucocorticoid barrier (Mark and Waddell, 2006). ABCB1 is expressed at the apical surface of the STB (Ni and Mao, 2011). In CTBs, the glucocorticoid drugs dexamethasone and betamethasone, significantly induce the expression of ABCB1 (Manceau et al., 2012). 11β-HSD2 and ABCB1 may thus act together to reduce fetal and placental exposure to maternal cortisol and thereby minimize the growth inhibitory action on the fetus (**Figure 8**).

11β-HSD1 and 2 are key molecules in the production and metabolism of glucocorticoids. Both are expressed in the human decidua and placenta and both are related to a number of pregnancy-associated complications. 11β-HSD1 is implicated in the pathogenesis of metabolic syndrome. 11β-HSD1 expression is altered in preeclampsia as well as IUGR and gene polymorphisms are associated with hypertensive disorders of pregnancy. Likewise, reduced 11β-HSD2 activity is related to preeclampsia, IUGR, and adverse pregnancy outcome (preterm birth). These interesting studies have been extensively reviewed in a recent publication (Konstantakou et al., 2017). Many of the underlying mechanisms causing altered expression of the enzymes remain to be explored, and additionally suspected correlations between altered enzyme expression and diseases such as GDM need to be confirmed. In addition, it remains to be demonstrated whether gene polymorphisms in 11β-HSD2 could serve as biomarkers for hypertensive disorders of pregnancy.

SUMMARY AND OUTLOOK

Cholesterol, progesterone, estrogens, and cortisol are required to establish and maintain pregnancy and ensure healthy fetal development. The human placenta, located at the interface of maternal and fetal circulation, has an active role in biosynthesis, metabolism, and transport of these molecules. Many enzymes and transporters are involved in these processes but our knowledge concerning their function and regulation is incomplete. The placental barrier is composed of trophoblast cells and pFECs. Few studies have addressed the role of pFECs in placental steroid handling. The functional interdependence of trophoblasts, pFECs, and fetal adrenal cells is incompletely understood. The use of co-culture systems may significantly broaden our understanding.

Diseases, but also external factors such as high fat diet or smoking alter the placental steroid metabolism. We need to explore these alterations and their potential consequences for fetus or mother. It should be kept in mind that the enzymes and transporters involved are regulated at multiple levels and by many endogenous molecules. Thus, whenever possible, mRNA levels, protein levels and posttranslational modifications should be examined (Hudon Thibeault et al., 2018). Likewise, when looking for changes in the concentration levels of steroids or other substances, subcellular fractionation should be considered in order not to miss important details (Lassance et al., 2015). Apart from diseases, we are facing an ever-growing number of toxic substances in the environment. As the steroid metabolism of the human placenta is crucial for life long health of fetus and mother, we should be interested to understand their influence on the function of the human placenta.

AUTHOR CONTRIBUTIONS

WC, KJ, and IE designed and wrote the article and met all criteria for authorship.

ACKNOWLEDGMENTS

We thank Adi Ellinger and Enna Schepelmann for careful reading of the manuscript and we gratefully acknowledge the support of Thomas Nardelli and Adi Ellinger in preparing part of the artwork.

REFERENCES

Acikgoz, S., Bayar, U. O., Can, M., Guven, B., Mungan, G., Dogan, S., et al. (2013). Levels of oxidized LDL, estrogens, and progesterone in placenta tissues and serum paraoxonase activity in preeclampsia. *Mediators Inflamm.* 2013:862982. doi: 10.1155/2013/862982

Albrecht, C., Soumian, S., Tetlow, N., Patel, P., Sullivan, M. H., Lakasing, L., et al. (2007). Placental ABCA1 expression is reduced in primary antiphospholipid syndrome compared to pre-eclampsia and controls. *Placenta* 28, 701–708. doi: 10.1016/j.placenta.2006.10.001

Albrecht, E. D., Babischkin, J. S., Koos, R. D., and Pepe, G. J. (1995). Developmental increase in low density lipoprotein receptor messenger ribonucleic acid levels in placental syncytiotrophoblasts during baboon pregnancy. *Endocrinology* 136, 5540–5546. doi: 10.1210/endo.136.12.7588306

Alsat, E., Bouali, Y., Goldstein, S., Malassine, A., Berthelier, M., Mondon, F., et al. (1984). Low-density lipoprotein binding sites in the microvillous membranes of human placenta at different stages of gestation. *Mol. Cell. Endocrinol.* 38, 197–203. doi: 10.1016/0303-7207(84)90118-7

Alsat, E., Bouali, Y., Goldstein, S., Malassine, A., Laudat, M. H., and Cedard, L. (1982). Characterization of specific low-density lipoprotein binding sites in human term placental microvillous membranes. *Mol. Cell. Endocrinol.* 28, 439–453. doi: 10.1016/0303-7207(82)90138-1

Alsat, E., and Malassine, A. (1991). High density lipoprotein interaction with human placenta: biochemical and ultrastructural characterization of binding to microvillous receptor and lack of internalization. *Mol. Cell. Endocrinol.* 77, 97–108. doi: 10.1016/0303-7207(91)90063-X

Arabin, B., and Baschat, A. A. (2017). Pregnancy: an underutilized window of opportunity to improve long-term maternal and infant health-an appeal for continuous family care and interdisciplinary communication. *Front. Pediatr.* 5:69. doi: 10.3389/fped.2017.00069

Aye, I. L., Singh, A. T., and Keelan, J. A. (2009). Transport of lipids by ABC proteins: interactions and implications for cellular toxicity, viability and function. *Chem. Biol. Interact.* 180, 327–339. doi: 10.1016/j.cbi.2009.04.012

Aye, I. L., Waddell, B. J., Mark, P. J., and Keelan, J. A. (2010). Placental ABCA1 and ABCG1 transporters efflux cholesterol and protect trophoblasts from oxysterol induced toxicity. *Biochim. Biophys. Acta* 1801, 1013–1024. doi: 10.1016/j.bbalip.2010.05.015

Aye, I. L., Waddell, B. J., Mark, P. J., and Keelan, J. A. (2011). Oxysterols inhibit differentiation and fusion of term primary trophoblasts by activating liver X receptors. *Placenta* 32, 183–191. doi: 10.1016/j.placenta.2010.12.007

Aye, I. L., Waddell, B. J., Mark, P. J., and Keelan, J. A. (2012). Oxysterols exert proinflammatory effects in placental trophoblasts via TLR4-dependent, cholesterol-sensitive activation of NF-kappaB. *Mol. Hum. Reprod.* 18, 341–353. doi: 10.1093/molehr/gas001

Baardman, M. E., Erwich, J. J., Berger, R. M., Hofstra, R. M., Kerstjens-Frederikse, W. S., Lutjohann, D., et al. (2012). The origin of fetal sterols in second-trimester amniotic fluid: endogenous synthesis or maternal-fetal transport? *Am. J. Obstet. Gynecol.* 207, 202.e19–225.e19. doi: 10.1016/j.ajog.2012.06.003

Baardman, M. E., Kerstjens-Frederikse, W. S., Berger, R. M. F., Bakker, M. K., Hofstra, R. M. W., and Plosch, T. (2013). The role of maternal-fetal cholesterol transport in early fetal life: current insights. *Biol. Reprod.* 88:24. doi: 10.1095/biolreprod.112.102442

Babischkin, J. S., Grimes, R. W., Pepe, G. J., and Albrecht, E. D. (1997a). Estrogen stimulation of P450 cholesterol side-chain cleavage activity in cultures of human placental syncytiotrophoblasts. *Biol. Reprod.* 56, 272–278. doi: 10.1095/biolreprod56.1.272

Babischkin, J. S., Pepe, G. J., and Albrecht, E. D. (1997b). Estrogen regulation of placental P-450 cholesterol side-chain cleavage enzyme messenger ribonucleic acid levels and activity during baboon pregnancy. *Endocrinology* 138, 452–459. doi: 10.1210/endo.138.1.4833

Bahn, R. S., Worsham, A., Speeg, K. V. Jr., Ascoli, M., and Rabin, D. (1981). Characterization of steroid production in cultured human choriocarcinoma cells. *J. Clin. Endocrinol. Metab.* 52, 447–450. doi: 10.1210/jcem-52-3-447

Baird, D. T., Cockburn, F., Galbraith, A., Kelly, R., and Livingstone, J. R. (1973). Formation of progesterone and pregnenolone from (4- 14 C) cholesterol by the intact mid-term human foeto-placental unit perfused in vitro. *J. Endocrinol.* 56, 187–202. doi: 10.1677/joe.0.0560187

Bansal, N., Cruickshank, J. K., McElduff, P., and Durrington, P. N. (2005). Cord blood lipoproteins and prenatal influences. *Curr. Opin. Lipidol.* 16, 400–408. doi: 10.1097/01.mol.0000174154.61307.16

Barker, D. J., and Thornburg, K. L. (2013). Placental programming of chronic diseases, cancer and lifespan: a review. *Placenta* 34, 841–845. doi: 10.1016/j.placenta.2013.07.063

Bartel, D. P. (2009). MicroRNAs: target recognition and regulatory functions. *Cell* 136, 215–233. doi: 10.1016/j.cell.2009.01.002

Baumann, M., Korner, M., Huang, X., Wenger, F., Surbek, D., and Albrecht, C. (2013). Placental ABCA1 and ABCG1 expression in gestational disease: pre-eclampsia affects ABCA1 levels in syncytiotrophoblasts. *Placenta* 34, 1079–1086. doi: 10.1016/j.placenta.2013.06.309

Belknap, W. M., and Dietschy, J. M. (1988). Sterol synthesis and low density lipoprotein clearance in vivo in the pregnant rat, placenta, and fetus. Sources for tissue cholesterol during fetal development. *J. Clin. Invest.* 82, 2077–2085. doi: 10.1172/jci113829

Belo, L., Caslake, M., Santos-Silva, A., Castro, E. M., Pereira-Leite, L., Quintanilha, A., et al. (2004). LDL size, total antioxidant status and oxidised LDL in normal human pregnancy: a longitudinal study. *Atherosclerosis* 177, 391–399. doi: 10.1016/j.atherosclerosis.2004.07.023

Benirschke, K., Burton, G. G. J., and Baergen, R. N. (2012). *Pathology of the Human Placenta*. ed. K. Benirschke, Heidelberg: Springer. doi: 10.1007/978-3-642-23941-0

Bhattacharjee, J., Ietta, F., Giacomello, E., Bechi, N., Romagnoli, R., Fava, A., et al. (2010). Expression and localization of ATP binding cassette transporter A1 (ABCA1) in first trimester and term human placenta. *Placenta* 31, 423–430. doi: 10.1016/j.placenta.2010.02.015

Bicknell, A. B. (2008). The tissue-specific processing of pro-opiomelanocortin. *J. Neuroendocrinol.* 20, 692–699. doi: 10.1111/j.1365-2826.2008.01709.x

Bilban, M., Tauber, S., Haslinger, P., Pollheimer, J., Saleh, L., Pehamberger, H., et al. (2010). Trophoblast invasion: assessment of cellular models using gene expression signatures. *Placenta* 31, 989–996. doi: 10.1016/j.placenta.2010.08.011

Bjorkhem, I. (2002). Do oxysterols control cholesterol homeostasis? *J. Clin. Invest.* 110, 725–730. doi: 10.1172/jci16388

Blassberg, R., and Jacob, J. (2017). Lipid metabolism fattens up hedgehog signaling. *BMC Biol.* 15:95. doi: 10.1186/s12915-017-0442-y

Bloch, K. (1965). The biological synthesis of cholesterol. *Science* 150, 19–28. doi: 10.1126/science.150.3692.19

Bloise, E., Ortiga-Carvalho, T. M., Reis, F. M., Lye, S. J., Gibb, W., and Matthews, S. G. (2016). ATP-binding cassette transporters in reproduction: a new frontier. *Hum. Reprod. Update* 22, 164–181. doi: 10.1093/humupd/dmv049

Blundell, C., Tess, E. R., Schanzer, A. S., Coutifaris, C., Su, E. J., Parry, S., et al. (2016). A microphysiological model of the human placental barrier. *Lab Chip* 16, 3065–3073. doi: 10.1039/c6lc00259e

Blundell, C., Yi, Y. S., Ma, L., Tess, E. R., Farrell, M. J., Georgescu, A., et al. (2018). Placental drug transport-on-a-chip: a microengineered in vitro model of transporter-mediated drug efflux in the human placental barrier. *Adv. Healthc. Mater.* 7:1700786. doi: 10.1002/adhm.201700786

Bodzek, P., Janoszka, B., Wielkoszynski, T., Bodzek, D., and Sieron, A. (2002a). Concentration of chosen oxycholesterols in plasma of pregnant women with pregnancy-induced hypertension. *Biomed. Chromatogr.* 16, 13–18. doi: 10.1002/bmc.114

Bodzek, P., Olejek, A., and Zamlynski, J. (2002b). [Concentration of the oxygenated derivates of cholesterol in pregnant women suffering from diabetes type I]. *Wiad Lek* 55(Suppl. 1), 50–53.

Boguslawski, W., and Sokolowski, W. (1984). HMG-CoA reductase activity in the microsomal fraction from human placenta in early and term pregnancy. *Int. J. Biochem.* 16, 1023–1026. doi: 10.1016/0020-711X(84)90120-4

Bokslag, A., van Weissenbruch, M., Mol, B. W., and de Groot, C. J. (2016). Preeclampsia; short and long-term consequences for mother and neonate. *Early Hum. Dev.* 102, 47–50. doi: 10.1016/j.earlhumdev.2016.09.007

Bonenfant, M., Provost, P. R., Drolet, R., and Tremblay, Y. (2000). Localization of type 1 17beta-hydroxysteroid dehydrogenase mRNA and protein in syncytiotrophoblasts and invasive cytotrophoblasts in the human term villi. *J. Endocrinol.* 165, 217–222. doi: 10.1677/joe.0.1650217

Bonet, B., Brunzell, J. D., Gown, A. M., and Knopp, R. H. (1992). Metabolism of very-low-density lipoprotein triglyceride by human placental cells: the role of lipoprotein lipase. *Metabolism* 41, 596–603. doi: 10.1016/0026-0495(92)90051-B

Bose, H. S., Whittal, R. M., Huang, M. C., Baldwin, M. A., and Miller, W. L. (2000). N-218 MLN64, a protein with StAR-like steroidogenic activity, is folded and cleaved similarly to StAR. *Biochemistry* 39, 11722–11731. doi: 10.1021/bi000911l

Bose, P. D., Das, B. C., Kumar, A., Gondal, R., Kumar, D., and Kar, P. (2011). High viral load and deregulation of the progesterone receptor signaling pathway: association with hepatitis E-related poor pregnancy outcome. *J. Hepatol.* 54, 1107–1113. doi: 10.1016/j.jhep.2010.08.037

Brett, K. E., Ferraro, Z. M., Yockell-Lelievre, J., Gruslin, A., and Adamo, K. B. (2014). Maternal-fetal nutrient transport in pregnancy pathologies: the role of the placenta. *Int. J. Mol. Sci.* 15, 16153–16185. doi: 10.3390/ijms150916153

Brownfoot, F. C., Hannan, N., Onda, K., Tong, S., and Kaitu'u-Lino, T. (2014). Soluble endoglin production is upregulated by oxysterols but not quenched by pravastatin in primary placental and endothelial cells. *Placenta* 35, 724–731. doi: 10.1016/j.placenta.2014.06.374

Burke, K. A., Jauniaux, E., Burton, G. J., and Cindrova-Davies, T. (2013). Expression and immunolocalisation of the endocytic receptors megalin and cubilin in the human yolk sac and placenta across gestation. *Placenta* 34, 1105–1109. doi: 10.1016/j.placenta.2013.08.003

Burke, K. T., Colvin, P. L., Myatt, L., Graf, G. A., Schroeder, F., and Woollett, L. A. (2009). Transport of maternal cholesterol to the fetus is affected by maternal plasma cholesterol concentrations in the golden Syrian hamster. *J. Lipid Res.* 50, 1146–1155. doi: 10.1194/jlr.M800538-JLR200

Burton, G. J., Charnock-Jones, D. S., and Jauniaux, E. (2009). Regulation of vascular growth and function in the human placenta. *Reproduction* 138, 895–902. doi: 10.1530/rep-09-0092

Burton, G. J., Fowden, A. L., and Thornburg, K. L. (2016). Placental origins of Chronic disease. *Physiol. Rev.* 96, 1509–1565. doi: 10.1152/physrev.00029.2015

Burton, G. J., Hempstock, J., and Jauniaux, E. (2001). Nutrition of the human fetus during the first trimester–a review. *Placenta* 22(Suppl. A), S70–S77. doi: 10.1053/plac.2001.0639

Busada, J. T., and Cidlowski, J. A. (2017). Mechanisms of glucocorticoid action during development. *Curr. Top. Dev. Biol.* 125, 147–170. doi: 10.1016/bs.ctdb.2016.12.004

Bussen, S., and Bussen, D. (2011). Influence of the vascular endothelial growth factor on the development of severe pre-eclampsia or HELLP syndrome. *Arch. Gynecol. Obstet.* 284, 551–557. doi: 10.1007/s00404-010-1704-x

Cao, C., Pressman, E. K., Cooper, E. M., Guillet, R., Westerman, M., and O'Brien, K. O. (2014). Placental heme receptor LRP1 correlates with the heme exporter FLVCR1 and neonatal iron status. *Reproduction* 148, 295–302. doi: 10.1530/rep-14-0053

Cao, G., Garcia, C. K., Wyne, K. L., Schultz, R. A., Parker, K. L., and Hobbs, H. H. (1997). Structure and localization of the human gene encoding SR-BI/CLA-1. Evidence for transcriptional control by steroidogenic factor 1. *J. Biol. Chem.* 272, 33068–33076. doi: 10.1074/jbc.272.52.33068

Cao, S., Ye, L., Wu, Y., Mao, B., Chen, L., Wang, X., et al. (2017). The effects of fungicides on human 3beta-Hydroxysteroid Dehydrogenase 1 and aromatase in human placental cell line JEG-3. *Pharmacology* 100, 139–147. doi: 10.1159/000475531

Cardoso, R. C., Puttabyatappa, M., and Padmanabhan, V. (2015). Steroidogenic versus metabolic programming of reproductive neuroendocrine, ovarian and metabolic dysfunctions. *Neuroendocrinology* 102, 226–237. doi: 10.1159/000381830

Carter, A. M. (2007). Animal models of human placentation–a review. *Placenta* 28(Suppl. A), S41–S47. doi: 10.1016/j.placenta.2006.11.002

Carter, A. M., and Enders, A. C. (2016). Placentation in mammals: definitive placenta, yolk sac, and paraplacenta. *Theriogenology* 86, 278–287. doi: 10.1016/j.theriogenology.2016.04.041

Castro, M., Elias, L. L., Elias, P. C. L., and Moreira, A. C. (2011). "Physiology and pathophysiology of the HPA Axis," in *Cushing's Syndrome: Pathophysiology, Diagnosis and Treatment*, ed. M. D. Bronstein (Totowa, NJ: Humana Press), 1–20.

Catov, J. M., Bodnar, L. M., Kip, K. E., Hubel, C., Ness, R. B., Harger, G., et al. (2007). Early pregnancy lipid concentrations and spontaneous preterm birth. *Am. J. Obstet. Gynecol.* 197,610.e1–617.e1. doi: 10.1016/j.ajog.2007.04.024

Cavender, C. P., Turley, S. D., and Dietschy, J. M. (1995). Sterol metabolism in fetal, newborn, and suckled lambs and their response to cholesterol after weaning. *Am. J. Physiol.* 269, E331–E340. doi: 10.1152/ajpendo.1995.269.2.E331

Cerqueira, N. M., Oliveira, E. F., Gesto, D. S., Santos-Martins, D., Moreira, C., Moorthy, H. N., et al. (2016). Cholesterol biosynthesis: a mechanistic overview. *Biochemistry* 55, 5483–5506. doi: 10.1021/acs.biochem.6b00342

Cha, S. H., Sekine, T., Kusuhara, H., Yu, E., Kim, J. Y., Kim, D. K., et al. (2000). Molecular cloning and characterization of multispecific organic anion transporter 4 expressed in the placenta. *J. Biol. Chem.* 275, 4507–4512. doi: 10.1074/JBC.275.6.4507

Challis, J. R., Matthews, S. G., Van Meir, C., and Ramirez, M. M. (1995). Current topic: the placental corticotrophin-releasing hormone-adrenocorticotrophin axis. *Placenta* 16, 481–502. doi: 10.1016/S0143-4004(05)80001-3

Chigusa, Y., Kondoh, E., Mogami, H., Nishimura, F., Ujita, M., Kawasaki, K., et al. (2013). ATP-binding cassette transporter A1 expression is decreased in preeclamptic placentas. *Reprod. Sci.* 20, 891–898. doi: 10.1177/1933719112468956

Collier, A. C., Miyagi, S. J., Yamauchi, Y., and Ward, M. A. (2009). Assisted reproduction technologies impair placental steroid metabolism. *J. Steroid Biochem. Mol. Biol.* 116, 21–28. doi: 10.1016/j.jsbmb.2009.04.005

Connor, W. E., and Lin, D. S. (1967). Placental transfer of cholesterol-4-14C into rabbit and guinea pig fetus. *J. Lipid Res.* 8, 558–564.

Costa, M. A. (2016). The endocrine function of human placenta: an overview. *Reprod. Biomed. Online* 32, 14–43. doi: 10.1016/j.rbmo.2015.10.005

Coukos, G., Gafvels, M. E., Wittmaack, F., Matsuo, H., Strickland, D. K., Coutifaris, C., et al. (1994). Potential roles for the low-density-lipoprotein receptor family of proteins in implantation and placentation. *Ann. N. Y. Acad. Sci.* 734, 91–102. doi: 10.1111/j.1749-6632.1994.tb21738.x

Cox, B., Leavey, K., Nosi, U., Wong, F., and Kingdom, J. (2015). Placental transcriptome in development and pathology: expression, function, and methods of analysis. *Am. J. Obstet. Gynecol.* 213, S138–S151. doi: 10.1016/j.ajog.2015.07.046

Cvitic, S., Longtine, M. S., Hackl, H., Wagner, K., Nelson, M. D., Desoye, G., et al. (2013). The human placental sexome differs between trophoblast epithelium and villous vessel endothelium. *PLoS One* 8:e79233. doi: 10.1371/journal.pone.0079233

Desforges, M., and Sibley, C. P. (2010). Placental nutrient supply and fetal growth. *Int. J. Dev. Biol.* 54, 377–390. doi: 10.1387/ijdb.082765md

Di Renzo, G. C., Giardina, I., Clerici, G., Brillo, E., and Gerli, S. (2016). Progesterone in normal and pathological pregnancy. *Horm. Mol. Biol. Clin. Investig.* 27, 35–48. doi: 10.1515/hmbci-2016-0038

Di Renzo, G. C., Giardina, I., Clerici, G., Mattei, A., Alajmi, A. H., and Gerli, S. (2012). The role of progesterone in maternal and fetal medicine. *Gynecol. Endocrinol.* 28, 925–932. doi: 10.3109/09513590.2012.730576

Drolet, R., Simard, M., Plante, J., Laberge, P., and Tremblay, Y. (2007). Human type 2 17 beta-hydroxysteroid dehydrogenase mRNA and protein distribution in placental villi at mid and term pregnancy. *Reprod. Biol. Endocrinol.* 5:30. doi: 10.1186/1477-7827-5-30

Drwal, E., Rak, A., and Gregoraszczuk, E. (2018). Co-culture of JEG-3, BeWo and syncBeWo cell lines with adrenal H295R cell line: an alternative model for examining endocrine and metabolic properties of the fetoplacental unit. *Cytotechnology* 70, 285–297. doi: 10.1007/s10616-017-0142-z

Dube, E., Ethier-Chiasson, M., and Lafond, J. (2013). Modulation of cholesterol transport by insulin-treated gestational diabetes mellitus in human full-term placenta. *Biol. Reprod.* 88:16. doi: 10.1095/biolreprod.112.105619

Duttaroy, A. K., and Basak, S. (2015). *Human Placental Trophoblasts: Impact of Maternal Nutrition.* Boca Raton, FL: CRC Press. doi: 10.1201/b19151

Eades, C. E., Cameron, D. M., and Evans, J. M. M. (2017). Prevalence of gestational diabetes mellitus in Europe: a meta-analysis. *Diabetes Res. Clin. Pract.* 129, 173–181. doi: 10.1016/j.diabres.2017.03.030

Edison, R. J., Berg, K., Remaley, A., Kelley, R., Rotimi, C., Stevenson, R. E., et al. (2007). Adverse birth outcome among mothers with low serum cholesterol. *Pediatrics* 120, 723–733. doi: 10.1542/peds.2006-1939

Elustondo, P., Martin, L. A., and Karten, B. (2017). Mitochondrial cholesterol import. *Biochim. Biophys. Acta* 1862, 90–101. doi: 10.1016/j.bbalip.2016.08.012

Enquobahrie, D. A., Meller, M., Rice, K., Psaty, B. M., Siscovick, D. S., and Williams, M. A. (2008). Differential placental gene expression in preeclampsia. *Am. J. Obstet. Gynecol.* 199, 566.e561–511.e11. doi: 10.1016/j.ajog.2008.04.020

Ermini, L., Post, M., and Caniggia, I. (2017). Statins, mevalonate pathway and its intermediate products in placental development and preeclampsia. *Curr. Mol. Pharmacol.* 10, 152–160. doi: 10.2174/1874467209666160112123457

Escobar, J. C., and Carr, B. R. (2011). The protein kinase a pathway regulates CYP17 expression and androgen production in the human placenta. *J. Clin. Endocrinol. Metab.* 96, 2869–2873. doi: 10.1210/jc.2011-0542

Escobar, J. C., Patel, S. S., Beshay, V. E., Suzuki, T., and Carr, B. R. (2011). The human placenta expresses CYP17 and generates androgens de novo. *J. Clin. Endocrinol. Metab.* 96, 1385–1392. doi: 10.1210/jc.2010-2504

Esparza-Perusquia, M., Olvera-Sanchez, S., Flores-Herrera, O., Flores-Herrera, H., Guevara-Flores, A., Pardo, J. P., et al. (2015). Mitochondrial proteases act on STARD3 to activate progesterone synthesis in human syncytiotrophoblast. *Biochim. Biophys. Acta* 1850, 107–117. doi: 10.1016/j.bbagen.2014.10.009

Esteve-Valverde, E., Ferrer-Oliveras, R., Gil-Aliberas, N., Baraldes-Farre, A., Llurba, E., and Alijotas-Reig, J. (2018). Pravastatin for preventing and treating preeclampsia: a systematic review. *Obstet. Gynecol. Surv.* 73, 40–55. doi: 10.1097/ogx.0000000000000522

Ethier-Chiasson, M., Duchesne, A., Forest, J. C., Giguere, Y., Masse, A., Mounier, C., et al. (2007). Influence of maternal lipid profile on placental protein expression of LDLr and SR-BI. *Biochem. Biophys. Res. Commun.* 359, 8–14. doi: 10.1016/j.bbrc.2007.05.002

Evain-Brion, D., and Malassine, A. (2003). Human placenta as an endocrine organ. *Growth Horm. IGF Res.* 13(Suppl. A), S34–S37. doi: 10.1016/S1096-6374(03)00053-4

Fahlbusch, F. B., Ruebner, M., Volkert, G., Offergeld, R., Hartner, A., Menendez-Castro, C., et al. (2012). Corticotropin-releasing hormone stimulates expression of leptin, 11beta-HSD2 and syncytin-1 in primary human trophoblasts. *Reprod. Biol. Endocrinol.* 10:80. doi: 10.1186/1477-7827-10-80

Favari, E., Chroni, A., Tietge, U. J., Zanotti, I., Escola-Gil, J. C., and Bernini, F. (2015). Cholesterol efflux and reverse cholesterol transport. *Handb. Exp. Pharmacol.* 224, 181–206. doi: 10.1007/978-3-319-09665-0_4

Florio, P., Franchini, A., Reis, F. M., Pezzani, I., Ottaviani, E., and Petraglia, F. (2000). Human placenta, chorion, amnion and decidua express different variants of corticotropin-releasing factor receptor messenger RNA. *Placenta* 21, 32–37. doi: 10.1053/plac.1999.0461

Forbes, K., Hurst, L. M., Aplin, J. D., Westwood, M., and Gibson, J. M. (2008). Statins are detrimental to human placental development and function; use of statins during early pregnancy is inadvisable. *J. Cell Mol. Med.* 12, 2295–2296. doi: 10.1111/j.1582-4934.2008.00466.x

Forbes, K., Shah, V. K., Siddals, K., Gibson, J. M., Aplin, J. D., and Westwood, M. (2015). Statins inhibit insulin-like growth factor action in first trimester placenta by altering insulin-like growth factor 1 receptor glycosylation. *Mol. Hum. Reprod.* 21, 105–114. doi: 10.1093/molehr/gau093

Fournier, T., Handschuh, K., Tsatsaris, V., Guibourdenche, J., and Evain-Brion, D. (2008). Role of nuclear receptors and their ligands in human trophoblast invasion. *J. Reprod. Immunol.* 77, 161–170. doi: 10.1016/j.jri.2007.05.004

Fowden, A. L., Forhead, A. J., Sferruzzi-Perri, A. N., Burton, G. J., and Vaughan, O. R. (2015). Review: endocrine regulation of placental phenotype. *Placenta* 36(Suppl. 1), S50–S59. doi: 10.1016/j.placenta.2014.11.018

French, A. P., and Warren, J. C. (1965). Steroid-3-beta-sulfatase in fetal and placental tissues. *Steroids* 6, 865–869. doi: 10.1016/0039-128X(65)90107-8

Frim, D. M., Robinson, B. G., Pasieka, K. B., and Majzoub, J. A. (1990). Differential regulation of corticotropin-releasing hormone mRNA in rat brain. *Am. J. Physiol.* 258(4 Pt 1), E686–E692. doi: 10.1152/ajpendo.1990.258.4.E686

Fukata, Y., Yu, X., Imachi, H., Nishiuchi, T., Lyu, J., Seo, K., et al. (2014). 17beta-Estradiol regulates scavenger receptor class BI gene expression via protein kinase C in vascular endothelial cells. *Endocrine* 46, 644–650. doi: 10.1007/s12020-013-0134-5

Furuhashi, M., Seo, H., Mizutani, S., Narita, O., Tomoda, Y., and Matsui, N. (1989). Expression of low density lipoprotein receptor gene in human placenta during pregnancy. *Mol. Endocrinol.* 3, 1252–1256. doi: 10.1210/mend-3-8-1252

Gafvels, M. E., Caird, M., Britt, D., Jackson, C. L., Patterson, D., and Strauss, J. F. III (1993). Cloning of a cDNA encoding a putative human very low density lipoprotein/apolipoprotein E receptor and assignment of the gene to chromosome 9pter-p23. *Somat. Cell Mol. Genet.* 19, 557–569. doi: 10.1007/BF01233382

Gafvels, M. E., Coukos, G., Sayegh, R., Coutifaris, C., Strickland, D. K., and Strauss, J. F. III (1992). Regulated expression of the trophoblast alpha 2-macroglobulin receptor/low density lipoprotein receptor-related protein. Differentiation and cAMP modulate protein and mRNA levels. *J. Biol. Chem.* 267, 21230–21234.

Gallo, L. A., Barrett, H. L., and Dekker Nitert, M. (2016). Review: placental transport and metabolism of energy substrates in maternal obesity and diabetes. *Placenta* 54, 59–67 doi: 10.1016/j.placenta.2016.12.006

Gangestad, S. W., Caldwell Hooper, A. E., and Eaton, M. A. (2012). On the function of placental corticotropin-releasing hormone: a role in maternal-fetal conflicts over blood glucose concentrations. *Biol. Rev. Camb. Philos. Soc.* 87, 856–873. doi: 10.1111/j.1469-185X.2012.00226.x

Gao, L., Lu, C., Xu, C., Tao, Y., Cong, B., and Ni, X. (2008). Differential regulation of prostaglandin production mediated by corticotropin-releasing hormone receptor type 1 and type 2 in cultured human placental trophoblasts. *Endocrinology* 149, 2866–2876. doi: 10.1210/en.2007-1377

Gao, L., Lv, C., Xu, C., Li, Y., Cui, X., Gu, H., et al. (2012). Differential regulation of glucose transporters mediated by CRH receptor type 1 and type 2 in human placental trophoblasts. *Endocrinology* 153(3), 1464-1471. doi: 10.1210/en.2011-1673

Geyer, J., Bakhaus, K., Bernhardt, R., Blaschka, C., Dezhkam, Y., Fietz, D., et al. (2017). The role of sulfated steroid hormones in reproductive processes. *J. Steroid Biochem. Mol. Biol.* 172, 207–221. doi: 10.1016/j.jsbmb.2016.07.002

Ghorashi, V., and Sheikhvatan, M. (2008). The relationship between serum concentration of free testosterone and pre-eclampsia. *Endokrynol. Pol.* 59, 390–392.

Giannopoulos, G., Jackson, K., and Tulchinsky, D. (1982). Glucocorticoid metabolism in human placenta, decidua, myometrium and fetal membranes. *J. Steroid Biochem.* 17, 371–374. doi: 10.1016/0022-4731(82)90628-8

Go, G. W., and Mani, A. (2012). Low-density lipoprotein receptor (LDLR) family orchestrates cholesterol homeostasis. *Yale J. Biol. Med.* 85, 19–28.

Gohner, C., Svensson-Arvelund, J., Pfarrer, C., Hager, J. D., Faas, M., Ernerudh, J., et al. (2014). The placenta in toxicology. Part IV: battery of toxicological test systems based on human placenta. *Toxicol. Pathol.* 42, 345–351. doi: 10.1177/0192623313482206

Goldkrand, J. W., Schulte, R. L., and Messer, R. H. (1976). Maternal and fetal plasma cortisol levels at parturition. *Obstet. Gynecol.* 47, 41–45.

Goodarzi, M. O., Dumesic, D. A., Chazenbalk, G., and Azziz, R. (2011). Polycystic ovary syndrome: etiology, pathogenesis and diagnosis. *Nat. Rev. Endocrinol.* 7:219. doi: 10.1038/nrendo.2010.217

Grammatopoulos, D. K., and Ourailidou, S. (2017). CRH receptor signalling: potential roles in pathophysiology. *Curr. Mol. Pharmacol.* 10, 296–310. doi: 10.2174/1874467210666170110125747

Gratton, A. M., Ye, L., Brownfoot, F. C., Hannan, N. J., Whitehead, C., Cannon, P., et al. (2016). Steroid sulfatase is increased in the placentas and whole blood of women with early-onset preeclampsia. *Placenta* 48(Suppl. C), 72–79. doi: 10.1016/j.placenta.2016.10.008

Grigsby, P. L. (2016). Animal models to study placental development and function throughout normal and dysfunctional human pregnancy. *Semin. Reprod. Med.* 34, 11–16. doi: 10.1055/s-0035-1570031

Grimes, R. W., Pepe, G. J., and Albrecht, E. D. (1996). Regulation of human placental trophoblast low-density lipoprotein uptake in vitro by estrogen. *J. Clin. Endocrinol. Metab.* 81, 2675–2679. doi: 10.1210/jcem.81.7.8675596

Grube, M., Kock, K., Karner, S., Reuther, S., Ritter, C. A., Jedlitschky, G., et al. (2006). Modification of OATP2B1-mediated transport by steroid hormones. *Mol. Pharmacol.* 70, 1735–1741. doi: 10.1124/mol.106.026450

Grube, M., Reuther, S., Meyer Zu Schwabedissen, H., Kock, K., Draber, K., Ritter, C. A., et al. (2007). Organic anion transporting polypeptide 2B1 and breast cancer resistance protein interact in the transepithelial transport of steroid sulfates in human placenta. *Drug Metab. Dispos.* 35, 30–35. doi: 10.1124/dmd.106.011411

Hafez, S. (2017). Comparative placental anatomy: divergent structures serving a common purpose. *Prog. Mol. Biol. Transl. Sci.* 145, 1–28. doi: 10.1016/bs.pmbts.2016.12.001

Hahnova-Cygalova, L., Ceckova, M., and Staud, F. (2011). Fetoprotective activity of breast cancer resistance protein (BCRP, ABCG2): expression and function throughout pregnancy. *Drug Metab. Rev.* 43, 53–68. doi: 10.3109/03602532.2010.512293

Hakkola, J., Raunio, H., Purkunen, R., Pelkonen, O., Saarikoski, S., Cresteil, T., et al. (1996). Detection of cytochrome P450 gene expression in human placenta in first trimester of pregnancy. *Biochem. Pharmacol.* 52, 379–383. doi: 10.1016/0006-2952(96)00216-X

Halasz, M., and Szekeres-Bartho, J. (2013). The role of progesterone in implantation and trophoblast invasion. *J. Reprod. Immunol.* 97, 43–50. doi: 10.1016/j.jri.2012.10.011

Hanukoglu, I. (1992). Steroidogenic enzymes: structure, function, and role in regulation of steroid hormone biosynthesis. *J. Steroid Biochem. Mol. Biol.* 43, 779–804. doi: 10.1016/0960-0760(92)90307-5

He, D., Meloche, C. A., Dumas, N. A., Frost, A. R., and Falany, C. N. (2004). Different subcellular localization of sulphotransferase 2B1b in human placenta and prostate. *Biochem. J.* 379(Pt 3), 533–540. doi: 10.1042/bj20031524

He, G., Xu, W., Chen, Y., Liu, X., and Xi, M. (2013). Abnormal apoptosis of trophoblastic cells is related to the up-regulation of CYP11A gene in placenta of preeclampsia patients. *PLoS One* 8:e59609. doi: 10.1371/journal.pone.0059609

Hellig, H., Gattereau, D., Lefebvre, Y., and Bolte, E. (1970). Steroid production from plasma cholesterol. I. Conversion of plasma cholesterol to placental progesterone in humans. *J. Clin. Endocrinol. Metab.* 30, 624–631. doi: 10.1210/jcem-30-5-624

Henderson, Y. C., Frederick, M. J., Wang, M. T., Hollier, L. M., and Clayman, G. L. (2008). LBP-1b, LBP-9, and LBP-32/MGR detected in syncytiotrophoblasts from first-trimester human placental tissue and their transcriptional regulation. *DNA Cell Biol.* 27, 71–79. doi: 10.1089/dna.2007.0640

Henson, M. C. (1998). Pregnancy maintenance and the regulation of placental progesterone biosynthesis in the baboon. *Hum. Reprod. Update* 4, 389–405. doi: 10.1093/humupd/4.4.389

Henson, M. C., Greene, S. J., Reggio, B. C., Shi, W., and Swan, K. F. (1997). Effects of reduced maternal lipoprotein-cholesterol availability on placental progesterone biosynthesis in the baboon. *Endocrinology* 138, 1385–1391. doi: 10.1210/endo.138.4.5039

Henson, M. C., Pepe, G. J., and Albrecht, E. D. (1991). Regulation of placental low-density lipoprotein uptake in baboons by estrogen: dose-dependent effects of the anti-estrogen ethamoxytriphetol (MER-25). *Biol. Reprod.* 45, 43–48. doi: 10.1095/biolreprod45.1.43

Hentschke, M. R., Poli-de-Figueiredo, C. E., da Costa, B. E., Kurlak, L. O., Williams, P. J., and Mistry, H. D. (2013). Is the atherosclerotic phenotype of preeclamptic placentas due to altered lipoprotein concentrations and placental lipoprotein receptors? Role of a small-for-gestational-age phenotype. *J. Lipid Res.* 54, 2658–2664. doi: 10.1194/jlr.M036699

Herman, B. E., Szabó, J., Bacsa, I., Wölfling, J., Schneider, G., Bálint, M., et al. (2016). Comparative investigation of the in vitro inhibitory potencies of 13-epimeric estrones and D-secoestrones towards 17β-hydroxysteroid dehydrogenase type 1. *J. Enzyme Inhib. Med. Chem.* 31(Suppl. 3), 61–69. doi: 10.1080/14756366.2016.1204610

Herrera, E. (2002). Lipid metabolism in pregnancy and its consequences in the fetus and newborn. *Endocrine* 19, 43–55. doi: 10.1385/ENDO:19:1:43

Herrera, E., Amusquivar, E., Lopez-Soldado, I., and Ortega, H. (2006). Maternal lipid metabolism and placental lipid transfer. *Horm. Res.* 65(Suppl. 3), 59–64. doi: 10.1159/000091507

Marseille-Tremblay, C., Gravel, A., Lafond, J., and Mounier, C. (2007). Effect of an enriched cholesterol diet during gestation on fatty acid synthase, HMG-CoA reductase and SREBP-1/2 expressions in rabbits. *Life Sci.* 81, 772–778. doi: 10.1016/j.lfs.2007.07.016

Maynard, S. E., Min, J.-Y., Merchan, J., Lim, K.-H., Li, J., Mondal, S., et al. (2003). Excess placental soluble fms-like tyrosine kinase 1 (sFlt1) may contribute to endothelial dysfunction, hypertension, and proteinuria in preeclampsia. *J. Clin. Invest.* 111, 649–658. doi: 10.1172/JCI200317189

Mesiano, S. (2001). *Roles of Estrogen and Progesterone in Human Parturition*, ed. R. Smith. Basel: Karger, 86–104. doi: 10.1159/000061038

Michael, A. E., and Papageorghiou, A. T. (2008). Potential significance of physiological and pharmacological glucocorticoids in early pregnancy. *Hum. Reprod. Update* 14, 497–517. doi: 10.1093/humupd/dmn021

Miki, Y., Nakata, T., Suzuki, T., Darnel, A. D., Moriya, T., Kaneko, C., et al. (2002). Systemic distribution of steroid sulfatase and estrogen sulfotransferase in human adult and fetal tissues. *J. Clin. Endocrinol. Metab.* 87, 5760–5768. doi: 10.1210/jc.2002-020670

Miller, W. L. (2013). Steroid hormone synthesis in mitochondria. *Mol. Cell. Endocrinol.* 379, 62–73. doi: 10.1016/j.mce.2013.04.014

Miller, W. L. (2017). Steroidogenesis: unanswered questions. *Trends Endocrinol. Metab.* 28, 771–793. doi: 10.1016/j.tem.2017.09.002

Miller, W. L., and Auchus, R. J. (2011). The molecular biology, biochemistry, and physiology of human steroidogenesis and its disorders. *Endocr. Rev.* 32, 81–151. doi: 10.1210/er.2010-0013

Miller, W. L., and Bose, H. S. (2011). Early steps in steroidogenesis: intracellular cholesterol trafficking. *J. Lipid Res.* 52, 2111–2135. doi: 10.1194/jlr.R016675

Miranda, A., and Sousa, N. (2018). Maternal hormonal milieu influence on fetal brain development. *Brain Behav.* 8:e00920. doi: 10.1002/brb3.920

Mistry, H. D., Kurlak, L. O., Mansour, Y. T., Zurkinden, L., Mohaupt, M. G., and Escher, G. (2017). Increased maternal and fetal cholesterol efflux capacity and placental CYP27A1 expression in preeclampsia. *J. Lipid Res.* 58, 1186–1195. doi: 10.1194/jlr.M071985

Moise, J., Ilekis, J., Scommegna, A., and Benveniste, R. (1986). The effect of dehydroepiandrosterone sulfate on de novo and low-density lipoprotein-stimulated progesterone secretion by human choriocarcinoma JEG-3 cells. *Am. J. Obstet. Gynecol.* 154, 1080–1085. doi: 10.1016/0002-9378(86)90755-6

Moisiadis, V. G., and Matthews, S. G. (2014a). Glucocorticoids and fetal programming part 1: Outcomes. *Nat. Rev. Endocrinol.* 10, 391–402. doi: 10.1038/nrendo.2014.73

Moisiadis, V. G., and Matthews, S. G. (2014b). Glucocorticoids and fetal programming part 2: Mechanisms. *Nat. Rev. Endocrinol.* 10, 403–411. doi: 10.1038/nrendo.2014.74

Monreal-Flores, J., Espinosa-Garcia, M. T., Garcia-Regalado, A., Arechavaleta-Velasco, F., and Martinez, F. (2017). The heat shock protein 60 promotes progesterone synthesis in mitochondria of JEG-3 cells. *Reprod. Biol.* 17, 154–161. doi: 10.1016/j.repbio.2017.04.001

Montoudis, A., Boileau, S., Simoneau, L., and Lafond, J. (2003). Impact of an enriched-cholesterol diet on enzymatic cholesterol metabolism during rabbit gestation. *Life Sci.* 73, 1463–1477. doi: 10.1016/S0024-3205(03)00436-3

Moon, J.-Y., Moon, M. H., Kim, K. T., Jeong, D. H., Kim, Y. N., Chung, B. C., et al. (2014). Cytochrome P450-mediated metabolic alterations in preeclampsia evaluated by quantitative steroid signatures. *J. Steroid Biochem. Mol. Biol.* 139(Suppl. C), 182–191. doi: 10.1016/j.jsbmb.2013.02.014

Murata, M., Kodama, H., Goto, K., Hirano, H., and Tanaka, T. (1996). Decreased very-low-density lipoprotein and low-density lipoprotein receptor messenger ribonucleic acid expression in placentas from preeclamptic pregnancies. *Am. J. Obstet. Gynecol.* 175, 1551–1556. doi: 10.1016/S0002-9378(96)70105-9

Mutemberezi, V., Guillemot-Legris, O., and Muccioli, G. G. (2016). Oxysterols: from cholesterol metabolites to key mediators. *Prog. Lipid Res.* 64, 152–169. doi: 10.1016/j.plipres.2016.09.002

Myllynen, P., and Vahakangas, K. (2013). Placental transfer and metabolism: an overview of the experimental models utilizing human placental tissue. *Toxicol. In Vitro* 27, 507–512. doi: 10.1016/j.tiv.2012.08.027

Nakamura, Y., Ikeda, S., Furukawa, T., Sumizawa, T., Tani, A., Akiyama, S., et al. (1997). Function of P-glycoprotein expressed in placenta and mole. *Biochem. Biophys. Res. Commun.* 235, 849–853. doi: 10.1006/bbrc.1997.6855

Naoum, H. G., De Chazal, R. C., Eaton, B. M., and Contractor, S. F. (1987). Characterization and specificity of lipoprotein binding to term human placental membranes. *Biochim. Biophys. Acta* 902, 193–199. doi: 10.1016/0005-2736(87)90295-1

Napoli, C., D'Armiento, F. P., Mancini, F. P., Postiglione, A., Witztum, J. L., Palumbo, G., et al. (1997). Fatty streak formation occurs in human fetal aortas and is greatly enhanced by maternal hypercholesterolemia. Intimal accumulation of low density lipoprotein and its oxidation precede monocyte recruitment into early atherosclerotic lesions. *J. Clin. Invest.* 100, 2680–2690. doi: 10.1172/JCI119813

Napoli, C., Glass, C. K., Witztum, J. L., Deutsch, R., D'Armiento, F. P., and Palinski, W. (1999). Influence of maternal hypercholesterolaemia during pregnancy on progression of early atherosclerotic lesions in childhood: Fate of Early Lesions in Children (FELIC) study. *Lancet* 354, 1234–1241. doi: 10.1016/s0140-6736(99)02131-5

Nardozza, L. M., Caetano, A. C., Zamarian, A. C., Mazzola, J. B., Silva, C. P., Marcal, V. M., et al. (2017). Fetal growth restriction: current knowledge. *Arch. Gynecol. Obstet.* 295, 1061–1077. doi: 10.1007/s00404-017-4341-9

Ni, X., Hou, Y., Yang, R., Tang, X., Smith, R., and Nicholson, R. C. (2004). Progesterone receptors A and B differentially modulate corticotropin-releasing hormone gene expression through a cAMP regulatory element. *Cell. Mol. Life Sci.* 61, 1114–1122. doi: 10.1007/s00018-004-4030-2

Ni, X. T., Duan, T., Yang, Z., Guo, C. M., Li, J. N., and Sun, K. (2009). Role of human chorionic gonadotropin in maintaining 11beta-hydroxysteroid dehydrogenase type 2 expression in human placental syncytiotrophoblasts. *Placenta* 30, 1023–1028. doi: 10.1016/j.placenta.2009.10.005

Ni, Z., and Mao, Q. (2011). ATP-binding cassette efflux transporters in human placenta. *Curr. Pharm. Biotechnol.* 12, 674–685. doi: 10.2174/138920111795164057

Nikitina, L., Wenger, F., Baumann, M., Surbek, D., Korner, M., and Albrecht, C. (2011). Expression and localization pattern of ABCA1 in diverse human placental primary cells and tissues. *Placenta* 32, 420–430. doi: 10.1016/j.placenta.2011.03.003

Noguchi, S., Nishimura, T., Fujibayashi, A., Maruyama, T., Tomi, M., and Nakashima, E. (2015). Organic anion transporter 4-mediated transport of olmesartan at basal plasma membrane of human placental barrier. *J. Pharm. Sci.* 104, 3128–3135. doi: 10.1002/jps.24434

Noyola-Martinez, N., Halhali, A., Zaga-Clavellina, V., Olmos-Ortiz, A., Larrea, F., and Barrera, D. (2017). A time-course regulatory and kinetic expression study of steroid metabolizing enzymes by calcitriol in primary cultured human placental cells. *J. Steroid Biochem. Mol. Biol.* 167, 98–105. doi: 10.1016/j.jsbmb.2016.11.015

Olvera-Sanchez, S., Espinosa-Garcia, M. T., Monreal, J., Flores-Herrera, O., and Martinez, F. (2011). Mitochondrial heat shock protein participates in placental steroidogenesis. *Placenta* 32, 222–229. doi: 10.1016/j.placenta.2010.12.018

Orendi, K., Kivity, V., Sammar, M., Grimpel, Y., Gonen, R., Meiri, H., et al. (2011). Placental and trophoblastic in vitro models to study preventive and therapeutic agents for preeclampsia. *Placenta* 32, S49–S54. doi: 10.1016/j.placenta.2010.11.023

Park, M. C., Cayatte, A., and Subbiah, M. T. (1988). Isolation and characterization of a novel lipoprotein particle from human placental extracts. *Biochem. Biophys. Res. Commun.* 153, 502–509. doi: 10.1016/S0006-291X(88)81123-9

Park, M. N., Park, K. H., Lee, J. E., Shin, Y. Y., An, S. M., Kang, S. S., et al. (2018). The expression and activation of sex steroid receptors in the preeclamptic placenta. *Int. J. Mol. Med.* 41, 2943–2951. doi: 10.3892/ijmm.2018.3474

Parker, C. R. Jr., Illingworth, D. R., Bissonnette, J., and Carr, B. R. (1986). Endocrine changes during pregnancy in a patient with homozygous familial hypobetalipoproteinemia. *N. Engl. J. Med.* 314, 557–560. doi: 10.1056/nejm198602273140906

Pasqualini, J. R., and Chetrite, G. S. (2016). The formation and transformation of hormones in maternal, placental and fetal compartments: biological implications. *Horm. Mol. Biol. Clin. Investig.* 27, 11–28. doi: 10.1515/hmbci-2016-0036

Patel, B., Elguero, S., Thakore, S., Dahoud, W., Bedaiwy, M., and Mesiano, S. (2015). Role of nuclear progesterone receptor isoforms in uterine pathophysiology. *Hum. Reprod. Update* 21, 155–173. doi: 10.1093/humupd/dmu056

Pavan, L., Hermouet, A., Tsatsaris, V., Therond, P., Sawamura, T., Evain-Brion, D., et al. (2004). Lipids from oxidized low-density lipoprotein modulate human trophoblast invasion: involvement of nuclear liver X receptors. *Endocrinology* 145, 4583–4591. doi: 10.1210/en.2003-1747

Pavek, P., and Smutny, T. (2014). Nuclear receptors in regulation of biotransformation enzymes and drug transporters in the placental barrier. *Drug Metab. Rev.* 46, 19–32. doi: 10.3109/03602532.2013.835819

Payne, A. H., and Hales, D. B. (2004). Overview of steroidogenic enzymes in the pathway from cholesterol to active steroid hormones. *Endocr. Rev.* 25, 947–970. doi: 10.1210/er.2003-0030

Pepe, G. J., and Albrecht, E. D. (1995). Actions of placental and fetal adrenal steroid hormones in primate pregnancy. *Endocr. Rev.* 16, 608–648. doi: 10.1210/edrv-16-5-608

Perez-Sepulveda, A., Monteiro, L. J., Dobierzewska, A., España-Perrot, P. P., Venegas-Araneda, P., Guzmán-Rojas, A. M., et al. (2015). Placental aromatase is deficient in placental ischemia and preeclampsia. *PLoS One* 10:e0139682. doi: 10.1371/journal.pone.0139682

Pezzi, V., Mathis, J. M., Rainey, W. E., and Carr, B. R. (2003). Profiling transcript levels for steroidogenic enzymes in fetal tissues. *J. Steroid Biochem. Mol. Biol.* 87, 181–189. doi: 10.1016/j.jsbmb.2003.07.006

Phillips, M. C. (2014). Molecular mechanisms of cellular cholesterol efflux. *J. Biol. Chem.* 289, 24020–24029. doi: 10.1074/jbc.R114.583658

Phillips, R. J., Fortier, M. A., and Lopez Bernal, A. (2014). Prostaglandin pathway gene expression in human placenta, amnion and choriodecidua is differentially affected by preterm and term labour and by uterine inflammation. *BMC Pregnancy Childbirth* 14:241. doi: 10.1186/1471-2393-14-241

Piltonen, T. T., Chen, J. C., Khatun, M., Kangasniemi, M., Liakka, A., Spitzer, T., et al. (2015). Endometrial stromal fibroblasts from women with polycystic ovary syndrome have impaired progesterone-mediated decidualization, aberrant cytokine profiles and promote enhanced immune cell migration in vitro. *Hum. Reprod.* 30, 1203–1215. doi: 10.1093/humrep/dev055

Pitkin, R. M., Connor, W. E., and Lin, D. S. (1972). Cholesterol metabolism and placental transfer in the pregnant Rhesus monkey. *J. Clin. Invest.* 51, 2584–2592. doi: 10.1172/JCI107075

Plosch, T., Gellhaus, A., van Straten, E. M., Wolf, N., Huijkman, N. C., Schmidt, M., et al. (2010). The liver X receptor (LXR) and its target gene ABCA1 are regulated upon low oxygen in human trophoblast cells: a reason for alterations in preeclampsia? *Placenta* 31, 910–918. doi: 10.1016/j.placenta.2010.07.009

Plosch, T., van Straten, E. M., and Kuipers, F. (2007). Cholesterol transport by the placenta: placental liver X receptor activity as a modulator of fetal cholesterol metabolism? *Placenta* 28, 604–610. doi: 10.1016/j.placenta.2006.10.009

Plotz, E. J., Kabara, J. J., Davis, M. E., LeRoy, G. V., and Gould, R. G. (1968). Studies on the synthesis of cholesterol in the brain of the human fetus. *Am. J. Obstet. Gynecol.* 101, 534–538. doi: 10.1016/0002-9378(68)90565-6

Pluchino, N., Russo, M., and Genazzani, A. R. (2016). The fetal brain: role of progesterone and allopregnanolone. *Horm Mol. Biol. Clin. Investig.* 27, 29X–34X. doi: 10.1515/hmbci-2016-0020

Pratt, J. P., Kaucher, M., Moyer, E., Richards, A. J., and Williams H. H. (1946). Composition of the human placenta; lipid content. *Am. J. Obstet. Gynecol.* 52, 665–668. doi: 10.1016/0002-9378(46)90135-4

Prouillac, C., and Lecoeur, S. (2010). The role of the placenta in fetal exposure to xenobiotics: importance of membrane transporters and human models for transfer studies. *Drug Metab. Dispos.* 38, 1623–1635. doi: 10.1124/dmd.110.033571

Qiu, C., Phung, T. T., Vadachkoria, S., Muy-Rivera, M., Sanchez, S. E., and Williams, M. A. (2006). Oxidized low-density lipoprotein (Oxidized LDL) and the risk of preeclampsia. *Physiol. Res.* 55, 491–500.

Rani, P. R., and Begum, J. (2016). Screening and diagnosis of gestational diabetes mellitus, where do we stand. *J. Clin. Diagn. Res.* 10, QE01–QE04. doi: 10.7860/JCDR/2016/17588.7689

Rantakari, P., Strauss, L., Kiviranta, R., Lagerbohm, H., Paviala, J., Holopainen, I., et al. (2008). Placenta defects and embryonic lethality resulting from disruption of mouse hydroxysteroid (17-β) dehydrogenase 2 gene. *Mol. Endocrinol.* 22, 665–675. doi: 10.1210/me.2007-0257

Rebourcet, R., Alsat, E., Mondon, F., Berthelier, M., Pastier, D., Cedard, L., et al. (1986). Detection of distinct receptors for native and acetylated low-density lipoproteins in human placental microvilli by ligand-immunoblotting. *Biochimie* 68, 1135–1140. doi: 10.1016/S0300-9084(86)80189-4

Reyes, L., Wolfe, B., and Golos, T. (2017). Hofbauer cells: placental macrophages of fetal origin. *Results Probl. Cell Differ.* 62, 45–60. doi: 10.1007/978-3-319-54090-0_3

Riley, S. C., Walton, J. C., Herlick, J. M., and Challis, J. R. (1991). The localization and distribution of corticotropin-releasing hormone in the human placenta and fetal membranes throughout gestation. *J. Clin. Endocrinol. Metab.* 72, 1001–1007. doi: 10.1210/jcem-72-5-1001

Rindler, M. J., Traber, M. G., Esterman, A. L., Bersinger, N. A., and Dancis, J. (1991). Synthesis and secretion of apolipoprotein E by human placenta and choriocarcinoma cell lines. *Placenta* 12, 615–624. doi: 10.1016/0143-4004(91)90496-3

Robinson, B. G., Emanuel, R. L., Frim, D. M., and Majzoub, J. A. (1988). Glucocorticoid stimulates expression of corticotropin-releasing hormone gene in human placenta. *Proc. Natl. Acad. Sci. U.S.A.* 85, 5244–5248. doi: 10.1073/pnas.85.14.5244

Rohrl, C., and Stangl, H. (2013). HDL endocytosis and resecretion. *Biochim. Biophys. Acta* 1831, 1626–1633. doi: 10.1016/j.bbalip.2013.07.014

Romano, A., Delvoux, B., Fischer, D.-C., and Groothuis, P. (2007). The PROGINS polymorphism of the human progesterone receptor diminishes the response to progesterone. *J. Mol. Endocrinol.* 38, 331–350. doi: 10.1677/jme.1.02170

Sacks, F. M. (2015). The crucial roles of apolipoproteins E and C-III in apoB lipoprotein metabolism in normolipidemia and hypertriglyceridemia. *Curr. Opin. Lipidol.* 26, 56–63. doi: 10.1097/mol.0000000000000146

Sati, L., Seval, Y., Yasemin Demir, A., Kosanke, G., Kohnen, G., and Demir, R. (2007). Cellular diversity of human placental stem villi: an ultrastructural and immunohistochemical study. *Acta Histochem.* 109, 468–479. doi: 10.1016/j.acthis.2007.04.006

Sattar, N., Greer, I. A., Galloway, P. J., Packard, C. J., Shepherd, J., Kelly, T., et al. (1999). Lipid and lipoprotein concentrations in pregnancies complicated by intrauterine growth restriction. *J. Clin. Endocrinol. Metab.* 84, 128–130. doi: 10.1210/jcem.84.1.5419

Schmid, K. E., Davidson, W. S., Myatt, L., and Woollett, L. A. (2003). Transport of cholesterol across a BeWo cell monolayer: implications for net transport of sterol from maternal to fetal circulation. *J. Lipid Res.* 44, 1909–1918. doi: 10.1194/jlr.M300126-JLR200

Schock, H., Surcel, H. M., Zeleniuch-Jacquotte, A., Grankvist, K., Lakso, H. A., Fortner, R. T., et al. (2014). Early pregnancy sex steroids and maternal risk of epithelial ovarian cancer. *Endocr. Relat. Cancer* 21, 831–844. doi: 10.1530/erc-14-0282

Schroepfer, G. J. Jr. (2000). Oxysterols: modulators of cholesterol metabolism and other processes. *Physiol. Rev.* 80, 361–554. doi: 10.1152/physrev.2000.80.1.361

Schweigmann, H., Sánchez-Guijo, A., Ugele, B., Hartmann, K., Hartmann, M. F., Bergmann, M., et al. (2014). Transport of the placental estriol precursor 16α-hydroxy-dehydroepiandrosterone sulfate (16α-OH-DHEAS) by stably transfected OAT4-, SOAT-, and NTCP-HEK293 cells. *J. Steroid Biochem. Mol. Biol.* 143(Suppl. C), 259–265. doi: 10.1016/j.jsbmb.2014.03.013

Sfakianaki, A. K., and Norwitz, E. R. (2006). Mechanisms of progesterone action in inhibiting prematurity. *J. Matern. Fetal Neonatal Med.* 19, 763–772. doi: 10.1080/14767050600949829

Shao, X., Liu, Y., Liu, M., Wang, Y., Yan, L., Wang, H., et al. (2017). Testosterone represses estrogen signaling by upregulating miR-22: a mechanism for imbalanced steroid hormone production in preeclampsia. *Hypertension* 69, 721–730. doi: 10.1161/hypertensionaha.116.08468

Sharifzadeh, F., Kashanian, M., and Fatemi, F. (2012). A comparison of serum androgens in pre-eclamptic and normotensive pregnant women during the third trimester of pregnancy. *Gynecol. Endocrinol.* 28, 834–836. doi: 10.3109/09513590.2012.683061

Shi, W., Swan, K. F., Lear, S. R., O'Neil, J. S., Erickson, S. K., and Henson, M. C. (1999). Regulation of pathways determining cholesterol availability in the baboon placenta with advancing gestation. *Biol. Reprod.* 61, 1499–1505. doi: 10.1095/biolreprod61.6.1499

Shimano, H., and Sato, R. (2017). SREBP-regulated lipid metabolism: convergent physiology - divergent pathophysiology. *Nat. Rev. Endocrinol.* 13, 710–730. doi: 10.1038/nrendo.2017.91

Shin, Y. Y., Jeong, J. S., Park, M. N., Lee, J. E., An, S. M., Cho, W. S., et al. (2018). Regulation of steroid hormones in the placenta and serum of women with preeclampsia. *Mol. Med. Rep.* 17, 2681–2688. doi: 10.3892/mmr.2017.8165

Siiteri, P. K., and MacDonald, P. C. (1966). Placental estrogen biosynthesis during human pregnancy. *J. Clin. Endocrinol. Metab.* 26, 751–761. doi: 10.1210/jcem-26-7-751

Simpson, E. R., Porter, J. C., Milewich, L., Bilheimer, D. W., and MacDonald, P. C. (1978). Regulation by plasma lipoproteins of progesterone biosynthesis and 3-hydroxy-3-methyl glutaryl coenzyme a reductase activity in cultured human choriocarcinoma cells. *J. Clin. Endocrinol. Metab.* 47, 1099–1105. doi: 10.1210/jcem-47-5-1099

Slominski, A., Semak, I., Wortsman, J., Zjawiony, J., Li, W., Zbytek, B., et al. (2006). An alternative pathway of vitamin D(2) metabolism cytochrome P450scc (CYP11A1)-mediated conversion to 20-hydroxyvitamin D(2) and 17,20-dihydroxyvitamin D(2). *FEBS J.* 273, 2891–2901. doi: 10.1111/j.1742-4658.2006.05302.x

Slominski, A., Semak, I., Zjawiony, J., Wortsman, J., Li, W., Szczesniewski, A., et al. (2005). The cytochrome P450scc system opens an alternate pathway of vitamin D3 metabolism. *FEBS J.* 272, 4080–4090. doi: 10.1111/j.1742-4658.2005.04819.x

Slominski, A. T., Kim, T.-K., Chen, J., Nguyen, M. N., Li, W., Yates, C. R., et al. (2012). Cytochrome P450scc-dependent metabolism of 7-dehydrocholesterol in placenta and epidermal keratinocytes. *Int. J. Biochem. Cell Biol.* 44, 2003–2018. doi: 10.1016/j.biocel.2012.07.027

Slominski, A. T., Kim, T. K., Li, W., Postlethwaite, A., Tieu, E. W., Tang, E. K., et al. (2015a). Detection of novel CYP11A1-derived secosteroids in the human epidermis and serum and pig adrenal gland. *Sci. Rep.* 5:14875. doi: 10.1038/srep14875

Slominski, A. T., Li, W., Kim, T.-K., Semak, I., Wang, J., Zjawiony, J. K., et al. (2015b). Novel activities of CYP11A1 and their potential physiological significance. *J. Steroid Biochem. Mol. Biol.* 151, 25–37. doi: 10.1016/j.jsbmb.2014.11.010

Slominski, A. T., Zmijewski, M. A., Semak, I., Sweatman, T., Janjetovic, Z., Li, W., et al. (2009). Sequential metabolism of 7-dehydrocholesterol to steroidal 5,7-dienes in adrenal glands and its biological implication in the skin. *PLoS One* 4:e4309. doi: 10.1371/journal.pone.0004309

Slominski, A. T., Zmijewski, M. A., Zbytek, B., Tobin, D. J., Theoharides, T. C., and Rivier, J. (2013). Key role of CRF in the skin stress response system. *Endocr. Rev.* 34, 827–884. doi: 10.1210/er.2012-1092

Snipes, G. J., and Suter, U. (1997). Cholesterol and myelin. *Subcell. Biochem.* 28, 173–204. doi: 10.1007/978-1-4615-5901-6_7

Soffientini, U., and Graham, A. (2016). Intracellular cholesterol transport proteins: roles in health and disease. *Clin. Sci.* 130, 1843–1859. doi: 10.1042/cs20160339

Stanley, E. L., Hume, R., Visser, T. J., and Coughtrie, M. W. (2001). Differential expression of sulfotransferase enzymes involved in thyroid hormone metabolism during human placental development. *J. Clin. Endocrinol. Metab.* 86, 5944–5955. doi: 10.1210/jcem.86.12.8081

Stefulj, J., Panzenboeck, U., Becker, T., Hirschmugl, B., Schweinzer, C., Lang, I., et al. (2009). Human endothelial cells of the placental barrier efficiently deliver cholesterol to the fetal circulation via ABCA1 and ABCG1. *Circ. Res.* 104, 600–608. doi: 10.1161/CIRCRESAHA.108.185066

Steinberg, M. L., and Robins, J. C. (2016). Cellular models of trophoblast differentiation. *Semin. Reprod. Med.* 34, 50–56. doi: 10.1055/s-0035-1570026

Stirrat, L. I., Sengers, B. G., Norman, J. E., Homer, N. Z. M., Andrew, R., Lewis, R. M., et al. (2018). transfer and metabolism of cortisol by the isolated perfused human placenta. *J. Clin. Endocrinol. Metab.* 103, 640–648. doi: 10.1210/jc.2017-02140

St-Pierre, M. V., Hagenbuch, B., Ugele, B., Meier, P. J., and Stallmach, T. (2002). Characterization of an organic anion-transporting polypeptide (OATP-B) in human placenta. *J. Clin. Endocrinol. Metab.* 87, 1856–1863. doi: 10.1210/jcem.87.4.8431

Sugawara, T., Holt, J. A., Driscoll, D., Strauss, J. F., Lin, D., Miller, W. L., et al. (1995). Human steroidogenic acute regulatory protein: functional activity in COS-1 cells, tissue-specific expression, and mapping of the structural gene to 8p11.2 and a pseudogene to chromosome 13. *Proc. Natl. Acad. Sci. U.S.A.* 92, 4778–4782. doi: 10.1073/pnas.92.11.4778

Sun, K., Adamson, S. L., Yang, K., and Challis, J. R. (1999). Interconversion of cortisol and cortisone by 11beta-hydroxysteroid dehydrogenases type 1 and 2 in the perfused human placenta. *Placenta* 20, 13–19. doi: 10.1053/plac.1998.0352

Sun, Y., Kopp, S., Strutz, J., Gali, C. C., Zandl-Lang, M., Fanaee-Danesh, E., et al. (2018). Gestational diabetes mellitus modulates cholesterol homeostasis in human fetoplacental endothelium. *Biochim. Biophys. Acta* 1863, 968–979. doi: 10.1016/j.bbalip.2018.05.005

Suzuki, T., Miki, Y., Nakata, T., Shiotsu, Y., Akinaga, S., Inoue, K., et al. (2003). Steroid sulfatase and estrogen sulfotransferase in normal human tissue and breast carcinoma. *J. Steroid Biochem. Mol. Biol.* 86, 449–454. doi: 10.1016/S0960-0760(03)00356-X

Takeyama, J., Sasano, H., Suzuki, T., Iinuma, K., Nagura, H., and Andersson, S. (1998). 17Beta-hydroxysteroid dehydrogenase types 1 and 2 in human placenta: an immunohistochemical study with correlation to placental development. *J. Clin. Endocrinol. Metab.* 83, 3710–3715. doi: 10.1210/jcem.83.10.5212

Tartakover-Matalon, S., Cherepnin, N., Kuchuk, M., Drucker, L., Kenis, I., Fishman, A., et al. (2007). Impaired migration of trophoblast cells caused by simvastatin is associated with decreased membrane IGF-I receptor, MMP2 activity and HSP27 expression. *Hum. Reprod.* 22, 1161–1167. doi: 10.1093/humrep/del464

Telegdy, G., Weeks, J. W., Lerner, U., Stakemann, G., and Diczfalusy, E. (1970). Acetate and cholesterol metabolism in the human foeto-placental unit at midgestation. 1. Sunthesis of cholesterol. *Acta Endocrinol.* 63, 91–104.

Thibeault, A. H., Sanderson, J. T., and Vaillancourt, C. (2018). Co-culture of H295R adrenocortical carcinoma and bewo choriocarcinoma cells to study feto-placental interactions: focus on estrogen biosynthesis. *Methods Mol. Biol.* 1710, 295–304. doi: 10.1007/978-1-4939-7498-6_23

Thomas, M. P., and Potter, B. V. (2013). The structural biology of oestrogen metabolism. *J. Steroid Biochem. Mol. Biol.* 137, 27–49. doi: 10.1016/j.jsbmb.2012.12.014

Thomson, M. (2013). The physiological roles of placental corticotropin releasing hormone in pregnancy and childbirth. *J. Physiol. Biochem.* 69, 559–573. doi: 10.1007/s13105-012-0227-2

Tint, G. S., Salen, G., Batta, A. K., Shefer, S., Irons, M., Elias, E. R., et al. (1995). Correlation of severity and outcome with plasma sterol levels in variants of the Smith-Lemli-Opitz syndrome. *J. Pediatr.* 127, 82–87. doi: 10.1016/S0022-3476(95)70261-X

Tiwari, D., Bose, P. D., Sultana, R., Das, C. R., and Bose, S. (2016). Preterm delivery and associated negative pregnancy outcome – A tale of faulty progesterone receptor signalling pathway and linked derailed immunomodulation: a study from Northeast India. *J. Reprod. Immunol.* 118(Suppl. C), 76–84. doi: 10.1016/j.jri.2016.10.001

Tomi, M., Eguchi, H., Ozaki, M., Tawara, T., Nishimura, S., Higuchi, K., et al. (2015). Role of OAT4 in uptake of estriol precursor 16α-hydroxydehydroepiandrosterone sulfate into human placental syncytiotrophoblasts from fetus. *Endocrinology* 156, 2704–2712. doi: 10.1210/en.2015-1130

Tomi, M., Miyata, Y., Noguchi, S., Nishimura, S., Nishimura, T., and Nakashima, E. (2014). Role of protein kinase A in regulating steroid sulfate uptake for estrogen production in human placental choriocarcinoma cells. *Placenta* 35, 658–660. doi: 10.1016/j.placenta.2014.06.003

Tranquilli, A. L., Dekker, G., Magee, L., Roberts, J., Sibai, B. M., Steyn, W., et al. (2014). The classification, diagnosis and management of the hypertensive disorders of pregnancy: a revised statement from the ISSHP. *Pregnancy Hypertens.* 4, 97–104. doi: 10.1016/j.preghy.2014.02.001

Trapani, L., and Pallottini, V. (2010). Age-related hypercholesterolemia and HMG-CoA reductase dysregulation: sex does matter (a gender perspective). *Curr. Gerontol. Geriatr. Res.* 2010:420139. doi: 10.1155/2010/420139

Trapani, L., Violo, F., and Pallottini, V. (2010). Hypercholesterolemia and 3-hydroxy-3-methylglutaryl coenzyme A reductase regulation in aged female rats. *Exp. Gerontol.* 45, 119–128. doi: 10.1016/j.exger.2009.10.014

Tuckey, R. C. (2005). Progesterone synthesis by the human placenta. *Placenta* 26, 273–281. doi: 10.1016/j.placenta.2004.06.012

Tuckey, R. C., Bose, H. S., Czerwionka, I., and Miller, W. L. (2004). Molten globule structure and steroidogenic activity of N-218 MLN64 in human placental mitochondria. *Endocrinology* 145, 1700–1707. doi: 10.1210/en.2003-1034

Ugele, B., Bahn, A., and Rex-Haffner, M. (2008). Functional differences in steroid sulfate uptake of organic anion transporter 4 (OAT4) and organic anion transporting polypeptide 2B1 (OATP2B1) in human placenta. *J. Steroid Biochem. Mol. Biol.* 111, 1–6. doi: 10.1016/j.jsbmb.2008.04.001

Ugele, B., St-Pierre, M. V., Pihusch, M., Bahn, A., and Hantschmann, P. (2003). Characterization and identification of steroid sulfate transporters of human placenta. *Am. J. Physiol. Endocrinol. Metab.* 284, E390–E398. doi: 10.1152/ajpendo.00257.2002

Uhr, M., Holsboer, F., and Muller, M. B. (2002). Penetration of endogenous steroid hormones corticosterone, cortisol, aldosterone and progesterone into the brain is enhanced in mice deficient for both mdr1a and mdr1b P-glycoproteins. *J. Neuroendocrinol.* 14, 753–759. doi: 10.1046/j.1365-2826.2002.00836.x

Ulrich, V., Gelber, S. E., Vukelic, M., Sacharidou, A., Herz, J., Urbanus, R. T., et al. (2016). ApoE receptor 2 mediation of trophoblast dysfunction and pregnancy complications induced by antiphospholipid antibodies in mice. *Arthritis Rheumatol.* 68, 730–739. doi: 10.1002/art.39453

Uzun, H., Benian, A., Madazli, R., Topcuoglu, M. A., Aydin, S., and Albayrak, M. (2005). Circulating oxidized low-density lipoprotein and paraoxonase activity in preeclampsia. *Gynecol. Obstet. Invest.* 60, 195–200. doi: 10.1159/000087205

Valbuena-Diez, A. C., Blanco, F. J., Oujo, B., Langa, C., Gonzalez-Nunez, M., Llano, E., et al. (2012). Oxysterol-induced soluble endoglin release and its involvement in hypertension. *Circulation* 126, 2612–2624. doi: 10.1161/circulationaha.112.101261

van Beek, J. P., Guan, H., Julan, L., and Yang, K. (2004). Glucocorticoids stimulate the expression of 11beta-hydroxysteroid dehydrogenase type 2 in cultured human placental trophoblast cells. *J. Clin. Endocrinol. Metab.* 89, 5614–5621. doi: 10.1210/jc.2004-0113

Vejux, A., Malvitte, L., and Lizard, G. (2008). Side effects of oxysterols: cytotoxicity, oxidation, inflammation, and phospholipidosis. *Braz. J. Med. Biol. Res.* 41, 545–556. doi: 10.1590/S0100-879X2008000700001

Voutilainen, R., and Miller, W. L. (1986). Developmental expression of genes for the stereoidogenic enzymes P450scc (20,22-desmolase), P450c17 (17 alpha-hydroxylase/17,20-lyase), and P450c21 (21-hydroxylase) in the human fetus. *J. Clin. Endocrinol. Metab.* 63, 1145–1150. doi: 10.1210/jcem-63-5-1145

Wadsack, C., Desoye, G., and Hiden, U. (2012). The feto-placental endothelium in pregnancy pathologies. *Wien. Med. Wochenschr.* 162, 220–224. doi: 10.1007/s10354-012-0075-2

Wadsack, C., Hammer, A., Levak-Frank, S., Desoye, G., Kozarsky, K. F., Hirschmugl, B., et al. (2003). Selective cholesteryl ester uptake from high density lipoprotein by human first trimester and term villous trophoblast cells. *Placenta* 24, 131–143. doi: 10.1053/plac.2002.0912

Wadsack, C., Tabano, S., Maier, A., Hiden, U., Alvino, G., Cozzi, V., et al. (2007). Intrauterine growth restriction is associated with alterations in placental lipoprotein receptors and maternal lipoprotein composition. *Am. J. Physiol. Endocrinol. Metab.* 292, E476–E484. doi: 10.1152/ajpendo.00547.2005

Walker, N., Filis, P., Soffientini, U., Bellingham, M., O'Shaughnessy, P. J., and Fowler, P. A. (2017). Placental transporter localization and expression in the human: the importance of species, sex, and gestational age differencesdagger. *Biol. Reprod.* 96, 733–742. doi: 10.1093/biolre/iox012

Walsh, M. T., and Hussain, M. M. (2017). Targeting microsomal triglyceride transfer protein and lipoprotein assembly to treat homozygous familial hypercholesterolemia. *Crit. Rev. Clin. Lab. Sci.* 54, 26–48. doi: 10.1080/10408363.2016.1221883

Wan, J., Hu, Z., Zeng, K., Yin, Y., Zhao, M., Chen, M., et al. (2018). The reduction in circulating levels of estrogen and progesterone in women with preeclampsia. *Pregnancy Hypertens.* 11, 18–25. doi: 10.1016/j.preghy.2017.12.003

Wang, C., Yang, J., Hao, Z., Gong, C., Tang, L., Xu, Y., et al. (2017). Suppression of progesterone synthesis in human trophoblast cells by fine particulate matter primarily derived from industry. *Environ. Pollut.* 231(Pt 1), 1172–1180. doi: 10.1016/j.envpol.2017.08.029

Wang, W., Li, J., Ge, Y., Li, W., Shu, Q., Guan, H., et al. (2012). Cortisol induces aromatase expression in human placental syncytiotrophoblasts through the cAMP/Sp1 pathway. *Endocrinology* 153, 2012–2022. doi: 10.1210/en.2011-1626

Wang, W. S., Liu, C., Li, W. J., Zhu, P., Li, J. N., and Sun, K. (2014). Involvement of CRH and hCG in the induction of aromatase by cortisol in human placental syncytiotrophoblasts. *Placenta* 35, 30–36. doi: 10.1016/j.placenta.2013.10.018

Warren, W. B., and Silverman, A. J. (1995). Cellular localization of corticotrophin releasing hormone in the human placenta, fetal membranes and decidua. *Placenta* 16, 147–156. doi: 10.1016/0143-4004(95)90003-9

Weedon-Fekjaer, M. S., Dalen, K. T., Solaas, K., Staff, A. C., Duttaroy, A. K., and Nebb, H. I. (2010a). Activation of LXR increases acyl-CoA synthetase activity through direct regulation of ACSL3 in human placental trophoblast cells. *J. Lipid Res.* 51, 1886–1896. doi: 10.1194/jlr.M004978

Weedon-Fekjaer, M. S., Johnsen, G. M., Anthonisen, E. H., Sugulle, M., Nebb, H. I., Duttaroy, A. K., et al. (2010b). Expression of liver X receptors in pregnancies complicated by preeclampsia. *Placenta* 31, 818–824. doi: 10.1016/j.placenta.2010.06.015

Weissgerber, T. L., and Wolfe, L. A. (2006). Physiological adaptation in early human pregnancy: adaptation to balance maternal-fetal demands. *Appl. Physiol. Nutr. Metab.* 31, 1–11. doi: 10.1139/h05-003

Wetendorf, M., and DeMayo, F. J. (2012). The progesterone receptor regulates implantation, decidualization, and glandular development via a complex paracrine signaling network. *Mol. Cell. Endocrinol.* 357, 108–118. doi: 10.1016/j.mce.2011.10.028

Wetendorf, M., and DeMayo, F. J. (2014). Progesterone receptor signaling in the initiation of pregnancy and preservation of a healthy uterus. *Int. J. Dev. Biol.* 58, 95–106. doi: 10.1387/ijdb.140069mw

Whirledge, S., and DeFranco, D. B. (2018). Glucocorticoid signaling in health and disease: insights from tissue-specific GR knockout mice. *Endocrinology* 159, 46–64. doi: 10.1210/en.2017-00728

Winkel, C. A., Gilmore, J., MacDonald, P. C., and Simpson, E. R. (1980a). Uptake and degradation of lipoproteins by human trophoblastic cells in primary culture. *Endocrinology* 107, 1892–1898. doi: 10.1210/endo-107-6-1892

Winkel, C. A., Snyder, J. M., Macdonald, P. C., and Simpson, E. R. (1980b). Regulation of cholesterol and progesterone synthesis in human placental cells in culture by serum lipoproteins. *Endocrinology* 106, 1054–1060. doi: 10.1210/endo-106-4-1054

Winkel, C. A., MacDonald, P. C., and Simpson, E. R. (1981). The role of receptor-mediated low-density lipoprotein uptake and degradation in the regulation of progesterone biosynthesis and cholesterol metabolism by human trophoblasts. *Placenta Suppl.* 3, 133–143.

Winkler, B. S., Pecks, U., Najjari, L., Kleine-Eggebrecht, N., Maass, N., Mohaupt, M., et al. (2017). Maternal 27-hydroxycholesterol concentrations during the course of pregnancy and in pregnancy pathologies. *BMC Pregnancy Childbirth* 17:106. doi: 10.1186/s12884-017-1287-7

Winkler, K., Wetzka, B., Hoffmann, M. M., Friedrich, I., Kinner, M., Baumstark, M. W., et al. (2000). Low density lipoprotein (LDL) subfractions during pregnancy: accumulation of buoyant LDL with advancing gestation. *J. Clin. Endocrinol. Metab.* 85, 4543–4550. doi: 10.1210/jcem.85.12.7027

Wittmaack, F. M., Gafvels, M. E., Bronner, M., Matsuo, H., Mccrae, K. R., Tomaszewski, J. E., et al. (1995). Localization and regulation of the human very-low-density lipoprotein apolipoprotein-e receptor - trophoblast expression predicts a role for the receptor in placental lipid transport. *Endocrinology* 136, 340–348. doi: 10.1210/en.136.1.340

Woo, C. S. J., Wan, M. L. Y., Ahokas, J., and El-Nezami, H. (2013). Potential endocrine disrupting effect of ochratoxin A on human placental 3β-hydroxysteroid dehydrogenase/isomerase in JEG-3 cells at levels relevant to human exposure. *Reprod. Toxicol.* 38, 47–52. doi: 10.1016/j.reprotox.2013.02.034

Woollett, L., and Heubi, J. E. (2000). "Fetal and neonatal cholesterol metabolism," in Endotext, eds L. J. De Groot, G. Chrousos, K. Dungan, K. R. Feingold, A. Grossman, J. M. Hershman, C. Koch, M. Korbonits, R. McLachlan, M. New, J. Purnell, R. Rebar, F. Singer, and A. Vinik (South Dartmouth MA: MDText.com Inc.).

Woollett, L. A. (1996). Origin of cholesterol in the fetal golden Syrian hamster: contribution of de novo sterol synthesis and maternal-derived lipoprotein cholesterol. *J. Lipid Res.* 37, 1246–1257.

Woollett, L. A. (2005). Maternal cholesterol in fetal development: transport of cholesterol from the maternal to the fetal circulation. *Am. J. Clin. Nutr.* 82, 1155–1161. doi: 10.1093/ajcn/82.6.1155

Woollett, L. A. (2011). Review: transport of maternal cholesterol to the fetal circulation. *Placenta* 32(Suppl. 2), S218–S221. doi: 10.1016/j.placenta.2011.01.011

Wu, L., Yan, J., Qu, S. C., Feng, Y. Q., and Jiang, X. L. (2012). Abnormal regulation for progesterone production in placenta with prenatal cocaine exposure in rats. *Placenta* 33, 977–981. doi: 10.1016/j.placenta.2012.10.001

Yang, H. Y., Lee, Q. P., Rettie, A. E., and Juchau, M. R. (1994). Functional cytochrome P4503A isoforms in human embryonic tissues: expression during organogenesis. *Mol. Pharmacol.* 46, 922–928.

Yang, Q., Wang, W., Liu, C., Wang, Y., and Sun, K. (2016). Compartmentalized localization of 11beta-HSD 1 and 2 at the feto-maternal interface in the first trimester of human pregnancy. *Placenta* 46, 63–71. doi: 10.1016/j.placenta.2016.08.079

Yang, R., You, X., Tang, X., Gao, L., and Ni, X. (2006). Corticotropin-releasing hormone inhibits progesterone production in cultured human placental trophoblasts. *J. Mol. Endocrinol.* 37, 533–540. doi: 10.1677/jme.1.02119

Yao, L., Jenkins, K., Horn, P. S., Lichtenberg, M. H., and Woollett, L. A. (2007). Inability to fully suppress sterol synthesis rates with exogenous sterol in embryonic and extraembyronic fetal tissues. *Biochim. Biophys. Acta* 1771, 1372–1379. doi: 10.1016/j.bbalip.2007.09.002

Yoshida, N., and Osawa, Y. (1991). Purification of human placental aromatase cytochrome P-450 with monoclonal antibody and its characterization. *Biochemistry* 30, 3003–3010. doi: 10.1021/bi00226a004

You, X., Yang, R., Tang, X., Gao, L., and Ni, X. (2006). Corticotropin-releasing hormone stimulates estrogen biosynthesis in cultured human placental trophoblasts. *Biol. Reprod.* 74, 1067–1072. doi: 10.1095/biolreprod.105.049361

Zabul, P., Wozniak, M., Slominski, A. T., Preis, K., Gorska, M., Korozan, M., et al. (2015). A Proposed molecular mechanism of high-dose vitamin D3 supplementation in prevention and treatment of preeclampsia. *Int. J. Mol. Sci.* 16, 13043–13064. doi: 10.3390/ijms160613043

Zarrouk, A., Vejux, A., Mackrill, J., O'Callaghan, Y., Hammami, M., O'Brien, N., et al. (2014). Involvement of oxysterols in age-related diseases and ageing processes. *Ageing Res. Rev.* 18, 148–162. doi: 10.1016/j.arr.2014.09.006

Zeybek, B., Costantine, M., Kilic, G. S., and Borahay, M. A. (2018). Therapeutic roles of statins in gynecology and obstetrics: the current evidence. *Reprod. Sci.* 25, 802–817. doi: 10.1177/1933719117750751

Zhang, E. G., Burton, G. J., Smith, S. K., and Charnock-Jones, D. S. (2002). Placental vessel adaptation during gestation and to high altitude: changes in diameter and perivascular cell coverage. *Placenta* 23, 751–762. doi: 10.1053/plac.2002.0856

Zhang, R., Dong, S., Ma, W. W., Cai, X. P., Le, Z. Y., Xiao, R., et al. (2017). Modulation of cholesterol transport by maternal hypercholesterolemia in human full-term placenta. *PLoS One* 12:e0171934. doi: 10.1371/journal.pone.0171934

Zhao, C., and Dahlman-Wright, K. (2010). Liver X receptor in cholesterol metabolism. *J. Endocrinol.* 204, 233–240. doi: 10.1677/joe-09-0271

Zhu, X. M., Han, T., Sargent, I. L., Yin, G. W., and Yao, Y. Q. (2009). Differential expression profile of microRNAs in human placentas from preeclamptic pregnancies vs normal pregnancies. *Am. J. Obstet. Gynecol.* 200, 661.e1–667.e1. doi: 10.1016/j.ajog.2008.12.045

8

The Significance of the Sulfatase Pathway for Local Estrogen Formation in Endometrial Cancer

*Maša Sinreih[1], Tamara Knific[1], Maja Anko[1], Neli Hevir[1], Katja Vouk[1], Aleš Jerin[2], Snježana Frković Grazio[3] and Tea Lanišnik Rižner[1]**

[1] Institute of Biochemistry, Faculty of Medicine, University of Ljubljana, Ljubljana, Slovenia, [2] Institute of Clinical Chemistry and Biochemistry, University Medical Centre, Ljubljana, Slovenia, [3] Division of Obstetrics and Gynecology, Department of Pathology, University Medical Centre, Ljubljana, Slovenia

***Correspondence:**
Tea Lanišnik Rižner
tea.lanisnik-rizner@mf.uni-lj.si

Endometrial cancer (EC) is the most common estrogen-dependent gynecological malignancy in the developed World. To investigate the local formation of estradiol (E2), we first measured the concentrations of the steroid precursor androstenedione (A-dione) and the most potent estrogen, E2, and we evaluated the metabolism of A-dione, estrone-sulfate (E1-S), and estrone (E1) in cancerous and adjacent control endometrium. Furthermore, we studied expression of the key genes for estradiol formation via the aromatase and sulfatase pathways. A-dione and E2 were detected in cancerous and adjacent control endometrium. In cancerous endometrium, A-dione was metabolized to testosterone, and no E2 was formed. Both, E1-S and E1 were metabolized to E2, with increased levels of E2 seen in cancerous tissue. There was no significant difference in expression of the key genes of the aromatase (*CYP19A1*) and the sulfatase (*STS*, *HSD17B1*, *HSD17B2*) pathways in cancerous endometrium compared to adjacent control tissue. The mRNA levels of *CYP19A1* and *HSD17B1* were low, and *HSD17B14,* which promotes inactivation of E2, was significantly down-regulated in cancerous endometrium, especially in patients with lymphovascular invasion. At the protein level, there were no differences in the levels of STS and HSD17B2 between cancerous and adjacent control tissue by Western blotting, and immunohistochemistry revealed intense staining for STS and HSD17B2, and weak staining for SULT1E1 and HSD17B1 in cancerous tissue. Our data demonstrate that in cancerous endometrium, E2 is formed from E1-S *via* the sulfatase pathway, and not from A-dione *via* the aromatase pathway.

Keywords: aromatase, 17β-hydroxysteroid dehydrogenases, aldo-keto reductase 1C3, sulfotransferases, sulfatase

INTRODUCTION

Endometrial cancer (EC) is the fifth-most-common cancer in women in Western Europe and the USA, with the majority of cases arising after menopause (Colombo et al., 2016; Morice et al., 2016). EC can be classified into estrogen-dependent type I, which comprises 80% of all cases, and the poorly differentiated, more aggressive, type II. Although, type II EC was considered to be estrogen independent (Inoue, 2001; Samarnthai et al., 2010), experimental data suggest involvement of estrogens (Berstein et al., 2003; Wan et al., 2016).

Local estrogen formation has an important role in the development of EC and increased estradiol (E2) concentrations have been detected in cancerous, as compared to normal endometrium (Berstein et al., 2003). Locally, E2 can be formed either via the so-called aromatase pathway from androstenedione (A-dione), which originates from dehydroepiandrosterone-sulfate (DHEA-S) and DHEA, or from testosterone (T), by the actions of aromatase and the reductive 17β-hydroxysteroid dehydrogenases (enzymes 17β-HSD, HSD17B; **Figure 1**). These are NADPH dependent enzymes, which due to high intracellular concentration ratio NADPH/$NADP^+$ act preferentially as reductases in a cellular context (Agarwal and Auchus, 2005). The most potent estrogen, E2 can also be formed from estrone-sulfate (E1-S) via the sulfatase pathway by the actions of sulfatase (STS) and the reductive enzymes HSD17B (**Figure 1**).

The aromatase pathway depends on availability of A-dione or T. A-dione, with 1–8 nM concentrations in blood, originates mainly from adrenal gland (zona reticularis), from ovaries in premenopausal women and also from conversions of DHEA-S and DHEA in peripheral tissues. Aromatase (CYP19A1) converts A-dione and T into estrone (E1) and E2, respectively (Krekels et al., 1991). As the plasma concentrations of A-dione in postmenopausal women are ~4-fold higher than those of T (Simpson, 2002; Keefe et al., 2014), aromatase mainly converts A-dione to E1. Currently, the data on aromatase expression in EC are controversial, with everything from high levels, to no significant differences between diseased and normal tissues, to no expression being reported (Yamamoto et al., 1993; Watanabe et al., 1995; Berstein et al., 2005; Jongen et al., 2005; Segawa et al., 2005; Lanišnik Rižner et al., 2006; Pathirage et al., 2006; Smuc and Rizner, 2009; Takahashi-Shiga et al., 2009; Lepine et al., 2010; Cornel et al., 2012).

E1 formed from A-dione should be further activated by the reductive estrogenic 17β-HSD type 1 (HSD17B1), to form E2. Although, several groups have failed to detect expression of *HSD17B1* in normal and cancerous endometrium, others have seen low mRNA levels in both tissues (Casey et al., 1994; Zeitoun et al., 1998; Utsunomiya et al., 2001; Lanišnik Rižner et al., 2006; Smuc and Rizner, 2009) with decreased mRNA levels in EC compared to adjacent control endometrial tissue (Smuc and Rizner, 2009; Lepine et al., 2010). In contrast Cornel et al. (2012) showed increased mRNA levels of *HSD17B1* in ERα positive grade 1 EC compared to control tissue.

In addition to HSD17B1, three other reductive estrogenic 17β-HSDs, types 7 and 12 (HSD17B7 and HSD17B12), and type 5 (aldo-keto reductase 1C3, AKR1C3), that can form E2 from E1, albeit with lower catalytic efficiencies, can contribute to E2 formation. Also the expression of these genes in EC is rather controversial as has been reviewed (Rižner, 2013). There were no significant differences in mRNA levels of *AKR1C3* (Rizner et al., 2006; Smuc and Rizner, 2009; Cornel et al., 2012), the expression of *HSD17B7* was reported as decreased (Smuc and Rizner, 2009) or unchanged (Lepine et al., 2010; Cornel et al., 2012) and expression of *HSD17B12* was unchanged (Smuc and Rizner, 2009; Cornel et al., 2012) or increased (Lepine et al., 2010) in EC compared to control tissue.

The expression of the oxidative NAD^+ dependent estrogenic 17β-HSDs, types 2, 4, 8, and 14 (HSD17B2, HSD17B4, HSD17B8, and HSD17B14), can also affect local E2 concentrations. These enzymes catalyze inactivation of E2 to E1. Previous studies by Lepine et al., and our group revealed increased mRNA levels of *HSD17B2* (Lepine et al., 2010; Sinreih et al., 2013) in EC, while Cornel et al. found no significant difference in ERα positive grade 1 EC (Cornel et al., 2012). For *HSD17B4* and *HSD17B8* we saw no changes in gene expression in EC compared to adjacent control tissue (Smuc and Rizner, 2009), while expression of *HSD17B14* has not yet been studied in EC.

E2 can also be formed *via* the sulfatase pathway from E1-S by the actions of STS and the reductive enzymes HSD17B1, HSD17B7, HSD17B12, and also AKR1C3. Unchanged (Smuc and Rizner, 2009), and increased (Lepine et al., 2010) expression of *STS* have previously been reported in EC. Sulfotransferase SULT1E1 catalyzes conjugation of estrogens and our previous studies show that gene encoding this enzyme is not differentially expressed in EC as compared to adjacent control tissue (Hevir et al., 2011b), while Lepine et al., reported borderline increased mRNA levels in cancer tissue (Lepine et al., 2010).

There is a great need for a better understanding of the local formation of E2 in cancerous endometrium, which may reveal novel targets for treatment of this most common gynecological malignancy. The aims of the present study were thus to investigate E2 formation in paired samples of EC and adjacent control endometrium at different levels. Our goals were: (i) to determine concentrations of steroid precursor A-dione and the most potent estrogen E2, (ii) to examine capacity for formation of A-dione, E1-S and E1; (iii) to re-examine the mRNA levels of individual genes involved in the aromatase pathway and the sulfatase pathway of E2 formation, (iv) to evaluate protein levels of the key players in the sulfatase pathway, STS, SULT1E1, HSD17B2, and HSD17B1 and their prognostic potential.

MATERIALS AND METHODS

Endometrial Tissue

The specimens of EC and paired adjacent control endometrium were obtained from 55 patients undergoing hysterectomies for histologically proven EC (**Table 1**, Supplementary Table 1). The study was approved by the National Medical Ethics Committee of the Republic of Slovenia with written informed consent required from all subjects involved. The patients were all treated in the Department of Gynecology and Obstetrics at the University Medical Centre Ljubljana, from 2003 to 2010. The samples used for steroid concentration measurements, metabolism studies, qPCR, Western blotting and immunohistochemical staining have been selected chronologically.

Steroid Concentration Measurements

Ten paired samples of EC and adjacent control tissue were frozen in liquid nitrogen and ground to a fine powder. Prior to extraction, 100–200 mg of homogenate was suspended in 0.1 M sodium phosphate buffer (pH 7.4). The extraction was

---

Abbreviations: A-dione, androstenedione; AKR, aldo-keto reductase; DHEA, dehydroepiandrosterone; DHEA-S, dehydroepiandrosterone sulfate; EC, endometrial cancer; E1, estrone; E1-S, estrone sulfate; E2, estradiol; ER, estrogen receptor; HSD, hydroxysteroid dehydrogenase; qPCR, quantitative real-time PCR; STS, sulfatase; SULT, sulfotransferase; T, testosterone.

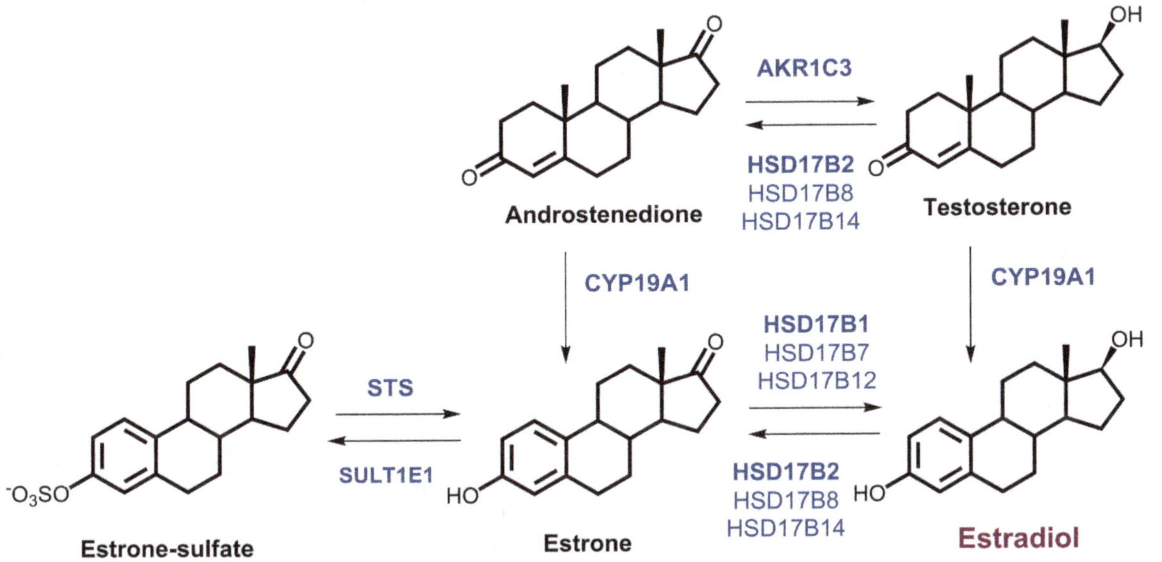

FIGURE 1 | Estrogen biosynthesis. Formation of estrogens via the aromatase pathway from androstenedione and testosterone, by the actions of aromatase (CYP19A1), and the reductive 17β-hydroxysteroid dehydrogenases types 1, 7, and 12 (HSD17B1, HSD17B7, HSD17B12) and type 5 (AKR1C3). Formation of estrogens via the sulfatase pathway from estrone-sulfate, by the action of sulfatase (STS), and the reductive HSD17B1, HSD17B7, and HSD17B12. The oxidative 17β-HSD types 2, 4, 8, and 14 (HSD17B2, HSD17B4, HSD17B8, HSD17B14) catalyze the inactivation of estradiol to estrone and sulfotransferase (SULT1E1) catalyzes conjugation of estrone.

performed three times with 4 mL of diethyl ether; the extracts were pooled and evaporated under a stream of nitrogen. Before analysis, the samples were resuspended in phosphate buffer. The levels of A-dione were measured using a double antibody radioimmunoassay with interassay CV < 10%, which uses a [^{125}I]-labeled tracer (Diagnostic Systems Laboratories, Webster, TX, USA). E2 was determined using an automated chemiluminescent immunoassay (Liaison, Diasorin, Saluggia, Italy) with interassay CV < 14%. Concentrations were calculated as pmol/g powdered tissue. The limit of detection was 0.1 pmol/g for A-dione and 0.4 pmol/g for E2.

RNA Isolation and qPCR

Total RNA was isolated from tissue samples using the Tri Reagent (Sigma Aldrich, St. Louis, MI, USA), according to the manufacturer instructions. The quality of the RNA samples was determined using an Agilent 2100 Bioanalyzer where they showed an average RIN of 7.7. The total RNA was reverse transcribed using SuperScript® VILO™ cDNA Synthesis kit (Invitrogen, Thermo Fisher Scientific, Carlsbad, CA, USA). One microgram of total RNA was converted into cDNA (20 μL) according to the manufacturer instructions, and then stored at −20°C. *CYP19A1*, *STS*, *HSD17B1*, and *HSD17B14* mRNA expression levels were determined with the exon-spanning hydrolysis probes (FAM or VIC dye labeled) that are commercially available as "Assay on Demand" (Applied Biosystems, Foster City, CA, USA). The qPCR analysis was performed in 27 samples of EC and adjacent control endometrium for *STS* and *HSD17B1*, in 22 paired samples for *CYP19A1* and 21 paired samples for *HSD17B14*. *PPIA*, *HPRT1*, and *POLR2A* were selected as the most stable reference genes, as described previously (Hevir et al., 2011a). The assay details are shown in Supplementary Table 2. The gene expression for each sample was calculated from the crossing point value (Cp) as E^{-Cp}, divided by the normalization factor and multiplied by 10^{14}. For *HSD17B14* and *CYP19A1*, only *PPIA* was used as the reference gene for the relative quantification with the comparative Ct method. Expression levels were multiplied by 10^{14}.

Western Blotting

Proteins were isolated from samples of EC tissue and the adjacent control endometrial tissue previously used for RNA isolation, following the Tri Reagent instructions. Protein concentrations were determined by Bradford assay and protein aliquots of 30 μg were separated by SDS PAGE on 10% Tris-glycine gels. The proteins were transferred from gels to polyvinylidene difluoride membranes (Millipore Corporation, Billerica, MA, USA) and incubated with 5% non-fat milk in Tris Buffered Saline buffer, with 0.1% Tween® 20 (TTBS) or with 5% BSA in TTBS, both for 2 h, when evaluating STS. The membranes were then incubated with antibodies against STS, HSD17B2, SULT1E1, and HSD17B1 and GAPDH, as normalization control, using antibodies and protocols described in Supplementary Table 3 (Dibbelt and Kuss, 1986; Dibbelt et al., 1989). Protein extracts from model cell lines of control endometrium (HIEEC), EC (HEC-1A), and liver cancer (HepG2) were used as controls.

Supersignal™ West Pico Chemiluminiscence Substrate (Thermo Fischer Scientific, Life Tecnologies, Carlsbad, CA, USA) was used for detection of the bound antibodies, according to the manufacturer instructions, using a Fujifilm LAS4000 image reader (Fujifilm, Tokyo, Japan). Detection of GAPDH was

TABLE 1 | Demographic and histopathological characteristics of the endometrial cancer patients.

Characteristics	Patient sample size	Mean ± *SD*
Age (years)	55	62.0 ± 13.7
Weight (kg)	53	82.2 ± 18.2
Height (cm)	49	163.1 ± 5.2
BMI (kg/m^2)	49	30.9 ± 7.0
MENOPAUSAL STATUS		
Premenopausal	16	
Postmenopausal	38	
NA	1	
Endometrioid adenocarcinoma	45	
Papillary serous carcinoma	6	
Carcinosarcoma	1	
Dedifferentiated	3	
GRADE		
G1	32	
G2	8	
G3	5	
INVASION OF MYOMETRIUM		
<50%	39	
≥50%	14	
NA	1	
PRESENCE OF LYMPHOVASCULAR INVASION		
No	39	
Yes	13	
NA	2	
FIGO STAGE		
IA	37	
IB	11	
II	1	
III	3	
IV	2	
NA	1	

G1–G3 endometrioid adenocarcinoma; NA, data not available.

used as the normalization control. Quantification of the Western blotting was carried out with ImageJ (National Institutes of Health, USA) or the Multi Gauge software (Fujifilm software, Fujifilm, Tokyo, Japan).

Steroid Hormone Metabolism Studies

A-dione Metabolism

From 60 to 85 mg of homogenized tissue from seven paired samples was resuspended in 470 μL of 50 mM sodium phosphate buffer pH 7.4 with protease inhibitor cocktail (Sigma Aldrich, St. Louis, MI, USA) added. This mixture was incubated with 80 nM androst-4-ene-3,[1,2,6,7-^{3}H(N)]-,17-dione in the presence of 2 mM NADPH in a reaction volume of 500 μL, for 20 h at 37°C. The steroids were extracted with ethyl acetate (3 × 500 μL), dried, resuspended in 40 μL ethyl acetate, and applied to Whatman Partisil® LK6DF silica gel TLC plates. The chromatograms were developed in cyclohexane/ethyl acetate (1:1, v/v), followed by autoradiography using Kodak BioMax MS-Films and LE Intensifying Screen (Sigma Aldrich, St. Louis, MI, USA) with incubation at −80°C for 6 days. The bands were identified by co-migration with authentic standards. Samples were next re-extracted from silica gel with ethyl acetate (3 × 500 μL), dried, resuspended in 40 μL ethyl acetate, applied to new silica gel TLC plates, and developed in cyclohexane/ethanol (95:5, v/v).

Additionally, 24 mg of homogenized tissue from three paired samples were incubated with 8 nM androst-4-ene-3,[1,2,6,7-^{3}H(N)], 17-dione in 50 mM sodium phosphate buffer, pH 7.4, with protease inhibitor cocktail (Sigma Aldrich, St. Louis, MI, USA) and 2.6 mM NADP$^+$, 5 mM Glucose-6-Phosphate, and 2.5 U of GAPDH. After 20 h incubation at 37°C the steroids were extracted from the medium with ethyl acetate (3 × 500 μL), dried in a SpeedVac™, and resuspended in 50% acetonitrile in water. The samples were then analyzed by HPLC using a Kinetex 2.6 μ XB-C18 column (150 × 4.6 mm; Phenomenex; Aschaffenburg, Germany) equipped with a Securityguard guard column and Securityguard cartridges (C18; 4 × 3.0 mm; Phenomenex, Aschaffenburg, Germany). The mobile phase was acetonitrile: water, 1:1, and the flow rate was 0.7 mL/min. The column temperature was 38°C. Conversion rates were obtained after integration of chromatograms and calculations to determine the percentages of transformation.

E1 and E1-S Metabolism

From 17 to 35 mg of homogenized tissue from 12 paired samples was resuspended in 50 mM sodium phosphate buffer (pH 7.4), with protease inhibitors (one tablet of Complete™ [Roche Molecular Biochemicals, Basel, Switzerland]/10 mL buffer). The tissue suspensions were incubated with 10 nM estrone, [2,4,6,7-^{3}H(N)]- and 6 mM NADPH in a reaction volume of 500 μL for 19 h at 37°C. The reaction was stopped with the addition of 100 μL 0.5 M ascorbic acid/1% acetic acid in methanol, and the mixture was centrifuged at 15,800 × g for 5 min. The supernatant was cleaned with solid phase extraction using Strata C-18E cartridges (Phenomenex, Aschaffenburg, Germany), according to the producer instructions, from which it was eluted with 2 × 350 μL methanol. The samples were then analyzed by HPLC (Beckman Coulter, Brea, CA, USA) using an Allure® Biphenyl Column [50 × 2.1 mm, particle size 3 μm (Restek Cooperation, Bellefonte, PA, USA)], with 55% (v/v) pure methanol mixed with 10% methanol, for 60 min at a flow rate of either 200 or 220 μL/min. Conversion rates were obtained after integration of chromatograms and evaluation with 24 Karat software (Beckman-Coulter, USA).

Additionally 24 mg of homogenized tissue from five paired samples was incubated with 16 nM ^{3}H E1-S in 50 mM phosphate buffer, pH 7.4 using the same procedure as described above for A-dione.

Immunohistochemistry

Pairs of tissue microarrays (TMA) with 3 mm cores of tumor and adjacent control endometrium were prepared from formalin-fixed, paraffin embedded tissues from 44 hysterectomy specimens. Five micrometers thick TMA sections were prepared, de-waxed in xylene and rehydrated. Immunohistochemical stainings for HSD17B2 and STS were performed on a fully automated Ventana BenchMark GX System (Ventana Medical Systems, Inc., Tuscon, AZ, USA). Protocol included a pretreatment step using Cell Conditioning Solution 1 (48 min at 37°C; Tris-based buffer pH 8.5) and incubation in H_2O_2 to block endogenous peroxidase. The anti-HSD17B2 (Solvay Pharmaceuticals, 1:100/Ventana diluent) and anti-STS antibodies (donated from prof. Dr. Gerhard Schuler 1:2,000/Ventana diluent; Supplementary Table 3) were added manually and the primary antibody incubation was set for 2 h. The Optiview DAB Detection Kit was used according to the manufacturer instructions. Placenta was used as a positive control.

Staining for SULT1E1 and HSD17B1 was done manually with Novolink Polymer Detection System (Leica Biosystems, Wetzlar, Germany) according to manufacturer instructions. For HSD17B1 detection two different antibodies were used (Supplementary Table 3). Antigen retrieval was performed with Tris-EDTA buffer (pH 9) in a pressure cooker for 20 min and TMA sections were incubated with anti-HSD17B1 polyclonal and monoclonal antibodies (Solvay Pharmaceuticals, 1:4,000, 1 h, room temperature and ab51045 EP1682Y; Abcam; Cambridge, UK, 1:70 in 1% BSA/PBS, overnight, 4°C). For SULT1E1 (Supplementary Table 3) antigen retrieval was done in citrate buffer (pH 6) in a pressure cooker for 20 min. The TMA sections were incubated with anti-SULT1E1 antibodies (HPA028728, R28328, Sigma Aldrich, Germany, 1:100, overnight, 4°C). DAB chromogen solution was used to detect the bound antibodies.

The immunohistochemical staining was assessed by a pathologist (SFG) based on the staining intensity (scored as: 1, weak; 2, moderate; 3, strong) and the percentage of stained cells. The immunohistochemical scores were calculated by multiplying the percentage of positive cells (P) by the intensities (I) (SCORING = P × I; maximum = 300).

Statistical Evaluation

The differences in expression levels of the selected genes were analyzed at the mRNA and protein levels in the cancerous endometrium, as compared to the adjacent control endometrium, using Wilcoxon matched-pair tests. Depending on the normality of sample distribution, the steroid concentration measurements in cancerous and control tissue were evaluated with either paired *t*-test or Wilcoxon matched pairs test. The statistical tests were two-tailed. Stratification analyses were done using repeated measures ANOVA. The differences in *p*-values of <0.05 were considered to be significant. The statistical calculations and tests were performed using GraphPad Prism software, version 5.00 (San Diego, CA, USA).

TABLE 2 | Androstenedione (A-dione) and estradiol (E2) concentrations in the cancer (Tumor) and adjacent control tissues (Control).

Sample	A-dione (pmol/g*)		E2 (pmol/g*)	
	Control	Tumor	Control	Tumor
49	0.63	0.41	2.24	3.47
50	5.08	6.54	13.00	4.71
51	<0.10	0.88	5.72	32.40
52	2.18	1.34	2.03	1.94
53	3.50	3.20	1.88	<0.40
54	17.19	9.22	3.76	3.06
55	1.69	0.30	<0.40	<0.40
56	0.20	<0.10	2.98	<0.40
57	5.27	1.45	11.73	7.67
58	1.53	1.34	0.78	0.97
Median	2.18	1.34	2.98	3.47
p-value	0.193		0.375	

*pmol/g of powdered tissue.

RESULTS

A-dione and E2 Are Present in Both Cancerous and Adjacent Control Endometrium

We measured A-dione and E2 concentrations in 10 paired samples of EC and adjacent control endometrium using radioimmunoassay and chemiluminescent immunoassay, respectively, which are still in routine clinical application for measuring blood concentrations (**Table 2**). A-dione was detected in 9 out of 10 samples, and E2 in seven of these samples. The variability in A-dione and E2 levels between patients was large and we found no significant differences in A-dione and E2 levels ($p = 0.193$ and 0.375, respectively) between EC and adjacent control tissue.

A-dione Is Metabolized to T in Cancerous and Adjacent Control Endometrium

A-dione formed locally in EC or A-dione from circulation might serve as precursor for E2 formation. We thus examined the ability of EC tissue for aromatization. We studied the metabolism of 80 nM ^3H labeled A-dione in seven paired samples of EC and adjacent control endometrium. In all of these samples, only conversion to T and much lower levels of 5α-androstanedione were detected by autoradiography after TLC in the first mobile phase (**Figure 2A**), while in the second mobile phase, 5α-dihydrotestosterone (5α-DHT) was also seen in two EC samples (**Figure 2B**). Aromatase activity was observed only in the control tissue, human placenta, where A-dione was metabolized to T, E1, and E2 (**Figures 2A,B**). As the first experiment included relatively high concentration of A-dione, we also examined the metabolism of 8 nM ^3H labeled A-dione in the presence of the NADPH regeneration system in three paired samples of EC and adjacent control endometrium. In this experiment the products

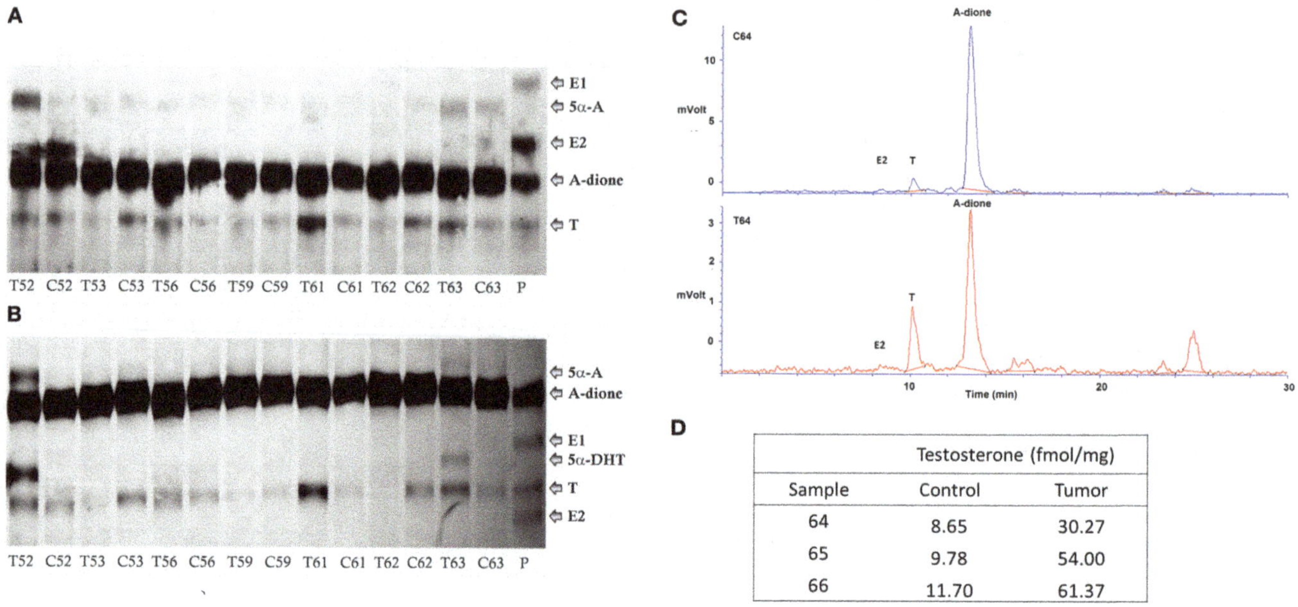

Sample	Testosterone (fmol/mg) Control	Tumor
64	8.65	30.27
65	9.78	54.00
66	11.70	61.37

FIGURE 2 | A-dione metabolism in the cancer and adjacent control endometrium. **(A)** Identification of the reaction products by autoradiography (TLC developed in cyclohexane/ ethyl acetate [1:1, v/v]) showing conversion of ^{3}H labeled A-dione (80 nM) to testosterone (T) and 5α-androstanedione (5α-A) in cancer, T, and corresponding control, C, tissues. In placenta, P, A-dione was metabolized to T, E1, and E2. **(B)** Autoradiography of the same samples that were extracted from silica gel and developed in cyclohexane/ ethanol (95:5, v/v), confirming the presence of 5α-dihydrotestosteone (5α-DHT) in two EC samples. **(C)** HPLC profiles demonstrates metabolism of ^{3}H labeled A-dione (8 nM) to T in control tissue and matched tumor tissue. **(D)** Formation of T (fmol/mg powdered tissue).

were separated by HPLC, where T was the major metabolite in all paired samples (**Figure 2C**) with increased formation of T seen in EC (**Figure 2D**). This is in agreement with our previous study in nine EC samples where 10 nM ^{3}H labeled A-dione was metabolized mainly to T with no E2 seen (Vouk and Rizner, Unpublished data; Supplementary Figure 1).

E1-S Is Metabolized to E2 in Cancerous and Adjacent Control Endometrium with Increased Formation of E2 Seen in Cancer Tissue

Since no E2 were formed by metabolism of A-dione in EC specimens, we next studied the ability of this tissue for metabolism of the major circulating estrogen, E1-S. This study was performed in five paired samples of EC and adjacent control tissue. Sixteen nM E1-S was metabolized to E1 and E2 in both, EC and adjacent control tissue, with significantly higher levels of E2 formed in cancerous tissue ($p = 0.0085$; **Figures 3A,B,D**). In addition to E2 and E1 also several unidentified polar metabolites were formed (**Figure 3C**). The metabolism of 10 nM E1 was further examined in 12 paired samples of EC and adjacent control endometrium. The formation of E2 was detected in all of the samples (**Figures 4A–C**); with a 2-fold, but non-significantly increased median levels seen in cancerous tissue ($p = 0.151$; **Figure 4A**). In seven samples of EC there was an increased E2 formation, in one sample there was no difference and in four samples of EC originating from one patient with serous EC and three patients with well-differentiated EC (G1) there was a decreased E2 formation as compared to adjacent control endometrial tissue (**Figure 4A**).

Genes for Local Formation of E2 via the Aromatase and Sulfatase Pathways Are Expressed in Cancerous Endometrium

Genes that are involved in local E2 formation from A-dione or E1S (**Figure 1**) are expressed in cancerous and adjacent control tissue. In the same cohort of EC patients, we previously reported no statistically significant differences in the expression of the majority of the genes involved in E2 formation: *CYP19A1*, *STS*, *HSD17B4*, *HSD17B8*, *HSD17B12*, and *SULT1E1*; however, *HSD17B1*, and *HSD17B7*, which promote E1 activation to E2, were down-regulated, and *HSD17B2*, which has the opposite role, was upregulated in the EC samples (Smuc and Rizner, 2009; Sinreih et al., 2013). In the present study, we re-examined the mRNA levels of *CYP19A1*, *STS*, and *HSD17B1* on a larger cohort of samples and found very low and unaltered mRNA levels of *CYP19A1* and *HSD17B1*. The mRNA levels of *STS* were about 1,000-fold higher than the levels of *HSD17B1*, but still unchanged in the EC and control tissues (**Figure 5**). With an arbitrary threshold of 1.2 for the ratio of mRNA levels in pairs of EC and adjacent control tissue we saw increased ratios in 8 out of 22 pairs for *CYP19A1*, 10 out of 27 pairs for *STS* and 9 out of 27 pairs for *HSD17B1*. We also investigated the mRNA levels of the oxidative *HSD17B14*, which has not yet been studied in EC and found high, but statistically significantly decreased levels ($p < 0.0001$) in cancer tissue, compared to control tissue.

A

E1-S metabolism (fmol/mg)				
Sample	Control	Tumor	Control	Tumor
	E1		E2	
61	131.15	160.56	15.41	90.66
63	136.35	148.53	6.49	38.32
64	191.84	106.53	22.32	51.43
65	109.47	127.99	14.03	92.91
66	152.60	159.80	18.14	106.99
Median	136.35	148.53	15.41	90.66
p value	0.8708		0.0085	

B

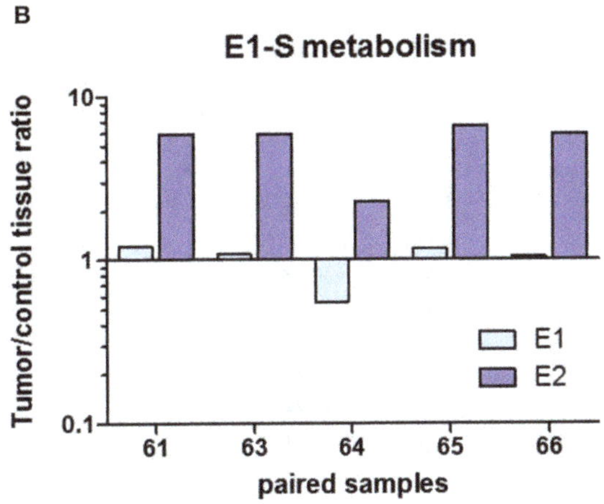

C

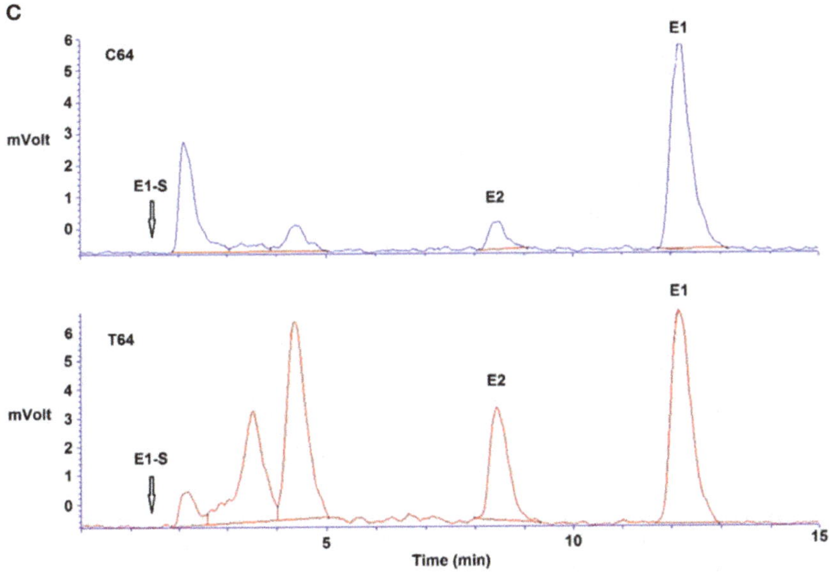

D

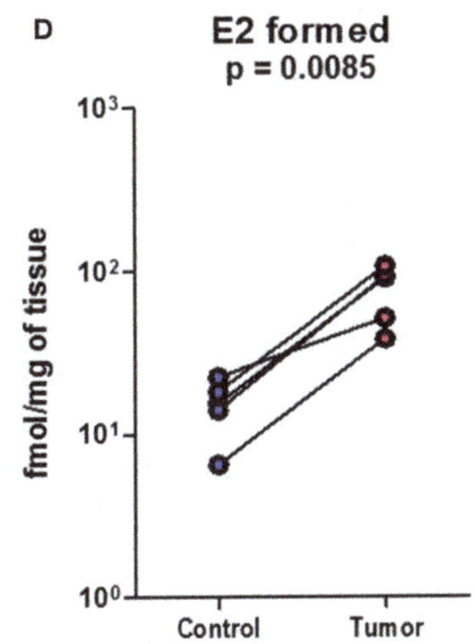

FIGURE 3 | E1-S metabolism in the EC and adjacent control endometrium. **(A)** Table for the conversion of E1-S to E1 and E2 (fmol/mg powdered tissue) in control and corresponding EC. **(B)** Histogram with logarithmic scale demonstrates increased tumor/ control tissue ratio for E2 formation in all paired samples. **(C)** HPLC elution profiles shows the formation of E2 and E1 from ^{3}H labeled E1-S (16 nM) for the representative samples of control (C64) and corresponding cancer (T64) tissues. Rf of E1-S and formation of several unidentified polar metabolites is also shown. **(D)** Before-and-after graph demonstrates levels of E2 formed in control endometrium (Control) and the corresponding EC (Tumor) for samples 61, 63, 64, 65, and 66.

Further, stratification according to clinical data (menopausal status and vital status of the patients' and FIGO stage) and histopathological data (histological type and grade of the tumor, depth of myometrial invasion, and presence of lymphovascular invasion) revealed differences in *STS*, *SULT1E1*, and *HSD17B14* expression (**Table 3**). *STS* was significantly downregulated ($p = 0.0439$) only in high grade tumors (G3) while in lower grade tumors (G1 and G2) *STS* levels did not differ between cancer and adjacent control tissue. The expression of *SULT1E1* was significantly downregulated ($p = 0.0392$) in cancer tissue from premenopausal women, with significantly lower levels seen in cancer and adjacent control tissue from postmenopausal women as compared to premenopausal women. The expression of *HSD17B14* changed in more invasive cancers, there was an extensive downregulation in cancer compared to adjacent control tissue form patients with lymphovascular invasion ($p = 0.0298$).

High Protein Levels of STS and HSD17B2 Are Seen in Cancerous and Adjacent Control Endometrium

As mRNA levels do not necessary correlate with protein levels and enzymatic activity, we also examined protein levels of STS, SULT1E1, HSD17B1, and HSD17B2. With the specific antibodies we performed Western blot analysis to evaluate protein levels of these enzymes in paired samples (**Figure 6**). We found high protein levels of STS, with increased levels in 12 EC samples out of 24, where this difference was not statistically significant (**Figures 6A–C**). SULT1E1 protein levels were very

A

Sample	E2 formation (fmol/mg)	
	Control	Tumor
49	34.36	27.43
50	0.06	410.78
52	9.56	38.15
53	45.31	98.47
54	23.52	82.23
55	50.55	6.68
56	30.63	35.63
58	19.38	166.43
59	7.90	14.06
61	14.77	53.21
62	19.71	3.72
63	29.52	20.07
Mean	23.77	79.74
p value	0.151	

B

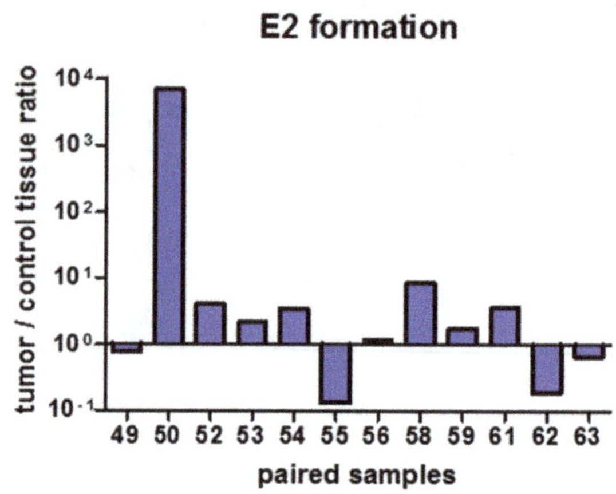

C

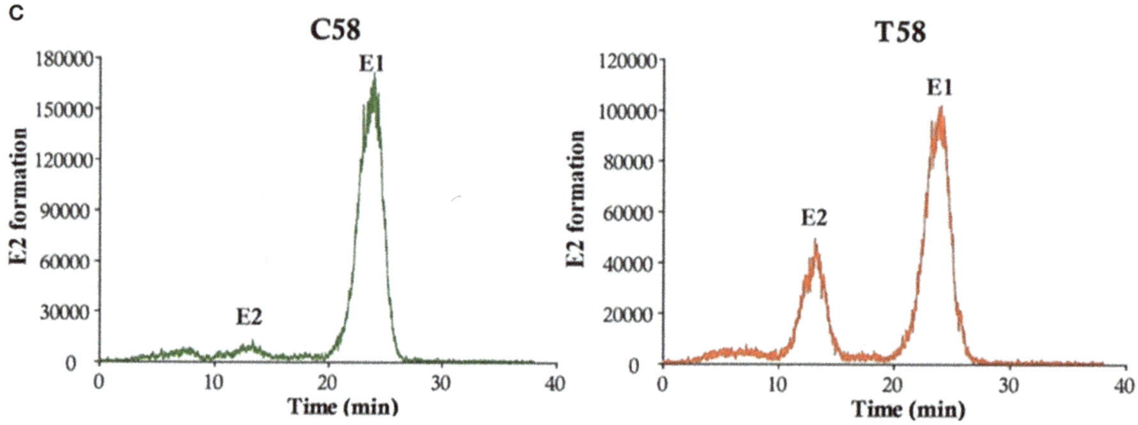

FIGURE 4 | E2 formation in the EC and adjacent control tissues. **(A)** Table showing the formation of E2 (fmol/mg powdered tissue) in control and corresponding cancer endometrium. **(B)** Histogram with logarithmic scale demonstrates increased tumor/ control tissue ratio for E2 in 7 of 12 paired samples. **(C)** HPLC elution profile shows the formation of E2 from E1 for representative control (C58) and cancer (T58) tissues.

low in all but one tumor sample (T53, **Figure 6D**) thus it was not possible to accurately estimate differences in protein levels between control compared to EC tissue. We were not able to detect HSD17B1 protein in EC tissues using two different antibodies (rabbit monoclonal antibody, EP1682Y, Abcam UK; and rabbit polyclonal antibodies from Solvay Pharmaceuticals; data not shown) although these antibodies recognized HSD17B1 in placenta tissue and in homogenates of *E. coli* overexpressing *HSD17B1*. Protein levels of HSD17B2 were seen in the majority of samples, with increased levels in 7 out of 17 pairs, but with no statistically significant difference between EC and adjacent control tissue (**Figures 6E–G**). The stratification according to clinical and histopathological data confirmed the effects of tumor differentiation on STS expression (**Table 4**). The significantly lower STS protein ($p = 0.0039$) levels in EC as compared to adjacent control tissue were seen only in high grade tumors (G3), while in well-differentiated tumors (G1, G2) there were no differences in STS levels between EC and control tissue (**Table 4**). However, this trend was not supported by further immunohistochemical staining.

With the same set of antibodies as previously used for Western blotting we performed immunohistochemical staining of tissue microarrays, which included 44 pairs of cancer and adjacent control tissue. We observed staining for STS, HSD17B2, HSD17B1, and SULT1E1 in EC and adjacent control tissue (**Figures 7A,C**). STS staining indicated clear cytoplasmic reaction with several samples showing distinct luminal accumulation of this protein. Scoring and further statistical analysis revealed overall significantly lower levels of STS ($p = 0.0219$) in cancer compared to adjacent control tissue but with unchanged levels in 12 pairs, increased levels in 10 pairs and decreased levels in 22 out of 44 pairs (**Figures 7A,B**, Supplementary Table 4). HSD17B2 showed granulated cytoplasmic reaction in all samples. Protein levels of HSD17B2 were in general significantly increased ($p = 0.0236$) in cancer as compared to adjacent control tissue with unchanged levels in 5 pairs, decreased levels in 11 pairs, and increased levels in 24 out of 40 pairs (**Figures 7A,B**, Supplementary Table 4). Staining for HSD17B1 with Abcam EP1682Y antibodies was weak but indicated distinct and clear cytoplasmic reaction with

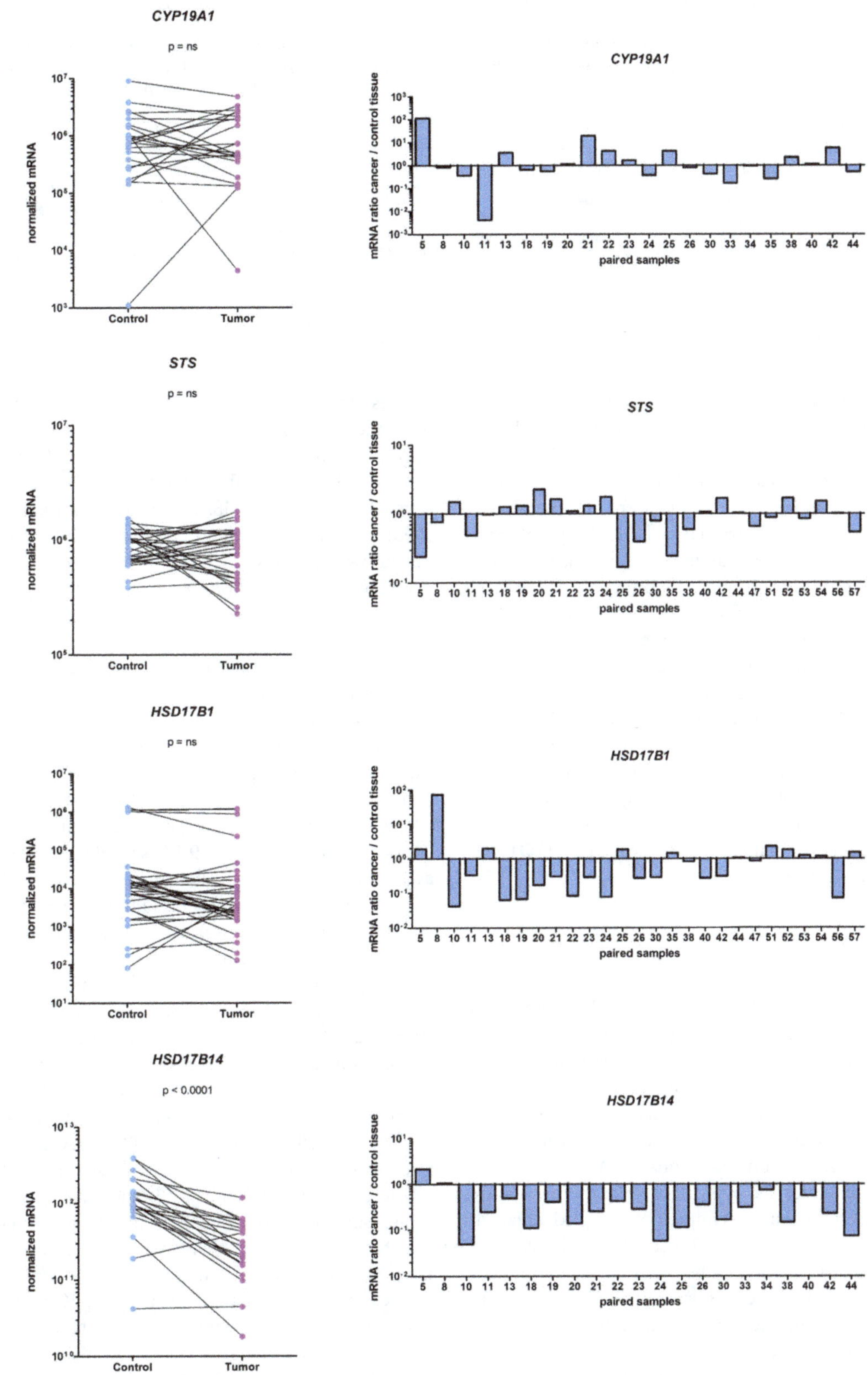

FIGURE 5 | Expression of *CYP19A1*, *STS*, *HSD17B1*, and *HSD17B14* in the EC and adjacent control tissues. On the left before-and-after graphs show the normalized expression levels of the genes investigated in control endometrium (Control) and the corresponding cancer endometrium (Tumor). The levels of gene expression are presented on a logarithmic scale. On the right are histograms with logarithmic scale shows mRNA ratio between cancer and control tissue.

TABLE 3 | Changes in expression of genes according to histopathological and clinical characteristics of endometrial cancer patients.

Gene	Tumor/control		Tumor differentiation (high grade vs. low grade)	Menopausal status	FIGO stage (IA vs. IB-IV)	Myometrial invasion (yes/no)	Lymphovascular invasion (yes/no)	Vital status
	Fold-change	*p*	*p*	*p*	*p*	*p*	*p*	*p*
CYP19A1	0.85	0.5203	0.1115	0.0615	0.0893	0.1830	0.1995	0.3106
STS	0.93	0.7639	**0.0439**	0.0868	0.4326	0.7682	0.3991	0.0529
HSD17B1	0.75	0.2110	0.1562	0.9748	0.6552	0.1273	0.1844	0.3882
HSD17B14	0.26	**<0.0001**	0.3136	0.2847	0.8550	0.4597	**0.0298**	0.4233
SULT1E1	0.43	0.1606	0.2128	**0.0392**	0.2615	0.7745	0.2252	0.3653

The differences in expression levels in tumor as compared to the adjacent control endometrium were analyzed using Wilcoxon matched-pair tests. Stratification analysis were done using 2-way ANOVA. The differences in p-values of < 0.05 were considered significant and are marked in bold.

clearly negative control staining and intense staining in placenta tissue, which served as a positive control (**Figure 7C**). Weak staining for HSD17B1 was seen in 38 control and 36 cancer samples out of 42 pairs investigated. With Solvay antibodies against HSD17B1 moderate staining was seen in control and cancer tissue in epithelial and stromal cells, with cytoplasmic but also some positive nuclear staining, and intense staining in placenta tissue (data not shown). Staining for SULT1E1 in EC and adjacent control endometrial tissue samples was cytoplasmic with no significant difference between cancer and the adjacent control tissue, but with decreased levels in 16 pairs, increased levels in six pairs and no staining in 8 out of 31 pairs (**Figures 7A,B**; Supplementary Table 4). The same antibody intensively stained small intestine and duodenum tissue, which served as positive controls and weakly lung tissue, which was a negative control (data not shown). Stratification of the experimental data according to clinical and histopathological characteristics of patients revealed no effects on STS, HSD17B2, and SULT1E1 levels (**Table 5**).

DISCUSSION

In postmenopausal EC patients estrogens can be formed in peripheral tissues, from inactive precursors of adrenal (DHEAS, DHEA) or ovarian origin (A-dione), or from circulating E1-S. However, the local formation of E2 in cancerous endometrium and especially the contributions of the sulfatase and aromatase pathways has not been clearly defined which called for further studies. We first measured concentrations of A-dione, which can serve as a precursor for E2 biosynthesis via the aromatase pathway and E2 itself in paired samples of EC and adjacent control endometrium. A-dione and E2 were detected almost in all samples, but with large variability between patients, similarly as reported previously for the measurements of mammary E2 (Chetrite et al., 2000; Geisler et al., 2000). Previously Berstein et al. (2003) detected significantly higher E2 levels by radioimmunological assay in 78 cases of cancer tissue compared to the macroscopically normal adjacent endometrium (mean levels 0.498 and 0.314 pmol/g wet tissue, respectively). We calculated the hormone levels per mass of powdered tissue and thus determined about 10-fold higher concentrations. Both studies used immunological assays which introduced certain methodological limitations. In the last decade the reliability of immunoassays has been questioned due to the potential cross-reactivity between different stereoisomers and low sensitivity, thus GC/MS and LC-MS/MS techniques are now recommended (Penning et al., 2010; Stanczyk and Clarke, 2010). To the best of our knowledge these methodologies have not yet been used for determination of A-dione and E2 concentrations in EC tissue. Although, the immunological assays used in this study might have not determined exact concentrations of A-dione and E2, they have confirmed presence of A-dione and E2 in the majority of cancer and adjacent control tissues, which supports local formation of E2.

Detection of A-dione in cancerous endometrium led us to examine its metabolism in paired samples of EC and adjacent control tissue. Our data show that A-dione at 80, 10, and 8 nM is reduced to T where no E2 is formed. These results were confirmed, altogether in 19 EC samples, by two methodological approaches (TLC with autoradiography and HPLC separations using radioactivity detector) also in the presence of regeneration system which provided sufficient levels of NADPH. Reduction of A-dione to T can be catalyzed by the reductive androgenic 17β-HSD type 5 (HSD17B5), better known as AKR1C3, which was shown to be expressed in EC samples from our cohort (Smuc and Rizner, 2009). The A-dione metabolism data using physiological steroid concentrations suggests a marginal role for aromatase in EC tissues, which is in agreement with the reports of Fournier and Poirier and our previous studies showing no E1 and E2 formation in four EC cell lines (Ishikawa, HEC-1A, HEC-1B and RL-95) after 24 h incubation with 8 nM A-dione (2009) (Fournier and Poirier, 2009; Hevir-Kene and Rižner, 2015).

As our data show that E2 cannot be formed from A-dione via the aromatase pathway, we next studied formation from E1-S via the sulfatase pathway. The E1-S and E1 metabolism studies in 5 and 12 paired samples of EC and adjacent control endometrium, respectively, support formation of E2 from both precursors with higher levels of E2 in EC. This data thus confirm that in EC the most potent estrogen E2 can be formed via the sulfatase pathway from circulating E1-S as also supported by increased E1-S plasma levels in EC patients compared to healthy postmenopausal women (Lepine et al., 2010; Audet-Walsh et al., 2011; Brinton et al., 2016). Our E1-S metabolism

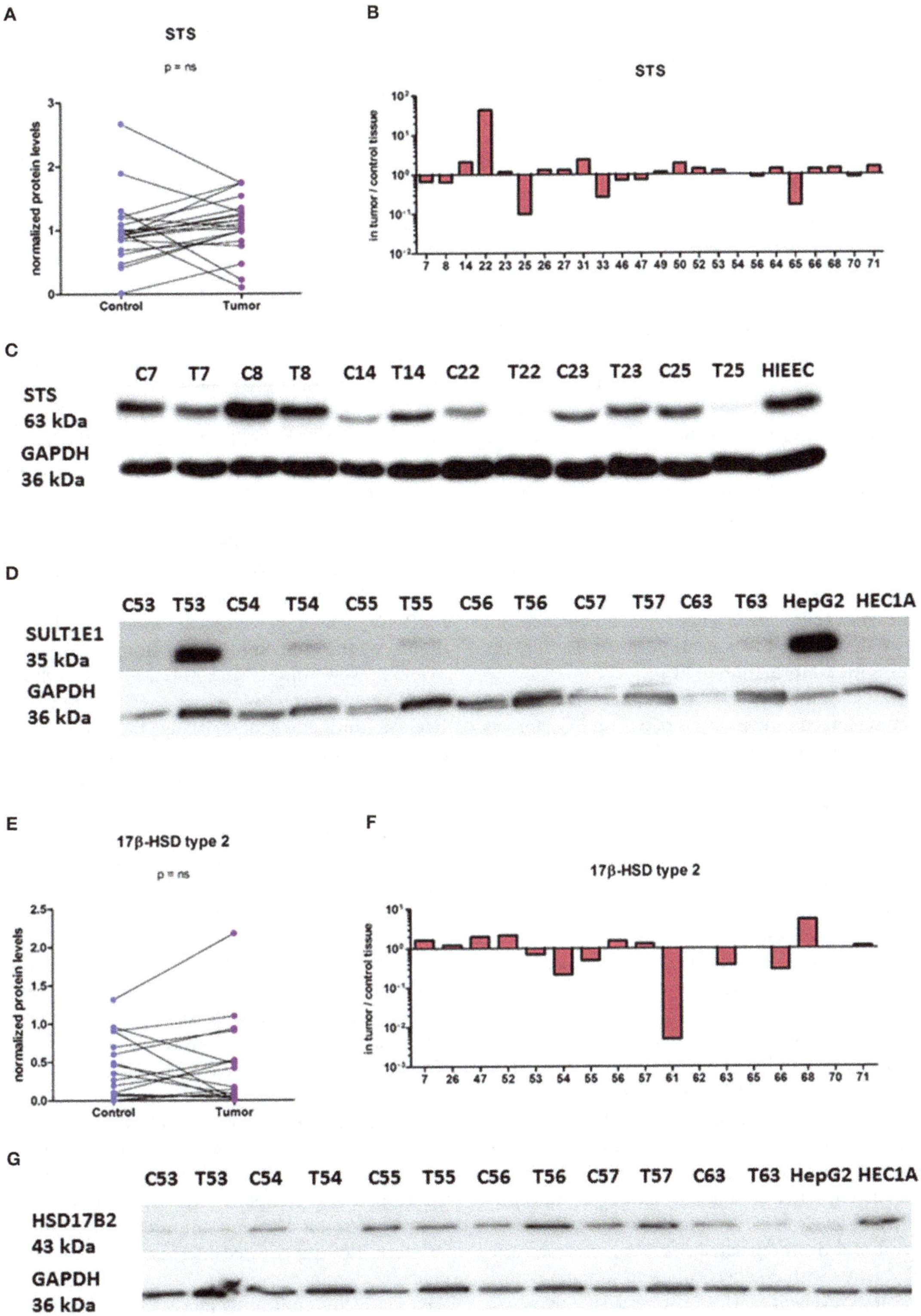

FIGURE 6 | Protein levels of STS, SULT1E1, and HSD17B2 in the EC and adjacent control tissue. **(A)** Before-and-after graph shows STS protein levels in 24 paired samples of control endometrium (Control) and corresponding cancer tissue (Tumor). The data was quantified and normalized to GAPDH levels. **(B)** Histogram with logarithmic scale demonstrates higher STS levels in cancer endometrium in 12 paired samples out of 24. **(C)** Representative membrane with STS and GAPDH staining. **(D)** Representative membrane with SULT1E1and GAPDH staining. **(E)** Before-and-after graph shows HSD17B2 protein levels in 17 paired samples of control endometrium (Control) and corresponding cancer tissue (Tumor). The data was quantified and normalized to GAPDH levels. **(F)** Histogram with logarithmic scale demonstrates protein ratio between paired samples of tumor and control tissue. **(G)** Representative membrane with HSD17B2 and GAPDH staining. C, control endometrium; T, EC tissue; HIEEC, control epithelial cell line of normal endometrium; HEC1A, endometrial cancer cell line; HepG2, liver cancer cell line.

TABLE 4 | Changes in protein levels according to histopathological and clinical characteristics of endometrial cancer patients.

Protein	Tumor/control		Histological differentiation (high grade vs. low grade)	Menopausal status	FIGO stage (IA vs. IB-IV)	Myometrial invasion (yes/no)	Lympho-vascular invasion (yes/no)	Vital status
	Fold-change	*p*	*p*	*p*	*P*	*p*	*p*	*p*
STS	1.09	0.2660	**0.0039**	0.9142	0.1013	0.7690	0.5050	0.5068
HSD17B2	1.03	0.8498	0.2891	0.0989	0.3028	0.5704	0.6941	0.6856

Protein levels were determined by Western blotting. The differences in expression levels in tumor as compared to the adjacent control endometrium were analyzed using Wilcoxon matched-pair tests. Stratification analysis were done using 2-way ANOVA. The differences in p-values of <0.05 were considered significant and are marked in bold.

data also show significantly increased levels of E2 in cancer tissue Similarly, Cornel et al., reported that reduction of E1 to E2 predominates over oxidation of E2 to E1 in EC compared to normal endometrial tissue and adjacent control tissue (Cornel et al., 2012).

The expression of the majority of these genes for local E2 formation via the aromatase and the sulfatase pathways has previously been studied in the same cohort of patients (Smuc and Rizner, 2009). Here, we re-examined expression of genes encoding the key enzymes of the aromatase and the sulfatase pathway, *CYP19A1*, *STS*, and *HSD17B1* on a larger number of samples. The very low and unchanged *CYP19A1* expression also reported by Cornel et al. (2012) support our A-dione metabolism data, which shows that aromatization of androgens is not the primary mechanism for E2 formation in EC.

On the other hand, high but unchanged expression of *STS* at the mRNA level, unchanged protein levels of STS in EC samples seen by Western blotting and significantly lower protein levels seen by IHC, imply that STS may have more important role in the adjacent control tissue as compared to EC. However, statistical analysis revealed that *STS* is downregulated in high grade cancers but not in low grade cancers, where similar levels were seen in EC and the adjacent control tissue (**Table 3**). Similar trend was seen also for protein levels of STS as determined by Western blotting (**Table 4**). However, due to a low number of high grade cancers, this association have to be considered with caution and the effect of high grade cancer should be reassessed on a higher number of samples.

The importance of the sulfatase pathway is also supported by the previously reported 5-fold lower expression of *SULT1E1* as compared to *STS* and decreased mRNA levels of *SULT1E1* in 27 out of 38 EC samples from the same cohort, where this difference did not reach statistical significance (Hevir et al., 2011b) and also by significantly increased ratio between *STS* and *SULT1E1* in EC. Furthermore, our current statistical analysis, showed significantly lower *SULT1E1* mRNA levels in EC samples from premenopausal women and several fold downregulated *SULT1E1* expression in postmenopausal patients with no effects of tumor differentiation (**Table 3**). The protein levels of SULT1E1 were very low, which is in line with mRNA levels, reports of others (Utsunomiya et al., 2004) and Human Protein Atlas (data obtained on April 28, 2017). Additionally, IHC staining for SULT1E1 was negative (>25% cases) or weak with a clear trend for decreased levels in EC (Supplementary Table 4). This data thus support the capacity of EC tissue for activation of E1-S to E1.

HSD17B1 is the most obvious candidate for reduction of E1 to E2. In this study, we saw low, but statistically unchanged mRNA levels of *HSD17B1* in EC as compared to control adjacent tissue. In 9 patients out of 27 these mRNA levels were increased in EC compared to adjacent control tissue. The gene expression of other reductive enzymes, as HSD17B7 and HSD17B12, was previously seen to be decreased and unchanged in the same cohort of EC, respectively (Smuc and Rizner, 2009). The average expression levels of *HSD17B7* were 5-fold higher than *HSD17B1*, while *HSD17B12* levels exceeded those of *HSD17B1* by more than 10^4-fold (Smuc and Rizner, 2009), implying that also HSD17B12 is important for E1 activation. Additionally, AKR1C3, which preferentially catalyzes the reduction of A-dione, might contribute to E2 formation, as shown after its overexpression in the MCF7 breast cancer cell line (Byrns et al., 2010). At the protein level we saw a weak specific cytoplasmic IHC staining for HSD17B1 in EC and control endometrial epithelial cells with no difference between cancer and adjacent control tissue. At the protein level Cornel et al., previously reported (Cornel et al., 2012) increased immunoreactivity in grade 1 EC and unchanged levels in high grade EC, whereas in their most recent study they reported very weak staining for HSD17B1 in EC (Cornel et al., 2016). Our results are in line with a low *HSD17B1* expression levels observed in cancer and adjacent control tissue. Due to the higher catalytic efficiency of HSD17B1 as compared to the other isoforms, low expression levels might still result in high conversion of E1 to E2 (Gangloff et al., 2001). Higher capacity of HSD17B1 for E2 formation, compared to other enzymes, was also confirmed by transient transfection of HSD17B1, HSD1712, and AKR1C3 in EC cell line ECC1 (Cornel et al., 2012).

HSD17B2 has the highest catalytic efficiency for oxidation of E2 to E1 and we recently reported significantly increased mRNA levels in EC compared to adjacent control tissue, where pairwise comparison showed increased levels in 32 EC samples out of 47 pairs (Sinreih et al., 2013). Our current Western blotting showed increased protein levels of HSD17B2 in cancer endometrium in 7 out of 17 paired samples while IHC revealed significantly increased protein levels in EC samples compared to adjacent control tissue but with lower levels seen in 11 EC samples out of 40 investigated (Supplementary Table 4). Among other oxidative HSD17Bs with lower catalytic efficiencies, we previously saw unchanged mRNA levels of *HSD17B4* and *HSD17B8* (Smuc and Rizner, 2009). In this study, *HSD17B14* was in general significantly downregulated at the

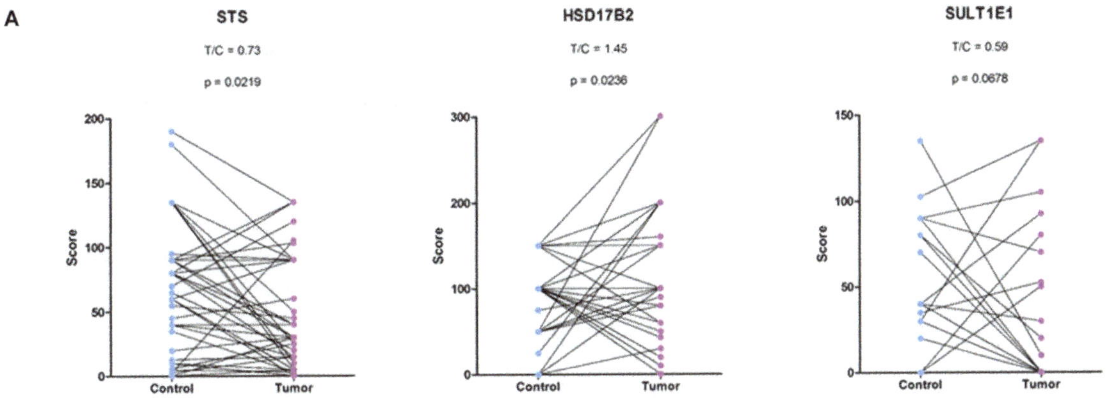

B

Number of EC	STS	HSD17B2	SULT1E1
increased levels	10	24	6
decreased levels	22	11	16
unchanged levels	12	5	9

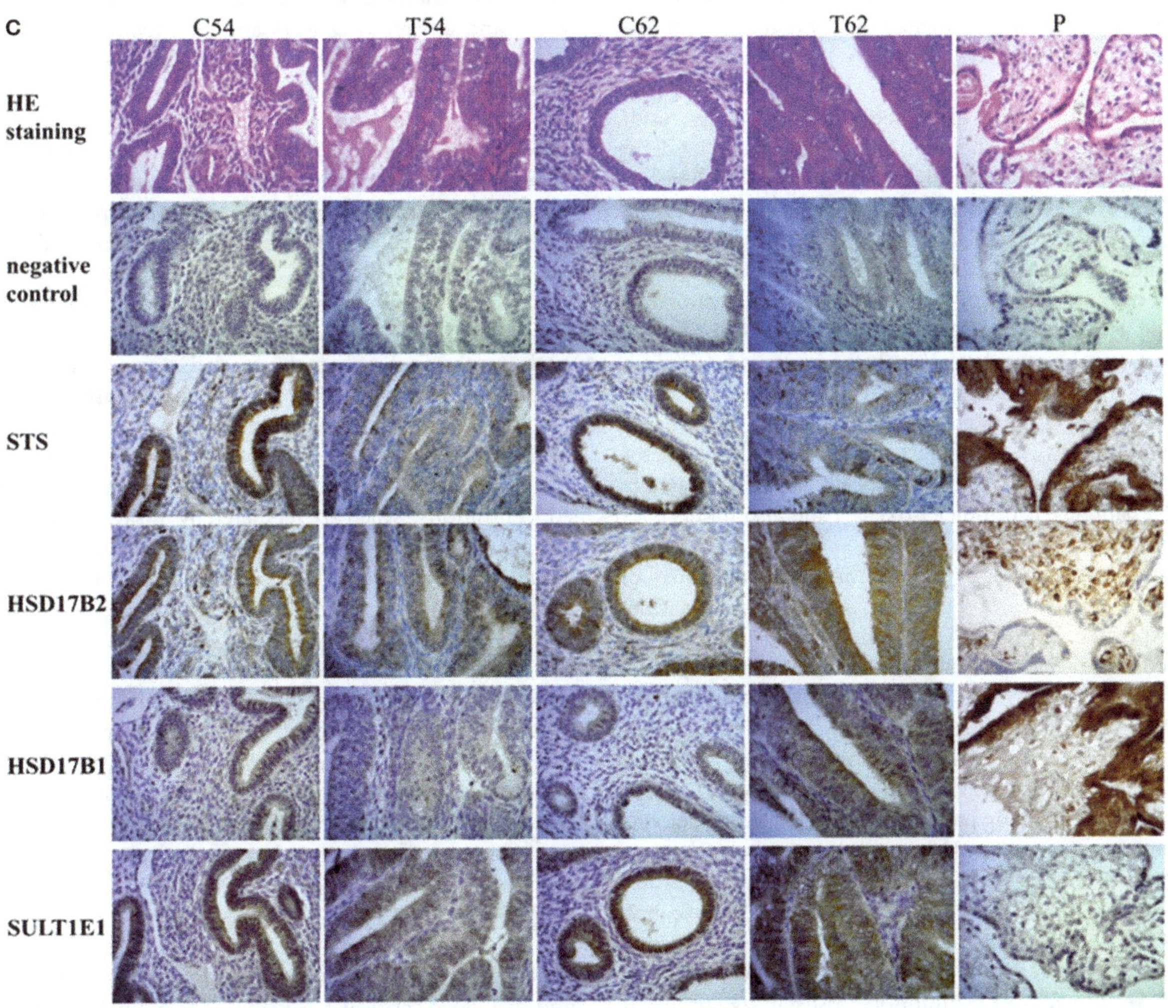

FIGURE 7 | Immunohistochemical staining for STS, HSD17B2, HSD17B1, and SULT1E1 in endometrial cancer. **(A)** Before-and-after graphs show scoring for STS, HSD17B2, and SULT1E1 in control endometrium (Control) and the corresponding cancer endometrium (Tumor). **(B)** Table with number of samples with increased, decreased or unchanged levels of protein in tumor tissue compared to adjacent control endometrium. **(C)** representative staining of adjacent control endometrium (C) and cancerous tissue (T) for STS, HSD17B2, HSD17B1, and SULT1E1 (samples 54 and 62), and placenta (P) as a positive control. Samples were stained with hematoxylin and eosin (HE staining) and with specific antibodies against STS, HSD17B2, HSD17B1, and SULT1E1. 400 × magnifications are shown.

TABLE 5 | Changes in immunohistochemical scoring according to histopathological and clinical characteristics of endometrial cancer patients.

Protein	Tumor/control		Tumor differentiation (high grade vs. low grade)	Menopausal status	FIGO stage (IA vs. IB-IV)	Myometrial invasion (yes/no)	Lympho-vascular invasion (yes/no)	Vital status
	Fold-change	*p*	*p*	*p*	*p*	*p*	*p*	*p*
STS	0.73	**0.0219**	0.6383	0.8962	0.8787	0.5752	0.693	0.7503
HSD17B2	1.45	**0.0236**	0.5055	0.5419	0.9576	0.45	0.7844	0.4178
SULT1E1	0.59	0.0678	0.657	0.0535	0.8447	0.6497	0.1287	0.3016

The differences in expression levels in tumor as compared to the adjacent control endometrium were analyzed using Wilcoxon matched-pair tests. Stratification analysis were done using 2-way ANOVA. The differences in p-values of <0.05 were considered significant and are marked in bold.

mRNA level and we saw lower expression in 19 out of 21 pairs of EC and adjacent control endometrium. Interestingly, more extensive downregulation of *HSD17B14* was seen in EC samples from patients with lymphovascular invasion (**Table 3**). Oxidation of E2 to E1 can be catalyzed by several isozymes. Although, HSD17B2 has the highest catalytic efficiency for oxidation of E2 to E1 also decreased expression of *HSD17B14* gene encoding the oxidative enzyme HSD17B14 may affect E2 levels.

The increased formation of E2 seen in EC certainly results from the disturbed balance between the reductive and oxidative isoforms of HSD17Bs. However, the unchanged mRNA levels of *HSD17B1* and *HSD17B12*, increased mRNA levels of *HSD17B2* and decreased mRNA levels of *HSD17B14* in EC do not fully explain higher capacity for E2 formation seen in EC tissue. Our results thus support studies in model cell lines, where individual inhibitors of HSD17B1, HSD17B5 (AKR1C3), HSD17B7, and HSD17B12 failed to completely block E2 formation (Fournier and Poirier, 2009). Our experimental data indicate that HSD17B1 might not be solely accountable for E2 formation and suggest that large differences in catalytic efficiencies of the reductive estrogenic HSD17B enzymes might partially be compensated by higher expression levels of other isozymes and also higher local concentration of E1 in EC tissue.

The local concentration of E1 and E2 depends on concentration of E1-S and especially activity of STS, which is highly expressed in EC tissue with unchanged protein levels in low grade cancers compared to adjacent control tissue, and is only weakly opposed by *SULT1E1*. The sulfatase pathway is thus clearly implicated in local estrogen formation, and concomitant enhanced estrogen actions in EC. It has to be stressed here that a great variabilities in gene expression at the mRNA and protein levels have been seen among patients. Also increased capacity for E2 formation in cancerous endometrium has not been observed in all patients.

STS inhibitors have been considered as novel anticancer agents where phase II clinical study has already been performed in ER-positive advanced/recurrent EC, however with no convincing results for STS inhibitor irosustat vs. progestin megestrol acetate (Pautier et al., 2017) with the progression free survival of 16 and 32 weeks, respectively. STS inhibitor thus performed worse as compared to the current medical treatment for recurrent EC. This suboptimal performance of STS inhibitor is not in contrast with the reported increased E2 formation in cancerous endometrium. Our cohort included EC patients with mostly well-differentiated low grade primary cancer. The situation in high grade cancers and especially advanced/recurrent cases may be different as suggested by decreased *STS* mRNA and protein levels seen in high grade vs. low grade cancers. It is clear that further studies including high grade and advanced cancers and also focusing on E1S uptake transporters are needed to clarify the clinical performance of STS inhibitor.

Altogether our study confirms the presence of E2 in cancerous endometrium, the capacity of this tissue for activation of E1S to E2 and reports expression of genes involved in local E2 formation via the sulfatase pathway at the mRNA and protein levels. This data is extended by a statistical evaluation of individual variables including histopathological and clinical characteristics that may affect the expression levels. Although the limitation of our study is a relatively low number of samples included in the individual analyses, the findings on the local E2 formation are supported by different methodological approaches and are substantiated by the protein levels and enzymatic activities of STS and HSD17B1 in EC tissue.

Formation of E2 in EC also depends on intracellular E1-S concentrations, which are regulated by the availability of Organic Anion Transporting Polypeptides (OATPs) and Organic Anion Transporters (OATs), where several OATPs and OATs catalyze the cellular uptake of E1-S (Mueller et al., 2015). However, the expression of genes encoding OATP and OAT transporters has not yet been examined in EC. As the concerted action of these transporters and intracellular enzymes is required for local E2 formation this lack of knowledge currently precludes the complete understanding of E2 formation in cancerous endometrium and calls for further studies. Especially, as these transporters may have crucial roles in local estrogen formation and may represent novel options for treatment.

AUTHOR CONTRIBUTIONS

TLR designed the study, contributed to writing of the manuscript and provided critical assessment and final approval of the manuscript. MS, TK, NH, MA, KV, and AJ carried out the experimental work, analyzed the results, and contributed to writing of the manuscript. SF assessed immunohistochemical staining, contributed to writing of the manuscript, and provided critical assessment of the manuscript.

ACKNOWLEDGMENTS

This work was supported by grants J3-4135 and J3-5510 to TLR and young researcher grants to NH, MS, and TK all from the Slovenian Research Agency. The authors thank Dr. J. Adamski from Helmholtz Zentrum München, Germany for hosting KV and NH to perform estrone metabolism studies in his laboratory; Dr. Gerhard Schuler from Faculty of Veterinary Medicine, Justus-Liebig-University, Giessen, Germany, for a kind gift of STS antiserum, Dr. Bettina Husen from Solvay Pharmaceuticals, Hannover, Germany for providing polyclonal antibodies against HSD17B1 and HSD17B2, Dr. Andrea Romano from School for Oncology & Developmental Biology, Department of Gynaecology, Maastricht University, The Netherlands for providing the protocol for immunohistochemical staining of HSD17B1, Dr. Špela Smrkolj from Department of Obstetrics and Gynecology, University Medical Centre Ljubljana for her help with gathering the clinical data and Špela Petelin from Institute of Biochemistry, Faculty of Medicine, Ljubljana, for technical support.

REFERENCES

Agarwal, A. K., and Auchus, R. J. (2005). Minireview: cellular redox state regulates hydroxysteroid dehydrogenase activity and intracellular hormone potency. *Endocrinology* 146, 2531–2538. doi: 10.1210/en.2005-0061

Audet-Walsh, E., Lépine, J., Grégoire, J., Plante, M., Caron, P., Têtu, B., et al. (2011). Profiling of endogenous estrogens, their precursors, and metabolites in endometrial cancer patients: association with risk and relationship to clinical characteristics. *J. Clin. Endocrinol. Metab.* 96, E330–E339. doi: 10.1210/jc.2010-2050

Berstein, L. M., Tchernobrovkina, A. E., Gamajunova, V. B., Kovalevskij, A. J., Vasilyev, D. A., Chepik, O. F., et al. (2003). Tumor estrogen content and clinico-morphological and endocrine features of endometrial cancer. *J. Cancer Res. Clin. Oncol.* 129, 245–249. doi: 10.1007/s00432-003-0427-9

Berstein, L., Kovalevskij, A., Zimarina, T., Maximov, S., Gershfeld, E., Vasilyev, D., et al. (2005). Aromatase and comparative response to its inhibitors in two types of endometrial cancer. *J. Steroid Biochem. Mol. Biol.* 95, 71–74. doi: 10.1016/j.jsbmb.2005.04.008

Brinton, L. A., Trabert, B., Anderson, G. L., Falk, R. T., Felix, A. S., Fuhrman, B. J., et al. (2016). Serum estrogens and estrogen metabolites and endometrial cancer risk among postmenopausal women. *Cancer Epidemiol. Biomarkers Prev.* 25, 1081–1089. doi: 10.1158/1055-9965.EPI-16-0225

Byrns, M. C., Duan, L., Lee, S. H., Blair, I. A., and Penning, T. M. (2010). Aldo-keto reductase 1C3 expression in MCF-7 cells reveals roles in steroid hormone and prostaglandin metabolism that may explain its over-expression in breast cancer. *J. Steroid Biochem. Mol. Biol.* 118, 177–187. doi: 10.1016/j.jsbmb.2009.12.009

Casey, M. L., MacDonald, P. C., and Andersson, S. (1994). 17 beta-Hydroxysteroid dehydrogenase type 2: chromosomal assignment and progestin regulation of gene expression in human endometrium. *J. Clin. Invest.* 94, 2135–2141. doi: 10.1172/JCI117569

Chetrite, G. S., Cortes-Prieto, J., Philippe, J. C., Wright, F., and Pasqualini, J. R. (2000). Comparison of estrogen concentrations, estrone sulfatase and aromatase activities in normal, and in cancerous, human breast tissues. *J. Steroid Biochem. Mol. Biol.* 72, 23–27. doi: 10.1016/S0960-0760(00)00040-6

Colombo, N., Creutzberg, C., Amant, F., Bosse, T., González-Martín, A., Ledermann, J., et al. (2016). ESMO-ESGO-ESTRO consensus conference on endometrial cancer: diagnosis, treatment and follow-up. *Int. J. Gynecol. Cancer* 26, 2–30. doi: 10.1097/IGC.0000000000000609

Cornel, K. M., Krakstad, C., Delvoux, B., Xanthoulea, S., Jori, B., Bongers, M. Y., et al. (2016). High mRNA levels of 17β-hydroxysteroid dehydrogenase type 1 correlate with poor prognosis in endometrial cancer. *Mol. Cell Endocrinol.* 442, 51–57. doi: 10.1016/j.mce.2016.11.030

Cornel, K. M., Kruitwagen, R. F., Delvoux, B., Visconti, L., Van de Vijver, K. K., Day, J. M., et al. (2012). Overexpression of 17β-hydroxysteroid dehydrogenase type 1 increases the exposure of endometrial cancer to 17β-estradiol. *J. Clin. Endocrinol. Metab.* 97, E591–E601. doi: 10.1210/jc.2011-2994

Dibbelt, L., and Kuss, E. (1986). Human placental steryl-sulfatase. Enzyme purification, production of antisera, and immunoblotting reactions with normal and sulfatase-deficient placentas. *Biol. Chem. Hoppe Seyler* 367, 1223–1229. doi: 10.1515/bchm3.1986.367.2.1223

Dibbelt, L., Herzog, V., and Kuss, E. (1989). Human placental sterylsulfatase: immunocytochemical and biochemical localization. *Biol. Chem. Hoppe Seyler* 370, 1093–1102. doi: 10.1515/bchm3.1989.370.2.1093

Fournier, M. A., and Poirier, D. (2009). Estrogen formation in endometrial and cervix cancer cell lines: involvement of aromatase, steroid sulfatase and 17β-hydroxysteroid dehydrogenases (types 1, 5, 7 and 12). *Mol. Cell Endocrinol.* 301, 142–145. doi: 10.1016/j.mce.2008.08.027

Gangloff, A., Garneau, A., Huang, Y. W., Yang, F., and Lin, S. X. (2001). Human oestrogenic 17β-hydroxysteroid dehydrogenase specificity: enzyme regulation through an NADPH-dependent substrate inhibition towards the highly specific oestrone reduction. *Biochem. J.* 356(Pt 1), 269–276. doi: 10.1042/bj3560269

Geisler, J., Berntsen, H., and Lonning, P. E. (2000). A novel HPLC-RIA method for the simultaneous detection of estrone, estradiol and estrone sulphate levels in breast cancer tissue. *J. Steroid Biochem. Mol. Biol.* 72, 259–264. doi: 10.1016/S0960-0760(00)00036-4

Hevir, N., Šinkovec, J., and Lanišnik Rižner, T. (2011a). Disturbed expression of phase I and phase II estrogen-metabolizing enzymes in endometrial cancer: lower levels of CYP1B1 and increased expression of S-COMT. *Mol. Cell Endocrinol.* 331, 158–167. doi: 10.1016/j.mce.2010.09.011

Hevir, N., Sinkovec, J., and Rižner, T. L. (2011b). Disturbed expression of phase I and phase II estrogen-metabolizing enzymes in endometrial cancer: lower levels of CYP1B1 and increased expression of S-COMT. *Mol. Cell Endocrinol.* 331, 158–167. doi: 10.1016/j.mce.2010.09.011

Hevir-Kene, N., and Rižner, T. L. (2015). The endometrial cancer cell lines Ishikawa and HEC-1A, and the control cell line HIEEC, differ in expression of estrogen biosynthetic and metabolic genes, and in androstenedione and estrone-sulfate metabolism. *Chem. Biol. Interact.* 234, 309–319. doi: 10.1016/j.cbi.2014.11.015

Inoue, M. (2001). Current molecular aspects of the carcinogenesis of the uterine endometrium. *Int. J. Gynecol. Cancer* 11, 339–348. doi: 10.1046/j.1525-1438.2001.01046.x

Jongen, V. H., Thijssen, J. H., Hollema, H., Donker, G. H., Santema, J. G., Van der Zee, A. G., et al. (2005). Is aromatase cytochrome P450 involved in the pathogenesis of endometrioid endometrial cancer?. *Int. J. Gynecol. Cancer* 15, 529–536. doi: 10.1111/j.1525-1438.2005.15320.x

Keefe, C. C., Goldman, M. M., Zhang, K., Clarke, N., Reitz, R. E., and Welt, C. K. (2014). Simultaneous measurement of thirteen steroid hormones in women with polycystic ovary syndrome and control women using liquid chromatography-tandem mass spectrometry. *PLoS ONE* 9:e93805. doi: 10.1371/journal.pone.0093805

Krekels, M. D., Wouters, W., De Coster, R., Van Ginckel, R., Leonaers, A., and Janssen, P. A. (1991). Aromatase in the human choriocarcinoma JEG-3: inhibition by R 76 713 in cultured cells and in tumors grown in nude mice. *J. Steroid Biochem. Mol. Biol.* 38, 415–422. doi: 10.1016/0960-0760(91)90329-4

Lanišnik Rižner, T., Šmuc, T., Rupreht, R., Sinkovec, J., and Penning, T. M. (2006). AKR1C1 and AKR1C3 may determine progesterone and estrogen ratios in endometrial cancer. *Mol. Cell Endocrinol.* 248, 126–135. doi: 10.1016/j.mce.2005.10.009

Lepine, J., Audet-Walsh, E., Gregoire, J., Tetu, B., Plante, M., Menard, V., et al. (2010). Circulating estrogens in endometrial cancer cases and their relationship with tissular expression of key estrogen biosynthesis and metabolic pathways. *J. Clin. Endocrinol. Metab.* 95, 2689–2698. doi: 10.1210/jc.2010-2648

Morice, P., Leary, A., Creutzberg, C., Abu-Rustum, N., and Darai, E. (2016). Endometrial cancer. *Lancet* 387, 1094–1108. doi: 10.1016/S0140-6736(15)00130-0

Mueller, J. W., Gilligan, L. C., Idkowiak, J., Arlt, W., and Foster, P. A. (2015). The regulation of steroid action by sulfation and desulfation. *Endocr. Rev.* 36, 526–563. doi: 10.1210/er.2015-1036

Pathirage, N., Di Nezza, L. A., Salmonsen, L. A., Jobling, T., Simpson, E. R., and Clyne, C. D. (2006). Expression of aromatase, estrogen receptors, and their coactivators in patients with endometrial cancer. *Fertil. Steril.* 86, 469–472. doi: 10.1016/j.fertnstert.2005.12.057

Pautier, P., Vergote, I., Joly, F., Melichar, B., Kutarska, E., Hall, G., et al. (2017). A phase 2, randomized, open-label study of irosustat versus megestrol acetate in advanced endometrial cancer. *Int. J. Gynecol. Cancer* 27, 258–266. doi: 10.1097/IGC.0000000000000862

Penning, T. M., Lee, S. H., Jin, Y., Gutierrez, A., and Blair, I. A. (2010). Liquid chromatography-mass spectrometry (LC-MS) of steroid hormone metabolites and its applications. *J. Steroid Biochem. Mol. Biol.* 121, 546–555. doi: 10.1016/j.jsbmb.2010.01.005

Rižner, T. L. (2013). Estrogen biosynthesis, phase I and phase II metabolism, and action in endometrial cancer. *Mol. Cell Endocrinol.* 381, 124–139. doi: 10.1016/j.mce.2013.07.026

Rizner, T. L., Smuc, T., Rupreht, R., Sinkovec, J., and Penning, T. M. (2006). AKR1C1 and AKR1C3 may determine progesterone and estrogen ratios in endometrial cancer. *Mol. Cell Endocrinol.* 248, 126–135. doi: 10.1016/j.mce.2005.10.009

Samarnthai, N., Hall, K., and Yeh, I. T. (2010). Molecular profiling of endometrial malignancies. *Obstet. Gynecol. Int.* 2010:162363. doi: 10.1155/2010/162363

Segawa, T., Shozu, M., Murakami, K., Kasai, T., Shinohara, K., Nomura, K., et al. (2005). Aromatase expression in stromal cells of endometrioid endometrial cancer correlates with poor survival. *Clin. Cancer Res.* 11, 2188–2194. doi: 10.1158/1078-0432.CCR-04-1859

Simpson, E. R. (2002). Aromatization of androgens in women: current concepts and findings. *Fertil. Steril.* 77(Suppl. 4), S6–S10. doi: 10.1016/S0015-0282(02)02984-9

Sinreih, M., Hevir, N., and Rižner, T. L. (2013). Altered expression of genes involved in progesterone biosynthesis, metabolism and action in endometrial cancer. *Chem. Biol. Interact.* 202, 210–217. doi: 10.1016/j.cbi.2012.11.012

Smuc, T., and Rizner, T. L. (2009). Aberrant pre-receptor regulation of estrogen and progesterone action in endometrial cancer. *Mol. Cell Endocrinol.* 301, 74–82. doi: 10.1016/j.mce.2008.09.019

Stanczyk, F. Z., and Clarke, N. J. (2010). Advantages and challenges of mass spectrometry assays for steroid hormones. *J. Steroid. Biochem. Mol. Biol.* 121, 491–495. doi: 10.1016/j.jsbmb.2010.05.001

Takahashi-Shiga, N., Utsunomiya, H., Miki, Y., Nagase, S., Kobayashi, R., Matsumoto, M., et al. (2009). Local biosynthesis of estrogen in human endometrial carcinoma through tumor-stromal cell interactions. *Clin. Cancer Res.* 15, 6028–6034. doi: 10.1158/1078-0432.CCR-09-1013

Utsunomiya, H., Ito, K., Suzuki, T., Kitamura, T., Kaneko, C., Nakata, T., et al. (2004). Steroid sulfatase and estrogen sulfotransferase in human endometrial carcinoma. *Clin. Cancer Res.* 10, 5850–5256. doi: 10.1158/1078-0432.CCR-04-0040

Utsunomiya, H., Suzuki, T., Kaneko, C., Takeyama, J., Nakamura, J., Kimura, K., et al. (2001). The analyses of 17β-hydroxysteroid dehydrogenase isozymes in human endometrial hyperplasia and carcinoma. *J. Clin. Endocrinol. Metab.* 86, 3436–3443. doi: 10.1210/jcem.86.7.7661

Wan, J., Gao, Y., Zeng, K., Yin, Y., Zhao, M., Wei, J., et al. (2016). The levels of the sex hormones are not different between type 1 and type 2 endometrial cancer. *Sci. Rep.* 6:39744. doi: 10.1038/srep39744

Watanabe, K., Sasano, H., Harada, N., Ozaki, M., Niikura, H., Sato, S., et al. (1995). Aromatase in human endometrial carcinoma and hyperplasia. Immunohistochemical, *in situ* hybridization, and biochemical studies. *Am. J. Pathol.* 146, 491–500.

Yamamoto, T., Kitawaki, J., Urabe, M., Honjo, H., Tamura, T., Noguchi, T., et al. (1993). Estrogen productivity of endometrium and endometrial cancer tissue; influence of aromatase on proliferation of endometrial cancer cells. *J. Steroid Biochem. Mol. Biol.* 44, 463–468. doi: 10.1016/0960-0760(93)90251-Q

Zeitoun, K., Takayama, K., Sasano, H., Suzuki, T., Moghrabi, N., Andersson, S., et al. (1998). Deficient 17beta-hydroxysteroid dehydrogenase type 2 expression in endometriosis: failure to metabolize 17beta-estradiol. *J. Clin. Endocrinol. Metab.* 83, 4474–4480.

9

Neurosteroid Transport in the Brain: Role of ABC and SLC Transporters

Markus Grube, Paul Hagen and Gabriele Jedlitschky*

Department of Pharmacology, Center of Drug Absorption and Transport, University Medicine Greifswald, Greifswald, Germany

***Correspondence:**
Gabriele Jedlitschky
jedlits@uni-greifswald.de

Neurosteroids, comprising pregnane, androstane, and sulfated steroids can alter neuronal excitability through interaction with ligand-gated ion channels and other receptors and have therefore a therapeutic potential in several brain disorders. They can be formed in brain cells or are synthesized by an endocrine gland and reach the brain by penetrating the blood–brain barrier (BBB). Especially sulfated steroids such as pregnenolone sulfate (PregS) and dehydroepiandrosterone sulfate (DHEAS) depend on transporter proteins to cross membranes. In this review, we discuss the involvement of ATP-binding cassette (ABC)- and solute carrier (SLC)-type membrane proteins in the transport of these compounds at the BBB and in the choroid plexus (CP), but also in the secretion from neurons and glial cells. Among the ABC transporters, especially BCRP (ABCG2) and several MRP/ABCC subfamily members (MRP1, MRP4, MRP8) are expressed in the brain and known to efflux conjugated steroids. Furthermore, several SLC transporters have been shown to mediate cellular uptake of steroid sulfates. These include members of the OATP/SLCO subfamily, namely OATP1A2 and OATP2B1, as well as OAT3 (SLC22A3), which have been reported to be expressed at the BBB, in the CP and in part in neurons. Furthermore, a role of the organic solute transporter OSTα-OSTβ (SLC51A/B) in brain DHEAS/PregS homeostasis has been proposed. This transporter was reported to be localized especially in steroidogenic cells of the cerebellum and hippocampus. To date, the impact of transporters on neurosteroid homeostasis is still poorly understood. Further insights are desirable also with regard to the therapeutic potential of these compounds.

Keywords: ATP-binding cassette transporters, blood–brain barrier, dehydroepiandrosterone, DHEAS, neuroactive steroids, pregnenolone sulfate, solute carriers

INTRODUCTION

Neurosteroids are cholesterol-derived compounds categorized in pregnane neurosteroids (e.g., allopregnanolone), androstane neurosteroids (e.g., androstanediol), and sulfated compounds [PregS and DHEAS] (Reddy, 2010). They can be synthesized in the central nervous system, or the compounds themselves or precursors can be taken up from the systemic circulation (Baulieu, 1997; Maninger et al., 2009). One of their main functions in the brain is to modulate

---

Abbreviations: ABC, ATP-binding cassette; BBB, blood–brain barrier; BCRP, breast cancer resistance protein; CP, choroid plexus; CSF, cerebrospinal fluid; DHEAS, dehydroepiandrosterone sulfate; E_1-3-S, estrone-3-sulfate; GABA, γ-aminobutyric acid; MRP, multidrug resistance protein; NMDA, *N*-methyl-D-aspartate; OATP, organic anion transporting polypeptide; OST, organic solute transporter; PregS, pregnenolone sulfate; SULT, sulfotransferase; TRP, transient receptor potential.

excitability by interaction with membrane receptors and ion channels (Reddy, 2010). Accordingly, a therapeutic potential of these compounds or synthetic analogs has been discussed for a variety of brain disorders (Reddy, 2010). Local steroid biosynthesis in rodent and human brain has been studied since 1990s (Baulieu, 1997). Expression of key enzymes (e.g., P450 side-chain cleavage enzyme, P450c17) has been demonstrated in the principal neurons of several brain areas and in the microglia and astrocytes (reviewed in: Maninger et al., 2009; Hojo et al., 2011; Porcu et al., 2016). However, the relative contributions of the local synthesis and uptake from blood to CNS levels have still to be clarified and may vary between different neurosteroids. In contrast to the lipophilic unconjugated compounds, especially DHEAS and PregS do not diffuse across membranes at a sufficient rate due to their hydrophilic sulfate moiety. Therefore, this review focuses on DHEAS/PregS membrane transporters in the brain. Both compounds play important roles in age-related memory and learning. They can be formed from the non-sulfated precursors by SULTs with SULT2B1b as a major isoform in the human brain (Salman et al., 2011). The ratio of sulfated versus non-sulfated neurosteroids in the brain may be decisive, since sulfation can change the direction of the neuromodulating activity. While for example some non-sulfated neurosteroids such as allopregnanolone are potent positive modulators of GABA type A receptors (for review see Chisari et al., 2010; Reddy, 2010), DHEAS and PregS have been shown to antagonize the GABA effect on the $GABA_A$ receptor (Seljeset et al., 2015) and to be potent allosteric agonists at NMDA receptors (Wu et al., 1991; Monnet et al., 1995). Furthermore, PregS has been shown to directly activate certain TRP channels (Harteneck, 2013).

DHEAS AND PREGS LEVELS IN PLASMA, BRAIN, AND CEREBROSPINAL FLUID (CSF) IN HUMANS

While the serum concentrations of the non-sulfated DHEA and pregnenolone are in the low nM range in men and women (Labrie et al., 1997; Kancheva et al., 2011), levels of DHEAS are much higher with a slight difference between men (2.3–11.5 μM) and women (1.6–6.2 μM). It should be noted that here total steroid concentrations were measured. Due to the high plasma protein binding (95% for DHEAS; Wang and Bulbrook, 1969) the concentration of the unbound steroids is accordingly lower. Generally, hormone levels decrease with age, exhibiting a maximum in young men and women (~20 years; Labrie et al., 1997). Total PregS serum levels in adolescence range between 40 and 140 nM, and increase during pregnancy and at birth (de Peretti and Mappus, 1983; Kancheva et al., 2011). In contrast to DHEAS and PregS serum levels, less information is available on their tissue concentrations in the brain and in the CSF. In the human brain, region-dependent PregS concentrations between 5 and 40 nmol/kg have been reported with the highest levels in the striatum and hypothalamus. DHEAS concentrations were detected in a similar range with the highest levels in the striatum and cerebellum (Weill-Engerer et al., 2002). The CSF concentrations of DHEAS and PregS were much lower compared to the respective serum levels [serum/CSF ratios: 584 (Preg-conjugates), 19849 (DHEA-conjugates); Kancheva et al., 2011]. These gradients are due to the fact that both compounds cannot cross the respective barriers by passive diffusion, but depend on selective uptake and efflux proteins. ABC- and solute carrier (SLC)-type transporters may not only be relevant for the transport at the BBB and the blood–CSF barrier in the CP, but also for secretion of these compounds from neurons and glial cells (**Figure 1**).

TRANSPORTERS THAT MAY PLAY A ROLE IN THE TRANSPORT OF NEUROSTEROIDS: ABC TRANSPORTERS

ATP-binding cassette proteins can mediate a unidirectional primary active transport of a variety of compounds across membranes. Among the ABC transporters especially ABCG2, also known as the BCRP, and several ABCC/MRP subfamily members are known efflux pumps for conjugated steroids (Suzuki et al., 2003; Haimeur et al., 2004).

BCRP/ABCG2

BCRP/ABCG2 was initially identified as a non-P-glycoprotein and non-MRP-type resistance factor from drug-selected cell lines (Doyle et al., 1998; Miyake et al., 1999). Besides anti-cancer drugs like mitoxantrone, BCRP actively transports sulfated steroids such as E_1-3-S and DHEAS, but not unconjugated or glucuronidated steroids (Imai et al., 2003; Grube et al., 2007). The K_m value for E_1-3-S calculated in isolated membrane vesicles was in the low μM range (**Table 1**). In addition, androgens such as dihydrotestosterone (DHT) have been identified as BCRP substrates (Huss et al., 2005). In human brain microvessels, ABCG2/BCRP transcript (Cooray et al., 2002; Warren et al., 2009) and protein was detected as one of the most abundant ABC transporters (Shawahna et al., 2011). Immunohistochemistry showed it primarily localized at the apical (luminal) side of the endothelial cells (Cooray et al., 2002; Aronica et al., 2005; Warren et al., 2009). In addition, it was detected in the apical membrane of the CP epithelium (Roberts et al., 2008a). Hence, BCRP could be involved in limiting the penetration of peripheral DHEAS and other steroids into the brain or facilitating the elimination of brain-derived DHEAS into blood. The apical localization in the CP, on the other hand, indicate that here BCRP is able to transport neurosteroids into the CSF.

Members of the MRP/ABCC Family

Anionic conjugates of lipophilic compounds are typical substrates for several members of the MRP family. As the founding member, MRP1 (ABCC1) was identified as second export pump conferring a multidrug resistance phenotype besides the MDR1/P-glycoprotein (ABCB1) (Cole et al., 1992). MRP1 was subsequently shown to preferentially transport amphiphilic anions, especially conjugates of lipophilic compounds with glutathione, glucuronate, or sulfate (Jedlitschky

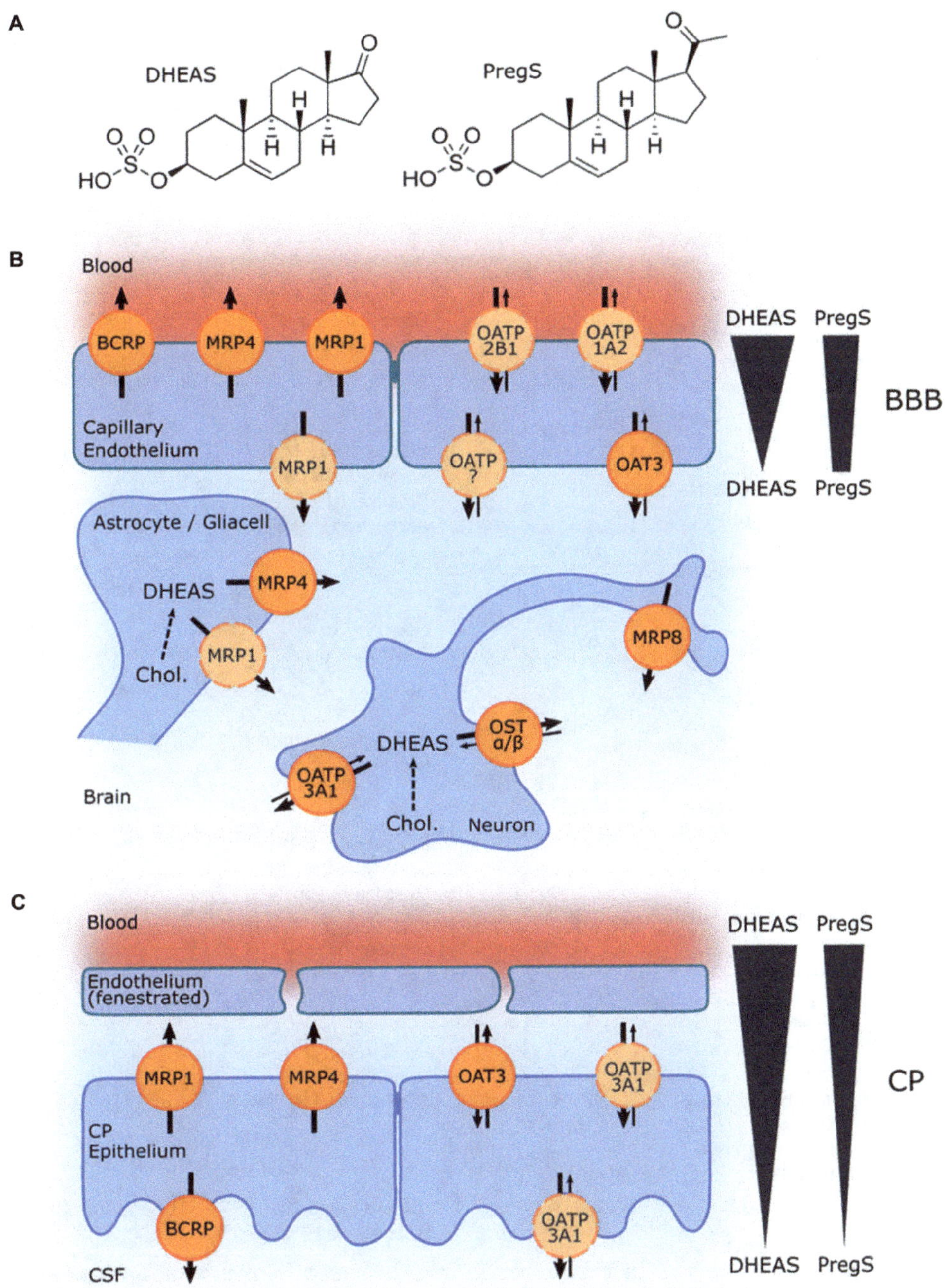

FIGURE 1 | Schematic illustration of ABC and SLC transporters putatively involved in DHEAS and PregS transport and their proposed localization. **(A)** Structures of DHEAS and PregS. **(B,C)** The ABC proteins BCRP (ABCG2), MRP1, MRP4, and MRP8 (ABCC1, ABCC4, and ABCC11), and the solute carriers OAT3 (SLC22A3), OATP1A2 (SLCO1A2), OATP2B1 (SLCO2B1), and OSTα/ß (SLC51A/B) may be involved in secretion of sulfated steroids from neurons and glial cells and/or in the transport across the BBB **(B)** as well as in transport at the blood–CSF barrier in the CP **(C)**. The arrows indicate the directions of substrate transport. Proteins for which there is little or controversial evidence for expression and localization in the basal or apical membrane are indicated in light orange and by a dashed line. Concentration gradients of DHEAS and PregS across the BBB and in the CP are schematically indicated at the right side.

et al., 1996; Loe et al., 1996). MRP1 transports in addition certain cationic or uncharged compounds, but only in co-transport with reduced glutathione (GSH; Loe et al., 1996). It also mediates the transport of E_1-3-S and of DHEAS in a glutathione-dependent manner (Qian et al., 2001; Zelcer et al., 2003) and is expressed in several tissues (Haimeur et al., 2004). It is also expressed in brain microvessels (Warren et al., 2009); however, the exact localization and function has not been finally clarified. It was detected to

TABLE 1 | ABC and SLC transporters possibly involved in neurosteroid transport in the brain.

Transporter	CNS expression (mRNA and protein analysis)	CNS localization (immunohistochemistry)	Steroid substrates (K_m value)
ABC Transporters			
BCRP (ABCG2)	mRNA: – Total brain[1] – Isolated brain microvessels (BMV)[2,3] Protein: – BMV (H, M, Mo, R, P)[4,5,6,7,8] – Isolated CP[9]	BBB: apical (luminal) (H, R); CP: apical (H, R)[2,10,11]	E_1-3-S (6.8 μM)[12,13] DHEAS[12] DHT[14]
MRP1 (ABCC1)	mRNA: – Total brain[1] – BMV[3] – Isolated CP[15] Protein: – Isolated CP (H, R)[9,16]	BBB: apical (H, B, M), Basal (abluminal) (R, M); CP: basal (H, R)[17,18,19,20]	E_1-3-S (+GSH)[21] DHEAS (+GSH) (5 μM)[22] E_2-17βG (1.5 μM)[23]
MRP4 (ABCC4)	mRNA: – Total brain[1] – BMV[3] – Isolated CP[15] Protein: – BMV (H, M, Mo, R)[4,5,6,7] – Isolated CP[9]	BBB: apical (H, M, R), Apical + basal (B); CP: basal (H, R); Astrocytes[3,11,19,20,24]	DHEAS (2 μM)[22] E_2-17βG (30 μM)[22,25]
MRP8 (ABCC11)	mRNA: – Total brain[1]	Neurons (axonal; cerebellum, cortex)[26]	E_1-3-S (>150 μM)[27] DHEAS (13–21 μM)[26,27] E_2-17βG (63 μM)[27]
SLC Transporters			
OATP1A2 (SLCO1A2)	mRNA: – Total brain[1] Protein: – BMV (M, Mo)[5,6]	BBB: luminal; amacrine neurons[28,29,30,31]	DHEAS (7 μM)[32] E_1-3-S (16 μM)[31]
OATP2B1 (SLCO2B1)	mRNA: – Total brain[1] Protein: – Brain capillary cells[31] – BMV (M)[6]	BBB: luminal; CP (ependymal cells) (R); amacrine neurons[11,29,30,33]	E_1-3-S (5–21 μM)[34,35] DHEAS (9 μM)[35] PregS[36]
OATP3A1 (SLCO3A1)	mRNA: – Total brain[1] Protein: – Isolated CP[9] – BMV (P)[8]	CP; neurons[37]	E_1-3-S[38]
OAT3 (SLC22A3)	mRNA: – Total brain[1] Protein: – Isolated CP[9] – BMV (R)[7]	BBB: basal (R); CP: basal (H, R)[39,40,11,41]	E_1-3-S (8.8 μM)[42] DHEAS[42]
OSTα-OSTβ (SLC51A/B)		Neurons (cerebellum, Hippocampus; Purkinje cells)[43]	DHEAS (1.5 μM)[43] PregS (6.9 μM)[43]

Unless otherwise specified, the data refer to human tissue and transporter protein. B, bovine; BBB, blood–brain barrier (capillary endothelial cells); BMV, isolated brain microvessels; CP, choroid plexus; DHEAS, dehydroepiandrosterone sulfate; DHT, dihydrotestosterone; E_1-3-S, estrone-3-sulfate; E_2-17βG, estradiol-17β-glucuronide; H, human; M, mouse; Mo, monkey; P, pig; R, rat; PregS, pregnenolone sulfate. [1]Nishimura and Naito, 2005; [2]Cooray et al., 2002; [3]Warren et al., 2009; [4]Shawahna et al., 2011; [5]Ito et al., 2011; [6]Uchida et al., 2011; [7]Hoshi et al., 2013; [8]Kubo et al., 2015; [9]Uchida et al., 2015; [10]Aronica et al., 2005; [11]Roberts et al., 2008a; [12]Grube et al., 2007; [13]Imai et al., 2003; [14]Huss et al., 2005; [15]Niehof and Borlak, 2009; [16]Gazzin et al., 2008; [17]Rao et al., 1999; [18]Wijnholds et al., 2000; [19]Nies et al., 2004; [20]Zhang et al., 2004; [21]Qian et al., 2001; [22]Zelcer et al., 2003; [23]Jedlitschky et al., 1996; [24]Leggas et al., 2004; [25]Chen et al., 2001; [26]Bortfeld et al., 2006; [27]Chen et al., 2005; [28]Gao et al., 2000; [29]Bronger et al., 2005; [30]Gao et al., 2015; [31]Lee et al., 2005; [32]Kullak-Ublick et al., 1998; [33]Ji et al., 2012; [34]Pizzagalli et al., 2003; [35]Hagenbuch and Stieger, 2013; [36]Grube et al., 2006; [37]Huber et al., 2007; [38]Tamai et al., 2000; [39]Alebouyeh et al., 2003; [40]Kikuchi et al., 2003; [41]Mori et al., 2003; [42]Burckhardt, 2012; [43]Fang et al., 2010.

be luminal in humans, bovine, and murine brain (Nies et al., 2004; Zhang et al., 2004), but also localization at the basolateral (abluminal) membrane was described in mice and rats (Kilic et al., 2008; Roberts et al., 2008a). Some groups did not detect MRP1 protein in human brain capillaries at all (Rao et al., 1999; Aronica et al., 2005). Because of the inconsistent and low-level expression, the relevance of this transporter at the BBB is so far unclear. It may play a more important role in the CP. Here, MRP1 mRNA was detected in rat and human tissue (Gazzin et al., 2008; Niehof and Borlak, 2009) and the protein was localized at the basolateral membrane (Rao et al., 1999; Wijnholds et al., 2000; Gazzin et al., 2008). Thus, it may be involved in the efflux of conjugated steroids from the CSF into blood. In addition, MRP1 mRNA was detected in cultured rat and human astrocytes (Hirrlinger et al., 2001; Spiegl-Kreinecker et al., 2002). However, the protein could not been detected in human glial cells or neurons in immunohistochemical studies (Nies et al., 2004; Aronica et al., 2005). MRP1 and MRP2 (ABCC2) share a similar substrate spectrum, but MRP2 is mainly expressed in polarized epithelial cells (Keppler, 2011). Immunostaining at the apical membrane in brain capillaries was described in rats (Miller et al., 2000), but was not observed in human and bovine brain (Nies et al., 2004; Zhang et al., 2004). Similarly, MRP3 (ABCC3) protein was not detected in human brain (Nies et al., 2004).

A more relevant efflux transporter for conjugated steroids in the brain may be MRP4/ABCC4, which exhibits a unique broad substrate specificity. MRP4 shows the remarkable capacity to transport cyclic nucleotides and MRP4 has been established as an independent regulator of intracellular cAMP levels in several cell types (Ritter et al., 2005; Jedlitschky et al., 2012; Belleville-Rolland et al., 2016). Furthermore, MRP4 transports lipid mediators such as prostanoids and conjugated steroids. DHEAS is transported by MRP4 in a glutathione-independent manner and with high affinity (K_m of 2 μM; Zelcer et al., 2003). It is expressed in several tissues especially in the prostate, kidney, blood cells, and brain (Kool et al., 1997; Haimeur et al., 2004; Nishimura and Naito, 2005; Niehof and Borlak, 2009; Warren et al., 2009; Shawahna et al., 2011). Here, it was localized apically in human, rodent and bovine capillaries (Nies et al., 2004; Leggas et al., 2004; Zhang et al., 2004; Roberts et al., 2008a). An additional detection at the basolateral membrane was only described in bovine brain (Zhang et al., 2004). MRP4 expression was also detected in human CP (Niehof and Borlak, 2009; Uchida et al., 2015) and it was localized to the basolateral membrane in human and murine tissue (Leggas et al., 2004). Moreover, it is expressed in glial cells. Immunofluorescence studies in the human brain revealed staining mainly in astrocytes of the subcortical white matter (Nies et al., 2004). Since glial cells are able to synthesize neurosteroids, MRP4 may account for the efflux of DHEAS and other neurosteroids from these cells for a paracrine action. Astrocytes play a critical role for the development and function of neurons and these cells in turn are regulated by steroid hormones as progesterone and DHEA (Acaz-Fonseca et al., 2016; Arbo et al., 2016). At the BBB and the CP, MRP4 may contribute to the transport of sulfated steroids from brain and CSF into blood.

A further member of the MRP family, the MRP8 (ABCC11) may be relevant with respect to neurosteroid transport. MRP8 was shown to transport DHEAS in isolated membrane vesicles with a K_m value of 13–21 μM, whereas the K_m was above 150 μM for MRP8-mediated transport of E_1-3-S (Chen et al., 2005; Bortfeld et al., 2006). In immunofluorescence studies, it was detected preferentially in the white matter of the cortex and cerebellum and co-localized with neurofilaments indicating localization in neuronal axons (Bortfeld et al., 2006). In addition, weak immunostaining was detected in the gray matter and also in the axons of peripheral neurons. The axonal localization implies that MRP8 can mediate presynaptic efflux of neurosteroids from neurons and thus could directly participate in modulating postsynaptic neurotransmitter receptors (Bortfeld et al., 2006).

Uptake (SLC) Transporters

Besides ABC-type efflux transporters, neurosteroid concentrations in the brain may also be modulated by uptake transporters. Since several members of the SLC superfamily have been identified as uptake transporters for steroid conjugates in general, these transporters are interesting candidates for the transport of neurosteroids. In fact, several SLCs have been shown to mediate cellular uptake of DHEAS and PregS.

Members of the OATP/SLCO Family

Among the SLC transporters, the OATP (SLCO) family is probably the most interesting one in this context. In humans, 11 SLCO transporters exist, organized in six families (Hagenbuch and Stieger, 2013). The physiological substrate profile of the OATP transporters comprises a wide variety of endogenous organic anions including bile acids, bilirubin, thyroid hormones, and prostaglandins (Hagenbuch and Stieger, 2013). In addition, OATPs transport steroid hormone conjugates like E_1-3-S (nearly all OATPs) or estradiol-17β-glucuronide (OATP1A2, OATP1B1, OATP1B3, OATP1C1, and OATP4A1) and the neurosteroid DHEAS (OATP1A2, OATP1B1, OATP1B3, and OATP2B1) (Hagenbuch and Stieger, 2013). The affinity of these transporters toward DHEAS was slightly above (OATP1B1 and OATP1B3) or in the range (OATP2B1 and OATP1A2) (**Table 1**) of the physiological plasma concentration (1.6–11.5 μM; Labrie et al., 1997) indicating an *in vivo* relevance of these findings. OATP1B1 and OATP1B3 are almost exclusively expressed in the human liver. Here, they are responsible for cellular uptake as a prerequisite for hepatic metabolism and elimination. In turn, the expression and function of these transporters affect systemic DHEAS levels as shown by enhanced DHEAS levels in monkeys and rats after treatment with the unspecific OATP inhibitor rifampicin (Watanabe et al., 2015; Nishizawa et al., 2017). Assuming a DHEAS transport/uptake from the blood into the brain/CSF (Kancheva et al., 2010), changes in DHEAS plasma concentration might indirectly influence the concentration in these compartments. Therefore, OATPs localized in the BBB and/ or the CP are of special interest. Indeed, OATP1A2, OATP1C1, OATP2B1, and OATP3A1 have been detected in these structures in humans (Kullak-Ublick et al., 1998; Pizzagalli et al., 2002; Huber et al., 2007; Roberts et al., 2008b; Ji et al., 2012). Since OATP1C1 is a thyroid hormone transporter and the function of OATP3A4 is only poorly understood, at present OATP1A2 and OATP2B1 are probably the most interesting members concerning neurosteroid transport in the brain. Both proteins are expressed in the endothelial cells of the BBB presumably in the luminal membrane predisposing them as transporters for uptake into the brain (Gao et al., 2000; Bronger et al., 2005; Lee et al., 2005). In addition, OATP1A2 and OATP2B1 are also expressed in other CNS cell types. While both transporters have been identified in amacrine neurons of the retina, OATP1A2 was additionally found in hippocampal pyramidal and granule cells (Gao et al., 2015). Besides DHEAS, PregS levels in the brain may also be influenced by uptake transporters in the BBB, even though plasma concentrations of PregS were up to two orders of magnitude below the

DHEAS levels (Sanchez-Guijo et al., 2015). Like for DHEAS, OATP-transporters are interesting candidates in this context. While PregS significantly inhibits OATP2B1 function (St Pierre et al., 2002; Grube et al., 2006) first reports indicated no direct transport of PregS by this transporter (Pizzagalli et al., 2003; Grube et al., 2006). Interestingly, OATP2B1-mediated transport of E_1-3-S and DHEAS was stimulated by steroid hormones like progesterone (Grube et al., 2006; Koenen et al., 2012). Under these conditions, PregS was also transported by OATP2B1 (Grube et al., 2006). PregS transport by other OATPs has not been studied so far. With regard to the CP only limited information is available about OATP expression and function in humans. In a recent LC-MS/MS-based study examining transporter protein expression in this structure, only OATP3A1 was detected, while OATP1A2 and OATP1C1 were below the detection limit and OATP2B1 was not analyzed (Ji et al., 2012). This finding was quite surprising, since in animal models several OATPs have been detected in the CP and shown to be involved in the neurosteroid transport into the liquor (Asaba et al., 2000; Choudhuri et al., 2003; Ji et al., 2012). Due to the limited information available, the significance of OATP3A1 in this context cannot be conclusively assessed. However, a transport of E_1-3-S has also been shown for the OATP3A1 and two splice variants of the transporter are selectively expressed in the apical and basal membrane of the ependymal cells of the CP (Tamai et al., 2000; Huber et al., 2007).

Other Organic Anion Transporters (OSTα-OSTβ, OATs)

Besides OATPs, an interaction of neurosteroids (mainly DHEAS and PregS) with several further organic anion transporters has been reported. For example, both sulfated neurosteroids have been shown to be transported with high affinity by the organic solute transporter OSTα-OSTβ [K_m: 1.5 μM (DHEAS) and 6.9 μM (PregS)] (Fang et al., 2010). The heterodimer OSTα-OSTβ is a relatively new member of the SLC family (SLC51) and encoded by two genes (SLC51A and SLC51B). Like OATPs, the transport mechanism is facilitated diffusion; therefore OSTα-OSTβ-mediated transport is dependent on the electrochemical gradient of its substrates (Ballatori et al., 2013). In the human brain, the transporter is expressed in Purkinje cells and hippocampal neurons (Fang et al., 2010). Both regions are well known for their function in the process of learning and memory, and hippocampal neurons have been suggested as a target site for PregS action (Akwa et al., 2001).

A third group of SLC transporters involved in the CNS distribution of sulfated neurosteroids are the organic anion transporters (OATs), which are part of the SLC22A branch (Burckhardt, 2012). The pivotal role of these transporters is the excretion of water-soluble organic anions in the kidney. However, selected members are also present in other organs including the brain (Burckhardt, 2012). In the brain OAT3, is probably the most interesting member of this family. The transporter is expressed in the BBB as well as the CP (Alebouyeh et al., 2003; Kikuchi et al., 2003; Uchida et al., 2015). In a mouse model, OAT3 was characterized as the DHEAS transporter in part responsible for the DHEAS efflux across the BBB (Miyajima et al., 2011). Besides OAT3, mRNA expression of OAT1 and OAT2 has also been shown for the human brain (Lopez-Nieto et al., 1997; Alebouyeh et al., 2003; Cropp et al., 2008); however, protein data for these transporters are limited.

CONCLUSION AND PERSPECTIVES

The detailed functions of the described ABC and SLC transporters in brain are still poorly understood. Even data on the expression and localization, e.g., at the BBB are often controversial. Knock-out mice of the ABC and some SLC transporters are available, but have been mainly used to study the role of these transporters for brain penetration of certain drugs (Dallas et al., 2006; Chaves et al., 2014). These studies are in part hampered by overlapping substrate specificities of several transporters and with respect to neurosteroids by the fact of negligible levels of sulfated steroids in rodent brain (Liu et al., 2003; Liere et al., 2009). Furthermore, a number of functional genetic variants in several transporter genes are known (Bruhn and Cascorbi, 2014); however, their impact on neurosteroid transport is so far largely unknown. Variations in transporter function may affect concentrations and action of several neurosteroids in brain. Therefore, a better understanding of these processes is an important aspect also in the context of a possible therapeutic use of these compounds.

AUTHOR CONTRIBUTIONS

MG and GJ conceived and wrote the manuscript. PH designed **Figure 1** and revised the manuscript. All authors read and approved the manuscript for publication.

REFERENCES

Acaz-Fonseca, E., Avila-Rodriguez, M., Garcia-Segura, L. M., and Barreto, G. E. (2016). Regulation of astroglia by gonadal steroid hormones under physiological and pathological conditions. *Prog. Neurobiol.* 144, 5–26. doi: 10.1016/j.pneurobio.2016.06.002

Akwa, Y., Ladurelle, N., Covey, D. F., and Baulieu, E. E. (2001). The synthetic enantiomer of pregnenolone sulfate is very active on memory in rats and mice, even more so than its physiological neurosteroid counterpart: distinct mechanisms? *Proc. Natl. Acad. Sci. U.S.A.* 98, 14033–14037. doi: 10.1073/pnas.241503698

Alebouyeh, M., Takeda, M., Onozato, M. L., Tojo, A., Noshiro, R., Hasannejad, H., et al. (2003). Expression of human organic anion transporters in the choroid plexus and their interactions with neurotransmitter metabolites. *J. Pharmacol. Sci.* 93, 430–436. doi: 10.1254/jphs.93.430

Arbo, B. D., Bennetti, F., and Ribeiro, M. F. (2016). Astrocytes as a target for neuroprotection: modulation by progesterone and dehydroepiandrosterone. *Prog. Neurobiol.* 144, 27–47. doi: 10.1016/j.pneurobio.2016.03.010

Aronica, E., Gorter, J. A., Redeker, S., van Vliet, E. A., Ramkema, M., Scheffer, G. L., et al. (2005). Localization of breast cancer resistance protein (BCRP) in microvessel endothelium of human control and epileptic brain. *Epilepsia* 46, 849–857. doi: 10.1111/j.1528-1167.2005.66604.x

Asaba, H., Hosoya, K., Takanaga, H., Ohtsuki, S., Tamura, E., Takizawa, T., and Terasaki, T. (2000). Blood-brain barrier is involved in the efflux transport of a neuroactive steroid, dehydroepiandrosterone sulfate, via organic anion transporting polypeptide 2. *J. Neurochem.* 75, 1907–1916. doi: 10.1046/j.1471-4159.2000.0751907.x

Ballatori, N., Christian, W. V., Wheeler, S. G., and Hammond, C. L. (2013). The heteromeric organic solute transporter, OSTalpha-OSTbeta/SLC51: a transporter for steroid-derived molecules. *Mol. Aspects Med.* 34, 683–692. doi: 10.1016/j.mam.2012.11.005

Baulieu, E. E. (1997). Neurosteroids: of the nervous system, by the nervous system, for the nervous system. *Recent Prog. Horm. Res.* 52, 1–32.

Belleville-Rolland, T., Sassi, Y., Decouture, B., Dreano, E., Hulot, J. S., Gaussem, P., et al. (2016). MRP4 (ABCC4) as a potential pharmacologic target for cardiovascular disease. *Pharmacol. Res.* 107, 381–389. doi: 10.1016/j.phrs.2016.04.002

Bortfeld, M., Rius, M., Konig, J., Herold-Mende, C., Nies, A. T., and Keppler, D. (2006). Human multidrug resistance protein 8 (MRP8/ABCC11), an apical efflux pump for steroid sulfates, is an axonal protein of the CNS and peripheral nervous system. *Neuroscience* 137, 1247–1257. doi: 10.1016/j.neuroscience.2005.10.025

Bronger, H., Konig, J., Kopplow, K., Steiner, H. H., Ahmadi, R., Herold-Mende, C., et al. (2005). ABCC drug efflux pumps and organic anion uptake transporters in human gliomas and the blood-tumor barrier. *Cancer Res.* 65, 11419–11428. doi: 10.1158/0008-5472.CAN-05-1271

Bruhn, O., and Cascorbi, I. (2014). Polymorphisms of the drug transporters ABCB1, ABCG2, ABCC2 and ABCC3 and their impact on drug bioavailability and clinical relevance. *Expert Opin. Drug Metab. Toxicol.* 10, 1337–1354. doi: 10.1517/17425255.2014.952630

Burckhardt, G. (2012). Drug transport by organic anion transporters (OATs). *Pharmacol. Ther.* 136, 106–130. doi: 10.1016/j.pharmthera.2012.07.010

Chaves, C., Shawahna, R., Jacob, A., Scherrmann, J. M., and Decleves, X. (2014). Human ABC transporters at blood-CNS interfaces as determinants of CNS drug penetration. *Curr. Pharm. Des.* 20, 1450–1462. doi: 10.2174/13816128113199990466

Chen, Z. S., Guo, Y., Belinsky, M. G., Kotova, E., and Kruh, G. D. (2005). Transport of bile acids, sulfated steroids, estradiol 17-beta-D-glucuronide, and leukotriene C4 by human multidrug resistance protein 8 (ABCC11). *Mol. Pharmacol.* 67, 545–557. doi: 10.1124/mol.104.007138

Chen, Z. S., Lee, K., and Kruh, G. D. (2001). Transport of cyclic nucleotides and estradiol 17-beta-D-glucuronide by multidrug resistance protein 4. Resistance to 6-mercaptopurine and 6-thioguanine. *J. Biol. Chem.* 276, 33747–33754. doi: 10.1074/jbc.M104833200

Chisari, M., Eisenman, L. N., Covey, D. F., Mennerick, S., and Zorumski, C. F. (2010). The sticky issue of neurosteroids and GABA(A) receptors. *Trends Neurosci.* 33, 299–306. doi: 10.1016/j.tins.2010.03.005

Choudhuri, S., Cherrington, N. J., Li, N., and Klaassen, C. D. (2003). Constitutive expression of various xenobiotic and endobiotic transporter mRNAs in the choroid plexus of rats. *Drug Metab. Dispos.* 31, 1337–1345. doi: 10.1124/dmd.31.11.1337

Cole, S. P., Bhardwaj, G., Gerlach, J. H., Mackie, J. E., Grant, C. E., Almquist, K. C., et al. (1992). Overexpression of a transporter gene in a multidrug-resistant human lung cancer cell line. *Science* 258, 1650–1654. doi: 10.1126/science.1360704

Cooray, H. C., Blackmore, C. G., Maskell, L., and Barrand, M. A. (2002). Localisation of breast cancer resistance protein in microvessel endothelium of human brain. *Neuroreport* 13, 2059–2063. doi: 10.1097/00001756-200211150-00014

Cropp, C. D., Komori, T., Shima, J. E., Urban, T. J., Yee, S. W., More, S. S., et al. (2008). Organic anion transporter 2 (SLC22A7) is a facilitative transporter of cGMP. *Mol. Pharmacol.* 73, 1151–1158. doi: 10.1124/mol.107.043117

Dallas, S., Miller, D. S., and Bendayan, R. (2006). Multidrug resistance-associated proteins: expression and function in the central nervous system. *Pharmacol. Rev.* 58, 140–161. doi: 10.1124/pr.58.2.3

de Peretti, E., and Mappus, E. (1983). Pattern of plasma pregnenolone sulfate levels in humans from birth to adulthood. *J. Clin. Endocrinol. Metab.* 57, 550–556. doi: 10.1210/jcem-57-3-550

Doyle, L. A., Yang, W., Abruzzo, L. V., Krogmann, T., Gao, Y., Rishi, A. K., et al. (1998). A multidrug resistance transporter from human MCF-7 breast cancer cells. *Proc. Natl. Acad. Sci. U.S.A.* 95, 15665–15670. doi: 10.1073/pnas.95.26.15665

Fang, F., Christian, W. V., Gorman, S. G., Cui, M., Huang, J., Tieu, K., et al. (2010). Neurosteroid transport by the organic solute transporter OSTalpha-OSTbeta. *J. Neurochem.* 115, 220–233. doi: 10.1111/j.1471-4159.2010.06920.x

Gao, B., Hagenbuch, B., Kullak-Ublick, G. A., Benke, D., Aguzzi, A., and Meier, P. J. (2000). Organic anion-transporting polypeptides mediate transport of opioid peptides across blood-brain barrier. *J. Pharmacol. Exp. Ther.* 294, 73–79.

Gao, B., Vavricka, S. R., Meier, P. J., and Stieger, B. (2015). Differential cellular expression of organic anion transporting peptides OATP1A2 and OATP2B1 in the human retina and brain: implications for carrier-mediated transport of neuropeptides and neurosteriods in the CNS. *Pflugers Arch.* 467, 1481–1493. doi: 10.1007/s00424-014-1596-x

Gazzin, S., Strazielle, N., Schmitt, C., Fevre-Montange, M., Ostrow, J. D., Tiribelli, C., et al. (2008). Differential expression of the multidrug resistance-related proteins ABCb1 and ABCc1 between blood-brain interfaces. *J. Comp. Neurol.* 510, 497–507. doi: 10.1002/cne.21808

Grube, M., Kock, K., Karner, S., Reuther, S., Ritter, C. A., Jedlitschky, G., et al. (2006). Modification of OATP2B1-Mediated transport by steroid hormones. *Mol. Pharmacol.* 70, 1735–1741. doi: 10.1124/mol.106.026450

Grube, M., Reuther, S., Meyer Zu Schwabedissen, H., Kock, K., Draber, K., et al. (2007). Organic anion transporting polypeptide 2B1 and breast cancer resistance protein interact in the transepithelial transport of steroid sulfates in human placenta. *Drug Metab. Dispos.* 35, 30–35. doi: 10.1124/dmd.106.011411

Hagenbuch, B., and Stieger, B. (2013). The SLCO (former SLC21) superfamily of transporters. *Mol. Aspects Med.* 34, 396–412. doi: 10.1016/j.mam.2012.10.009

Haimeur, A., Conseil, G., Deeley, R. G., and Cole, S. P. (2004). The MRP-related and BCRP/ABCG2 multidrug resistance proteins: biology, substrate specificity and regulation. *Curr. Drug Metab.* 5, 21–53. doi: 10.2174/1389200043489199

Harteneck, C. (2013). Pregnenolone sulfate: from steroid metabolite to TRP channel ligand. *Molecules* 18, 12012–12028. doi: 10.3390/molecules181012012

Hirrlinger, J., Konig, J., Keppler, D., Lindenau, J., Schulz, J. B., and Dringen, R. (2001). The multidrug resistance protein MRP1 mediates the release of glutathione disulfide from rat astrocytes during oxidative stress. *J. Neurochem.* 76, 627–636. doi: 10.1046/j.1471-4159.2001.00101.x

Hojo, Y., Higo, S., Kawato, S., Hatanaka, Y., Ooishi, Y., Murakami, G., et al. (2011). Hippocampal synthesis of sex steroids and corticosteroids: essential for modulation of synaptic plasticity. *Front. Endocrinol.* 2:43. doi: 10.3389/fendo.2011.00043

Hoshi, Y., Uchida, Y., Tachikawa, M., Inoue, T., Ohtsuki, S., and Terasaki, T. (2013). Quantitative atlas of blood-brain barrier transporters, receptors, and tight junction proteins in rats and common marmoset. *J. Pharm. Sci.* 102, 3343–3355. doi: 10.1002/jps.23575

Huber, R. D., Gao, B., Sidler, P., fandler, M. A., Zhang-Fu, W., Leuthold, S., et al. (2007). Characterization of two splice variants of human organic anion transporting polypeptide 3A1 isolated from human brain. *Am. J. Physiol. Cell Physiol.* 292, C795–C806. doi: 10.1152/ajpcell.00597.2005

Huss, W. J., Gray, D. R., Greenberg, N. M., Mohler, J. L., and Smith, G. J. (2005). Breast cancer resistance protein-mediated efflux of androgen in putative benign and malignant prostate stem cells. *Cancer Res.* 65, 6640–6650. doi: 10.1158/0008-5472.CAN-04-2548

Imai, Y., Asada, S., Tsukahara, S., Ishikawa, E., Tsuruo, T., and Sugimoto, Y. (2003). Breast cancer resistance protein exports sulfated estrogens but not free estrogens. *Mol. Pharmacol.* 64, 610–618. doi: 10.1124/mol.64.3.610

Ito, K., Uchida, Y., Ohtsuki, S., Aizawa, S., Kawakami, H., Katsukura, Y., et al. (2011). Quantitative membrane protein expression at the blood-brain barrier of adult and younger cynomolgus monkeys. *J. Pharm. Sci.* 100, 3939–3950. doi: 10.1002/jps.22487

Jedlitschky, G., Greinacher, A., and Kroemer, H. K. (2012). Transporters in human platelets: physiologic function and impact for pharmacotherapy. *Blood* 119, 3394–3402. doi: 10.1182/blood-2011-09-336933

Jedlitschky, G., Leier, I., Buchholz, U., Barnouin, K., Kurz, G., and Keppler, D. (1996). Transport of glutathione, glucuronate, and sulfate conjugates by the MRP gene-encoded conjugate export pump. *Cancer Res.* 56, 988–994.

Ji, C., Tschantz, W. R., Pfeifer, N. D., Ullah, M., and Sadagopan, N. (2012). Development of a multiplex UPLC-MRM MS method for quantification of human membrane transport proteins OATP1B1, OATP1B3 and OATP2B1 in in vitro systems and tissues. *Anal. Chim. Acta* 717, 67–76. doi: 10.1016/j.aca.2011.12.005

Kancheva, R., Hill, M., Novak, Z., Chrastina, J., Kancheva, L., and Starka, L. (2011). Neuroactive steroids in periphery and cerebrospinal fluid. *Neuroscience* 191, 22–27. doi: 10.1016/j.neuroscience.2011.05.054

Kancheva, R., Hill, M., Novak, Z., Chrastina, J., Velikova, M., Kancheva, L., et al. (2010). Peripheral neuroactive steroids may be as good as the steroids in the cerebrospinal fluid for the diagnostics of CNS disturbances. *J. Steroid Biochem. Mol. Biol.* 119, 35–44. doi: 10.1016/j.jsbmb.2009.12.006

Keppler, D. (2011). Multidrug resistance proteins (MRPs, ABCCs): importance for pathophysiology and drug therapy. *Handb. Exp. Pharmacol.* 201, 299–323. doi: 10.1007/978-3-642-14541-4_8

Kikuchi, R., Kusuhara, H., Sugiyama, D., and Sugiyama, Y. (2003). Contribution of organic anion transporter 3 (Slc22a8) to the elimination of p-aminohippuric acid and benzylpenicillin across the blood-brain barrier. *J. Pharmacol. Exp. Ther.* 306, 51–58. doi: 10.1124/jpet.103.049197

Kilic, E., Spudich, A., Kilic, U., Rentsch, K. M., Vig, R., Matter, C. M., et al. (2008). ABCC1: a gateway for pharmacological compounds to the ischaemic brain. *Brain* 131, 2679–2689. doi: 10.1093/brain/awn222

Koenen, A., Kock, K., Keiser, M., Siegmund, W., Kroemer, H. K., and Grube, M. (2012). Steroid hormones specifically modify the activity of organic anion transporting polypeptides. *Eur. J. Pharm. Sci.* 47, 774–780. doi: 10.1016/j.ejps.2012.08.017

Kool, M., de Haas, M., Scheffer, G. L., Scheper, R. J., van Eijk, M. J., Juijn, J. A., et al. (1997). Analysis of expression of cMOAT (MRP2), MRP3, MRP4, and MRP5, homologues of the multidrug resistance-associated protein gene (MRP1), in human cancer cell lines. *Cancer Res.* 57, 3537–3547.

Kubo, Y., Ohtsuki, S., Uchida, Y., and Terasaki, T. (2015). Quantitative determination of luminal and abluminal membrane distributions of transporters in porcine brain capillaries by plasma membrane fractionation and quantitative targeted proteomics. *J. Pharm. Sci.* 104, 3060–3068. doi: 10.1002/jps.24398

Kullak-Ublick, G. A., Fisch, T., Oswald, M., Hagenbuch, B., Meier, P. J., Beuers, U., et al. (1998). Dehydroepiandrosterone sulfate (DHEAS): identification of a carrier protein in human liver and brain. *FEBS Lett.* 424, 173–176. doi: 10.1016/S0014-5793(98)00168-9

Labrie, F., Belanger, A., Cusan, L., Gomez, J. L., and Candas, B. (1997). Marked decline in serum concentrations of adrenal C19 sex steroid precursors and conjugated androgen metabolites during aging. *J. Clin. Endocrinol. Metab.* 82, 2396–2402. doi: 10.1210/jcem.82.8.4160

Lee, W., Glaeser, H., Smith, L. H., Roberts, R. L., Moeckel, G. W., Gervasini, G., et al. (2005). Polymorphisms in human organic anion-transporting polypeptide 1A2 (OATP1A2): implications for altered drug disposition and central nervous system drug entry. *J. Biol. Chem.* 280, 9610–9617. doi: 10.1074/jbc.M411092200

Leggas, M., Adachi, M., Scheffer, G. L., Sun, D., Wielinga, P., Du, G., et al. (2004). Mrp4 confers resistance to topotecan and protects the brain from chemotherapy. *Mol. Cell. Biol.* 24, 7612–7621. doi: 10.1128/MCB.24.17.7612-7621.2004

Liere, P., Pianos, A., Eychenne, B., Cambourg, A., Bodin, K., Griffiths, W., et al. (2009). Analysis of pregnenolone and dehydroepiandrosterone in rodent brain: cholesterol autoxidation is the key. *J. Lipid Res.* 50, 2430–2444. doi: 10.1194/jlr.M900162-JLR200

Liu, S., Sjovall, J., and Griffiths, W. J. (2003). Neurosteroids in rat brain: extraction, isolation, and analysis by nanoscale liquid chromatography-electrospray mass spectrometry. *Anal. Chem.* 75, 5835–5846. doi: 10.1021/ac0346297

Loe, D. W., Almquist, K. C., Deeley, R. G., and Cole, S. P. (1996). Multidrug resistance protein (MRP)-mediated transport of leukotriene C4 and chemotherapeutic agents in membrane vesicles. Demonstration of glutathione-dependent vincristine transport. *J. Biol. Chem.* 271, 9675–9682. doi: 10.1074/jbc.271.16.9675

Lopez-Nieto, C. E., You, G., Bush, K. T., Barros, E. J., Beier, D. R., and Nigam, S. K. (1997). Molecular cloning and characterization of NKT, a gene product related to the organic cation transporter family that is almost exclusively expressed in the kidney. *J. Biol. Chem.* 272, 6471–6478. doi: 10.1074/jbc.272.10.6471

Maninger, N., Wolkowitz, O. M., Reus, V. I., Epel, E. S., and Mellon, S. H. (2009). Neurobiological and neuropsychiatric effects of dehydroepiandrosterone (DHEA) and DHEA sulfate (DHEAS). *Front. Neuroendocrinol.* 30, 65–91. doi: 10.1016/j.yfrne.2008.11.002

Miller, D. S., Nobmann, S. N., Gutmann, H., Toeroek, M., Drewe, J., and Fricker, G. (2000). Xenobiotic transport across isolated brain microvessels studied by confocal microscopy. *Mol. Pharmacol.* 58, 1357–1367. doi: 10.1124/mol.58.6.1357

Miyajima, M., Kusuhara, H., Fujishima, M., Adachi, Y., and Sugiyama, Y. (2011). Organic anion transporter 3 mediates the efflux transport of an amphipathic organic anion, dehydroepiandrosterone sulfate, across the blood-brain barrier in mice. *Drug Metab. Dispos.* 39, 814–819. doi: 10.1124/dmd.110.036863

Miyake, K., Mickley, L., Litman, T., Zhan, Z., Robey, R., Cristensen, B., et al. (1999). Molecular cloning of cDNAs which are highly overexpressed in mitoxantrone-resistant cells: demonstration of homology to ABC transport genes. *Cancer Res.* 59, 8–13.

Monnet, F. P., Mahe, V., Robel, P., and Baulieu, E. E. (1995). Neurosteroids, via sigma receptors, modulate the [3H]norepinephrine release evoked by N-methyl-D-aspartate in the rat hippocampus. *Proc. Natl. Acad. Sci. U.S.A.* 92, 3774–3778. doi: 10.1073/pnas.92.9.3774

Mori, S., Takanaga, H., Ohtsuki, S., Deguchi, T., Kang, Y. S., Hosoya, K., et al. (2003). Rat organic anion transporter 3 (rOAT3) is responsible for brain-to-blood efflux of homovanillic acid at the abluminal membrane of brain capillary endothelial cells. *J. Cereb. Blood Flow Metab.* 23, 432–440. doi: 10.1097/01.WCB.0000050062.57184.75

Niehof, M., and Borlak, J. (2009). Expression of HNF4alpha in the human and rat choroid plexus: implications for drug transport across the blood-cerebrospinal-fluid (CSF) barrier. *BMC Mol. Biol.* 10:68. doi: 10.1186/1471-2199-10-68

Nies, A. T., Jedlitschky, G., Konig, J., Herold-Mende, C., Steiner, H. H., Schmitt, H. P., et al. (2004). Expression and immunolocalization of the multidrug resistance proteins, MRP1-MRP6 (ABCC1-ABCC6), in human brain. *Neuroscience* 129, 349–360. doi: 10.1016/j.neuroscience.2004.07.051

Nishimura, M., and Naito, S. (2005). Tissue-specific mRNA expression profiles of human ATP-binding cassette and solute carrier transporter superfamilies. *Drug Metab. Pharmacokinet.* 20, 452–477. doi: 10.2133/dmpk.20.452

Nishizawa, K., Nakanishi, T., and Tamai, I. (2017). Comparative evaluation of dehydroepiandrosterone sulfate potential to predict hepatic organic anion transporting polypeptide transporter-based drug-drug interactions. *Drug Metab. Dispos.* 45, 224–227. doi: 10.1124/dmd.116.072355

Pizzagalli, F., Hagenbuch, B., Stieger, B., Klenk, U., Folkers, G., and Meier, P. J. (2002). Identification of a novel human organic anion transporting polypeptide as a high affinity thyroxine transporter. *Mol. Endocrinol.* 16, 2283–2296. doi: 10.1210/me.2001-0309

Pizzagalli, F., Varga, Z., Huber, R. D., Folkers, G., Meier, P. J., and St Pierre, M. V. (2003). Identification of steroid sulfate transport processes in the human mammary gland. *J. Clin. Endocrinol. Metab.* 88, 3902–3912. doi: 10.1210/jc.2003-030174

Porcu, P., Barron, A. M., Frye, C. A., Walf, A. A., Yang, S. Y., He, X. Y., et al. (2016). Neurosteroidogenesis today: novel targets for neuroactive steroid synthesis and action and their relevance for translational research. *J. Neuroendocrinol.* 28:12351. doi: 10.1111/jne.12351

Qian, Y. M., Song, W. C., Cui, H., Cole, S. P., and Deeley, R. G. (2001). Glutathione stimulates sulfated estrogen transport by multidrug resistance protein 1. *J. Biol. Chem.* 276, 6404–6411. doi: 10.1074/jbc.M008251200

Rao, V. V., Dahlheimer, J. L., Bardgett, M. E., Snyder, A. Z., Finch, R. A., Sartorelli, A. C., et al. (1999). Choroid plexus epithelial expression of MDR1 P glycoprotein and multidrug resistance-associated protein contribute to the blood-cerebrospinal-fluid drug-permeability barrier. *Proc. Natl. Acad. Sci. U.S.A.* 96, 3900–3905. doi: 10.1073/pnas.96.7.3900

Reddy, D. S. (2010). Neurosteroids: endogenous role in the human brain and therapeutic potentials. *Prog. Brain Res.* 18, 113–137. doi: 10.1016/B978-0-444-53630-3.00008-7

Ritter, C. A., Jedlitschky, G., Meyer Zu Schwabedissen, H., Grube, M., Kock, K., and Kroemer, H. K. (2005). Cellular export of drugs and signaling molecules by the ATP-binding cassette transporters MRP4 (ABCC4) and MRP5 (ABCC5). *Drug Metab. Rev.* 37, 253–278. doi: 10.1081/DMR-200047984

Roberts, L. M., Black, D. S., Raman, C., Woodford, K., Zhou, M., Haggerty, J. E., et al. (2008a). Subcellular localization of transporters along the rat blood-brain barrier and blood-cerebral-spinal fluid barrier by in vivo biotinylation. *Neuroscience* 155, 423–438. doi: 10.1016/j.neuroscience.2008.06.015

Roberts, L. M., Woodford, K., Zhou, M., Black, D. S., Haggerty, J. E., Tate, E. H., et al. (2008b). Expression of the thyroid hormone transporters monocarboxylate transporter-8 (SLC16A2) and organic ion transporter-14 (SLCO1C1) at the blood-brain barrier. *Endocrinology* 149, 6251–6261. doi: 10.1210/en.2008-0378

Salman, E. D., Faye-Petersen, O., and Falany, C. N. (2011). Hydroxysteroid sulfotransferase 2B1b expression and localization in normal human brain. *Horm. Mol. Biol. Clin. Investig.* 8, 445–454. doi: 10.1515/HMBCI.2011.117

Sanchez-Guijo, A., Oji, V., Hartmann, M. F., Traupe, H., and Wudy, S. A. (2015). Simultaneous quantification of cholesterol sulfate, androgen sulfates, and progestagen sulfates in human serum by LC-MS/MS. *J. Lipid Res.* 56, 1843–1851. doi: 10.1194/jlr.D061499

Seljeset, S., Laverty, D., and Smart, T. G. (2015). Inhibitory neurosteroids and the GABAA receptor. *Adv. Pharmacol.* 72, 165–187. doi: 10.1016/bs.apha.2014.10.006

Shawahna, R., Uchida, Y., Decleves, X., Ohtsuki, S., Yousif, S., Dauchy, S., et al. (2011). Transcriptomic and quantitative proteomic analysis of transporters and drug metabolizing enzymes in freshly isolated human brain microvessels. *Mol. Pharm.* 8, 1332–1341. doi: 10.1021/mp200129p

Spiegl-Kreinecker, S., Buchroithner, J., Elbling, L., Steiner, E., Wurm, G., Bodenteich, A., et al. (2002). Expression and functional activity of the ABC-transporter proteins P-glycoprotein and multidrug-resistance protein 1 in human brain tumor cells and astrocytes. *J. Neurooncol.* 57, 27–36. doi: 10.1023/A:1015735815111

St Pierre, M. V., Hagenbuch, B., Ugele, B., Meier, P. J., and Stallmach, T. (2002). Characterization of an organic anion-transporting polypeptide (OATP-B) in human placenta. *J. Clin. Endocrinol. Metab.* 87, 1856–1863. doi: 10.1210/jcem.87.4.8431

Suzuki, M., Suzuki, H., Sugimoto, Y., and Sugiyama, Y. (2003). ABCG2 transports sulfated conjugates of steroids and xenobiotics. *J. Biol. Chem.* 278, 22644–22649. doi: 10.1074/jbc.M212399200

Tamai, I., Nezu, J., Uchino, H., Sai, Y., Oku, A., Shimane, M., et al. (2000). Molecular identification and characterization of novel members of the human organic anion transporter (OATP) family. *Biochem. Biophys. Res. Commun.* 273, 251–260. doi: 10.1006/bbrc.2000.2922

Uchida, Y., Ohtsuki, S., Katsukura, Y., Ikeda, C., Suzuki, T., Kamiie, J., et al. (2011). Quantitative targeted absolute proteomics of human blood-brain barrier transporters and receptors. *J. Neurochem.* 117, 333–345. doi: 10.1111/j.1471-4159.2011.07208.x

Uchida, Y., Zhang, Z., Tachikawa, M., and Terasaki, T. (2015). Quantitative targeted absolute proteomics of rat blood-cerebrospinal fluid barrier transporters: comparison with a human specimen. *J. Neurochem.* 134, 1104–1115. doi: 10.1111/jnc.13147

Wang, D. Y., and Bulbrook, R. D. (1969). The binding of steroids to plasma proteins in normal women and women with breast cancer. *Eur. J. Cancer* 5, 247–253. doi: 10.1016/0014-2964(69)90074-7

Warren, M. S., Zerangue, N., Woodford, K., Roberts, L. M., Tate, E. H., Feng, B., et al. (2009). Comparative gene expression profiles of ABC transporters in brain microvessel endothelial cells and brain in five species including human. *Pharmacol. Res.* 59, 404–413. doi: 10.1016/j.phrs.2009.02.007

Watanabe, M., Watanabe, T., Yabuki, M., and Tamai, I. (2015). Dehydroepiandrosterone sulfate, a useful endogenous probe for evaluation of drug-drug interaction on hepatic organic anion transporting polypeptide (OATP) in cynomolgus monkeys. *Drug Metab. Pharmacokinet.* 30, 198–204. doi: 10.1016/j.dmpk.2014.12.009

Weill-Engerer, S., David, J. P., Sazdovitch, V., Liere, P., Eychenne, B., Pianos, A., et al. (2002). Neurosteroid quantification in human brain regions: comparison between Alzheimer's and nondemented patients. *J. Clin. Endocrinol. Metab.* 87, 5138–5143. doi: 10.1210/jc.2002-020878

Wijnholds, J., deLange, E. C., Scheffer, G. L., van den Berg, D. J., Mol, C. A., van, D. V, et al. (2000). Multidrug resistance protein 1 protects the choroid plexus epithelium and contributes to the blood-cerebrospinal fluid barrier. *J. Clin. Invest.* 105, 279–285. doi: 10.1172/JCI8267

Wu, F. S., Gibbs, T. T., and Farb, D. H. (1991). Pregnenolone sulfate: a positive allosteric modulator at the N-methyl-D-aspartate receptor. *Mol. Pharmacol.* 40, 333–336.

Zelcer, N., Reid, G., Wielinga, P., Kuil, A., van, D. H. I., Schuetz, J. D., et al. (2003). Steroid and bile acid conjugates are substrates of human multidrug-resistance protein (MRP) 4 (ATP-binding cassette C4). *Biochem. J.* 371, 361–367. doi: 10.1042/bj20021886

Zhang, Y., Schuetz, J. D., Elmquist, W. F., and Miller, D. W. (2004). Plasma membrane localization of multidrug resistance-associated protein homologs in brain capillary endothelial cells. *J. Pharmacol. Exp. Ther.* 311, 449–455. doi: 10.1124/jpet.104.068528

10

Estrone Sulfate Transport and Steroid Sulfatase Activity in Colorectal Cancer: Implications for Hormone Replacement Therapy

*Lorna C. Gilligan[1], Ali Gondal[1], Vivien Tang[1], Maryam T. Hussain[1], Anastasia Arvaniti[1], Anne-Marie Hewitt[1] and Paul A. Foster[1,2]**

[1] Institute of Metabolism and Systems Research, Centre for Endocrinology, Diabetes, and Metabolism, University of Birmingham, Birmingham, UK, [2] Centre for Endocrinology, Diabetes, and Metabolism, Birmingham Health Partners, Birmingham, UK

Correspondence:
Paul A. Foster
p.a.foster@bham.ac.uk

Hormone replacement therapy (HRT) affects the incidence and potential progression of colorectal cancer (CRC). As HRT primarily consists of estrone sulfate (E_1S), understanding whether this conjugated estrogen is transported and metabolized in CRC will define its potential effect in this malignancy. Here, we show that a panel of CRC cell lines (Colo205, Caco2, HCT116, HT-29) have steroid sulfatase (STS) activity, and thus can hydrolyze E_1S. STS activity is significantly higher in CRC cell lysate, suggesting the importance of E_1S transport in intracellular STS substrate availability. As E_1S transport is regulated by the expression pattern of certain solute carrier organic anion transporter polypeptides, we show that in CRC OATP4A1 is the most abundantly expressed transporter. All four CRC cell lines rapidly transported E_1S into cells, with this effect significantly inhibited by the competitive OATP inhibitor BSP. Transient knockdown of OATP4A1 significantly disrupted E_1S uptake. Examination of estrogen receptor status showed ERα was present in Colo205 and Caco2 cells. None of the cells expressed ERβ. Intriguingly, HCT116 and HT29 cells strongly expressed the G protein coupled estrogen receptor (GPER), and that stimulation of this receptor with estradiol (E_2) and G1, a GPER agonist, significantly ($p < 0.01$) increased STS activity. Furthermore, tamoxifen and fulvestrant, known GPER agonist, also increased CRC STS activity, with this effect inhibited by the GPER antagonist G15. These results suggest that CRC can take up and hydrolyze E_1S, and that subsequent GPER stimulation increases STS activity in a potentially novel positive feedback loop. As elevated STS expression is associated with poor prognosis in CRC, these results suggest HRT, tamoxifen and fulvestrant may negatively impact CRC patient outcomes.

Keywords: estrogen, colorectal cancer, steroid sulfatase, OATP, SLCO, GPER, tamoxifen

---

Abbreviations: BPS, bromsulphthalein; CRC, colorectal cancer; E_1, estrone; E_2, estradiol; E_1S, estrone sulfate; ER, estrogen receptor; FBS, fetal bovine serum; GPER, G-protein coupled estrogen receptor; HRT, hormone replacement therapy; OATP, organic anion transporter polypeptides; sFBS, charcoal-stripped fetal bovine serum; SLCO, solute carrier organic transporter family; STS, steroid sulfatase; SULT, sulfotransferase.

INTRODUCTION

Estrogens play an important role in the etiology of CRC (Foster, 2013). Pre-menopausal women are protected against CRC compared to age-matched men (Farquhar et al., 2005), and data from the Women's Health Initiative suggests post-menopausal women on HRT, a combination of estrone sulfate (E_1S) and progestins, have a 40% reduced incidence of developing CRC compared to women not on HRT (Chlebowski et al., 2004).

Despite this epidemiological evidence suggesting HRT as protective against CRC, evidence also exists showing estrogens influence CRC proliferation. For example, the CRC cell line Lovo increases proliferation, via a FASN-mediated mechanism, when exposed to estradiol (E_2) (Santolla et al., 2012). Indeed, E_2 increases the proliferation of the CRC cell line Caco2 (Di Domenico et al., 1996) and T84 (Hennessy et al., 2005), and inhibits apoptosis in DLD-1 cells (Messa et al., 2005). CRC patients on HRT present at a later and more advanced stage of disease (Chlebowski et al., 2004), suggesting estrogens as mitogenic in CRC. Thus, the ability of CRC to take up and consequently metabolize E_1S will define local concentrations of active estrogens and subsequent action.

Steroid sulfatase is the key enzyme involved in hydrolyzing E_1S to E_1 (**Figure 1**) (Mueller et al., 2015), and its activity is known to directly increase the proliferation of estrogen-dependent breast cancer (Foster et al., 2006) and endometrial cancer (Foster et al., 2008b). Inhibition of STS has shown significant promise against ERα positive breast cancer (Stanway et al., 2006; Foster et al., 2008a). Intriguingly, STS expression, elevated E_1 and E_2 intratumoural concentrations, are associated with a poor prognosis in CRC patients (Sato et al., 2009). This suggests that colonic estrogen metabolism may play an important role in CRC patient outcomes.

However, very little is known about whether E_1S is transported into CRC. Sulfated steroids require transport into cells via solute carrier organic anion transporting polypeptides (SLCO/OATP); membrane bound proteins that transport a plethora of organic anions (Roth et al., 2012). Six different SLCO/OATP (OATP1A2, OATP1B1, OATP1B3, OATP2B1, OATP3A1, OATP4A1) are known to effectively transport E_1S (Mueller et al., 2015), although their expression and action in CRC is poorly defined. Other OATPs are known to transport E_1S (OATP4C1 and OATP1C1), however OATP4C1 is primarily expressed in the kidney (Mikkaichi et al., 2004), and microarray analysis shows it may have some expression in the liver but not the human colon (Bleasby et al., 2006). OATP1C1 is localized to human brain and testis (Pizzagalli et al., 2002), and is not evident in human colorectal tissue, as measure by microarray (Bleasby et al., 2006).

Here, we investigate STS activity and E_1S transport kinetics in four CRC cell lines. We demonstrate that OATP4A1 is most likely the principle E_1S transporter in CRC and that all cell lines have the ability to hydrolyze E_1S. We also show that STS activity in CRC may be regulated by local E_2 availability via a novel GPER mechanism.

MATERIALS AND METHODS

Compounds

STX64 (Irosustat, 667COUMATE) was kindly supplied by Prof. Barry Potter (University of Oxford, UK). G1 and G15 were purchased from Torcis Bioscience (Abingdon, UK). E_2, tamoxifen, fulvestrant, and BSP were purchased from Sigma-Aldrich (Dorset, UK).

Cell Culture

The CRC cell lines Colo205, HCT116, and HT29 were purchased from the American Type Culture Collection, USA; Caco2 and JEG3 cells were purchased from The European Collection of Cell Cultures (ECACC). Prior to experiments, all cell lines were authenticated by short tandem repeat profiling and were used between passages 10 and 35. Furthermore, all experiments were performed during the exponential growth phase of the cell line. HCT116 and HT29 were routinely cultured in McCoy's 5a modified medium (Gibco, Life Technologies, USA) with 10% v/v heat inactivated FBS (Sigma-Aldrich, UK). Colo205 cells were culture in RPMI with 10% FBS; Caco2 cells were cultured in MEM with 10% FBS. JEG3 cells were cultured in DM-F12 (Gibco, USA) with 10% FBS. All culture mediums were supplemented with 2 mM L-glutamine (Sigma-Aldrich, UK) and 1% PenStrep (Gibco, USA). JEG3 cells were used as control as they exhibit high STS activity.

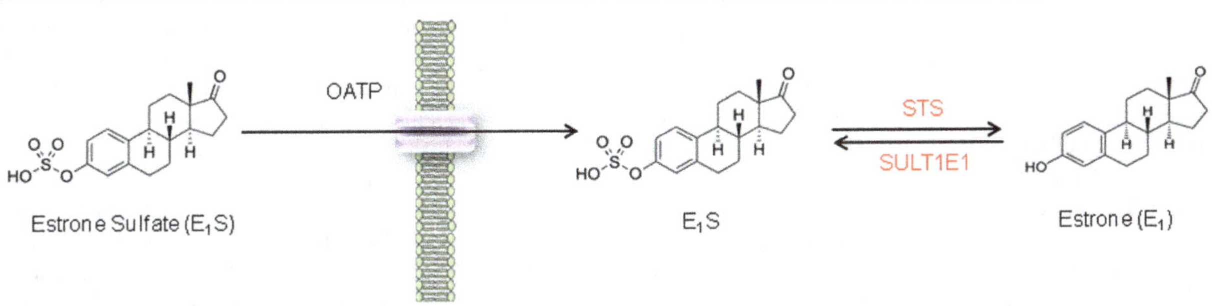

FIGURE 1 | Steroid sulfatase activity in CRC cell lines. E_1S is transported across the cell membrane by OATPs and once intracellular E_1S can be hydrolyzed by STS to form E_1.

For experimental conditions, cells were initially starved of estrogens for 72 h by placing them in their appropriate phenol-red free medium plus 10% charcoal stripped FBS (sFBS) (Sigma-Aldrich, UK). After starvation, HCT116 and HT29 cells were treated with E_2 (100 nM), G1 (100 nM), G15 (1 μM), Tamoxifen (10 nM) or fulvestrant (1 μM) in stripped medium for 24 h prior to measuring STS activity.

STS Activity Assay

In vitro STS activities of cell lines were measured as previously described (Purohit et al., 1997). Briefly, in intact cell assays, cells were incubated with appropriate medium containing [6,7-^{3}H] E_1S (4 × 10^5 dpm, Perkin-ElmerLS, Boston, MA, USA) adjusted to a final concentration of 20 μM with unlabeled E_1S (Sigma-Aldrich, UK). [4-^{14}C] E_1 (1 × 10^4 dpm, Perkin-Elmer) was also included in the reaction mixture to monitor procedural losses. Samples were incubated for 18 h at 37°C after which the product, E_1, was separated from E_1S by partition with toluene. A toluene aliquot was removed and ^{3}H and ^{14}C radioactivity measured by liquid scintillation spectrometry. The mass of E_1S hydrolyzed was calculated from the ^{3}H counts detected corrected for procedural losses. A protein measurement was obtained for the cells by lysing the cells with RIPA buffer (Sigma-Aldrich, UK) followed by a BCA assay (Thermo Fisher Scientific, UK).

To determine STS activity in cell lysates, cells were first lysed with RIPA buffer and protein content determined using a BCA assay. Subsequently, 100 μg of cell protein was incubated for 4 h with PBS containing [6,7-^{3}H] E_1S (4 × 10^5 dpm) adjusted to a final concentration of 20 μM with unlabeled E_1S. [4-^{14}C] E_1 (1 × 10^4 dpm) was again used to monitor procedural losses. E_1 was separated from E_1S by partition with toluene and ^{3}H and ^{14}C radioactivity measured by liquid scintillation spectrometry. Results for both intact and cell lysates were determined as pmol E_1 formed/h/mg protein.

qRT-PCR Analysis

From cells mRNA was purified from T75 flasks or six well plates at approximately 80% confluency using RNeasy kits (QIAGEN, Crawley, UK) and stored at −80°C. Aliquots containing 5 μg of mRNA were reverse transcribed in a final volume of 20 μl to form cDNA using Tetro cDNA Synthesis Kit (Bioline Reagents, Ltd, UK). RT-PCR reactions were performed in a 'Rotor Gene 2000 Real-Time Cycler' (Corbett Life Science, Cambridge, UK) with 1 μl cDNA in a final volume of 12 μl, using Taqman universal PCR master mix and Taqman expression assays containing primers and probes for OATP1A2, OATP1B1, OATP1B3, OATP2B1, OATP3A1, OATP4A1, and for the endogenous control gene, RPLP0 (Applied Biosystems, UK). In CRC, RPLPO is considered the most reliable single standard gene to examine (Sørby et al., 2010). The conditions were as follows: 95°C for 10 min; followed by 40 cycles of 95°C for 15 s, and 60°C for 60 s. Relative mRNA expression was calculated using the comparative quantisation algorithm in the Rotor Gene 6 software (Corbett Life Science).

E_1S Uptake Studies

Cells were seeded at 200,000 cells per well in 6-well plates and allowed to acclimatize for 24 h. Appropriate phenol red free medium containing 10% sFBS plus [6,7-^{3}H] E_1S (4 × 10^5 dpm) was placed on the cells and was subsequently removed after 2, 5, 10, 15, 20, 30 min. For OATP inhibition studies, the competitive OATP inhibitor BSP (at 1 μM) was added to the medium and therefore was present throughout the 30 min uptake time. The cells were then washed twice in PBS, lysed using RIPA buffer, and the intracellular ^{3}H radioactivity measured by liquid scintillation spectrometry. Cell protein content was also determined with a BCA assay. Results are expressed as E_1S uptake pmol/mg protein.

Immunoblotting

Protein concentration was determined from cell lysates using the BCA assay, and 15 μg samples were separated by electrophoresis under reducing conditions on 4–12% Bis-Tris 10% SDS-PAGE gels (Invitrogen, Paisley, UK) before being transferred to PVDF membranes. Membranes were immunoblotted with either ERα (1:1000), ERβ (1:1000), GPER (1:800) (all from Santa Cruz, UK), or β-actin (1:50,000) (Sigma-Aldrich, UK) monoclonal antibodies in incubation buffer containing 0.1% milk (Marvel; Premier Brands UK Ltd, Lincolnshire, UK) in TBST. For full details of antibodies and conditions used see **Table 1**. Bound antibody was detected with horseradish peroxidase-conjugated anti-mouse or anti-rabbit secondary antibodies and chemiluminescence detection.

siRNA Transfection

Twenty four hours after seeding HCT116 cultures were transfected with OATP-specific and control siRNA (Thermo Fisher Scientific, UK) by lipofectamine-2000 (Invitrogen) using standard protocols. 72 h post-transfection, E_1S uptake studies were performed over 30 min and total E_1S uptake calculated.

RESULTS

STS Activity in Intact and Lysed CRC Cell Lines

The panel of four CRC cell lines, plus the positive control JEG3, were investigated and demonstrate a wide range of STS activity (**Figures 2A,B**). In intact (not lysed) cells, Caco2 exhibited the highest STS activity (65.47 ± 28.51 pmol/mg/h), with HCT116 cells having the lowest activity (1.65 ± 0.14 pmol/mg/h). STS activity could be almost completely inhibited in intact cells using 1 μM of the specific STS inhibitor STX64 (**Figure 2A**).

When lysed, the intracellular STS activity was much greater in all cell lines examined compared to their intact state (**Figure 2B**). STS activity was again greatest in the Caco2 cell lines (452.90 ± 56.34 pmol/mg/h) with HCT116 cell showing the lowest STS activity (11.87 ± 6.41 pmol/mg/h). These results demonstrate that E_1S uptake kinetics most likely dictate the ability of CRC to hydrolyze E_1. Therefore, as E_1S is transported through the cell membrane by OATPs the expression of these transporters was next determined.

TABLE 1 | Information regarding antibodies and conditions used for immunoblotting.

Antibody	Manufacturer, Cat. #, Lot #	Peptide/protein target	Species raised, monoclonal/polyclonal	Dilution used	Positive control
ERα	Santa Cruz, sc-130072, C2910	aa 301–595	Mouse, monoclonal	1:1000, 1% milk	MCF-7
ERβ	Abcam, ab288, GR79420-5	aa 1–153	Mouse, monoclonal	1:1000, 1% milk	MCF-7
GPER	Santa Cruz, sc-48525-R, F2414	N-terminus	Rabbit, Polyclonal	1:800, 5% milk	MCF-7
β-actin	Sigma, A228	slightly modified β-cytoplasmic actin N-terminal peptide	Mouse, Monoclonal	1:50,000	

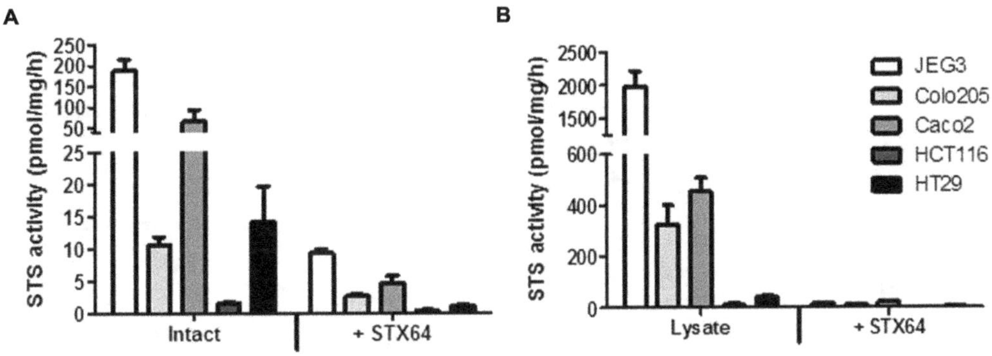

FIGURE 2 | (A) Steroid sulfatase activity (E_1S conversion in pmol/mg/h) and inhibition by STX64 (1 μM) in intact CRC cell lines. **(B)** STS activity and inhibition by STX64 (1 μM) in CRC cell lysate. JEG3 cells were used as a positive control in all experiments. Data represents mean ± SD. n = 3 independent experiments.

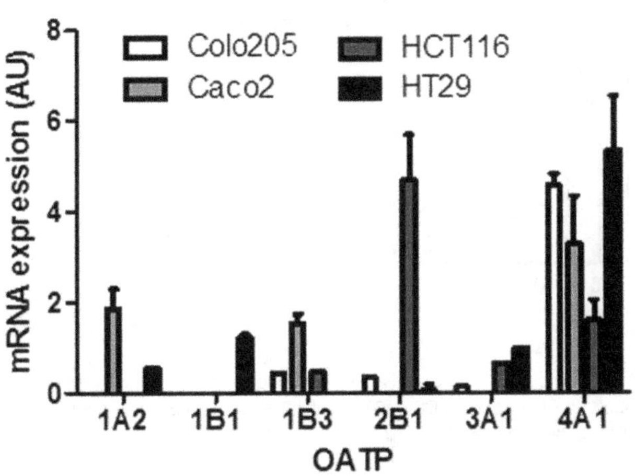

FIGURE 3 | Organic anion transporter polypeptide mRNA expression in Colo205, Caco2, HCT116, and HT-29 cells. OATP4A1 expression was the highest in all cell lines. Data represents mean ± SD. n = 3 independent experiments.

OATP Expression and E_1S Uptake in CRC Cell Lines

The mRNA expression of OATPs known to transport E_1S across the plasma membrane was determined in the panel of CRC cell lines (**Figure 3**). Of the six OATPs examined only OATP4A1 was present in all four cell lines. OATP2B1 expression was also notably high in Caco2 cells. The HT29 cells expressed five of the six OATPs determined (OATP1B3 was not present in HT29 cells), with the Caco2 cells expressing four (OATP1A1, OATP1B3, OATP2B1, OATP4A1) out of six. Our results are roughly consistent with the expression patterns obtained from the CellMiner database[1], as shown by average transcript $\log^2$ intensities (see **Table 2**).

When the ability of CRC cells to transport E_1S into the cells was determined, Colo205 demonstrated the quickest uptake rate, with HCT116 cells having the slowest uptake (**Figure 4A**). Inhibition of OATP transport with the non-specific OATP inhibitor BSP significantly reduced E_1S uptake in all four cell lines (**Figures 4B–E**). Caco2 cells had the most rapid with HCT116 cells exhibited the slowest E_1S transport. E_1S uptake after 30 min demonstrated that Colo205 (89.41 ± 16.80 pmol/mg) and Caco2 (61.78 ± 10.80 pmol/mg) cells exhibited the most intracellular E_1S transport, with HCT116 (16.73 ± 6.80 pmol/mg) and HT29 (34.59 ± 5.63 pmol/mg) cells showing lower E_1S transport (**Figure 4F**). BSP

[1]https://discover.nci.nih.gov/cellminer/

TABLE 2 | Average transcript $\log^2$ intensities determined from the National Cancer Institute (NCI) CellMiner database (https://discover.nci.nih.gov/cellminer/).

	1A2	1B1	1B3	2B1	3A1	4A1
Colo205	3.24	3.22	5.50	7.29	4.76	8.38
HCT116	2.96	3.23	5.75	5.34	4.61	8.19
HT29	2.84	2.89	4.02	5.39	6.54	8.04

Average $\log^2$ determined from mRNA various probes/probe sets.

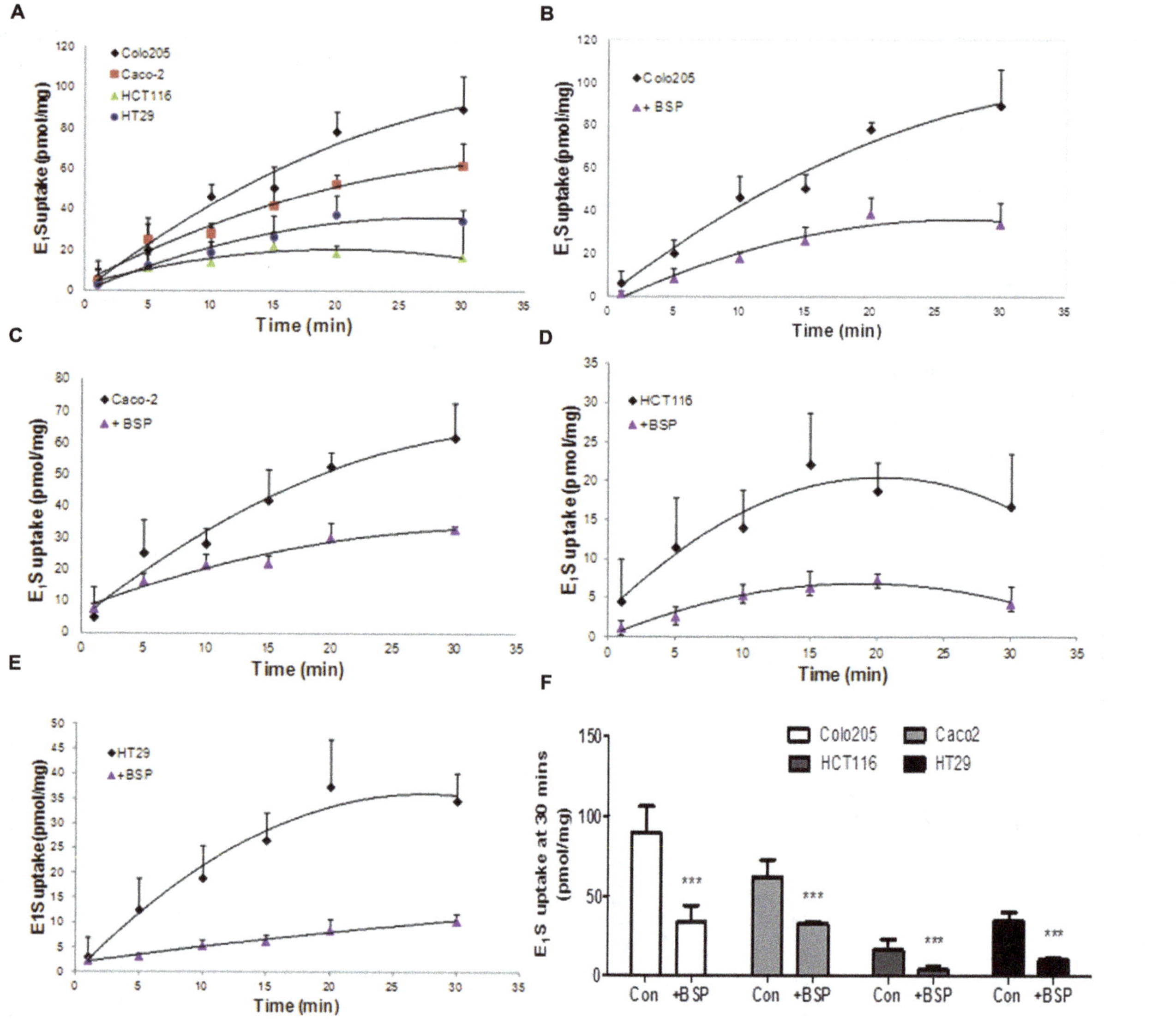

FIGURE 4 | Estrone sulfate transport in Colo205, Caco2, HCT116 and HT-29 cells. (A) Comparison of the different uptake kinetics of E_1S over 30 min in four CRC cell lines. **(B)** Inhibition of Colo205 E_1S transport by BSP (1 mM). **(C)** Inhibition of Caco2 E_1S transport by BSP. **(D)** Inhibition of HCT116 E_1S transport by BSP. **(E)** Inhibition of HT-29 E_1S transport by BSP. **(F)** Total E_1S uptake over 30 min by four CRC cell lines and the total inhibition caused by BSP. Data represents mean ± SD. $n = 3$ independent experiments. ***$p < 0.001$ compared to control.

significantly ($p < 0.001$) inhibited E_1S transport in all four cell lines.

To examine if OATP inhibition by BSP reduces E_1S intracellular substrate availability to STS, we examined the effect of BSP on STS activity in intact cells and cell lysates. We selected Caco2 and HCT116 cells as representative of CRC cells with high and low STS activity, respectively. In intact cells, treatment with BPS (1 μM) non-significantly reduced STS activity in Caco2 cells but had no effect on HCT116 STS activity (**Figure 5A**). When BPS (1 μM) was tested in cell lysates it had no effect on STS activity in both Caco2 and HCT116 cells, suggesting it does not directly inhibit the STS enzyme (**Figure 5B**). These results imply that OATP transport into cells plays a rate-limiting step on E_1S STS hydrolysis. The discrepancy between Caco2 and HCT116 cells in response to BSP most likely represents the difference between the STS activity in the cell lines. When STS activity is high (Caco2), limiting E_1S OATP transport limits intracellular E_1S availability thus reducing E_1 hydrolysis. When STS activity is low (HCT116), limiting E_1S OATP transport does not directly translate to decreased hydrolysis as there is less STS activity, and thus limiting substrate availability via OATP inhibition and where enzyme activity is already low does not translate to reduced E_1S hydrolysis.

As OATP2B1 and OATP4A1 were expressed at the highest concentrations compared to the other OATPs, we next performed siRNA knockdown of these two transporters in HCT116 cells to

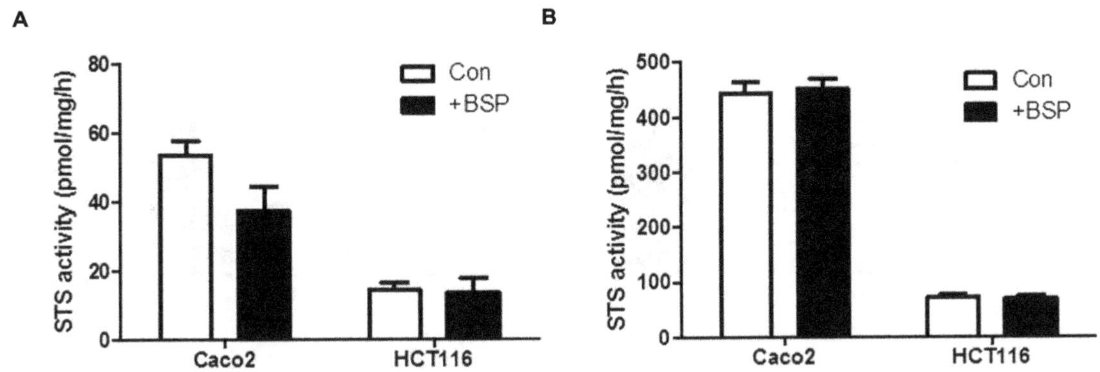

FIGURE 5 | Bromsulfthalein has limited effect on STS activity Caco2 and HCT116 cells. (A) In intact cells, STS activity is non-significantly reduced by BSP (1 μM) in Caco2 cells and has no effect on HCT116 cells. **(B)** In cell lysates, BSP (1 μM) has no effect on STS activity in Caco2 or HCT116 lysates. Data represents mean ± SD. $n = 3$ independent experiments.

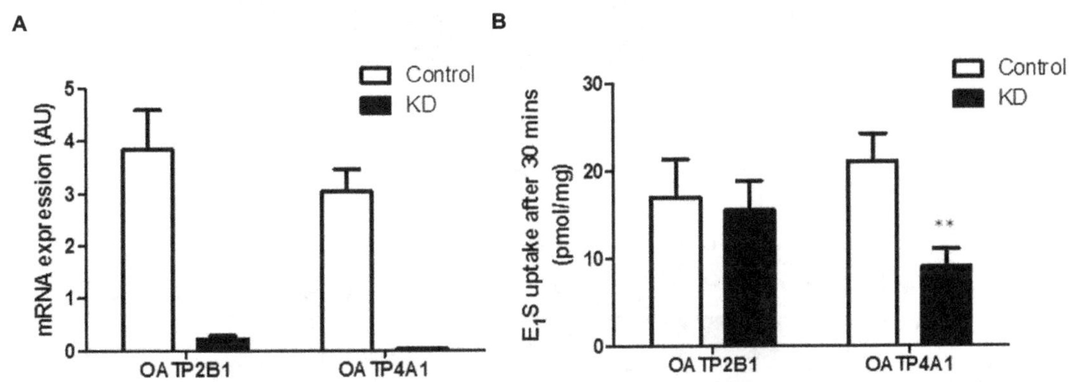

FIGURE 6 | OATP4A1 knockdown in HCT116 cells blocks E_1S transport. (A) siRNA knockdown of OATP2B1 and OATP4A1 reduced transporter expression by over 95%. **(B)** In HCT116 cells OATP2B1 knockdown has no effect on E_1S transport, however OATP4A1 knockdown inhibited E_1S transport by 52.4%. Data represents mean ± SD. $n = 3$ independent experiments. $^{**}p < 0.01$ compared to control.

determine their importance on E_1S uptake. We used HCT116 cells as they had high OATP2B1 and OATP4A1 expression without high expression of any other OATPs. Furthermore, HCT116 cells are readily transfected by lipofectamine for siRNA delivery. For both OATPs siRNA gave $<$ 95% knockdown as measured by qRT-PCR (**Figure 6A**). OATP2B1 knockdown did not significantly affect E_1S uptake (**Figure 6B**), however OATP4A1 knockdown significantly reduced E_1S uptake from 21.02 ± 3.12 to 8.93 ± 2.07 pmol/mg/h ($p < 0.01$), suggesting this transporter may play a key role in E_1S transport in CRC.

STS Activity is Regulated by E_2 Availability and GPER Action in CRC

As steroid metabolism and estrogen action in the colon is poorly defined we next speculated whether estrogens may influence steroid sulfatase activity, as it has been reported to do in other malignancies (Zaichuk et al., 2007). Thus we next examined how E_2 starvation and subsequent E_2 supplementation effects STS activity. HT29 cell treated with sFBS medium (i.e., estrogen starvation) demonstrated a trend toward reduction in STS activity, with this effect reversed when supplemented with E_2 (**Figure 7A**). In HCT116 cells, 24 h of E_2 (100 nM) treatment significantly ($p < 0.01$) induced STS activity compared to sFBS controls (**Figure 7B**).

We next attempted to inhibit this E_2-induced increase in STS activity by treating HCT116 with Tamoxifen or fulvestrant co-administered with E_2. Surprisingly, both Tamoxifen and fulvestrant significantly increased STS activity in HCT116 cells (**Figure 7C**) and neither compound had any effect on E_2-induced STS activity. Tamoxifen (at 10 nM) increased STS activity to 6.43 ± 0.95 pmol/mg/h and fulvestrant (1 μM) increase activity to 7.84 ± 1.36 pmol/mg/h compared to 2.43 ± 0.31 pmol/mg/h.

Examination of the CRC cell lines ER status demonstrated that ERα protein expression was present in Caco2 cells, and lowly expressed in Colo205 cells. HCT116 and HT29 cells did not express ERα (**Figure 7D**). None of the cell lines expressed ERβ (**Figure 7D**). We also assessed the GPER status in our CRC cell lines. HCT116 and HT29 cells expressed GPER (**Figure 7E**), as did Caco2 and Colo205 (data not shown). Unedited immunoblots are shown in Supplementary Figure 1. As both Tamoxifen and fulvastrant have been shown to be GPER agonist (Prossnitz and Barton, 2014) we next examined whether the increased STS

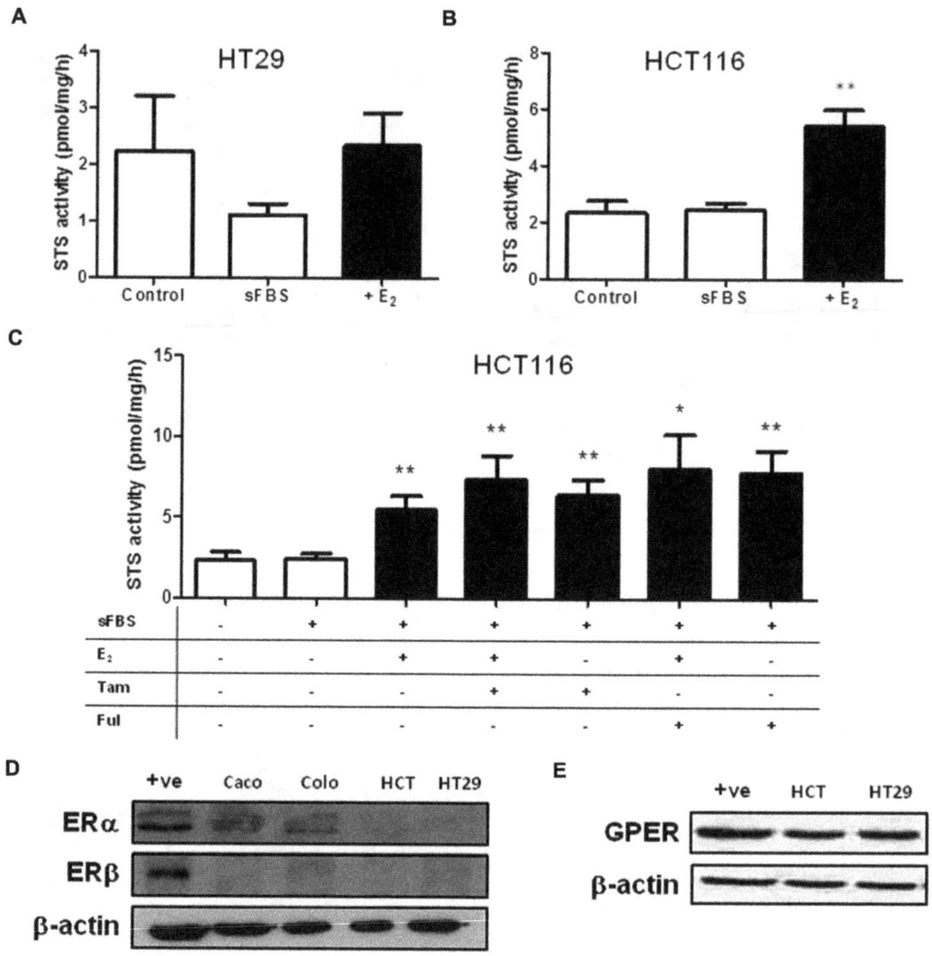

FIGURE 7 | Steroid sulfatase activity is regulated by estrogen availability in CRC cell lines. (A) E_2 (100 nM) does not increase STS activity in HT29. **(B)** E_2 (100 nM) significantly increase STS activity in HCT116 cells. **(C)** 24 h treatment of Tamoxifen (10 nM) and fulvestrant (1 mM) increases STS activity in HCT116 cells. **(D)** Colo205 and Caco2 cells express ERα, but not ERβ. HCT116 and HT29 cells do not express ERα or ERβ. The +ive control is MCF-7 protein. **(E)** GPER is expressed in HCT116 and HT29 cells. Data represents mean ± SD. $n = 3$ independent experiments. $^*p < 0.05$, $^{**}p < 0.01$ compared to sFBS control.

activity induced by these compounds could be inhibited by G15, a specific GPER antagonist (Dennis et al., 2009). In HCT116 cells, G15 (1 μM) significantly inhibited the increase of STS activity induced by 24 h treatment with E_2 (100 nM), the GPER agonist G1 (100 nM), Tamoxifen (10 nM), and fulvestrant (1 μM) (**Figure 8**). This suggests a potential novel positive estrogen metabolism feedback loop through GPER stimulation is present in CRC.

DISCUSSION

Hormone replacement therapy, usually a combination of equine E_1S and progestins, may play a dual role in the incidence and progression of CRC. Initially protective against the development of CRC (Chlebowski et al., 2004), once the malignancy is formed CRC may be estrogen responsive (Foster, 2013). Thus, defining how CRC transports and metabolizes estrogens, and the ER status of CRC, may define how this tissue responds to HRT. Here we demonstrate that CRC cell lines possess STS activity (see **Figure 2**) and are able to transport E_1S (see **Figure 4**), most likely through OATP4A1 (see **Figure 6**), into cells. Furthermore, we show that STS activity is elevated by local E_2 concentrations (see **Figure 7**) via GPER action. Finally we show that tamoxifen and fulvestrant, both GPER agonists, also elevate STS activity (see **Figure 8**) indicating that its use in breast cancer patients may have unwanted consequences in the colon.

Elevated STS expression has been demonstrated in breast (Pasqualini et al., 1996), prostate (Nakamura et al., 2006) endometrial (Lepine et al., 2010), and epithelial ovarian cancer (Ren et al., 2015). We demonstrate here for the first time that STS activity is present in both intact and lysed CRC cells, and this activity could be inhibited with STX64 (**Figure 2**). Although the role of STS activity and estrogens in CRC is not yet defined, our results, combined with evidence showing increased STS expression as a poor prognostic indicator in CRC patients (Sato et al., 2009), suggests STX64 as a potential therapeutic

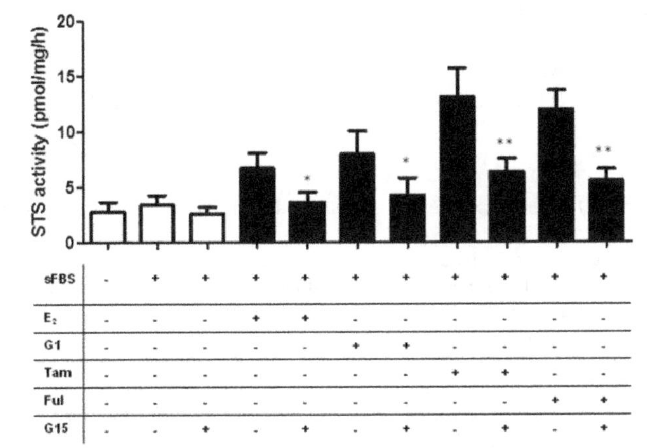

FIGURE 8 | Stimulation of GPER increases STS activity in HCT116 cells. E_2 (100 nM), G1 (100 nM), Tamoxifen (10 nM), and fulvestrant (1 mM) induce increased STS activity in HCT116 cells. These effects are inhibited by the addition of the GPER antagonist G15 (1 mM). Data represents mean ± SD. $n = 3$ independent experiments. $^*p < 0.05$, $^{**}p < 0.01$.

option for this disease. Indeed, STX64 has shown significant promise in hormone-dependent breast cancer patients (Stanway et al., 2006, 2007) with limited adverse events (Stanway et al., 2006). Further Phase II trials of STX64 are currently ongoing in patients with hormone-dependent breast cancer.

Cell protein (from cell lysates) exhibited significantly greater STS activity compared to intact cells suggesting E_1S cell membrane transport as the limiting factor in estrogen hydrolysis. Thus, OATP expression patterns in CRC may be a key regulator of E_1S transport and subsequent estrogen action. Our results demonstrate OATP4A1, followed by OATP2B1, as the most abundantly expressed E_1S transporters in CRC cell lines (**Figure 3**). OATP4A1 is up-regulated and hypomethylated in CRC compared to normal colon tissue (Rawluszko-Wieczorek et al., 2015), suggesting its importance in disease progression, and implying that E_1S uptake through this transporter may influence tumor proliferation. Furthermore, OATP3A1 is down-regulated in CRC (Rawluszko-Wieczorek et al., 2015), and reflected in our results as low expression of this transporter is evident in all four cell lines. OATP1B3 correlates to the Gleason score as a marker of CRC dedifferentiation: higher OATP1B3 expression in the colon is associated with earlier tumor stage and improved tumor differentiation (Pressler et al., 2011). We demonstrate low OATP1B3 expression in our cell lines, supporting a role for this transporter in early tumor stage as all four cell lines examined were derived from latter-stage tumors.

Once transported, E_1S requires hydrolysis to form E_1, and subsequently E_2 via 17β-hydroxysteroid dehydrogenase activity. However, controversy surrounds how estrogens act in CRC. Evidence suggests ERα is either lowly expressed (Cavallini et al., 2002) or not present (Witte et al., 2001), and ERβ is down-regulated during CRC development from colon adenomas (Konstantinopoulos et al., 2003). Thus, we determined ER status in four CRC cell lines, showing that Caco2 and Colo205 cells have some ERα immunoreactivity (**Figure 7**). None of the cell lines expressed ERβ. As they did not express either ERα or ERβ, we selected HCT116 and HT29 cells and determined that they expressed GPER. As ERα and ERβ are not present in CRC, this suggests that estrogens may primarily act through GPER in CRC. Indeed, estrogen binding to GPER increases colonic transit time (Li et al., 2016) and is associated with pain severity in irritable bowel disease (Qin et al., 2014). However, this is the first report of GPER stimulation having a functional molecular consequence in STS activity.

Intriguingly, E_2 and G1, a specific GPER agonist, increased STS activity in HCT116 cell lines (**Figure 7**), suggesting a potential novel positive estrogen feedback loop is present within CRC. In theory, greater STS activity should result in increased local E_1 and E_2 synthesis. Little is known about the regulation of STS activity. STS can undergo various post-translational modifications resulting in greater activity (Stengel et al., 2008), and this effect may be NF-κB regulated (Jiang et al., 2016). However, there are no other reports that estrogen availability impacts STS activity. In breast cancer, GPER stimulation by tamoxifen does elevate the expression of aromatase (Catalano et al., 2014), the enzyme involved in estrogen synthesis from androgen pre-cursors. It is with some interest then to see that tamoxifen also increased STS activity in HCT116 cell lines. As a selective ER modulator, tamoxifen is a first line therapy against hormone-dependent breast cancer. However, it has recently been shown that tamoxifen may act as a GPER agonist in tamoxifen-resistant tumors (Mo et al., 2013). Thus, tamoxifen-induced increase of STS activity, and therefore increasing local estrogen availability, in CRC and potentially other malignancies may represent a novel GPER-stimulated pathway regulating STS action. It will be of importance to further examine whether tamoxifen and fulvestrant induce STS activity via GPER stimulation, as this may represent a novel route for tamoxifen and fulvestrant resistance.

CONCLUSION

We have demonstrated here that CRC cell lines can transport E_1S and have sufficient STS activity to liberate E_1. STS activity is possibly regulated by local estrogen availability through GPER stimulation, and this represents a novel positive estrogen feedback loop within CRC. These results have direct consequences for HRT therapy, suggesting that HRT may increase STS activity in the colon leading to potentially undesired effects through GPER action.

AUTHOR CONTRIBUTIONS

LG performed qRT-PCR and analysis on cell lines and wrote the manuscript, AG and VT performed STS activity assays, MH performed qRT-PCR analysis and ran the E1S uptake studies, A-MH performed qRT-PCR on cell lines, AA, performed immunoblotting, PF performed E1S uptake studies, STS activity assays, analyzed data, and wrote the manuscript.

ACKNOWLEDGMENT

This work was supported by the Society for Endocrinology (UK) Early Careers Grant given to PF, and by a MRC Ph.D. stipend awarded to LG.

REFERENCES

Bleasby, K., Castle, J. C., Roberts, C. J., Cheng, C., Bailey, W. J., Sina, J. F., et al. (2006). Expression profiles of 50 xenobiotic transporter genes in humans and pre-clinical species: a resource for investigations into drug disposition. *Xenobiotica* 36, 963–988. doi: 10.1080/00498250600861751

Catalano, S., Giordano, C., Panza, S., Chemi, F., Bonofiglio, D., Lanzino, M., et al. (2014). Tamoxifen through GPER upregulates aromatase expression: a novel mechanism sustaining tamoxifen-resistant breast cancer cell growth. *Breast Cancer Res. Treat.* 146, 273–285. doi: 10.1007/s10549-014-3017-4

Cavallini, A., Messa, C., Pricci, M., Caruso, M. L., Barone, M., and Di Leo, A. (2002). Distribution of estrogen receptor subtypes, expression of their variant forms, and clinicopathological characteristics of human colorectal cancer. *Dig. Dis. Sci.* 47, 2720–2728. doi: 10.1023/A:1021053105096

Chlebowski, R. T., Wactawski-Wende, J., Ritenbaugh, C., Hubbell, F. A., Ascensao, J., Rodabough, R. J., et al. (2004). Estrogen plus progestin and colorectal cancer in postmenopausal women. *N. Engl. J. Med.* 350, 991–1004. doi: 10.1056/NEJMoa032071350/10/991

Dennis, M. K., Burai, R., Ramesh, C., Petrie, W. K., Alcon, S. N., Nayak, T. K., et al. (2009). In vivo effects of a GPR30 antagonist. *Nat. Chem. Biol.* 5, 421–427. doi: 10.1038/nchembio.168nchembio.168

Di Domenico, M., Castoria, G., Bilancio, A., Migliaccio, A., and Auricchio, F. (1996). Estradiol activation of human colon carcinoma-derived Caco-2 cell growth. *Cancer Res.* 56, 4516–4521.

Farquhar, C. M., Marjoribanks, J., Lethaby, A., Lamberts, Q., and Suckling, J. A. (2005). Long term hormone therapy for perimenopausal and postmenopausal women. *Cochrane Database Syst. Rev.* 3:CD004143. doi: 10.1002/14651858.CD004143.pub2

Foster, P. A. (2013). Oestrogen and colorectal cancer: mechanisms and controversies. *Int. J. Colorectal. Dis.* 28, 737–749. doi: 10.1007/s00384-012-1628-y

Foster, P. A., Chander, S. K., Parsons, M. F., Newman, S. P., Woo, L. W., Potter, B. V., et al. (2008a). Efficacy of three potent steroid sulfatase inhibitors: pre-clinical investigations for their use in the treatment of hormone-dependent breast cancer. *Breast Cancer Res. Treat.* 111, 129–138. doi: 10.1007/s10549-007-9769-3

Foster, P. A., Newman, S. P., Chander, S. K., Stengel, C., Jhalli, R., Woo, L. L., et al. (2006). In vivo efficacy of STX213, a second-generation steroid sulfatase inhibitor, for hormone-dependent breast cancer therapy. *Clin. Cancer Res.* 12, 5543–5549. doi: 10.1158/1078-0432.CCR-06-0632

Foster, P. A., Woo, L. W., Potter, B. V., Reed, M. J., and Purohit, A. (2008b). The use of steroid sulfatase inhibitors as a novel therapeutic strategy against hormone-dependent endometrial cancer. *Endocrinology* 149, 4035–4042. doi: 10.1210/en.2008-0223en.2008-0223

Hennessy, B. A., Harvey, B. J., and Healy, V. (2005). 17beta-Estradiol rapidly stimulates c-fos expression via the MAPK pathway in T84 cells. *Mol. Cell. Endocrinol.* 229, 39–47. doi: 10.1016/j.mce.2004.10.001

Jiang, M., Klein, M., Zanger, U. M., Mohammad, M. K., Cave, M. C., Gaikwad, N. W., et al. (2016). Inflammatory regulation of steroid sulfatase: a novel mechanism to control estrogen homeostasis and inflammation in chronic liver disease. *J. Hepatol.* 64, 44–52. doi: 10.1016/j.jhep.2015.07.022S0168-8278(15)00513-9

Konstantinopoulos, P. A., Kominea, A., Vandoros, G., Sykiotis, G. P., Andricopoulos, P., Varakis, I., et al. (2003). Oestrogen receptor beta (ERbeta) is abundantly expressed in normal colonic mucosa, but declines in colon adenocarcinoma paralleling the tumour's dedifferentiation. *Eur. J. Cancer* 39, 1251–1258. doi: 10.1016/S0959-8049(03)00239-9

Lepine, J., Audet-Walsh, E., Gregoire, J., Tetu, B., Plante, M., Menard, V., et al. (2010). Circulating estrogens in endometrial cancer cases and their relationship with tissular expression of key estrogen biosynthesis and metabolic pathways. *J. Clin. Endocrinol. Metab.* 95, 2689–2698. doi: 10.1210/jc.2010-2648jc.2010-2648

Li, Y., Xu, J., Jiang, F., Jiang, Z., Liu, C., Li, L., et al. (2016). G protein-coupled estrogen receptor is involved in modulating colonic motor function via nitric oxide release in C57BL/6 female mice. *Neurogastroenterol. Motil.* 28, 432–442. doi: 10.1111/nmo.12743

Messa, C., Notarnicola, M., Russo, F., Cavallini, A., Pallottini, V., Trentalance, A., et al. (2005). Estrogenic regulation of cholesterol biosynthesis and cell growth in DLD-1 human colon cancer cells. *Scand. J. Gastroenterol.* 40, 1454–1461. doi: 10.1080/00365520510024007

Mikkaichi, T., Suzuki, T., Tanemoto, M., Ito, S., and Abe, T. (2004). The organic anion transporter (OATP) family. *Drug Metab. Pharmacokinet.* 19, 171–179. doi: 10.2133/dmpk.19.171

Mo, Z., Liu, M., Yang, F., Luo, H., Li, Z., Tu, G., et al. (2013). GPR30 as an initiator of tamoxifen resistance in hormone-dependent breast cancer. *Breast Cancer Res.* 15, R114. doi: 10.1186/bcr3581bcr3581

Mueller, J. W., Gilligan, L. C., Idkowiak, J., Arlt, W., and Foster, P. A. (2015). The regulation of steroid action by sulfation and desulfation. *Endocr. Rev.* 36, 526–563. doi: 10.1210/er.2015-1036

Nakamura, Y., Suzuki, T., Fukuda, T., Ito, A., Endo, M., Moriya, T., et al. (2006). Steroid sulfatase and estrogen sulfotransferase in human prostate cancer. *Prostate* 66, 1005–1012. doi: 10.1002/pros.20426

Pasqualini, J. R., Chetrite, G., Blacker, C., Feinstein, M. C., Delalonde, L., Talbi, M., et al. (1996). Concentrations of estrone, estradiol, and estrone sulfate and evaluation of sulfatase and aromatase activities in pre- and postmenopausal breast cancer patients. *J. Clin. Endocrinol. Metab.* 81, 1460–1464. doi: 10.1210/jcem.81.4.8636351

Pizzagalli, F., Hagenbuch, B., Stieger, B., Klenk, U., Folkers, G., and Meier, P. J. (2002). Identification of a novel human organic anion transporter polypeptide as a high affinity thyroxine transporter. *Mol. Endocrinol.* 16, 2283–2296. doi: 10.1210/me.2001-0309

Pressler, H., Sissung, T. M., Venzon, D., Price, D. K., and Figg, W. D. (2011). Expression of OATP family members in hormone-related cancers: potential markers of progression. *PLoS ONE* 6, e20372. doi: 10.1371/journal.pone.0020372PONE-D-11-01633

Prossnitz, E. R., and Barton, M. (2014). Estrogen biology: new insights into GPER function and clinical opportunities. *Mol. Cell. Endocrinol.* 389, 71–83. doi: 10.1016/j.mce.2014.02.002S0303-7207(14)00039-2

Purohit, A., Froome, V. A., Wang, D. Y., Potter, B. V., and Reed, M. J. (1997). Measurement of oestrone sulphatase activity in white blood cells to monitor in vivo inhibition of steroid sulphatase activity by oestrone-3-O-sulphamate. *J. Steroid Biochem. Mol. Biol.* 62, 45–51. doi: 10.1016/S0960-0760(97)00018-6

Qin, B., Dong, L., Guo, X., Jiang, J., He, Y., Wang, X., et al. (2014). Expression of G protein-coupled estrogen receptor in irritable bowel syndrome and its clinical significance. *Int. J. Clin. Exp. Pathol.* 7, 2238–2246.

Rawluszko-Wieczorek, A. A., Horst, N., Horbacka, K., Bandura, A. S., Swiderska, M., Krokowicz, P., et al. (2015). Effect of DNA methylation profile on OATP3A1 and OATP4A1 transcript levels in colorectal cancer. *Biomed. Pharmacother.* 74, 233–242. doi: 10.1016/j.biopha.2015.08.026S0753-3322(15)00211-5

Ren, X., Wu, X., Hillier, S. G., Fegan, K. S., Critchley, H. O., Mason, J. I., et al. (2015). Local estrogen metabolism in epithelial ovarian cancer suggests novel targets for therapy. *J. Steroid Biochem. Mol. Biol.* 150, 54–63. doi: 10.1016/j.jsbmb.2015.03.010S0960-0760(15)00095-3

Roth, M., Obaidat, A., and Hagenbuch, B. (2012). OATPs, OATs and OCTs: the organic anion and cation transporters of the SLCO and SLC22A gene superfamilies. *Br. J. Pharmacol.* 165, 1260–1287. doi: 10.1111/j.1476-5381.2011.01724.x

Santolla, M. F., Lappano, R., De Marco, P., Pupo, M., Vivacqua, A., Sisci, D., et al. (2012). G protein-coupled estrogen receptor mediates the up-regulation of fatty acid synthase induced by 17beta-estradiol in cancer cells and cancer-associated fibroblasts. *J. Biol. Chem.* 287, 43234–43245. doi: 10.1074/jbc.M112.417303M112.417303

Sato, R., Suzuki, T., Katayose, Y., Miura, K., Shiiba, K., Tateno, H., et al. (2009). Steroid sulfatase and estrogen sulfotransferase in colon carcinoma: regulators of intratumoral estrogen concentrations and potent prognostic factors. *Cancer Res.* 69, 914–922. doi: 10.1158/0008-5472.CAN-08-09060008-5472.CAN-08-0906

Sørby, L. A., Anderson, S. N., Bukholm, I. R., and Jacobsen, M. B. (2010). Evaluation of suitable reference genes for normalization of real-time reverse transcription PCR analysis in colon cancer. *J. Exp. Clin. Cancer Res.* 29:144. doi: 10.1186/1756-9966-29-144

Stanway, S. J., Delavault, P., Purohit, A., Woo, L. W., Thurieau, C., Potter, B. V., et al. (2007). Steroid sulfatase: a new target for the endocrine therapy of breast cancer. *Oncologist* 12, 370–374. doi: 10.1634/theoncologist.12-4-370

Stanway, S. J., Purohit, A., Woo, L. W., Sufi, S., Vigushin, D., Ward, R., et al. (2006). Phase I study of STX 64 (667 Coumate) in breast cancer patients: the first study of a steroid sulfatase inhibitor. *Clin. Cancer Res.* 12, 1585–1592. doi: 10.1158/1078-0432.CCR-05-1996

Stengel, C., Newman, S. P., Day, J. M., Tutill, H. J., Reed, M. J., and Purohit, A. (2008). Effects of mutations and glycosylations on STS activity: a site-directed mutagenesis study. *Mol. Cell. Endocrinol.* 283, 76–82. doi: 10.1016/j.mce.2007.11.012S0303-7207(07)00430-3

Witte, D., Chirala, M., Younes, A., Li, Y., and Younes, M. (2001). Estrogen receptor beta is expressed in human colorectal adenocarcinoma. *Hum. Pathol.* 32, 940–944. doi: 10.1053/hupa.2001.27117

Zaichuk, T., Ivancic, D., Scholtens, D., Schiller, C., and Khan, S. A. (2007). Tissue-specific transcripts of human steroid sulfatase are under control of estrogen signaling pathways in breast carcinoma. *J. Steroid Biochem. Mol. Biol.* 105, 76–84. doi: 10.1016/j.jsbmb.2006.12.101

11

Antiproliferative Properties of Newly Synthesized 19-Nortestosterone Analogs without Substantial Androgenic Activity

*András Gyovai[1], Renáta Minorics[1], Anita Kiss[2], Erzsébet Mernyák[2], Gyula Schneider[2], András Szekeres[3], Erika Kerekes[3], Imre Ocsovszki[4] and István Zupkó[1,5]**

[1] Department of Pharmacodynamics and Biopharmacy, University of Szeged, Szeged, Hungary, [2] Department of Organic Chemistry, University of Szeged, Szeged, Hungary, [3] Department of Microbiology, University of Szeged, Szeged, Hungary, [4] Department of Biochemistry, University of Szeged, Szeged, Hungary, [5] Interdisciplinary Centre for Natural Products, University of Szeged, Szeged, Hungary

***Correspondence:**
István Zupkó
zupko@pharm.u-szeged.hu

19-Nortestosterone C-17 epimers with prominent antiproliferative properties have been previously described. In our present study, five novel 17α-19-nortestosterones (**3–7**) were synthesized to increase their beneficial biological activities with no associated undesired hormonal effects. The compounds were screened by a viability assay against a panel of human adherent gynecological cancer cell lines. Three of the tested derivatives (**3–5**) exhibited a remarkable inhibitory effect on the proliferation of HeLa cells with IC_{50} values lower than that of our reference agent cisplatin (CIS). These three active agents also displayed considerable cancer selectivity as evidenced by their weaker growth inhibitory effect on non-cancerous fibroblast cells compared to CIS. The most potent newly synthesized 17α-chloro derivative (**3**) was selected for additional experiments in order to characterize its mechanism of action. Since nandrolone (19-nortestosterone, **1**) is a structural analog with selective antiproliferative action on cervical carcinoma cells, it was utilized as a positive control in these studies. A lactate dehydrogenase (LDH) assay demonstrated a moderate cytotoxic effect of the test compounds. Cell cycle disturbance and the elevation of the hypodiploid population elicited by the test agents were detected by flow cytometry following propidium staining. The proapoptotic effects of the tested steroids were confirmed by fluorescent microscopy and a caspase-3 activity assay. Treatment-related caspase-9 activation without a substantial change in caspase-8 activity indicates the induction of the intrinsic apoptotic pathway. The selected agents directly influence the rate of tubulin assembly as evidenced by a polymerization assay. Yeast-based reporter gene assay revealed that the androgenic activity of the novel 19-nortestosterone derivative **3** is by multiple orders of magnitude weaker than that of the reference agent **1**. Based on the behavior of the examined compounds it can be concluded that a halogen substitution of the 19-nortestosterone scaffold at the 17α position may produce compounds with unique biological activities. The results of the present study support that structurally modified steroids with negligible hormonal activity are a promising basis for the research and development of novel anticancer agents.

Keywords: 19-nortestosterone analogs, antiproliferative action, HeLa Cells, tubulin polymerization, androgenic activity, cell cycle, caspase

INTRODUCTION

Cancer is the second leading cause of death globally: in 2015 malignancies were responsible for 8.7 million deaths, and 17.5 million new cancer cases were registered worldwide. Based on incidence estimates the number of new cases is expected to rise by about 70% over the next two decades (Fitzmaurice et al., 2017). Besides numerous preventive strategies and early diagnosis, the research for and development of innovative anticancer agents is one of the most important approaches to decrease global cancer burden.

Steroidal agents used in oncological practice are typically administered for their endocrine disruptor properties (e.g., estrogen antagonists, aromatase inhibitors). Synthetic analogs of naturally occurring steroids are widely utilized in the treatment of cancers of the reproductive system (Lin et al., 2010; Sharifi et al., 2010).

Besides the well-known endocrine disruptors several other steroids have been reported to exert pronounced anticancer effects in a hormone-independent manner. 2-Methoxyestradiol, an endogenous metabolite of estradiol without hormonal activity, exhibits a potent antiproliferative action against various tumor cell lines *in vitro*, and inhibits tumor growth *in vivo* (Fotsis et al., 1994). It is also demonstrated to induce programmed cell death in endothelial cells and suppresses cancer-related angiogenesis (Yue et al., 1997; LaVallee et al., 2002).

Cardiac glycosides are a group of steroidal compounds traditionally utilized in the management of congestive heart failure. Epidemiological studies have revealed that many of them, including digitoxin, oleandrin, bufalin, and calotropin exert a potent anticancer effect against different malignancies via the inhibition of proliferation and apoptosis induction involving complex cell signal transduction mechanisms (Mijatovic et al., 2007; Newman et al., 2008).

Steroidal alkaloids are nitrogen containing secondary metabolites found in many plant families (e.g., Liliaceae, Solanaceae), and many of them are well characterized as potent anticancer agents against human malignant cell lines (Koduru et al., 2007). Solasodine glycosides have been investigated in the clinical setting against basal cell carcinoma, and a locally applied cream was found to be effective in a substantial proportion of patients (Punjabi et al., 2008).

Androstanes and their structural analogs are regarded as a promising skeleton for the development of steroid-based anticancer agents. A large body of evidence indicates the outstanding importance of these compounds and their versatile antitumor effects. A considerable antiproliferative action of several sets of innovative androstane analogs have been reported against a broad variety of cell lines, including prostate, breast, cervix, ovarium, leukemia, melanoma, colon, and gastric cancers (Iványi et al., 2012; Ajdukovic et al., 2013, 2015; Acharya and Bansal, 2014; Cui et al., 2015; Jakimov et al., 2015). 19-Nortestosterone derivatives, e.g., levonorgestrel, desogestrel, and dienogest, an important division of testosterone-derived molecules are widely utilized in hormone replacement therapy (Campagnoli et al., 2005), contraception (Minami et al., 2013; Royer and Jones, 2014), and treatment of endometriosis (Minami et al., 2013; Miyashita et al., 2014). Beyond these well-established clinical applications, several 19-nortestosterone derivatives have recently been reported as potential anticancer agents. Mibolerone (7α,17α-dimethyl-19-nortestosterone), a metabolically stable synthetic member of this class has been demonstrated to effectively inhibit estrogen-stimulated breast cancer cell proliferation *in vitro* (Cops et al., 2008).

Tibolone, a selective regulator of tissue estrogen activity for postmenopausal women, is also known to induce apoptosis in breast cancer cells *in vitro*, and has been demonstrated to suppress tumor growth in animal models (Franke and Vermes, 2003; Erel et al., 2006). Further, 19-nortestosterones, such as gestodene and 3-ketodesogestrel exhibit antitumor activity against several breast cancer cell lines *in vitro*, as well as *in vivo*, in rat model of breast cancer (Kloosterboer et al., 1994). Additional, 19-nortestosterone derivatives as potential proliferation inhibitors in brain, prostate, and renal cancer cell lines have also been described (Mohamed et al., 2015).

Although several analogs truly possess a promising anticancer effect, their actions are mainly mediated by their hormonal activity, hindering a wide-scale utilization of these compounds in cancer therapy.

Since the 17β-hydroxy function of endogen androgens play a crucial role in the molecule's interaction with its hormone receptors, modifications of this group reduce hormonal activity. The lack of the C-19 methyl group also decreases the hormonal properties of such analogs substantially (Fragkaki et al., 2009). In a previous research, we have reported on the synthesis of a series of 17-substituted 19-nortestosterone derivatives and demonstrated their antiproliferative properties against human ovarium, cervix, and breast cancer cell lines. Nandrolone (19-nortestosterone, **1**) was found to exhibit a selective proliferation inhibitory effect against cervical cancer cells (HeLa) at low concentrations (Schneider et al., 2016). As an extension of this previous research a set of novel 19-nortestosterone analogs with various substituents at position C-17 have been synthesized. Recent reports about halogen-substituted androstane-derivatives with an increased *in vitro* anticancer activity encouraged us to introduce halogens in order to enhance the antiproliferative activity (Banday et al., 2010; Iványi et al., 2012). The aims of our current study were to assess the antiproliferative properties of these analogs, including tumor selectivity, as well as to characterize the mechanism of action of the most potent compound. Since, the endocrine actions of steroid-based drug candidates are exceptionally relevant, the androgenic potentials of the compounds were also tested.

MATERIALS AND METHODS

Synthesis and Chemicals

The exact conditions applied for the preparation processes of the synthesized 19-nortestosterone analogs **2–7** and their detailed characterization are provided as Supplementary Material. 10 mM stock solutions of the tested agents were prepared with dimethyl sulfoxide (DMSO) for all *in vitro* experiments. The medium with the highest DMSO concentration (0.3%) did not exert any notable effect on cell proliferation. Unless otherwise specified, all other chemicals and kits were purchased from Sigma-Aldrich Ltd. (Budapest, Hungary).

Cell Cultures

Gynecological cancer cell lines, including ovarian (A2780), cervical (HeLa), and breast cancer cell lines (MCF7, T47D, MDA-MB-231, and MDA-MB-361) were purchased from the European Collection of Authenticated Cell Cultures (ECACC, Salisbury, United Kingdom). Additional cervical cell lines (SiHa and C33A) and a non-cancerous immortalized, mammary gland epithelial cell line (hTERT-HME1) were purchased from LGC Standards GmbH (Wesel, Germany). Non-cancerous fibroblast cells (MRC-5) were also obtained from the ECACC. All cells were cultured in minimal essential medium supplemented with 10% fetal bovine serum, 1% non-essential amino acids, and 1% antibiotic-antimycotic mixture, in humidified air containing 5% CO_2 at 37°C. Immortalized hTERT-HME1 cells were maintained in serum-free mammary epithelial cell growth medium (MEGM) supplemented with insulin, human epidermal growth factor (hEGF), hydrocortisone, bovine pituitary extract, and an antibiotic-antimycotic mixture. All the medium and supplements were purchased from Lonza Group Ltd. (Basel, Switzerland).

Assessing the Antiproliferative Effect

The antiproliferative properties of the compounds were assessed by an MTT assay (Mosmann, 1983). Cells were seeded onto 96-well microplates at a density of 10,000 cells/well (MDA-MB-361 and C33A) or 5,000 cells/well (all other cell lines). After an overnight incubation, fresh medium containing the test compounds (at a concentration of 10 or 30 μM) was added. After incubation for 72 h at 37°C in humidified air, [3-(4,5-dimethylthiazol-2-yl)-2,5-diphenyltetrazolium bromide] (MTT) solution (5 mg/mL) was added. Purple formazan crystals were formed by the living cells during a 4 h contact period, which were assayed by spectrophotometry after having been dissolved in 100 μL DMSO. Untreated cells served as control, and cisplatin (CIS) (Ebewe Pharma GmbH, Unterach, Austria) was used as a reference compound. When a test agent elicited over 50% growth inhibition at the 30 μM concentration, the assay was repeated with a series of dilutions (0.1–30 μM) and IC_{50} values were calculated (GraphPad Prism 5.0, GraphPad Software, San Diego, CA, United States). Two independent measurements were performed with five parallel wells. To present preliminary data concerning tumor selectivity of the potent compounds, the procedure was repeated on MRC-5 fibroblast and hTERT-HME1 immortalized mammary gland epithelial cells under the same experimental conditions.

Assessing the Cytotoxic Effect

The direct cytotoxic effects of the test agents were determined by a lactate dehydrogenase (LDH) assay. Cells were seeded onto 96-well microplates at a density of 5,000 cells/well and were incubated overnight, after which the medium containing the test compounds at proper concentrations was added. After incubation for 24 h, the activity of LDH released by the treated cells was determined by a commercially available colorimetric kit according to the manufacturer's instructions (Hoffmann-La Roche Ltd., Basel, Switzerland). Untreated cells served as control, while detergent Triton X-100 and CIS were used as reference agents.

Flow Cytometric Analysis of Cell Cycle and Apoptosis

The distribution of cells in different cell cycle phases (subG1, G1, S and G2/M) was analyzed via the measurement of cellular DNA content by flow cytometry. HeLa cells were seeded onto 6-well plates and allowed to stand for an overnight. The cells were treated with the selected compounds for 24, 48, or 72 h. Then cells were harvested, washed and fixed in ice cold 70% ethanol and stored at −20°C at least for an hour. Next, a DNA staining solution (containing distilled water, propidium-iodide, Triton-X100, sodium citrate, and ribonuclease-A) was added to each sample and stored in the dark at room temperature for an hour. Stained cells were analyzed by flow cytometry (Partec CyFlow, Partec GmbH, Munster, Germany) with at least 20,000 cells being evaluated for each analysis. Data processing was performed using the ModFit LT 3.3.11 software (Verity Software House, Topsham, ME, United States).

Morphological Studies Using Fluorescent Microscopy

Fluorescent double staining was performed in order to detect apoptosis induction and morphological changes using fluorescent microscopy. HeLa cells were seeded into a 96-well plate at the density of 3,000–5,000 cells per well. After an overnight incubation, the cells were treated with various concentrations of the test compounds for 24 h. The treated cells were then incubated with a fluorescent staining solution (containing Hoechst 33258 and propidium iodide, 500 and 300 μg/mL, respectively) for an hour. After staining, the cells were analyzed using a fluorescent microscope (Nikon ECLIPSE 146 TS100, Nikon Instruments Europe, Amstelveen, Netherlands) equipped with appropriate optical filters. For all different conditions, at least six fields were recorded with an attached QCapture CCD camera. This way cells with an intact, apoptotic or necrotic morphology can be distinguished based on their different nuclear morphological appearance and distinct membrane integrity.

Caspase Activity Measurements

In order to detect, whether the test compounds induce programmed cell death, the activity of caspase-3 was determined by a colorimetric assay. To elucidate the exact pathway of apoptosis, activities of caspase-8 and caspase-9 were additionally determined by colorimetric kits. In all cases approximately 12 million cells were treated with appropriate concentrations of the compounds for 24 or 72 h. After the treatment, the cells were scraped and the enzyme activities were determined by means of colorimetric assays mentioned above. All kits were purchased from Abnova Corp. (Taipei, Taiwan) and used in accordance with the instructions of the manufacturer.

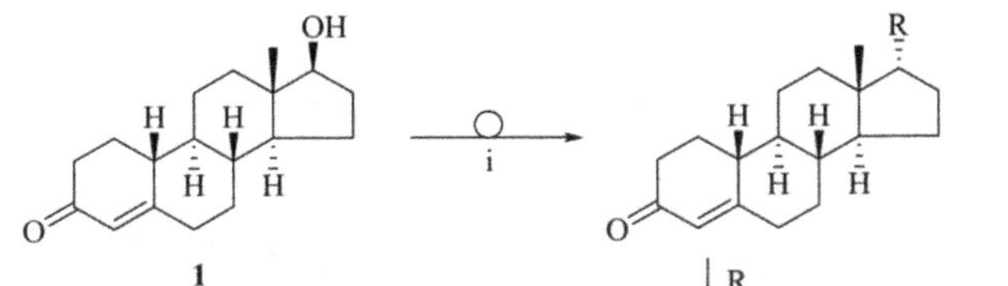

	R
2	OH
3	Cl
4	Br
5	I
6	$(2,4\text{-}NO_2)C_6H_3COO$
7	$(3,5\text{-}NO_2)C_6H_3COO$

FIGURE 1 | Chemical structures of the synthesized 19-nortestosterone derivatives. Applied reagents and conditions: (i) Ph_3P, aryl acids or alkyl halogenides, diethyl azodicarboxylate, toluene, 80°C.

Tubulin Polymerization Assay

In order to determine the direct action of the test compounds on the microtubular system, an *in vitro* tubulin polymerization assay was performed using a commercially available kit (Cytoskeleton Inc., Denver, CO, United States) in accordance with the provider's instructions. The assay reactions were performed on a pre-warmed (37°C), UV-transparent 96-well microplate. Ten microliters of the test solutions were placed on the wells supplemented with 2 mM $MgCl_2$, 0.5 mM ethylene glycol tetraacetic acid (EGTA), 1 mM guanosine triphosphate (GTP) and 10.2% glycerol. Ten microliters of general tubulin buffer was used as untreated control, and paclitaxel (PAC) served as the reference compound. The polymerization reaction was initiated by adding 100 μL of 3.0 mg/mL tubulin in 80 mM PIPES, pH 6.9, to each sample. Absorbance of the samples was measured per minute, at 340 nm, using a 60-min kinetic measurement protocol. Each sample was prepared in two parallels. To characterize the process, polymerization curves were fitted to the measured data. The highest difference between the absorbances measured at two consecutive time points was regarded as V_{max} (Δabsorbance/min) for the tested compound. A clinically applied reference agent, PAC was used at a relatively high concentration (10 μM) as recommended by the manufacturer. This concentration is approximately 1,000-fold higher than the IC_{50} value of PAC on HeLa cells (Jordan et al., 1996). Since similarly high concentrations of the tested compounds were not possible to be applied because of the limited solubility of the substances in the recommended buffer, we used the highest concentrations reflecting the differences in the efficacies of the tested compounds.

Assessing Hormonal Effect

An endocrine bioassay kit (Xenometrix AG, Allschwil, Switzerland) was used to test for a potential residual androgenic

TABLE 1 | Antiproliferative effects of the synthesized compounds (1–7) on human cell lines.

Comp.	Conc. (μM)	Growth inhibition (%) ± SEM [calculated IC_{50} value (μM)][a]									
		HeLa	SiHa	C33A	A2780	MCF-7	MDA-MB-231	MDA-MB-361	T47D	MRC-5	hTERT-HME1
1[b]	10	99.5 ± 0.2	–[c]	–	–	–	–	–	–	5.4 ± 1.2	16.9 ± 1.2
	30	99.5 ± 0.3 [0.65]	20.7 ± 2.6	25.2 ± 1.7	–	–	21.4 ± 1.2	–	–	11.3 ± 0.5	37.1 + 1.0
2[b]	10	28.1 ± 4.0	–	–	–	–	–	–	–	n.d.[d]	n.d.
	30	37.9 ± 3.4	–	–	–	27.7 ± 3.7	–	–	–		
3	10	95.9 ± 0.3	–	–	–	–	–	–	–	4.3 ± 3.7	76.2 ± 0.5
	30	95.1 ± 0.5 [1.21]	26.0 ± 2.3	61.7 ± 1.7	32.7 ± 1.0	36.9 ± 2.0	–	21.8 ± 2.5	–	8.0 ± 2.3	99.9 ± 0.1 [4.63]
4	10	94.4 ± 0.7	–	–	–	–	–	–	–	11.9 ± 2.3	n.d.
	30	94.1 ± 0.5 [1.69]	–	–	54.4 ± 1.6	–	–	–	–	20.4 ± 2.1	
5	10	95.2 ± 0.4	–	–	27.7 ± 1.3	–	–	–	–	13.1 ± 1.9	n.d.
	30	95.8 ± 0.2 [1.49]	–	–	61.6 ± 1.8	–	–	–	–	13.8 ± 2.0	
6	10	32.0 ± 2.9	–	–	–	–	–	–	–	n.d.	n.d.
	30	26.5 ± 2.3	–	–	31.9 ± 2.6	35.9 ± 1.4	–	–	47.2 ± 2.6		
7	10	26.6 ± 1.8	–	–	49.2 ± 0.9	25.9 ± 3.1	–	–	–	n.d.	n.d.
	30	21.5 ± 1.9	–	–	58.1 ± 2.0	37.7 ± 3.4	–	22.0 ± 1.6	–		
CIS[e]	10	42.6 ± 2.3	88.6 ± 0.5	83.8 ± 0.8	83.6 ± 1.2	66.9 ± 1.8	–	67.5 ± 1.0	51.0 ± 2.0	60.3 ± 3.3	97.7 ± 0.3
	30	99.9 ± 0.3	90.2 ± 1.8	93.9 ± 0.6	95.0 ± 0.3	96.8 ± 0.4	71.5 ± 1.2	87.8 ± 1.1	55.0 ± 1.5	61.9 ± 1.0	99.1 ± 0.3
		12.43	7.84	1.77	1.30	5.78	19.13	3.74	9.78	6.19	[2.45]

[a] *IC_{50} values were calculated when the growth inhibition value for a compound exceeded 75% at a concentration of 30 μM. See Supplementary Figure S1 for representative concentration-response curves.* [b] *Data previously reported (Schneider et al., 2016).* [c] *Inhibition values less than 20% are not presented.* [d] *n.d., not determined.* [e] *Reference agent cisplatin.*

activity of the selected agents. Genetically modified yeast cells (*Saccharomyces cerevisiae*) containing the human androgenic receptor gene integrated into a yeast chromosome, as well as an expression plasmid with the sequences of both the androgen responsive element and a lacZ reporter gene were cultured in humidified air at 31°C with agitation for 2 days. The appropriate concentrations of the test compounds and a CPRG substrate solution (chlorophenol red-β-D-galactopyranoside) for β-galactosidase were added into a 96-well microplate according to the instructions of the manufacturer. Androgen agonistic and antagonistic properties of the test compounds were determined by a colorimetric assay. For the antagonistic measurements the medium was supplemented with 5α-dihydrotestosterone (DHT). Once the reporter gene is expressed, β-galactosidase is secreted into the medium, and converts the yellow CPRG substrate into a red product, which can be quantified at 570 nm. Quantities of this red product correlate with the liberation of β-galactosidase, which is increased when an agonistic effect is present, while it is decreased when the test compound exerts an antagonistic effect. For the agonistic and antagonistic assays, nandrolone (**1**) and flutamide were used as reference agents, respectively.

Statistical Analysis

In all experiments, the statistical evaluation of the results was performed by one-way analysis of variance followed by the Dunnett posttest, using the GraphPad Prism 5 software (GraphPad Software; San Diego, CA, United States). Mean values and the SEM were calculated in all cases.

RESULTS

Synthetic Studies

The Mitsunobu reaction is widely employed for the inversion of stereogenic centers of secondary alcohols including steroid alcohols. The reaction allows the conversion of alcohols with alkyl or aryl carboxylic acids in the presence of diethyl azodicarboxylate and triphenylphosphine (Ph_3P). The result is an alkyl- or aryl carboxylic ester of the alcohol with inverted configuration (Mitsunobu, 1981). Here, we describe the Mitsunobu reaction for 19-nortestosterone (**1**) utilizing 2,4-, or 3,5-dinitrobenzoic acid in the presence of diethyl azodicarboxylate and Ph_3P in toluene at 80°C leading to the corresponding 17α-19-nortestosterone-17-yl 2′,4′- or 3′,5′-dinitrobenzoate (**6** or **7**, respectively; **Figure 1**). Reacting compound **1** with isopropyl halides under the same conditions produces the corresponding 17α-chloro-, bromo-, and iodo-19-nortestosterone (**3–5**, respectively). Hydrolyzing compounds **6** or **7** in methanol, in the presence of $NaOCH_3$ yields 17α-19-nortestosterone (**2**).

Antiproliferative Properties of 19-Nortestosterone Derivatives

The antiproliferative activities of the test compounds were determined by MTT assay on a panel of adherent gynecological cancer cell lines (**Table 1**). Nandrolone (**1**) as reported previously, exerted a considerable antiproliferative effect against HeLa cells. Compounds **2**, **6**, and **7** exerted no remarkable antiproliferative action against the gynecological cancer cell lines. 17α-Halogen derivatives (**3–5**) exerted a pronounced antiproliferative effect against HeLa cells, while they did not elicit any notable influence on the remaining cell lines including fibroblasts. These derivatives had lower IC_{50} values on HeLa cells than that of the reference agent CIS. Compound **3** proved to be the most potent antiproliferative agent, characterized by an effect size comparable to that of **1**. Cancer selectivity of the potent compounds was determined by the same method using human fibroblasts (MRC-5) and non-cancerous immortalized, mammary gland derived epithelial (hTERT-HME1) cells. None of the test agents exhibited a considerable growth inhibitory effect against intact fibroblasts up to a concentration of 30 μM. Compound **1** had no pronounced action on immortalized epithelial cells, while compound **3** inhibited the growth of these cells with an IC_{50} value approximately four times higher than that obtained on HeLa cells. Compound **3** exerted the most explicit tumor selectivity, showing a substantially weaker effect on non-cancerous cells than CIS. Due to their potent and selective antiproliferative actions, compound **3** and nandrolone (**1**) were selected for further investigations to characterize their mechanism of action and assess their hormonal effect.

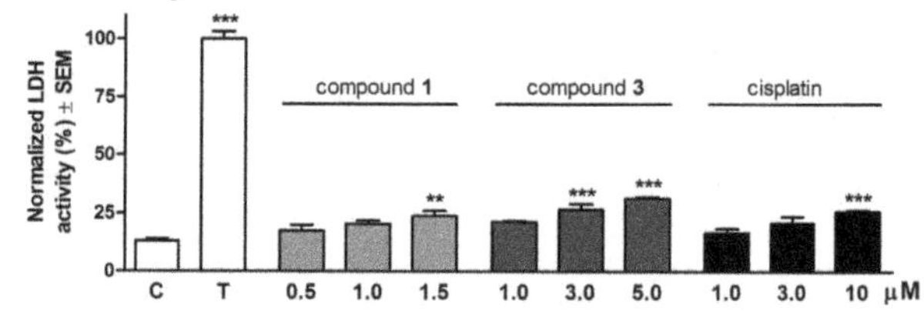

FIGURE 2 | Cytotoxic effects of compounds 1, 3 and cisplatin on HeLa cells after 24 h treatment. The effect of Triton X-100 (T) was considered 100%. Results are mean values ± SEM of the data from two separate measurements, $n = 4$. *$p < 0.05$, **$p < 0.01$, and ***$p < 0.001$ compared to untreated control (C).

Cytotoxic Activity

Cytotoxic properties of the selected compounds were ascertained by measuring LDH activity resulting from cell membrane damage. Each molecule exerted a concentration-dependent increase of LDH activity compared to the untreated control after 24 h treatment (**Figure 2**). Compound **1** elicited a substantial LDH release at a concentration of 1.5 μM. The effect of compound **3** proved to be significant when applied at concentrations above its IC_{50} values (3.0 or 5.0 μM). None of the test agents induced an LDH activity comparable to the maximum LDH release triggered by detergent Triton X-100.

Cell Cycle Analysis

Alterations in cell cycle and apoptotic fragmentations were determined by flow cytometry after treatment with the test compounds for 24 and 48 h. Since **1** elicited no change in the subG1 population at these time points this agent was

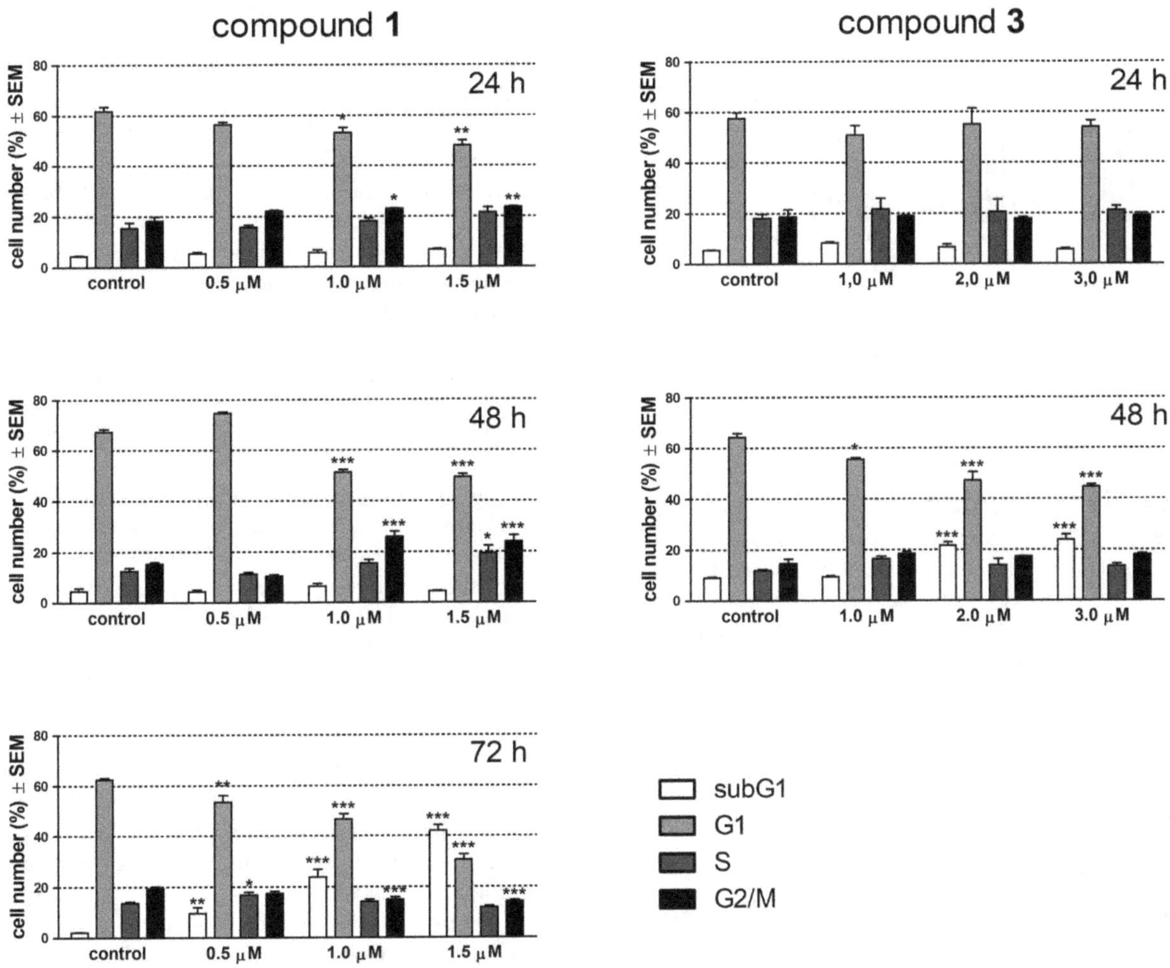

FIGURE 3 | Effects of compounds 1 and 3 on cell cycle phase distribution of HeLa cells determined by flow cytometry after incubation for 24, 48, or 72 h. Results are mean values ± SEM of the data from two independent measurements, $n = 6$. $^*p < 0.05$, $^{**}p < 0.01$, and $^{***}p < 0.001$ compared to untreated control.

re-tested after 72 h incubation. Treatment with **1** for 24 h resulted in a concentration-dependent and significant decrease in the G1 and a moderate but significant increase in the G2/M phase cell population (**Figure 3**). After 48 h of exposure these changes became more pronounced, and completed with the elevated ratio of the S phase cell population in the presence of 1.5 μM of **1**. A longer incubation time (72 h) with **1** elicited a substantial disturbance in the cell phase distribution and a concentration-dependent accumulation of hypodiploid cells indicating apoptotic nuclear fragmentation. Compound **3** did not have any remarkable effect on cell cycle after 24 h exposure, while a longer incubation time (48 h) resulted in a substantially elevated increase of the subG1 population at the expense of G1 cells.

Morphological Changes

To characterize the morphological features of the apoptosis induced by compounds **1** and **3** HeLa cells were examined by fluorescent microscopy after 24 h treatment with three different concentrations (1.0, 3.0, or 5.0 μM) of the test compounds. For the quantitative analysis, cells with intact, apoptotic and necrotic morphological features were labeled, and the ratios of different morphologies were calculated. Treatments with **1** and **3** resulted in a substantial and concentration-dependent increase in both the apoptotic and necrotic cell populations, at the expense of the intact population (**Figure 4**).

Induction of Apoptotic Enzymes

Based on the above results, changes of the activities of caspase-3, caspase-8, and caspase-9 were determined using a colorimetric assay. After treatment with **1** for 72 h, the activity of executive caspase-3 increased significantly and in a concentration-dependent manner (**Figure 5**). Under the same experimental conditions **1** also activated the initiator caspases, although the induction of caspase-8 was less pronounced. Compound **3** enhanced caspase-3 activity at 5.0 μM even after a shorter incubation period (24 h). Caspase-9 activity was also significantly elevated, while there was no change in the function of caspase-8.

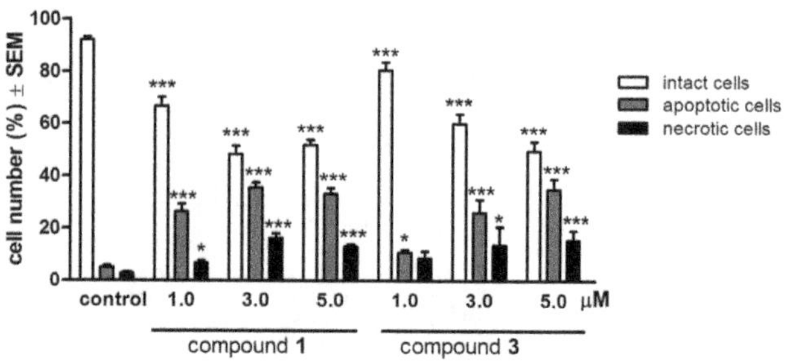

FIGURE 4 | Qualitative evaluation of fluorescent double staining of HeLa cells after 24 h treatment with compounds 1 or 3. $^{*}p < 0.05$ and $^{***}p < 0.001$ compared to untreated control (C). See Supplementary Figure S2 for representative pictures.

Tubulin Polymerization

The direct effect of the test compounds on microtubule formation was determined by a specific photometric assay in a cell-free system. The tested concentrations of the compounds were chosen based on their calculated IC_{50} values according to the recommendation of the manufacturer. Both compounds **1** and **3** induced a significant acceleration of tubulin polymerization compared to untreated control samples (**Figure 6**). Calculated values of maximal rate of tubulin polymerization (V_{max}) were elevated compared to control, although none of these V_{max} values were comparable to that of the reference agent PAC.

Hormonal Effect

Since residual hormonal activity of a potential sterane lead compound is a crucial aspect of further drug development, the androgenic properties of the most promising agents were investigated by a yeast-based reporter assay. As **1** is a well-characterized androgen, it was used as a reference agent (Bergink et al., 1985). According to our results **3** exerts a substantially lower hormonal activity, with no relevant action unless applied in extremely high concentrations (**Figure 7**). Calculated EC_{50} values of **1** and **3** differed by approximately 2 orders of magnitude (3.43×10^{-8} and 3.80×10^{-6} M, respectively). Compound **3** exhibited no antagonistic activity in the assay system (data not shown).

DISCUSSION

Various biological effects of compounds with an androstane skeleton mostly stem from their endocrine disruptor properties, thus the medical use of androgens is mainly limited to androgen replacement and androgen deprivation therapies, including the management of some hormone dependent malignancies (Wadosky and Koochekpour, 2016). Beyond their approved medical applications, numerous androgenic anabolic steroids are utilized illegally to enhance physical performance, a risky use often accompanied by serious adverse effects. Recently, numerous androstanes with anticancer potential have been described, and the importance of androstane compounds and their derivatives in the research and development of steroid-based anticancer agents for hormone-independent malignancies is continuously increasing (Frank and Schneider, 2013; Wadosky and Koochekpour, 2016). Although several 19-nortestosterone derivatives have been identified as potent anticancer agents (e.g., mibolerone, tibolone, gestodene), most of them have pronounced hormonal properties involved in their therapeutic action, as well as in their undesired adverse effects (Saito et al., 2016). In a previous research, we investigated a set of newly synthesized 19-nortestosterone analogs, and reported that some of them exhibited a moderate antiproliferative activity. That study of our research group revealed that the widely known 19-nortestosterone analog **1** (nandrolone) has a potent and selective antiproliferative effect against cervical carcinoma cells positive for type 18 of human papilloma virus (HPV-18) (Schneider et al., 2016).

The aim of our present study was to synthesize and investigate a set of novel 19-nortestosterone derivatives with improved antiproliferative properties and limited hormonal activities. Three of the novel compounds (**3–5**) were found to exhibit a pronounced antiproliferative effect against HeLa cells (calculated IC_{50} values: 1.21–1.69 μM), while exerting a negligible or lower impact on other cell lines including intact fibroblasts (MRC-5) and the immortalized mammary gland epithelial cell line (hTERT-HME1). In contrast, dinitrobenzoates (**6** and **7**) appeared to be ineffective in terms of growth inhibition of cancer cells. The most potent compound, **3** was further investigated to describe its possible mechanism of action. A well-known androgen, **1** a with similar antiproliferative capacity was utilized as a steroidal reference agent.

The antiproliferative property of a compound is typically reflected by a disturbance induced in cell cycle distribution. These changes in cell cycle phases inform about the probable mechanism of the antiproliferative action. Both **1** and **3** caused a cell cycle disturbance characterized by the accumulation of hypodiploid (subG1) cells at the expense of the G1 population.

The increase of hypodiploid cell populations can be regarded as an evidence for proapoptotic properties of the test compounds. Alterations in cell cycle during physiological conditions usually lead to induction of programmed cell death. Activation of the apoptotic machinery, selectively in cancer cells without a substantial necrotizing effect is one of the most desirable characteristics of a promising anticancer agent (Tolomeo and Simoni, 2002). Some steroidal compounds with anticancer activity (e.g., 2-methoxyestradiol, D-homoestrone, a D-secoestrone-triazole analog) have been described as efficacious inducers of programmed cell death in cancer cells (Li et al., 2004; Minorics et al., 2015; Bózsity et al., 2017). Therefore, the demonstration of apoptosis induction was a basic feature of our study. We utilized fluorescent microscopy and observed the characteristic features of apoptosis elicited by the test agents in a concentration-dependent manner.

Caspase enzymes are crucial implementers of the apoptotic program executed by downstream effector caspases such as caspase-3. Caspase-9 is the major enzyme involved in the initiation of the intrinsic apoptotic pathway, while caspase-8 plays an essential role in the extrinsic pathway of the

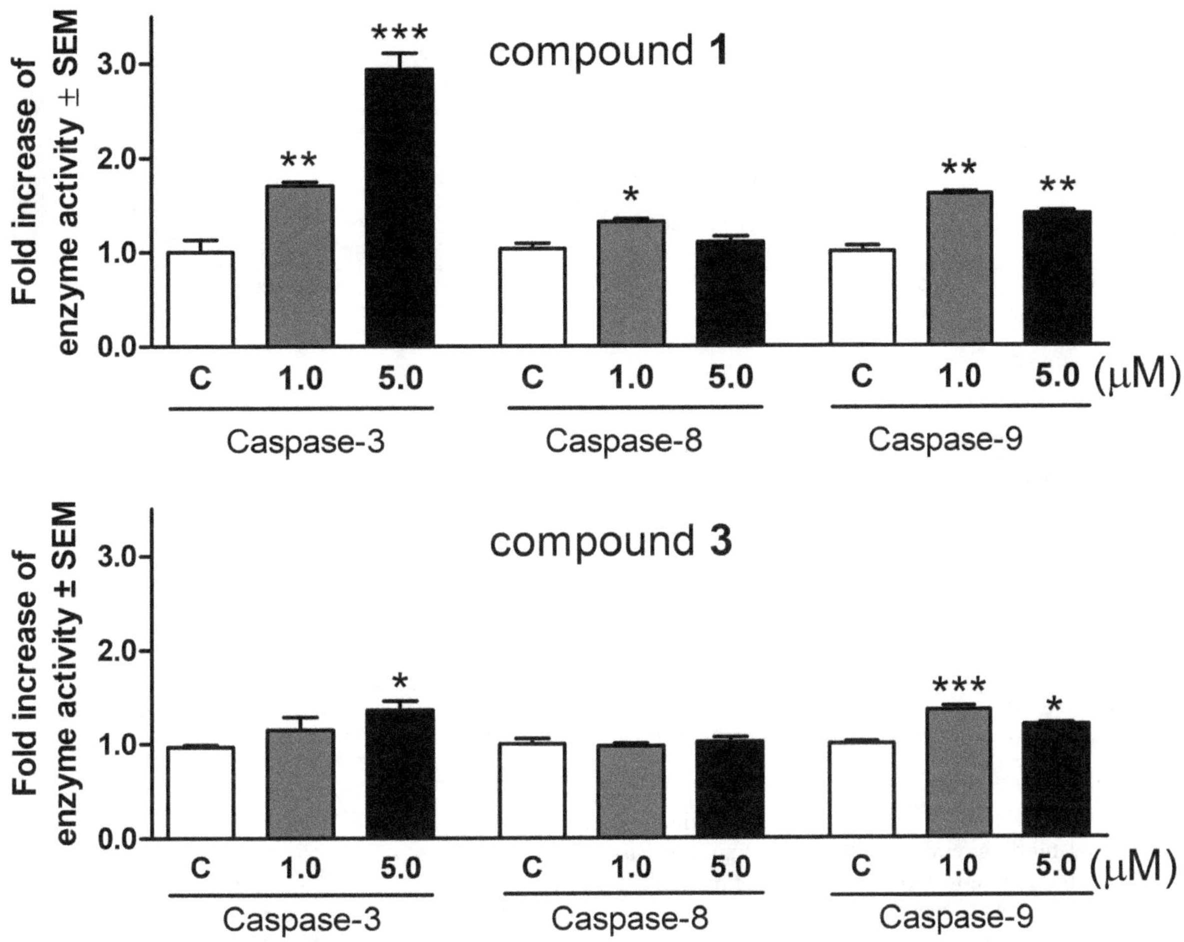

FIGURE 5 | Activation of caspase-3, caspase-8, and caspase-9 enzymes in HeLa cells after incubation with compounds 1 and 3 for 72 or 24 h, respectively. Results are mean values ± SEM of the data from two independent measurements, $n = 6$. $^{*}p < 0.05$, $^{**}p < 0.01$, and $^{***}p < 0.001$ compared to untreated control.

apoptotic process (Hajra and Liu, 2004). Treatments with the test compounds resulted in a significant elevation in the activity of caspase-3, reflecting the activation of apoptotic cell death. Both agents elicited a considerable increase in activity of caspase-9 at both concentrations tested (1 and 5 μM) without expected concentration-dependency. The exact reason for this is not elucidated, but based on the results of our fluorescent microscopy analysis, necrotic cell death induced by the higher concentration could be a plausible explanation. Based on these findings activation of the intrinsic apoptotic pathway is hypothesized. Although, the activity of caspase-8 was slightly but significantly increased by **1** at a concentration of 1 μM, this limited change seems to be inefficient to indicate a dominant role of the extrinsic apoptotic pathway.

Previous studies revealed that some proapoptotic steroidal compounds induced a pronounced cell cycle arrest via a direct influence on tubulin polymerization during mitosis. The inhibitory effect of 2-methoxyestradiol on microtubule formation resulting from its interaction with the colchicine-binding site of β-tubulin has also been reported (Peyrat et al., 2012). Thus, a possible direct influence of **1** and **3** on the polymerization of tubulin heterodimers in a cell-free system was also investigated.

Both of our test agents elicited a concentration-dependent acceleration of the polymerization reaction as reflected by significantly increased V_{max} values. This molecular behavior indicates a possible PAC-like microtubule stabilizing effect of the test compounds which may contribute to cell cycle arrest and lead to the induction of the apoptotic machinery.

The possible androgenic activity of a novel steroid-based agent may implicate a source of potential adverse reactions limiting its therapeutic value. Receptor binding properties of **1** and 5α-dihydrotestosterone are indistinguishable by a radio ligand assay using androgen receptors prepared from rat prostate and MCF-t cells (Bergink et al., 1985). Therefore, **1** can be utilized as a reference agent when novel compounds with possible androgenic properties are characterized. Compound **3** was detected to possess a substantially lower androgenic activity compared to **1**.

Moreover, **3** had no androgen antagonistic properties when tested in the presence 5α-dihydrotestosterone. This hormonal neutrality of **3** could be explained by the α-position of chlorine

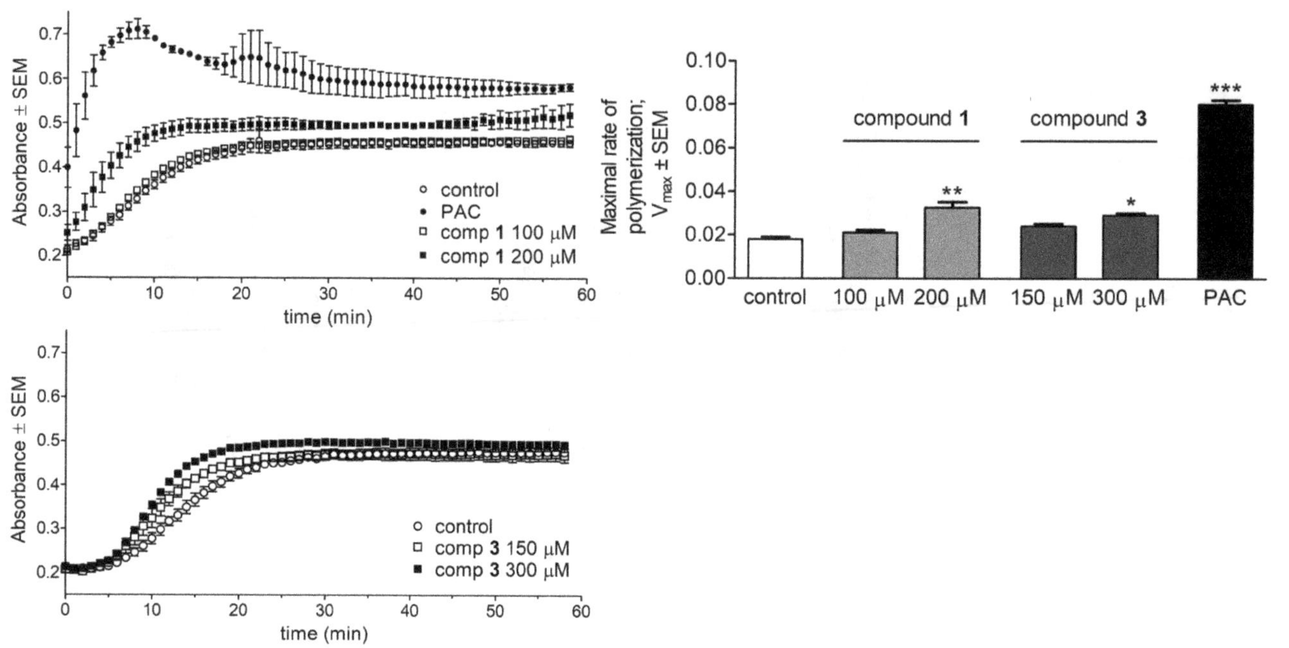

FIGURE 6 | Direct effects of compounds 1 and 3 on tubulin polymerization. Kinetic curves characterizing tubulin polymerization in the presence of 1, 3 or paclitaxel (PAC) were recorded after 58 min kinetic measurements (Left). Direct effects of the test agents on the maximal rate of polymerization were evaluated (Right). Results are mean values ± SEM of the data from two independent measurements, $n = 4$. *$p < 0.05$, **$p < 0.01$, and ***$p < 0.001$ compared to untreated control sample.

on the ring D of the skeleton. The substituent at position 17 determines receptor binding, and only the β configuration is favored. Consequently, 17α-testosterone has virtually no affinity for the receptor (Fragkaki et al., 2009).

Although mediated by the same nuclear receptor, androgenic and anabolic actions of a ligand can be partially dissociated depending on the tissue expression of crucial metabolic enzymes including 5α-reductase. While the androgenic action may be disadvantageous and may limit the development of a drug candidate, an anabolic or "myotropic" property could theoretically be advantageous when a chronic or devastating disease is treated (Tóth and Zakár, 1982).

Beside the well-characterized action of androgens mediated via androgen response elements within the DNA, the presented 19-nortestosterone analogs may also interact with membrane-associated androgen receptors (Kampa et al., 2006). This latter action could be of special importance since the stimulation of these receptors elicits an increase in the intracellular free zinc concentration accompanied by induction of apoptosis in cancer cell (Thomas et al., 2014).Two further membrane-bound proteins have been recently reported as potential non-genomic receptors for androgens and related steroids. One of them is the putative G-protein coupled receptor GPRC6A, an amino acid, calcium, and osteocalcin sensing receptor. The interaction of this receptor with testosterone is reported to result in increased phosphorylation of extracellular signal-regulated kinases in human embryonic kidney cells expressing the GPRC6A protein (Pi et al., 2010).

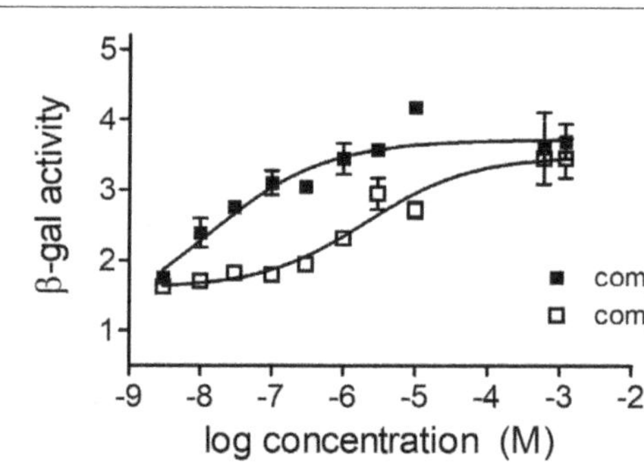

FIGURE 7 | Effects of compounds 1 and 3 in the yeast-based androgenic reporter assay. Results are mean values ± SEM of the data from two independent measurements, $n = 4$.

Oxoeicosanoid receptor 1 (OXER1) is a membrane receptor for the arachidonic acid metabolite 5-oxoeicosatetraenoic acid (5-oxoETE) and serves as a binding site for testosterone in prostate cancer cells. The steroid testosterone is reported to antagonize the action of the natural agonist 5-oxoETE on the intracellular cAMP production, and the interaction between testosterone and OXER1 was confirmed by an *in silico* molecular docking study as well (Kalyvianaki et al., 2017).

Since apoptosis and cell growth are indirectly involved in the signal mechanism of these non-genomic receptors, an action mediated by membrane-bound steroid receptors may contribute to the overall effects of the presented compounds.

In summary, our present results demonstrated that three of a set of newly synthesized 19-nortestosterone exhibit a pronounced antiproliferative activity against cervical carcinoma cells with lower influence on fibroblasts and a modest action on non-cancerous immortalized epithelial cells. The most potent agent **3** is characterized by a moderate cytotoxic effect, elicits cell cycle disturbance and induces the mitochondrial pathway of apoptosis. As a possible molecular mechanism of these actions, a PAC-like microtubule-stabilizing property is suggested based on its direct effect on the microtubular system.

Based on our present findings, the 19-nortestosterone backbone with a 17α-halogen substitution provides an excellent skeleton for designing novel antiproliferative steroidal compounds with negligible androgenic activity.

AUTHOR CONTRIBUTIONS

AG, AK, and EK performed the experiments. IO and AS analyzed the data. RM, EM, GS, and IZ were involved in experiment planning and supervision. AG, GS, and IZ wrote the manuscript.

FUNDING

The authors are grateful for financial support from the Hungarian Scientific Research Fund (OTKA K109293 and K113150). Financial support from the Economic Development and Innovation Operational Programme (GINOP-2.3.2-15-2016-00012 and GINOP-2.3.2-15-2016-00038) is gratefully acknowledged.

ACKNOWLEDGMENTS

The authors thank Dora Bokor, PharmD, for proof-reading the manuscript.

REFERENCES

Acharya, P. C., and Bansal, R. (2014). Synthesis and antiproliferative activity of some androstene oximes and their O-Alkylated derivatives. *Arch. Pharm.* 347, 193–199. doi: 10.1002/ardp.201300216

Ajdukovic, J. J., Djurendic, E. A., Petri, E. T., Klisuric, O. R., Celic, A. S., Sakac, M. N., et al. (2013). 17(E)-picolinylidene androstane derivatives as potential inhibitors of prostate cancer cell growth: antiproliferative activity and molecular docking studies. *Bioorg. Med. Chem.* 21, 7257–7266. doi: 10.1016/j.bmc.2013.09.063

Ajdukovic, J. J., Penov Gasi, K. M., Jakimov, D. S., Klisuric, O. R., Jovanovic-Santa, S. S., Sakac, M. N., et al. (2015). Synthesis, structural analysis and antitumor activity of novel 17alpha-picolyl and 17(E)-picolinylidene A-modified androstane derivatives. *Bioorg. Med. Chem.* 23, 1557–1568. doi: 10.1016/j.bmc.2015.02.001

Banday, A. H., Mir, B. P., Lone, I. H., Suri, K. A., and Kumar, H. M. (2010). Studies on novel D-ring substituted steroidal pyrazolines as potential anticancer agents. *Steroids* 75, 805–809. doi: 10.1016/j.steroids.2010.02.014

Bergink, E. W., Janssen, P. S., Turpijn, E. W., and van der Vies, J. (1985). Comparison of the receptor binding properties of nandrolone and testosterone under in vitro and in vivo conditions. *J. Steroid Biochem.* 22, 831–836. doi: 10.1016/0022-4731(85)90293-6

Bózsity, N., Minorics, R., Szabó, J., Mernyák, E., Schneider, G., Wölfling, J., et al. (2017). Mechanism of antiproliferative action of a new d-secoestrone-triazole derivative in cervical cancer cells and its effect on cancer cell motility. *J. Steroid Biochem. Mol. Biol.* 165, 247–257. doi: 10.1016/j.jsbmb.2016.06.013

Campagnoli, C., Clavel-Chapelon, F., Kaaks, R., Peris, C., and Berrino, F. (2005). Progestins and progesterone in hormone replacement therapy and the risk of breast cancer. *J. Steroid Biochem. Mol. Biol.* 96, 95–108. doi: 10.1016/j.jsbmb.2005.02.014

Cops, E. J., Bianco-Miotto, T., Moore, N. L., Clarke, C. L., Birrell, S. N., Butler, L. M., et al. (2008). Antiproliferative actions of the synthetic androgen, mibolerone, in breast cancer cells are mediated by both androgen and progesterone receptors. *J. Steroid Biochem. Mol. Biol.* 110, 236–243. doi: 10.1016/j.jsbmb.2007.10.014

Cui, J. G., Liu, L., Zhao, D. D., Gan, C. F., Huang, X., Xiao, Q., et al. (2015). Synthesis, characterization and antitumor activities of some steroidal derivatives with side chain of 17-hydrazone aromatic heterocycle. *Steroids* 95, 32–38. doi: 10.1016/j.steroids.2015.01.002

Erel, C. T., Senturk, L. M., and Kaleli, S. (2006). Tibolone and breast cancer. *Postgrad. Med. J.* 82, 658–662. doi: 10.1136/pgmj.2005.037184

Fitzmaurice, C., Allen, C., Barber, R. M., Barregard, L., Bhutta, Z. A., Brenner, H., et al. (2017). Global, regional, and national cancer incidence, mortality, years of life lost, years lived with disability, and disability-adjusted life-years for 32 cancer groups, 1990 to 2015: a systematic analysis for the global burden of disease study. *JAMA Oncol.* 3, 524–548. doi: 10.1001/jamaoncol.2016.5688

Fotsis, T., Zhang, Y., Pepper, M. S., Adlercreutz, H., Montesano, R., Nawroth, P. P., et al. (1994). The endogenous oestrogen metabolite 2-methoxyoestradiol inhibits angiogenesis and suppresses tumour growth. *Nature* 368, 237–239. doi: 10.1038/368237a0

Fragkaki, A. G., Angelis, Y. S., Koupparis, M., Tsantili-Kakoulidou, A., Kokotos, G., and Georgakopoulos, C. (2009). Structural characteristics of anabolic androgenic steroids contributing to binding to the androgen receptor and to their anabolic and androgenic activities. Applied modifications in the steroidal structure. *Steroids* 74, 172–197. doi: 10.1016/j.steroids.2008.10.016

Frank, E., and Schneider, G. (2013). Synthesis of sex hormone-derived modified steroids possessing antiproliferative activity. *J. Steroid Biochem. Mol. Biol.* 137, 301–315. doi: 10.1016/j.jsbmb.2013.02.018

Franke, H. R., and Vermes, I. (2003). Differential effects of progestogens on breast cancer cell lines. *Maturitas* 46(Suppl. 1), S55–S58. doi: 10.1016/j.maturitas.2003.09.019

Hajra, K. M., and Liu, J. R. (2004). Apoptosome dysfunction in human cancer. *Apoptosis* 9, 691–704. doi: 10.1023/B:APPT.0000045786.98031.1d

Iványi, Z., Szabó, N., Huber, J., Wölfling, J., Zupkó, I., Szécsi, M., et al. (2012). Synthesis of D-ring-substituted (5'R)- and (5'S)-17b-pyrazolinylandrostene epimers and comparison of their potential anticancer activities. *Steroids* 77, 566–574. doi: 10.1016/j.steroids.2012.02.001

Jakimov, D. S., Kojic, V. V., Aleksic, L. D., Bogdanovic, G. M., Ajdukovic, J. J., Djurendic, E. A., et al. (2015). Androstane derivatives induce apoptotic death in MDA-MB-231 breast cancer cells. *Bioorg. Med. Chem.* 23, 7189–7198. doi: 10.1016/j.bmc.2015.10.015

Jordan, M. A., Wendell, K., Gardiner, S., Derry, W. B., Copp, H., and Wilson, L. (1996). Mitotic block induced in HeLa cells by low concentrations of paclitaxel (Taxol) results in abnormal mitotic exit and apoptotic cell death. *Cancer Res.* 56, 816–825.

Kalyvianaki, K., Gebhart, V., Peroulis, N., Panagiotopoulou, C., Kiagiadaki, F., Pediaditakis, I., et al. (2017). Antagonizing effects of membrane-acting androgens on the eicosanoid receptor OXER1 in prostate cancer. *Sci. Rep.* 7:44418. doi: 10.1038/srep44418

Kampa, M., Kogia, C., Theodoropoulos, P. A., Anezinis, P., Charalampopoulos, I., Papakonstanti, E. A., et al. (2006). Activation of membrane androgen receptors potentiates the antiproliferative effects of paclitaxel on human prostate cancer cells. *Mol. Cancer Ther.* 5, 1342–1351. doi: 10.1158/1535-7163.MCT-05-0527

Kloosterboer, H. J., Schoonen, W. G., Deckers, G. H., and Klijn, J. G. (1994). Effects of progestagens and Org OD14 in in vitro and in vivo tumor models. *J. Steroid Biochem. Mol. Biol.* 49, 311–318. doi: 10.1016/0960-0760(94)90273-9

Koduru, S., Grierson, D. S., van de Venter, M., and Afolayan, A. J. (2007). Anticancer activity of steroid alkaloids isolated from *Solanum aculeastrum*. *Pharm. Biol.* 45, 613–618. doi: 10.1080/13880200701538690

LaVallee, T. M., Zhan, X. H., Herbstritt, C. J., Kough, E. C., Green, S. J., and Pribluda, V. S. (2002). 2-Methoxyestradiol inhibits proliferation and induces apoptosis independently of estrogen receptors alpha and beta. *Cancer Res.* 62, 3691–3697.

Li, L., Bu, S., Backstrom, T., Landstrom, M., Ulmsten, U., and Fu, X. (2004). Induction of apoptosis and G2/M arrest by 2-methoxyestradiol in human cervical cancer HeLaS3 cells. *Anticancer Res.* 24, 873–880.

Lin, S. X., Chen, J., Mazumdar, M., Poirier, D., Wang, C., Azzi, A., et al. (2010). Molecular therapy of breast cancer: progress and future directions. *Nat. Rev. Endocrinol.* 6, 485–493. doi: 10.1038/nrendo.2010.92

Mijatovic, T., Van Quaquebeke, E., Delest, B., Debeir, O., Darro, F., and Kiss, R. (2007). Cardiotonic steroids on the road to anti-cancer therapy. *Biochim. Biophys. Acta* 1776, 32–57. doi: 10.1016/j.bbcan.2007.06.002

Minami, T., Kosugi, K., Suganuma, I., Yamanaka, K., Kusuki, I., Oyama, T., et al. (2013). Antiproliferative and apoptotic effects of norethisterone on endometriotic stromal cells in vitro. *Eur. J. Obstet. Gynecol. Reprod. Biol.* 166, 76–80. doi: 10.1016/j.ejogrb.2012.08.023

Minorics, R., Bózsity, N., Molnár, J., Wölfling, J., Mernyák, E., Schneider, G., et al. (2015). A molecular understanding of d-homoestrone-induced G2/M cell cycle arrest in HeLa human cervical carcinoma cells. *J. Cell Mol. Med.* 19, 2365–2374. doi: 10.1111/jcmm.12587

Mitsunobu, O. (1981). The use of diethyl azodicarboxylate and triphenylphosphine in synthesis and transformation of natural products. *Synthesis* 1981, 1–28. doi: 10.1055/s-1981-29317

Miyashita, M., Koga, K., Takamura, M., Izumi, G., Nagai, M., Harada, M., et al. (2014). Dienogest reduces proliferation, aromatase expression and angiogenesis, and increases apoptosis in human endometriosis. *Gynecol. Endocrinol.* 30, 644–648. doi: 10.3109/09513590.2014.911279

Mohamed, Z. H., El-Koussi, N. A., Mahfouz, N. M., Youssef, A. F., Abdel Jaleel, G. A., and Shouman, S. A. (2015). Cu (I) catalyzed alkyne-azide 1,3-dipolar cycloaddition (CuAAC): synthesis of 17alpha-[1-(substituted phenyl)-1,2,3-triazol-4-yl]-19-nor-testosterone-17beta-yl acetates targeting progestational and antipro-liferative activities. *Eur. J. Med. Chem.* 97, 75–82. doi: 10.1016/j.ejmech.2015.04.045

Mosmann, T. (1983). Rapid colorimetric assay for cellular growth and survival: application to proliferation and cytotoxicity assays. *J. Immunol. Methods* 65, 55–63. doi: 10.1016/0022-1759(83)90303-4

Newman, R. A., Yang, P., Pawlus, A. D., and Block, K. I. (2008). Cardiac glycosides as novel cancer therapeutic agents. *Mol. Interv.* 8, 36–49. doi: 10.1124/mi.8.1.8

Peyrat, J. F., Brion, J. D., and Alami, M. (2012). Synthetic 2-methoxyestradiol derivatives: structure-activity relationships. *Curr. Med. Chem.* 19, 4142–4156. doi: 10.2174/092986712802430072

Pi, M., Parrill, A. L., and Quarles, L. D. (2010). GPRC6A mediates the non-genomic effects of steroids. *J. Biol. Chem.* 285, 39953–39964. doi: 10.1074/jbc.M110.158063

Punjabi, S., Cook, L. J., Kersey, P., Marks, R., and Cerio, R. (2008). Solasodine glycoalkaloids: a novel topical therapy for basal cell carcinoma. A double-blind, randomized, placebo-controlled, parallel group, multicenter study. *Int. J. Dermatol.* 47, 78–82. doi: 10.1111/j.1365-4632.2007.03363.x

Royer, P. A., and Jones, K. P. (2014). Progestins for contraception: modern delivery systems and novel formulations. *Clin. Obstet. Gynecol.* 57, 644–658. doi: 10.1097/GRF.0000000000000072

Saito, F., Tashiro, H., Yamaguchi, M., Honda, R., Ohba, T., Suzuki, A., et al. (2016). Development of a mouse model for testing therapeutic agents: the anticancer effect of dienogest on endometrial neoplasms. *Gynecol. Endocrinol.* 32, 403–407. doi: 10.3109/09513590.2015.1124411

Schneider, G., Kiss, A., Mernyák, E., Benke, Z., Wölfling, J., Frank, É., et al. (2016). Stereocontrolled synthesis of the four 16-hydroxymethyl-19-nortestosterone isomers and their antiproliferative activities. *Steroids* 105, 113–120. doi: 10.1016/j.steroids.2015.12.003

Sharifi, N., Gulley, J. L., and Dahut, W. L. (2010). An update on androgen deprivation therapy for prostate cancer. *Endocr. Relat. Cancer* 17, R305–R315. doi: 10.1677/ERC-10-0187

Thomas, P., Pang, Y., Dong, J., and Berg, A. H. (2014). Identification and characterization of membrane androgen receptors in the ZIP9 zinc transporter subfamily: II. Role of human ZIP9 in testosterone-induced prostate and breast cancer cell apoptosis. *Endocrinology* 155, 4250–4265. doi: 10.1210/en.2014-1201

Tolomeo, M., and Simoni, D. (2002). Drug resistance and apoptosis in cancer treatment: development of new apoptosis-inducing agents active in drug resistant malignancies. *Curr. Med. Chem. Anticancer Agents* 2, 387–401. doi: 10.2174/1568011024606361

Tóth, M., and Zakár, T. (1982). Relative binding affinities of testosterone, 19-nortestosterone and their 5 alpha-reduced derivatives to the androgen receptor and to other androgen-binding proteins: a suggested role of 5 alpha-reductive steroid metabolism in the dissociation of "myotropic" and "androgenic" activities of 19-nortestosterone. *J. Steroid Biochem.* 17, 653–660. doi: 10.1016/0022-4731(82)90567-2

Wadosky, K. M., and Koochekpour, S. (2016). Molecular mechanisms underlying resistance to androgen deprivation therapy in prostate cancer. *Oncotarget* 7, 64447–64470. doi: 10.18632/oncotarget.10901

Yue, T. L., Wang, X., Louden, C. S., Gupta, S., Pillarisetti, K., Gu, J. L., et al. (1997). 2-Methoxyestradiol, an endogenous estrogen metabolite, induces apoptosis in endothelial cells and inhibits angiogenesis: possible role for stress-activated protein kinase signaling pathway and Fas expression. *Mol. Pharmacol.* 51, 951–962. doi: 10.1124/mol.51.6.951

12

miR-9-5p as a Regulator of the Androgen Receptor Pathway in Breast Cancer Cell Lines

Erika Bandini[1], Francesca Fanini[1], Ivan Vannini[1], Tania Rossi[1], Meropi Plousiou[1], Maria Maddalena Tumedei[1], Francesco Limarzi[2], Roberta Maltoni[2], Francesco Fabbri[1], Silvana Hrelia[3], William C. S. Cho[4] and Muller Fabbri[5]*

[1] Biosciences Laboratory, Istituto Scientifico Romagnolo per lo Studio e la Cura dei Tumori (IRST) IRCCS, Meldola, Italy, [2] Istituto Scientifico Romagnolo per lo Studio e la Cura dei Tumori (IRST) IRCCS, Meldola, Italy, [3] Department for Life Quality Studies, Alma Mater Studiorum - University of Bologna, Rimini, Italy, [4] Department of Clinical Oncology, Queen Elizabeth Hospital, Kowloon, Hong Kong, [5] Cancer Biology Program, University of Hawai'i Cancer Center, Hawaii, HI, United States

***Correspondence:**
Francesca Fanini
francesca.fanini@irst.emr.it*

Breast cancer (BC) is the most diagnosed carcinoma and the leading cause of cancer death in female over 100 countries. Thanks to the advance in therapeutic strategies, patients' survival has improved. However, the lack of response to treatments and drug resistance are still a main concern, demanding for new therapeutic approaches, in particular for the advanced stages of the disease. Androgen receptor (AR) is gaining increasing interest as a fourth targetable receptor in BC, however, its regulation in BC cells is still poorly understood. MicroRNAs (miRNAs) regulate gene expression post-transcriptionally. Here, we identified miR-9-5p as an inhibitor of AR expression, we validated the inverse correlation between miR-9-5p and AR in primary BC samples and we further identified a feedback loop in which androgen agonists of AR up-regulate miR-9-5p. We also provided evidence that miR-9-5p elicits anti-proliferative effects in BC cell lines regardless of their estrogen receptor status. Finally, we showed that miR-9-5p can revert AR-downstream signaling even in presence of AR-agonists, highlighting the role of this miR in the hormonal response of BC. In conclusion, this study supports the role of miR-9-5p as an anti-proliferative miR in BC and as a central modulator of AR-signaling response to circulating androgens in BC.

Keywords: microRNAs, miR-9-5p, androgen receptor, breast, cancer

INTRODUCTION

Despite progresses in its global management approaches, breast cancer (BC) still remains the most diagnosed carcinoma and the leading cause of cancer death in women over 100 countries (Bray et al., 2018). In 2020 it was estimated an incidence of 276,480 cases and 42,170 deaths in women due to BC in the United States (Siegel et al., 2020). Although several therapeutic approaches have provided remarkable improvements in survival, drug resistance and the lack of response to treatments are still a main issue, suggesting a great need to exploit novel therapeutic strategies in

---

Abbreviations: AR, Androgen receptor; BC, Breast cancer; EMT, Epithelial mesenchymal transition; FFPE, Formalin-fixed paraffin-embedded; miRNAsmicroRNAs; DHT, Dihydrotestosterone; DHEA, Dehydroepiandrosterone.

particular in the advanced stages (Zhao et al., 2019). Androgen receptor (AR) is a member of the steroid nuclear receptors family that mediates the biological effects of androgens. It is considered an emerging target in the treatment of patients characterized by the lack of expression of hormone receptors (the so called "Triple-Negative Breast Cancer" or TNBC), and in other BC subtypes, despite its role is still controversial (Takagi et al., 2018; Vidula et al., 2019). In recent years, several molecules have been investigated as crucial regulators of transcription, and translation of genes involved in carcinogenesis, and microRNAs (miRNAs) are among the most studied. They belong to a large family of small non-coding RNAs and deserve great attention since they can modulate the expression of tumor suppressor genes and oncogenes, affecting the signal pathways in cancer cells. However, little is known about miRNA regulation of hormonal signaling, especially androgen signaling, in BC, and how this affects hormone-therapy. Several studies have been performed in order to identify a miRNA signature that could predict their potential role as prognostic or predictive biomarkers for patient management. In particular, miR-9-5p dysregulation has been reported in many cancer types, but its role as a tumor suppressor gene or as an oncomiR remains unclear, especially in BC. Some studies reported miR-9-5p as a negative prognostic marker related to more aggressive clinical pathological features and as involved in epithelial-mesenchymal transition (EMT) (Almeida et al., 2010; Gwak et al., 2014; van Schooneveld et al., 2015; Bastos et al., 2016; Jang et al., 2017; Cheng et al., 2018). AR has emerged as a fourth receptor in BC and as a promising target, especially for those patients who do not respond to current hormone receptor-targeted therapies. In this study, we investigated the role of miR-9-5p in the AR pathway. We showed that AR is a target of miR-9-5p and we identified a novel miR-9-5p/AR feedback loop with important implications for the response of BC to anti-androgen therapy.

MATERIALS AND METHODS

Cell Cultures

The human breast carcinoma cell lines MDA-MB-453 and MCF-7 were purchased from the American Type Culture Collection (ATCC; Manassas, Virginia, United States), and the cell line T-47D was purchased from Zooprophylactic Institute of Genova (Italy). MDA-MB-453 were maintained in Leibovitz's L-15 medium (ATCC 30-2008, United States) supplemented with fetal bovine serum (FBS) (Gibco, Thermo Fisher Scientific, United States) to a final concentration of 10%, according to the manufacturer's information sheet. MCF-7 was maintained in Eagle's Minimum Essential Medium (EMEM) medium (ATCC 30-2003, United States) supplemented with FBS to a final concentration of 10%. T-47D were maintained in Dulbecco's Modified Eagle's Medium (DMEM) High Glucose (Euroclone, Italy), and FBS to a final concentration of 10%. One percent of Penicillin-streptomycin (PAA, Carlo Erba Reagents, Italy), and 0.002% of MycoZap Prophylactic (Lonza Group Ltd., Switzerland) were added to all mediums. The cultures were maintained in a Heraeus incubator, in atmosphere composed of 95% air, and 5% CO_2, except for MDA-MB-453 that required a free gas exchange with atmospheric air. Every 4 days we proceeded to sub-cultivation of cell lines by using Trypsin-EDTA (Life Technologies, United States). Cell lines were tested every 2 months with MycoAlert™ Mycoplasma Detection Kit (Lonza Group Ltd., Switzerland) to check a possible contamination by mycoplasma. In experiments where hormonal treatments were performed, medium phenol red free added of FBS charcoal stripped was used (Gibco, Thermo Fisher Scientific, United States).

Patient Sample

Paired FFPE tumor and adjacent non-tumor tissue from 11 BC patients (5 Triple Negative Breast Cancers TNBCs, and 6 Luminal A) were obtained at the Istituto Scientifico Romagnolo per lo Studio e la Cura dei Tumori IRST, S.r.l, IRCCS, in Meldola (FC), Italy. Histological and clinical characteristics are listed in **Supplementary Table S1**. Written informed consent was obtained from all patients before sample analyses. The study was approved by the Ethical Committee of our institute and conducted in accordance with the Declaration of Helsinki. Written informed consent was obtained from all patients before the first sampling.

Drug Treatments

Dihydrotestosterone (DHT) was purchased from Sigma-Aldrich (Merck, Germany) in powder formulation and a 10 μM working solution was obtained by resuspending it in dimethyl sulfoxide (DMSO); DHT was then used at 10 nM and DMSO never exceeded 0.1%. Dehydroepiandrosterone (DHEA) was provided by the Pharmacy of our Institute at a concentration of 7.6 mM dissolved in sterile water, and 50 μM solution was used to perform experiments.

Pre-miRNAs Transfection

Pre-miRNAs (pre-miRNA miR precursors, Ambion, Life Technologies, United States), and the corresponding negative control, SCR (Pre-miR miRNA precursor scrambled negative control #1, Ambion, Life Technologies, United States) were used to transfect BC cell lines at a final concentration of 100 nM through TransIT-X2® Dynamic Delivery System (Mirus Bio LLC, United States), in accordance with the instructions provided by the manufacturer. Opti-Mem Medium (Gibco, Thermo Fisher Scientific, United States) was used for transfection complex. Depending on the type of final analysis, transfections were stopped and pellets collected at 24–48–72 h. MiRNA transfection efficiencies were evaluated by Real-time quantitative PCR (qRT-PCR).

AR Silencing

SMARTpool siGENOME AR siRNA (Dharmacon), and the corresponding negative control, siGENOME Non-Targeting siRNA #1 (Dharmacon), were transfected into BC cell lines at a final concentration of 50 nM, through TransIT-X2® Dynamic Delivery System (Mirus Bio LLC, United States), in accordance with the instructions provided by the manufacturer. Opti-Mem

Medium (Gibco, Thermo Fisher Scientific, United States) was used for transfection complex. Transfections were stopped and pellets collected at 48 h. AR transfection efficiencies and miR-9-5p expression were evaluated by qRT-PCR.

Extraction of RNA and Proteins

RNA was isolated from BC cells with mirVana™ miRNA Isolation Kit (Invitrogen, Thermo Fisher Scientific, United States), following the manufacturer's instruction. RNA isolation from 2-to-4 10 μm thick slices FFPE was performed by using RecoverAll Total Nucleic Acid Isolation Kit for FFPE (Invitrogen, Thermo Fisher Scientific, United States) following the protocol provided by the manufacturer. The quantification of extracted RNA was carried out using NanoDrop ND-1,000 (Thermo Fisher Scientific, United States). Total proteins were extracted, keeping samples on ice, with 1X RIPA lysis buffer (Santa Cruz Biotechnology, United States) with the addition of 10 μl of PMSF, 10 μl of sodium orthovanadate and 15 μl of protease inhibitors per ml of 1X RIPA lysis buffer, as recommended by the datasheet. The lysates were centrifuged at 4°C for 30 min. Then, supernatant was transferred to another tube. Proteins were quantified through BCA Protein Assay (Pierce, Thermo Fisher Scientific, United States), and using a Multiscan EX microplate reader (Thermo Fisher Scientific, United States), at a wavelength of 490 nm.

Protein Expression Analysis

Western blotting was used to evaluate the expression of AR. Proteins (50 μg) were denatured and separated by electrophoresis using a gel Criterion TGX Stain Free Gel Precast 4–20% (Bio-Rad Laboratories, CA, United States), and Laemmli Sample Buffer (Bio-Rad Laboratories, CA, United States) with 5% of β-mercaptoethanol (Carlo Erba Reagents, Italy), in 1:1 ratio with the sample. Electrophoretic run was performed at a constant voltage of 180V in a TRIS/Glycine/SDS 1X buffer (Bio-Rad Laboratories, CA, United States). Trans-Blot Transfer Turbo midi-format 0.2 μm PVDF membrane (Bio-Rad Laboratories, CA, United States) using the Trans Blot Turbo System (Bio-Rad Laboratories, CA, United States). The membrane was subsequently incubated for at least 2 h at room temperature in a solution of Tween 20 (Bio-Rad) at 0.1% and 1X Dulbecco's phosphate buffered saline (DPBS) (Invitrogen, Thermo Fisher Scientific, United States) supplemented with 5% nonfat dry milk (Bio-Rad Laboratories, CA, United states) in order to facilitate the saturation of non-specific binding sites. Primary antibodies and dilutions used are the following: anti-Androgen Receptor (1:1,000; ab133273, Abcam, United States), anti-Vinculin clone FB11 (1:1,000; Biohit, United Kingdom), anti-β-actin Antibody HRP (1:50,000; ab49900, Abcam, United States). Secondary antibodies HRP-conjugated goat anti-mouse and anti-rabbit (1:5,000; Santa Cruz, United States) and Precision Plus Protein Western C Strep Tactin-HRP Conjugate (1:10,000; Bio-Rad Laboratories, CA, United States) were used. The secondary HRP-conjugated antibodies were used for 1 h at room temperature. The membranes, after washes with T-PBS, were developed using Clarity Western ECL reagent (Bio-Rad Laboratories), and images acquired through Chemidoc (Bio-Rad Laboratories), and analyzed using ImageJ Software (Wayne Rasband, NIH, United States).

miRNA and mRNA Expression Analysis

MiRNAs expression analysis was performed using the TaqMan miRNA Assays (Applied Biosystems, Thermo Fisher Scientific, United States). Briefly, the molecule of complementary DNA (cDNA) was synthesized using 10 ng of RNA as template, specific primer and TaqMan MicroRNA Reverse Transcription Kit (Applied Biosystems, Thermo Fisher Scientific, United States). mRNAs expression was evaluated with the use of the TaqMan Gene Expression Assays (Applied Biosystems, Lifetechnologies, United States). The cDNA was synthesized using 80 ng of RNA as a template and the TaqMan RT PCR Kit (Applied Biosystems, Thermo Fisher Scientific, United States). qRT-PCR was performed with Applied Biosystems 7500 Real-Time PCR System (Thermo Fisher Scientific, United States) using cDNA, TaqMan probes and TaqMan Universal PCR Master Mix (Applied Biosystems, Thermo Fisher Scientific, United States). To determine the basal expression of miR-9-5p in BC cell lines, a reference RNA composed of total RNA from nine human tissues or cell lines was used (Total RNA Breast Human, #750500, Agilent Technologies, United States). Experiments were conducted in triplicate and normalized to RNU48, RNU44 and GAPDH, used as endogenous controls. Relative expression levels were calculated using the method of comparative Ct ($2^{-\Delta\Delta Ct}$ method).

Immunohistochemistry

During surgery some tumor samples were obtained and fixed in neutral buffered formalin, then embedded in paraffin. For each patient, 5 μm thickness sections were mounted on positive-charged slides (Bio Optica, Milan, Italy). AR expression was performed using the Ventana Benchmark ULTRA staining system (Ventana Medical Systems, Tucson, AZ, United States) with the Optiview DAB Detection Kit (Ventana Medical Systems). AR (SP107 Cell Marque, Ventana Medical Systems) antibody pre-diluted by the supplier was used. The slides were incubated for 16 min and automatically counterstained with hematoxylin II (Ventana Medical Systems). AR positivity was detected and semiquantitatively quantified as the percentage ratio between immunopositive tumor cells and the total number of tumor cells. All samples were evaluated by two independent observers. Any disagreement (>10% of positive cells for the different markers) was resolved by consensus after joint review using a multihead microscope. Biomarker determination was performed according to European Quality Assurance guidelines

CellTiter-Glo Luminescent Cell Viability Assay

CellTiter-Glo Luminescent Cell Viability Assay (Promega, United States) was used to determine the number of viable cells after hormone treatments and transfections. It is based on the quantification of present ATP that indicates the existence of metabolically active cells. The procedure, according to the instructions provided by the manufacturer, requires the adding of a single reagent (CellTiter-Glo Reagent) directly to cultured cells. This system produces a cell lysis and the generation of a luminescent signal, captured through a GloMax luminometer (Promega, United States), proportional to the ATP content, which, in turn, is directly proportional to the number of viable cells.

Flow Cytometry

All samples were analyzed by using a FACSCanto^{TM} cytofluorimeter (BD Biosciences). Data acquisition (10,000 events were collected for each sample) was performed by using the FACS Diva^{TM} software (BD Biosciences), as recommended by the manufacturer. After cells were seeded in 6-well plates and treated with DHT 10 nM or DHEA 50 μM, or after miR-9-5p transfection they underwent different protocols.

Bromodeoxyuridine assay was used to determine the percentage of S-phase cells. Cells were incubated with a 60 μM Bromodeoxyuridine (BrdU) solution in 1 ml of medium and then centrifuged and fixed with 70% cold ethanol. The day after cells were washed in PBS 1X and incubated with the following reagents in this order: HCL 2M (Carlo Erba Reagents, Italy), sodium tetraborate (Sigma-Aldrich, Merck, Germany), and Tween 20 0.5% (Bio-Rad Laboratories, CA, United States) + BSA 1% (Thermo Fisher Scientific, United States). Finally, cells were incubated with a 1:50 dilution of anti-BrdU antibody (Thermo

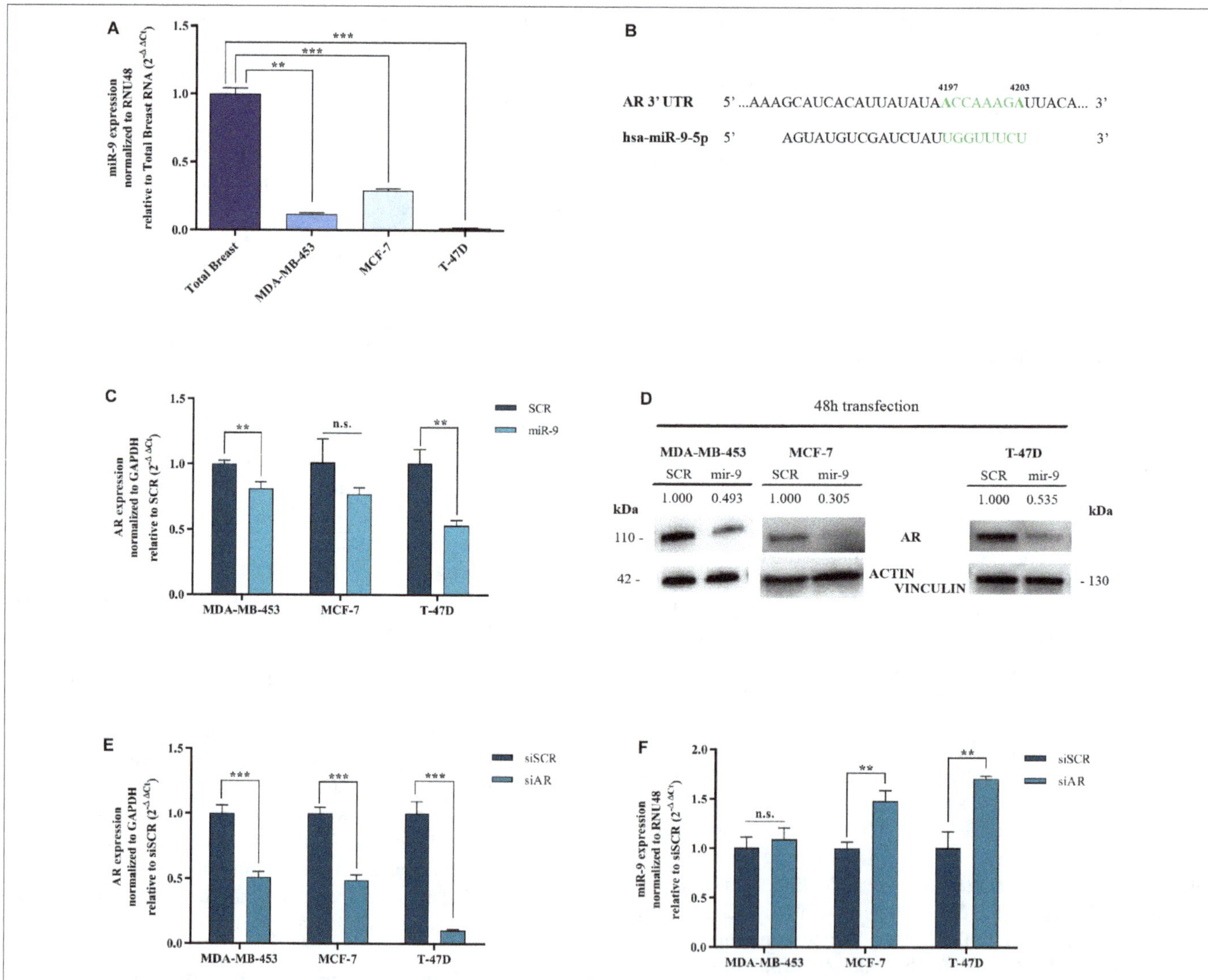

FIGURE 1 | MiR-9-5p is downregulated in BC cell lines and down-regulates AR. **(A)** MiR-9-5p (mir-9) expression was measured by qRT-PCR in three BC cell lines and compared to Total Breast RNA. **(B)** Predicted miR-9-5p target sites in the AR 3′UTR mRNA, as shown by the Software TargetScan Human Release v6.2. in green, the seed region of miR-9::AR mRNA predicted interaction. **(C)** mRNA expression level of AR in MDA-MB-453, MCF-7, and T-47D cell lines, 48 h after transfection with pre-miR-9-5p (miR-9), or scrambled (SCR). **(D)** Protein expression level of AR in MDA-MB-453, MCF-7 and T-47D cell lines, 48 h after transfection with pre-miR-9-5p (miR-9), or scrambled (SCR). **(E)** AR levels after transfection of MDA-MB-453, MCF-7, and T-47D cell lines with AR siRNA (siAR) compared to scrambled (siSCR). **(F)** MiR-9-5p (miR-9) expression in MDA-MB-453, MCF-7, and T-47D cell lines after 48 h transfection with AR siRNA (siAR) or scrambled (siSCR). $^{**}p < 0.01$, $^{***}p < 0.001$, n.s., not significant. Multiple *t*-test, corrected for multiple comparison using the Holm-Sidak method in **(A–D)**.

Fisher Scientific, United States) for 1 h, followed by 1 h of a FITC-conjugated secondary antibody (Dako, Agilent Technologies, United States) diluted 1:250. After antibody incubation, cells were washed with PBS 1X, stained with propidium iodide solution and incubated overnight at 4°C. Samples were processed and analyzed the day after.

For cell cycle evaluation, cells were harvested after each treatment timepoint, fixed in 70% ethanol, and stained in a solution containing 10µg ml/1 of propidium iodide (Sigma-Aldrich), 10,000 U ml/1 of RNase (Sigma-Aldrich), and 0.01% of NP40 (Sigma-Aldrich). After 30–60 min, the samples were analyzed. Data were elaborated using the ModFit LT^{TM} software v.4.1.7 (Verity Software House), and expressed as fractions of cells in the different cell-cycle phases.

Cignal Reporter Assay

Cignal Reporter Assay Kit (Qiagen, United States) was used to assess the activation of AR transduction pathway, by measuring the activities of downstream AR transcription factors (both increases and decreases). One microgram of AR-responsive reporter (a mixture of inducible transcription factor responsive construct and constitutively expressing Renilla luciferase construct) and negative control (a mixture of non-inducible reporter construct and constitutively expressing Renilla luciferase construct), along with pre-miR-9-5p and the corresponding negative control SCR (100 nM), were diluted in Opti-Mem Medium (Gibco, Thermo Fisher Scientific, United States). The diluted nucleic acids were mixed with TransIT-X2 Mirus (Temaricerca, Italy). Following 24 h transfection, cells were treated with DHT 10 nM for additional 24 h, so that 48 h post-transfection cells were harvested into cell lysis buffer (Promega, United States). Luciferase activity was measured using the Dual-Luciferase Assay System (Promega, United States). The change in the activity of AR signaling pathway was determined by comparing the normalized luciferase activities of the reporter in treated *versus* untreated transfectants (SCR vs. miR-9-5p and SCR + DHT vs. miR-9-5p + DHT). The activity ratio Firefly:Renilla was calculated from experimental and control transfections. Then, ratios from AR responsive reporter transfections were divided by ratios from negative controls to obtain relative luciferase units (RLU).

Data Analysis

Data obtained from qRT-PCR were analyzed by Life Technologies TM 7500 Software v2.0.6 for 7500 Fast Real Time PCR System (Life Technologies, Thermo Fisher Scientific, United States). Relative expression levels were calculated using the method of comparative Ct ($2^{-\Delta\ \Delta\ Ct}$). The images of the Western Blot, acquired through Chemidoc, were analyzed using ImageJ Software (Wayne Rasband, NIH, United States). Viability experiments were conducted in 96 wells plate, using 8 wells for every sample. Statistical analyses were performed using GraphPad Prism 8 (version 8.4.2) statistical software (GraphPad

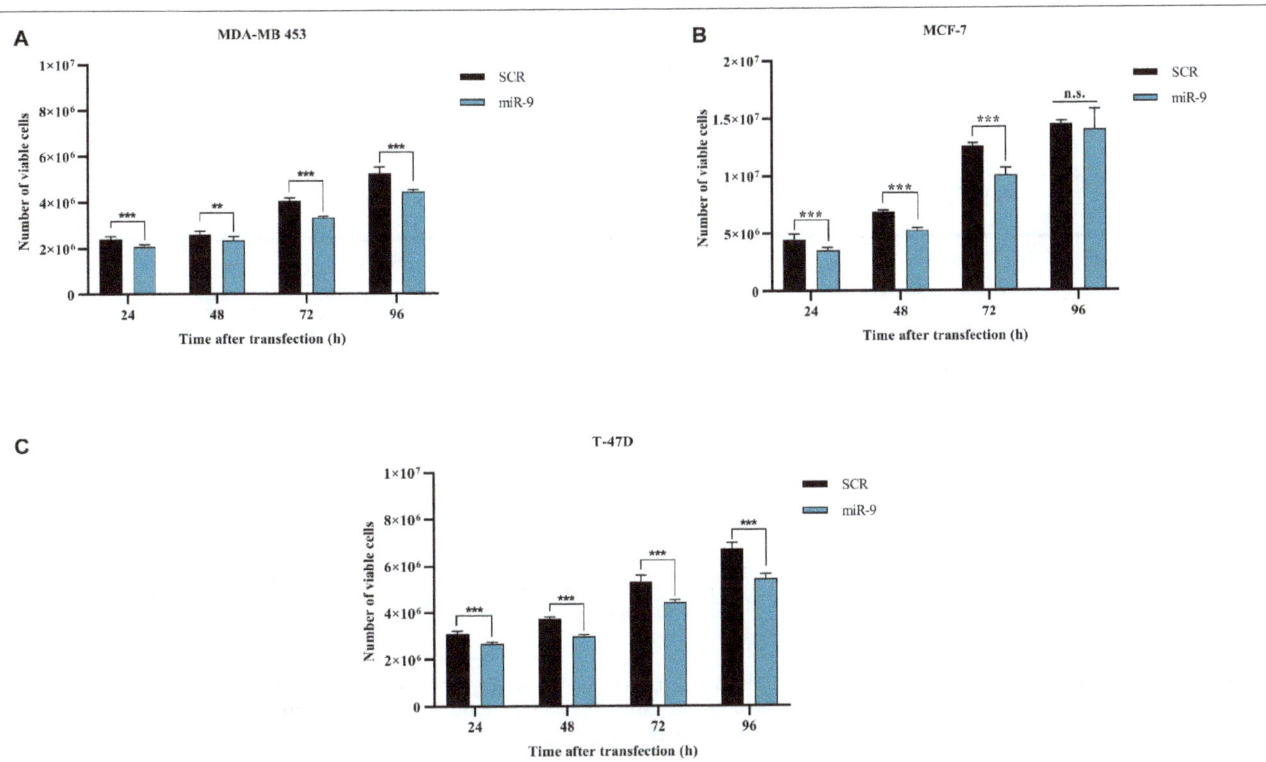

FIGURE 2 | Effects of miR-9-5p (mir-9) on proliferation of BC cell lines **(A)** MDA-MB-453 **(B)** MCF-7 **(C)** T-47D. $^{**}p < 0.01$, $^{***}p < 0.001$, n.s., not significant. Multiple *t*-test, corrected for multiple comparison using the Holm-Sidak method in **(A–C)**.

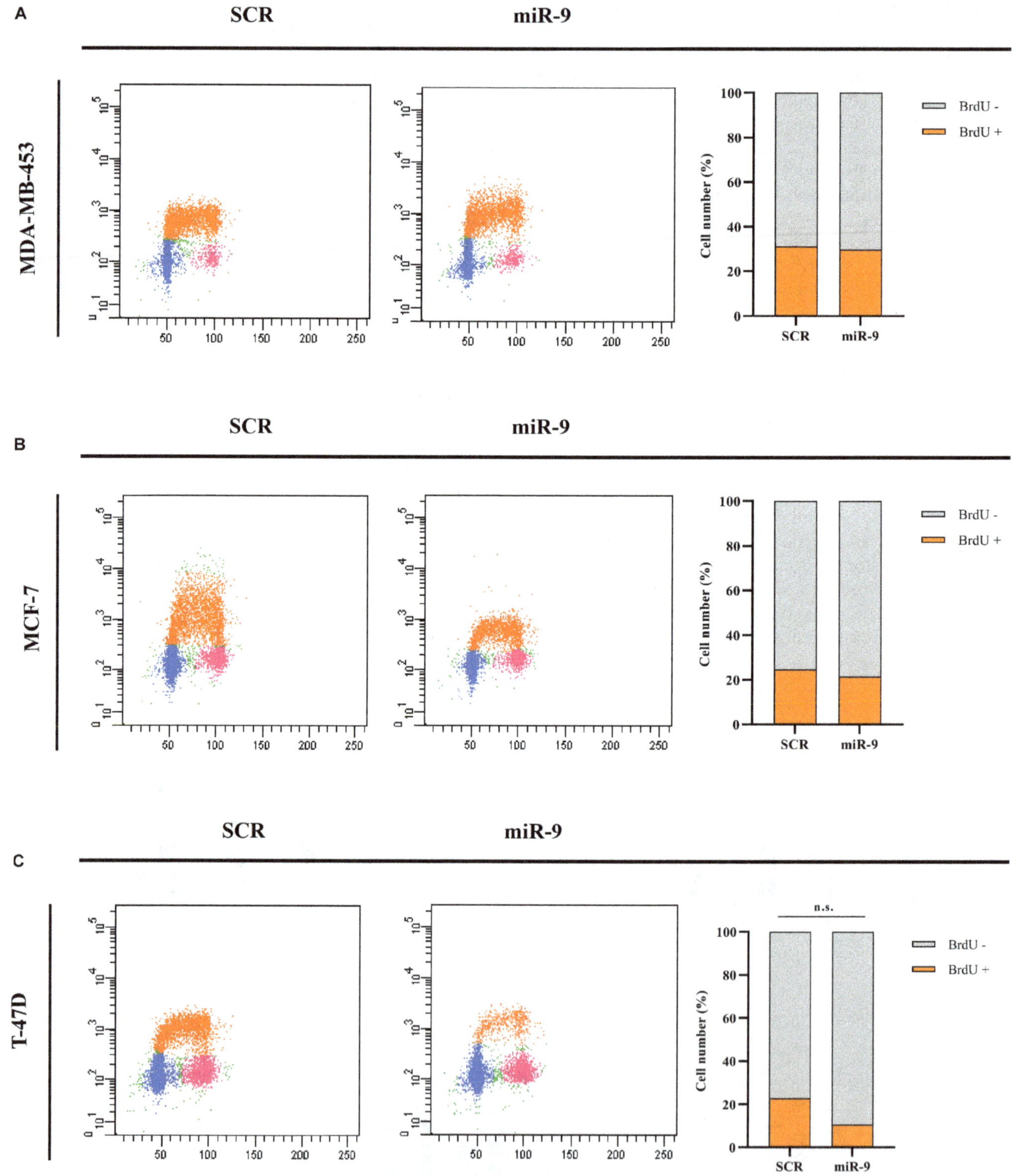

FIGURE 3 | Cytofluorimetric evaluation of the effects of miR-9-5p (miR-9) on DNA replication at 72 h post-transfection. Cytofluorimetric dot plots of proliferating MDA-MB-453 **(A)**, MCF-7 **(B)**, and T-47D **(C)** BC cell lines, following BrdU incorporation, and anti-BrdU antibody incubation. The percentage of cells in S phase, which results in BrdU positive cells (BrdU+) was presented in the histograms on the right.

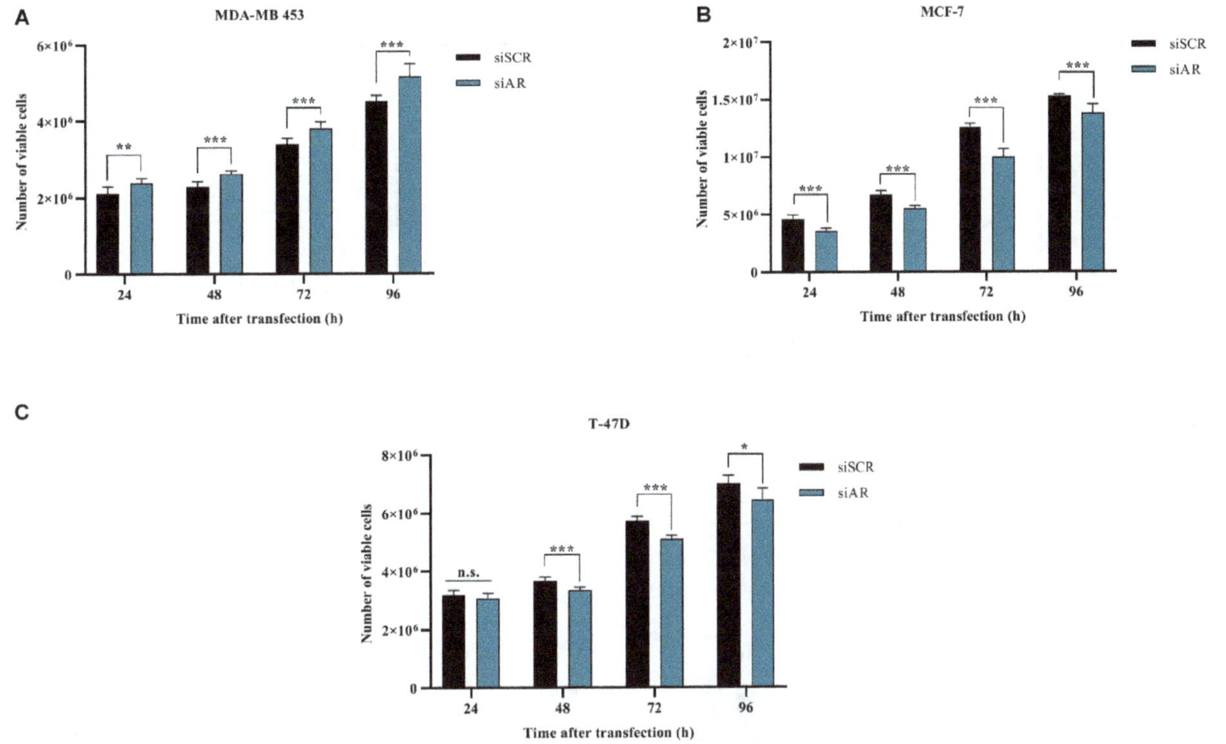

FIGURE 4 | Effects of AR silencing (siAR) on proliferation of BC cell lines **(A)** MDA-MB-453 **(B)** MCF-7 **(C)** T-47D. *$p < 0.05$, **$p < 0.01$, ***$p < 0.001$, n.s., not significant. Multiple *t*-test, corrected for multiple comparison using the Holm-Sidak method in **(A–C)**.

Software, United States). Statistical significance was indicated as follows: *$p < 0.05$; **$p < 0.01$; ***$p < 0.001$.

RESULTS

MicroRNA-9-5p Is Downregulated in BC Cell Lines

MDA-MB-453 are molecular apocrine BC cell lines (AR^+, ER^-) (Robinson et al., 2011). MCF-7 and T-47D are luminal A BC cell lines (AR^+, ER^+) (Dai et al., 2017). We performed qRT-PCR for miR-9-5p to assess the endogenous expression of miR-9-5p in these 3 different BC cells lines, compared to human Total Normal Breast RNA (Agilent Technologies). All cell lines show a low endogenous expression of miR-9-5p when compared to Total Normal Breast RNA (**Figure 1A**).

MicroRNA-9-5p Silences AR

AR is an emerging target for hormone therapy in BC. However, the factors regulating its expression are not understood. Intriguingly, miR-9-5p is predicted to target AR by TargetScan Software v7.2 (Agarwal et al., 2015) and miRWalk database (Medical Faculty Mannheim of the University of Heidelberg) (**Figure 1B**). To assess whether miR-9-5p silences AR, MDA-MB-453, MCF-7 and T-47D cells were transfected with miR-9-5p or a scrambled oligonucleotide as a control (SCR) and the expression of AR was measured both at the mRNA and at the protein level by qRT-PCR and immunoblotting, respectively. We observed a significant down-regulation of AR expression in all three tested BC cell lines both at the mRNA (**Figure 1C**) and at the protein level (**Figure 1D**).

AR Silencing Upregulates miR-9-5p in ER+ Cell Lines

Intriguingly, when we silenced AR endogenous expression with a pool of siRNAs (a mixture of 4 siRNA provided as a single reagent) (**Figure 1E**), upregulation of miR-9-5p was observed (compared to a siRNA negative control) but only in ER+ BC cell lines MCF-7 and T-47D, with no effects on the ER- cell line MDA-MB-453 (**Figure 1F**). Overall, these data indicate that while miR-9-5p downregulates AR expression regardless of the ER status of BC cell lines, AR silencing up-regulates miR-9 only in ER^+ cell lines.

MicroRNA-9-5p Reduces BC Cell Growth

BC cells were transfected with the pre-miR-9-5p mimic, or a scrambled miRNA as a control (SCR), and *in vitro* cell growth at 24–48–72–96 h post-transfection was evaluated. MiR-9-5p increased expression significantly reduced the proliferation of all three BC cells at all tested times (**Figures 2A–C**). Overexpression of miR-9-5p was verified by qRT-PCR (**Supplementary Figures S1A–C**). In order to study the effects of mir-9-5p on cell proliferation, we further quantified replicating

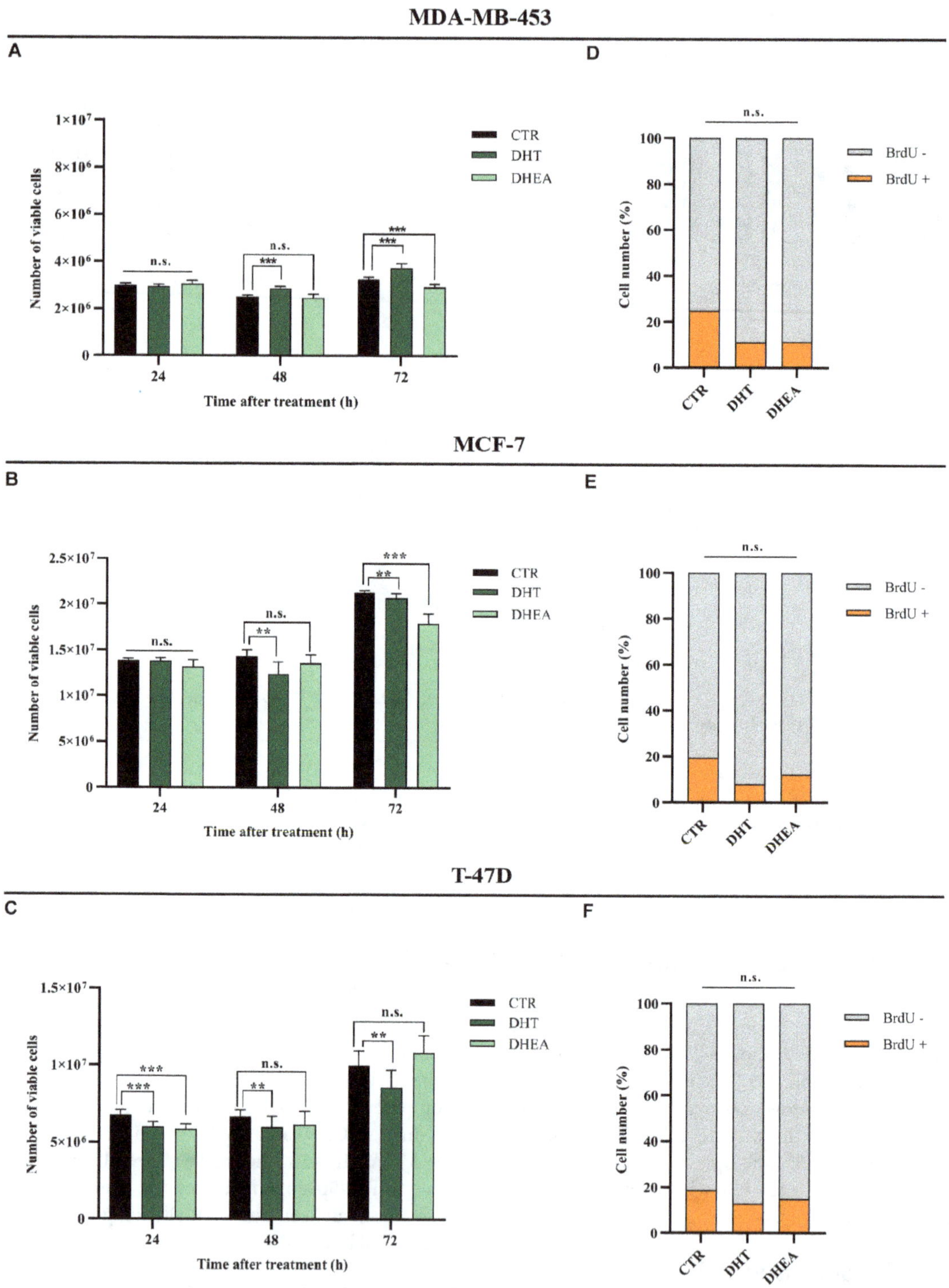

FIGURE 5 | Effect of DHT and DHEA on proliferation of BC cell lines at the indicated time points **(A–C)** and on DNA replication at 48 h post-transfection **(D–F)**. $^{**}p < 0.01$, $^{***}p < 0.001$, n.s., not significant. Multiple *t*-test, corrected for multiple comparison using the Holm-Sidak method in **(A–F)**.

DNA by performing a BrdU assay. While only little difference was observed in MDA-MB-453 and MCF-7 cell lines at 72 h (**Figures 3A,B**), we observed a notable reduction of DNA replication in T-47D cell line transfected with pre-miR-9-5p compared to scrambled (25 vs. 6.2%) at 72 h (**Figure 3C**) which persisted even at 96 h (**Supplementary Figure S2**), suggesting that cells did not enter S phase. These results were confirmed also by cell cycle analysis using propidium iodide, which showed a

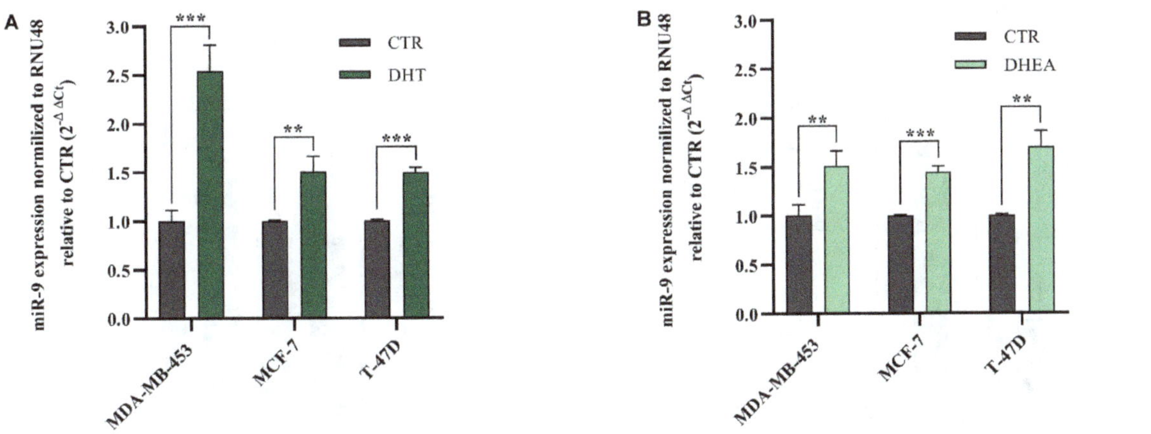

FIGURE 6 | Effects of DHT and DHEA on miR-9-5p (miR-9) expression at 24 h post-transfection **(A,B)**. $^{**}p < 0.01$, $^{***}p < 0.001$. Multiple *t*-test, corrected for multiple comparison using the Holm-Sidak method in **(A,B)**.

reduction of T-47D cells in S-phase and a block in G1-phase when miR-9-5p was overexpressed (**Supplementary Figures S3–S5**).

AR Silencing Reduces Proliferation of ER+ Cells Lines

BC cells were transfected with a pool of AR siRNAs (a mixture of 4 siRNA provided as a single reagent) (**Figure 1E**) and *in vitro* cell growth at 24–48–72–96 h post-transfection was assessed. AR silencing did not reduce the proliferation of ER- MDA-MB-453 (**Figure 4A**), but significantly reduced the proliferation of the two ER+ cell lines MCF-7 and T-47D (**Figures 4B,C**). These data are consistent with the inhibitory effect of miR-9-5p on BC proliferation and with the fact that silencing of AR expression up-regulates miR-9-5p only in ER+ cells and not in the ER- MDA-MB-453 BC cells.

DHT and DHEA Reduce Growth of BC Cell Lines

MDA-MB-453, MCF-7, and T-47D cell lines express AR (**Figure 1D**). In order to assess the effects of circulating AR-agonists on BC cell proliferation, we treated BC cells with DHT and DHEA, respectively. DHT showed a cell growth promoting effect only in MDA-MB-453 at 48 and 72 h (**Figure 5A**), while it displayed a significant inhibitory effect in MCF-7 at 48 and 72 h (**Figure 5B**) and in T-47D at all tested time-points (**Figure 5C**). Nevertheless, BrdU assay indicated a reduction trend in percentage of cells in S phase for all three cell lines tested, although the statistical analysis did not yield any significant differences between treated and untreated group (**Figures 5D–F**). DHEA showed inhibition of cell growth in MDA-MB-453 and MCF-7 cell lines at 72 h (**Figures 5A,B**) and in T-47D only at 24 h after treatment (**Figure 5C**). Similarly to DHT-treated cells, also for DHEA-treated cells the BrdU assay showed a decrease of cell number in S phase for all three tested cell lines although the statistical analysis did not yield any significant differences between the two groups (**Figures 5D–F**).

DHT and DHEA Up-Regulate miR-9-5p

Next, we decided to assess whether AR agonists DHT and DHEA were able to modulate miR-9-5p expression, which is endogenously low in the three BC cell lines included in this study, compared to normal breast cells (**Figure 1A**). We treated MDA-MB-453, MCF-7, and T-47D cells with DHT or DHEA, and we observed that miR-9-5p was significantly upregulated in all cell lines both by DHT (**Figure 6A**) and DHEA (**Figure 6B**). Since miR-9-5p down-regulates AR protein expression (**Figure 1D**), we conclude that a feedback loop occurs between miR-9-5p and AR, in which AR agonists can induce miR-9-5p expression which, in turn, inhibits AR protein levels in all three BC cell lines and regardless of their ER status.

MicroRNA-9 Inhibits AR Transcriptional Activity

It has been shown that miR-9-5p silences AR in BC cell lines. In order to assess whether this reflects in an effect of miR-9-5p on AR-mediated downstream signaling, we performed the AR Cignal Reporter Assay. We observed that while miR-9-5p over-expression had minimal effects on the AR signaling (as measured by the luciferase activity of the Cignal reporter plasmid) and in absence of AR agonists (DHT and DHEA), miR-9-5p over-expression was able to reverse the activation of AR signaling even in presence of AR agonists (**Figures 7A–C**). These findings suggest that miR-9-5p has a leading effect in shaping AR-mediated downstream pathway and that the effects of miR-9-5p on the AR downstream signaling mostly occur in presence of the AR agonists (**Figures 7A–C**).

MicroRNA-9 and AR Expression Show an Inverse Correlation in BC Patients

In order to evaluate if miR-9-5p was downregulated in BC patients, we performed a qRT-PCR analysis in 11 primary BC samples. Results showed that miR-9-5p was significantly downregulated in tumor tissues (T) compared to healthy adjacent ones (N) in all patients (**Figure 8A**), and an inverse correlation

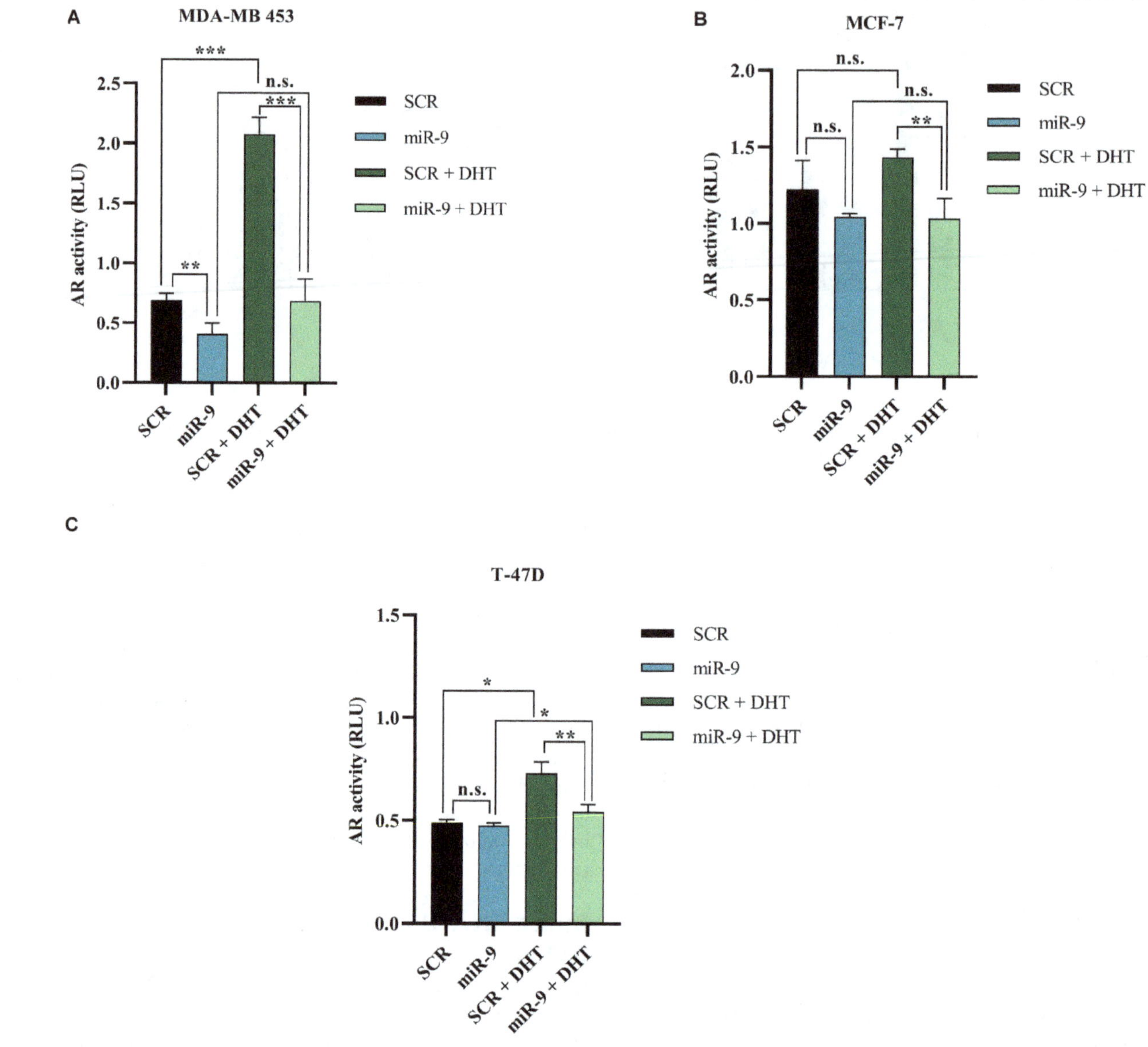

FIGURE 7 | Effects of miR-9-5p (mir-9) on AR signaling. AR transcriptional activity as measured with the AR Cignal reporter assay at 48 h in MDA-MB-453 **(A)**, MCF7 **(B)**, and T47D **(C)** cells. The modulation of AR transcription factor was determined by comparing the normalized luciferase activities of the reporter in treated vs. untreated transfectants (SCR vs. miR-9, SCR vs. SCR + DHT, miR-9 vs. miR-9+DHT, and SCR+DHT vs. miR-9+DHT), in all the BC cell lines MDA-MB-453 **(A)**, MCF-7 **(B)**, and T-47D **(C)**. Firefly: Renilla activity ratios were calculated from experimental and control transfections. Then, ratios from AR responsive reporter transfections were divided by ratios from negative controls to obtain relative luciferase units (RLU). $^{*}p < 0.05$, $^{**}p < 0.01$, $^{***}p < 0.001$, n.s., not significant. Multiple *t*-test, corrected for multiple comparison using the Holm-Sidak method in **(A–C)**.

between miR-9-5p and AR expression was observed in tumor tissues (**Figure 8B**) validating in patient samples our findings that miR-9-5p is a regulator of AR expression in BC. Expression of AR in FFPE samples was confirmed by immunohistochemistry (IHC) (**Supplementary Figures S6A,B**).

DISCUSSION

In the last few years, AR has emerged as a new potential target for the treatment of BC patients. Indeed, circulating androgens are present at physiological conditions in women, and their levels vary depending on hormonal needs and in relation to pre- or post-menopausal state (Giovannelli et al., 2018). Approximately 50–80% of BCs are positive for AR, but the prognostic and predictive value of its expression in BC is still controversial (Yang et al., 2020). MiRNAs are increasingly implicated in regulating tumorigenesis of BC, and among them miR-9-5p is attracting great attention. Its role is currently still debated since it has shown functions both as an oncomir and as a tumor suppressor gene (Gravgaard et al., 2012; Selcuklu et al., 2012; Orangi and Motovali-Bashi, 2019; Sporn et al., 2019).

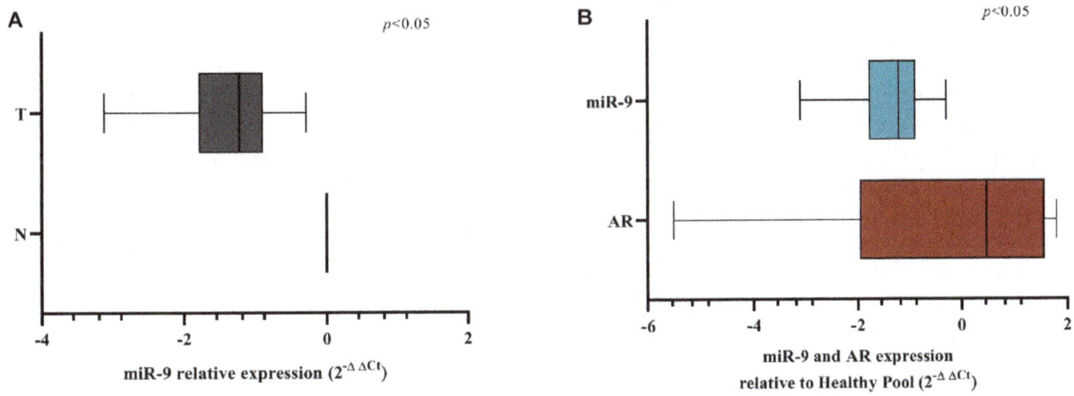

FIGURE 8 | MiR-9-5p is downregulated in BC FFPE samples. **(A)** Box-plot representation of the miR-9-5p (miR-9) qRT-PCR expression in adjacent normal (N) vs. tumoral (T) samples for all FFPE samples examined ($n = 11$). **(B)** Box-plot representation of the miR-9-5p (miR-9) and AR qRT-PCR expression in all FFPE samples examined ($n = 11$). The expression of AR and miR-9 have been normalized to GAPDH and RNU44, respectively. A non-parametric unpaired *t*-test (Kolmogorov-Smirnov test) method in **(A,B)**. Box-plots have been presented on a ln-scale.

The current evidence points toward a BC stage-dependent role of miR-9-5p: as a tumor suppressor gene in the early stage of BC, and as a promoter of the metastatic progression, essentially playing as an oncogene, at later stages (Li et al., 2020). For instance, Gravgaard et al. (2012) observed that miR-9-5p may be involved in the metastatic process, with a higher expression in distant metastases compared to the corresponding primary tumor. Low miR-9-5p expression was also found to be associated with a better prognosis, smaller tumors, earlier stage and ER+ cancers (Sporn et al., 2019). Controversial studies attributed downregulated miR-9-5p to anti-proliferative and pro-apoptotic functions in BC cells compared to healthy ones (Selcuklu et al., 2012; Orangi and Motovali-Bashi, 2019). Others described an unclear role of miR-9-5p in tumor tissues and BC cells, suggesting that its function may depend on different subtypes of BC or progression level (Krell et al., 2012; Hasanzadeh et al., 2016; Shi et al., 2017). Curiously, a group reported different expression levels of miR-9-5p in tissues compared to serum of BC patients (Tavakolian et al., 2019). Previous findings revealed that miR-9-5p expression can be influenced by steroid hormone receptors, and that it is implicated in a regulatory mechanism signaling in BC, besides being involved in affecting the biology of the tumor microenvironment (Zhuang et al., 2012; Pillai et al., 2014; Baroni et al., 2016; Barbano et al., 2017). Interestingly, Baldassari et al. (2018) demonstrated that a combined treatment with miRNAs, including miR-9-5p, enhances the activity of specific anti-BC drugs *in vitro*, even on the most aggressive HER2+ and TNBC subtype. However, the functional implications of miR-9-5p in AR signaling have not yet been deeply explored in BC. Today, among the main therapies for advanced BC in Tamoxifen-resistant BCs and TNBCs, are Bicalutamide and Enzalutamide, first and second generation AR-directed antagonists (Salvi et al., 2019). One of the first phase II trials involving Bicalutamide revealed evidence of androgen blockade and good tolerance in patients with AR+, ER− metastatic BC (Gucalp et al., 2013). Later, a phase II study enrolling patients with locally advanced or metastatic AR+ TNBC, confirmed the antitumor activity and safety of Enzalutamide (Traina et al., 2018). Other studies, including the one by Lu et al. (2019), described the combination of Bicalutamide and Aromatase inhibitor in patients with ER+/AR+ advanced BC. However, in this cohort, it was not reported a synergistic activity, suggesting that more large-sample clinical trials should be managed in this population to better understand how to overcome endocrine resistance (Lu et al., 2019). At present, there are no standard targeted therapies for the treatment of AR+ patients, given that AR is recognized as a protein whose regulation is still under discussion. Targeting the AR signaling could represent one of the challenging approaches to overcome the lack of response to current available therapies, and miRNAs belong to the most appealing candidates to be used for such therapeutic purposes. Here we show that miR-9-5p, which is downregulated in BC cell lines and in primary BC FFPE samples compared to healthy counterparts, downregulates AR, both at the mRNA and at the protein level, and that it is upregulated after androgens stimulation, regardless of the ER status. These findings suggest a possible feedback loop in which AR stimulation induces miR-9-5p in BC cells, which in turn silences AR expression and prevents AR downstream signaling even in presence of AR agonists. To our knowledge, this is the first evidence that demonstrates such an intertwined loop between androgens, miR-9-5p and AR in BC (**Supplementary Figure S7**). While the pro- or anti-proliferative effect of miR-9-5p in BC is still debated, in our cell line models miR-9-5p elicits an anti-proliferative effect (3 different cell lines and 3 different time points). Interestingly, the anti-tumoral effect of miR-9-5p is independent of the ER status, providing the rationale for the study of this miRNA as a possible therapeutics especially in subtypes of BC such as TNBC, currently with a dismal prognosis. Cell Titer-Glo assay was used to assess the number of viable cells based on the number of metabolically active cells, whereas BrdU incorporation assay was used to obtain quantitative information on cells that are actively replicating their DNA. The different results obtained with the two methods should be interpreted in light of the intrinsic differences between the two assays. We observed a significant decrease of cell proliferation in

ER+ cells MCF-7 and T-47D, after DHT exposure, while in ER- cell line MDA-MB-453 although it induced a slight increase of cell metabolic activity, it seemed to decrease the percentage of cells in S phase, overall supporting an antiproliferative effect. It is believed that the androgen/estrogen imbalance can promote tumor progression depending on the predominant hormone. In addition, aromatizable androgens such as androstenedione and testosterone may have both anti-proliferative or pro-proliferative effect depending on several variables, i.e., the activity of estrogen- or androgen- synthesizing enzymes (aromatase and 5α-reductase, respectively), the intracellular ER/AR expression ratio, and the concentration of circulating androgens (Secreto et al., 2019). About the latter, it has been suggested that they could have a role as independent molecules but also as a substrate for estrogen synthesis albeit limited to AR+/ER+ BC (Giovannelli et al., 2018). Interestingly, in the absence of ER-α more than a half of AR binding events had a pattern analogous to that of ER-α in ER+ cells, promoting ER target genes expression and cell growth, thus suggesting a role of AR as a ER-α mimic (Robinson et al., 2011). All together, these findings highlight the need to better understand the androgen/estrogen network, in order to clarify the different behaviors observed in BC subtypes and patients, especially in relation to the presence or absence of ER, as we showed in our data. Since miR-9-5p over-expression decreases BC cell proliferation, our findings rise the very provocative question whether AR antagonists might actually weaken the anti-proliferative effects of miR-9-5p, by preventing androgen-induced up-regulation of miR-9-5p in BC cells. Certainly further studies should be conducted to better understand this point and clarify how miR-9-5p levels and modulation could affect anti-AR treatments in AR+ BC. In support to a possible correlation between miR-9-5p and AR, we further reported an inverse correlation between miR-9-5p and AR expression in a set of paired FFPE tumor and adjacent non-tumor BC patients. Obviously, the small size of our patient cohort represents a limitation of this study, together with the fact that we did not interrogate the effects of miR-9-5p in AR regulation in an *in vivo* model. Future studies will cover these limitations but the fact that an inverse correlation between miR-9-5p and AR expression in primary samples was achieved already in such a small number of patients, should be interpreted as encouraging and superior to any animal model data. In summary, we identified miR-9-5p as a tumor suppressor gene in BC, regardless of ER status, capable of down-regulating AR in BC cells and to inhibit AR downstream signaling even in presence of androgen agonists. We finally report that miR-9-5p is induced by AR agonists, supporting the existence of an androgen/miR-9-5p/AR feedback circuitry that should be accounted for when exploiting AR antagonists as therapeutics for BC patients.

AUTHOR CONTRIBUTIONS

MF: conceptualization, supervision. EB and FF: data curation, writing–original draft. FF: formal analysis. EB, IV, TR, MP, and FFb: investigation. RM: patients enrollement. MT and FL: immunoistochemistry and slide evaluation. EB: methodology. EB and MF: project administration. FF, IV, FFb, SH, WC, and MF: writing–review and editing. All authors have read and agreed to the published version of the manuscript.

FUNDING

This research was partially supported by Alma Mater Studiorum – University of Bologna for the Erika Bandini's Ph.D. study and research (Bandini, 2015). MF was the recipient of a Pablove Accelerator award. MF was supported by the National Institutes of Health (NIH/NCI) grant 5P30CA071789-20. Work in MF's lab was supported by the NIH/NCI grants R01CA215753 and R01CA219024.

ACKNOWLEDGMENTS

We thank Michela Tebaldi for the bioinformatic assistance.

REFERENCES

Agarwal, V., Bell, G. W., Nam, J.-W., and Bartel, D. P. (2015). Predicting effective microRNA target sites in mammalian mRNAs. *Elife* 4:e05005. doi: 10.7554/eLife.05005

Almeida, M. I., Reis, R. M., and Calin, G. A. (2010). MYC-microRNA-9-metastasis connection in breast cancer. *Cell Res.* 20, 603–604. doi: 10.1038/cr.2010.70

Baldassari, F., Zerbinati, C., Galasso, M., Corrà, F., Minotti, L., Agnoletto, C., et al. (2018). Screen for MicroRNA and Drug Interactions in Breast Cancer Cell Lines Points to miR-126 as a Modulator of CDK4/6 and PIK3CA Inhibitors. *Front. Genet.* 9:174. doi: 10.3389/fgene.2018.00174

Bandini, E. (2015). *Involvement of microRNAs in Androgen Receptor-dependent Breast Cancers.* Dissertation thesis, Bologna: Alma mater studiorum università di bologna.

Barbano, R., Pasculli, B., Rendina, M., Fontana, A., Fusilli, C., Copetti, M., et al. (2017). Stepwise analysis of MIR9 loci identifies miR-9-5p to be involved in Oestrogen regulated pathways in breast cancer patients. *Sci. Rep.* 7:45283. doi: 10.1038/srep45283

Baroni, S., Romero-Cordoba, S., Plantamura, I., Dugo, M., D'Ippolito, E., Cataldo, A., et al. (2016). Exosome-mediated delivery of miR-9 induces cancer-associated fibroblast-like properties in human breast fibroblasts. *Cell Death Dis.* 7, e2312–e2312. doi: 10.1038/cddis.2016.224

Bastos, E. P., Brentani, H., Pereira, C. A. B., Polpo, A., Lima, L., Puga, R. D., et al. (2016). A Set of miRNAs. *PLoS One* 11:e0154325. doi: 10.1371/journal.pone.0154325

Bray, F., Ferlay, J., Soerjomataram, I., Siegel, R. L., Torre, L. A., and Jemal, A. (2018). Global cancer statistics 2018: GLOBOCAN estimates of incidence and mortality worldwide for 36 cancers in 185 countries. *CA. Cancer J. Clin.* 68, 394–424. doi: 10.3322/caac.21492

Cheng, C.-W., Yu, J.-C., Hsieh, Y.-H., Liao, W.-L., Shieh, J.-C., Yao, C.-C., et al. (2018). Increased Cellular Levels of MicroRNA-9 and MicroRNA-221 Correlate with Cancer Stemness and Predict Poor Outcome in Human Breast Cancer. *Cell. Physiol. Biochem.* 48, 2205–2218. doi: 10.1159/000492561

Dai, X., Cheng, H., Bai, Z., and Li, J. (2017). Breast Cancer Cell Line Classification and Its Relevance with Breast Tumor Subtyping. *J. Cancer* 8, 3131–3141. doi: 10.7150/jca.18457

Giovannelli, P., Di Donato, M., Galasso, G., Di Zazzo, E., Bilancio, A., and Migliaccio, A. (2018). The Androgen Receptor in Breast Cancer. *Front. Endocrinol.* 9:492. doi: 10.3389/fendo.2018.00492

Gravgaard, K. H., Lyng, M. B., Laenkholm, A.-V., Søkilde, R., Nielsen, B. S., Litman, T., et al. (2012). The miRNA-200 family and miRNA-9 exhibit differential expression in primary versus corresponding metastatic tissue in breast cancer. *Breast Cancer Res. Treat.* 134, 207–217. doi: 10.1007/s10549-012-1969-9

Gucalp, A., Tolaney, S., Isakoff, S. J., Ingle, J. N., Liu, M. C., Carey, L. A., et al. (2013). Phase II Trial of Bicalutamide in Patients with Androgen Receptor-Positive, Estrogen Receptor-Negative Metastatic Breast Cancer. *Clin. Cancer Res.* 19, 5505–5512. doi: 10.1158/1078-0432.CCR-12-3327

Gwak, J. M., Kim, H. J., Kim, E. J., Chung, Y. R., Yun, S., Seo, A. N., et al. (2014). MicroRNA-9 is associated with epithelial-mesenchymal transition, breast cancer stem cell phenotype, and tumor progression in breast cancer. *Breast Cancer Res. Treat.* 147, 39–49. doi: 10.1007/s10549-014-3069-5

Hasanzadeh, A., Mesrian Tanha, H., Ghaedi, K., and Madani, M. (2016). Aberrant expression of miR-9 in benign and malignant breast tumors. *Mol. Cell. Probes.* 30, 279–284. doi: 10.1016/j.mcp.2016.10.005

Jang, M. H., Kim, H. J., Gwak, J. M., Chung, Y. R., and Park, S. Y. (2017). Prognostic value of microRNA-9 and microRNA-155 expression in triple-negative breast cancer. *Hum. Pathol.* 68, 69–78. doi: 10.1016/j.humpath.2017.08.026

Krell, J., Frampton, A. E., Jacob, J., Pellegrino, L., Roca-Alonso, L., Zeloof, D., et al. (2012). The clinico-pathologic role of microRNAs miR-9 and miR-151-5p in breast cancer metastasis. *Mol. Diagn. Ther.* 16, 167–172. doi: 10.1007/bf03262205

Li, X., Zeng, Z., Wang, J., Wu, Y., Chen, W., Zheng, L., et al. (2020). MicroRNA-9 and breast cancer. *Biomed. Pharmacother.* 122:109687. doi: 10.1016/j.biopha.2019.109687

Lu, Q., Xia, W., Lee, K., Zhang, J., Yuan, H., Yuan, Z., et al. (2019). Bicalutamide Plus Aromatase Inhibitor in Patients with Estrogen Receptor–Positive/Androgen Receptor–Positive Advanced Breast Cancer. *Oncologist* 25:21–e15. doi: 10.1634/theoncologist.2019-0564

Orangi, E., and Motovali-Bashi, M. (2019). Evaluation of miRNA-9 and miRNA-34a as potential biomarkers for diagnosis of breast cancer in Iranian women. *Gene* 687, 272–279. doi: 10.1016/j.gene.2018.11.036

Pillai, M. M., Gillen, A. E., Yamamoto, T. M., Kline, E., Brown, J., Flory, K., et al. (2014). HITS-CLIP reveals key regulators of nuclear receptor signaling in breast cancer. *Breast Cancer Res. Treat.* 146, 85–97. doi: 10.1007/s10549-014-3004-9

Robinson, J. L. L., MacArthur, S., Ross-Innes, C. S., Tilley, W. D., Neal, D. E., Mills, I. G., et al. (2011). Androgen receptor driven transcription in molecular apocrine breast cancer is mediated by FoxA1. *EMBO J.* 30, 3019–3027. doi: 10.1038/emboj.2011.216

Salvi, S., Bonafè, M., and Bravaccini, S. (2019). Androgen receptor in breast cancer: A wolf in sheep's clothing? A lesson from prostate cancer. *Semin. Cancer Biol.* 60, 132-137.doi: 10.1016/j.semcancer.2019.04.002

Secreto, G., Girombelli, A., and Krogh, V. (2019). Androgen excess in breast cancer development: implications for prevention and treatment. *Endocr. Relat. Cancer* 26, R81–R94. doi: 10.1530/ERC-18-0429

Selcuklu, S. D., Donoghue, M. T. A., Rehmet, K., de Souza Gomes, M., Fort, A., Kovvuru, P., et al. (2012). MicroRNA-9 Inhibition of Cell Proliferation and Identification of Novel miR-9 Targets by Transcriptome Profiling in Breast Cancer Cells. *J. Biol. Chem.* 287, 29516–29528. doi: 10.1074/jbc.M111.335943

Shi, Y., Ye, P., and Long, X. (2017). Differential Expression Profiles of the Transcriptome in Breast Cancer Cell Lines Revealed by Next Generation Sequencing. *Cell. Physiol. Biochem.* 44, 804–816. doi: 10.1159/000485344

Siegel, R. L., Miller, K. D., and Jemal, A. (2020). Cancer statistics, 2020. *CA. Cancer J. Clin.* 70, 7–30. doi: 10.3322/caac.21590

Sporn, J. C., Katsuta, E., Yan, L., and Takabe, K. (2019). Expression of MicroRNA-9 is Associated With Overall Survival in Breast Cancer Patients. *J. Surg. Res.* 233, 426–435. doi: 10.1016/j.jss.2018.08.020

Takagi, K., Miki, Y., Ishida, T., Sasano, H., and Suzuki, T. (2018). The interplay of endocrine therapy, steroid pathways and therapeutic resistance: Importance of androgen in breast carcinoma. *Mol. Cell. Endocrinol.* 466, 31–37. doi: 10.1016/j.mce.2017.09.011

Tavakolian, S., Goudarzi, H., Torfi, F., and Faghihloo, E. (2019). Evaluation of microRNA-9 and -192 expression levels as biomarkers in patients suffering from breast cancer. *Biomed. Rep.* 12, 30–34. doi: 10.3892/br.2019.1257

Traina, T. A., Miller, K., Yardley, D. A., Eakle, J., Schwartzberg, L. S., O'Shaughnessy, J., et al. (2018). Enzalutamide for the Treatment of Androgen Receptor–Expressing Triple-Negative Breast Cancer. *J. Clin. Oncol.* 36, 884–890. doi: 10.1200/JCO.2016.71.3495

van Schooneveld, E., Wildiers, H., Vergote, I., Vermeulen, P. B., Dirix, L. Y., and Van Laere, S. J. (2015). Dysregulation of microRNAs in breast cancer and their potential role as prognostic and predictive biomarkers in patient management. *Breast Cancer Res.* 17:21. doi: 10.1186/s13058-015-0526-y

Vidula, N., Yau, C., Wolf, D., and Rugo, H. S. (2019). Androgen receptor gene expression in primary breast cancer. *NPJ Breast Cancer* 5:47. doi: 10.1038/s41523-019-0142-6

Yang, Y., Min, A., Lee, K.-H., Ryu, H. S., Kim, T.-Y., Woo, G., et al. (2020). Prognostic Role of Androgen Receptor Expression in Surgically Resected Early Breast Cancer Patients. *J. Breast Cancer* 23:182. doi: 10.4048/jbc.2020.23.e28

Zhao, L., Zhou, S., and Gustafsson, J. Å (2019). Nuclear receptors: recent drug discovery for cancer therapies. *Endocr. Rev.* 40, 1207–1249.doi: 10.1210/er.2018-00222

Zhuang, G., Wu, X., Jiang, Z., Kasman, I., Yao, J., Guan, Y., et al. (2012). Tumour-secreted miR-9 promotes endothelial cell migration and angiogenesis by activating the JAK-STAT pathway. *EMBO J.* 31, 3513–3523. doi: 10.1038/emboj.2012.183

13

Glucocorticoid Therapy in Inflammatory Bowel Disease: Mechanisms and Clinical Practice

*Stefano Bruscoli**, *Marta Febo*, *Carlo Riccardi* and *Graziella Migliorati*

Section of Pharmacology, Department of Medicine and Surgery, University of Perugia, Perugia, Italy

***Correspondence:**
Stefano Bruscoli
stefano.bruscoli@unipg.it

Inflammatory bowel disease (IBD) comprises ulcerative colitis (UC) and Crohn's disease (CD). IBD etiopathology is multifactorial and involves alteration of immune cells and chronic activation of the inflammatory cascade against yet unknown environmental factors that trigger the disease. IBD therapy aims at improving the quality of life and reducing the risk of disease-related complications to avoid the need for surgery. There is no specific cure for IBDs, and the focus of therapy is supportive measures and use of anti-inflammatory and immunosuppressive drugs. Glucocorticoids (GCs) are powerful anti-inflammatory and immunomodulatory agents used to treat many acute and chronic inflammatory diseases. GCs remain basic treatment for moderate-to-severe IBD, but their use is limited by several important adverse drug effects. Topical administration of a second-generation of GCs, such as budesonide and beclomethasone dipropionate (BDP), represents a valid alternative to use of older, systemic GCs. Administration of second-generation GCs shows promisingly high topical activity and less systemic toxicity, but maintenance therapy with these new GCs in IBD patients is associated with multiple adverse effects. In this review, we make a comparative analysis of the efficacy of first-generation and second-generation GCs in IBD treatment. Unraveling GC biology at the molecular level to uncouple their clinical benefits from detrimental effects is important. One approach is to consider new GC mediators, such as glucocorticoid-induced leucine zipper, which may have similar anti-inflammatory properties, but avoids the side effects of GCs. This in-depth analysis can help to improve the development and the clinical outcomes of GC therapies in IBD.

Keywords: glucocorticoids, IBD, GILZ, inflammation, drug delivery

INTRODUCTION

Inflammatory bowel disease (IBD) comprises Crohn's disease (CD) and ulcerative colitis (UC). These are chronic and progressive diseases affecting the gastrointestinal tract. They arise as a consequence of a complex multifactorial etiopathogenesis that is incompletely understood, but which includes genetic predisposition and various environmental factors (1, 2). Oral systemic corticosteroids (e.g., prednisone, prednisolone) have been used to induce remission in IBD patients for more than 60 years due to their powerful anti-inflammatory effects. Second generation glucocorticoids (GCs), such as budesonide and beclomethasone dipropionate (BDP), which are characterized by high anti-inflammatory activity, with low systemic bioavailability due to a significant first-pass effect and higher affinity for the glucocorticoid receptor (GR) compared to first generation GCs, represent an important alternative approach for IBD therapy (3). The possible advantage derives mainly from the lower adverse effects following treatment with these second-generation GCs. Nevertheless, the increase in IBD incidence and lack of long-term treatment alternatives have led to a search for new strategies and approaches.

In this review, we discuss the medical uses of synthetic GCs (e.g., second-generation GCs). We also report new perspectives in the study of GCs, focusing especially on the role of the glucocorticoid-induced leucine zipper (GILZ) protein in the clinical outcome of IBD.

GCs

GCs are endogenous molecules (cortisol, cortisone, corticosterone) that can also be synthesized in the laboratory and widely used as treatments for several diseases. GC secretion is mediated by the hypothalamic–pituitary–adrenal (HPA) axis and is regulated by the circadian rhythm and stress, but also by inflammatory stimuli. For example, upon activation by cytokines such as interleukin (IL)-1, tumor necrosis factor, (TNF) and IL-6 (which can lead to extreme tissue damage due to uncontrollable inflammation), the HPA triggers the production and secretion of GCs. The HPA acts on inflammation by regulating genomic and non-genomic pathways, thereby blocking the activation, migration, and proliferation of immune cells of the innate and adaptive immune system (**Figure 1**) (4). Their action is mediated mainly by the GR, which is present predominantly in the cell cytoplasm, bound to a multi-protein complex of heat-shock proteins, immunophilins, kinases, and phospholipases (receptosome). After GC/GR interaction and the consequent conformational changes, the GR dissociates from the receptosome and translocates to the nucleus. The genomic action of the activated GR is elicited by a DNA-binding sequence with two zinc finger motifs. This sequence targets specific glucocorticoid-responsive elements (GREs) to control expression of many genes, such as proinflammatory mediators

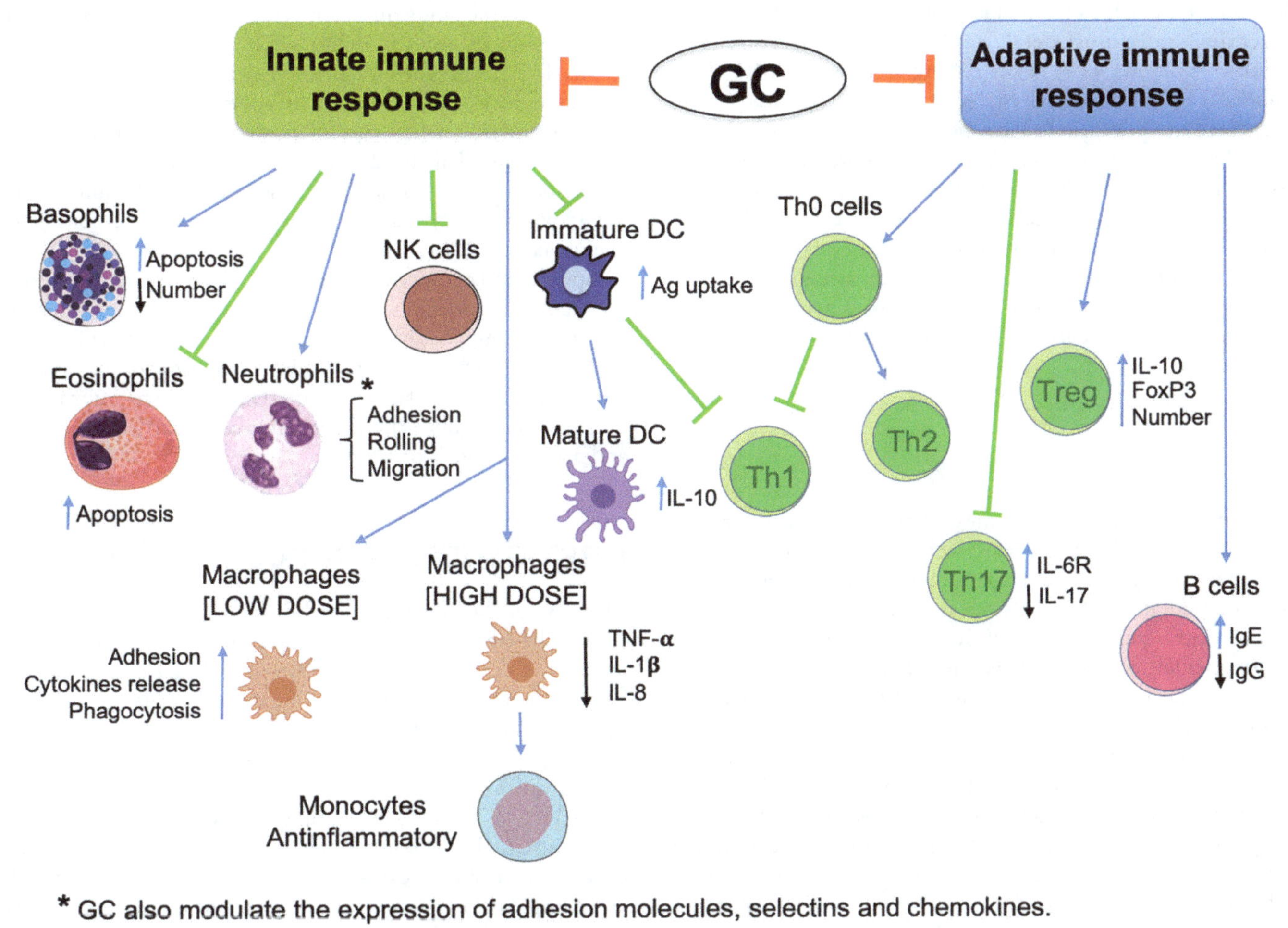

FIGURE 1 | Glucocorticoid effects in innate and adaptive immune response (schematic).

and transcription factors [e.g., activator protein-1, nuclear factor-kappa B (NF-κB)] (5, 6). Conversely, GC/GR upregulate expression of lipocortin-1, IL-1 receptor antagonists, and Iκ-B. These transcriptional effects contribute to the anti-inflammatory and immunoregulatory actions of GCs. An important target of GC/GR transcriptional activity is GILZ, which interferes with the mitogen-activated protein kinase (MAPK) pathway and NF-kB transcriptional activity and, consequently, regulates inflammatory and immune-mediated reactions (7–10).

Nonetheless, GRE presence is not the only mechanism by which the GR regulates its transcriptional activity. The cell type-specific activities of GCs are dependent upon several other factors, including the chromatin accessibility of target genes, which modulates the availability of DNA sequences (11). Non-genomic actions also contribute to the complexity of GC/GR signaling. These are characterized mainly by a short delay of action and often involve generation of intracellular second messengers and various signal-transduction cascades, such as phospholipase activation, modulation of cyclic adenosine monophosphate, protein kinase pathways, and Ca^{2+} mobilization (12, 13).

GCs have an essential role in controlling the metabolism of carbohydrates, lipids, proteins, water, Ca^{2+}, and other electrolytes, as well as maintaining the optimal function of the endocrine, musculoskeletal, cardiovascular, nervous, and immune systems (14–16). Prolonged therapy with GCs amplifies the physiological effects of endogenous GCs, which often lead to deleterious side effects such as hypertension, hyperglycemia, osteoporosis, Cushing's syndrome, and mood disorders (17, 18). Therefore, the anti-inflammatory and immunosuppressive clinical effects of GCs, even if they are considerable, are transitory. The influence of GCs on the complex control of cellular responses to stress and in the regulation of inflammatory processes is linked markedly also to the adverse effects that accompany their chronic use, and therapy must be discontinued.

IBD

IBD represents a hypernym for the chronic remission and relapse of an immunologically mediated chronic and lifelong disease characterized by gastrointestinal-tract inflammation. IBD is caused by the interaction between the genetic predisposition of the individual and activation of the immune response. Various environmental factors also have important roles in IBD onset. UC and CD are chronic and debilitating diseases that are incurable (19, 20). T-helper type 2 (Th2) cells have been demonstrated to have a pathogenic role. An imbalance in Th17/T regulatory cells has been linked to UC. CD is characterized by an imbalance in the number of Th1 cells (21). However, recent researches reported a number of novel immune cell populations that correlate with disease in IBD patients indicating that there is no clean cut that UC and CD could be separated according to Th1 and Th2 action (22). The role of B cells is less clear because they mainly control mucosal homeostasis, antibody production, and co-stimulation of T lymphocytes. Experimental evidence suggests that cytokine production by B cells may also affect immune regulation (23, 24).

UC and CD show heterogeneity in terms of clinical and pathological features, and can be distinguished by their location and the nature of inflammation they cause. UC attacks mainly the colonic mucosa, whereas CD can affect the gastrointestinal tract at any level. UC causes inflammation and ulceration of the inner lining of the colon and rectum, and usually manifests with diarrhea, loss of appetite/weight, abdominal pain, fatigue, and anemia. The level of inflammation determines disease severity and the subsequent therapeutic strategy. CD is a chronic inflammatory disorder that can affect all parts of the gastrointestinal tract, but mainly influences the terminal ileum, caecum, perianal area, and colon. Several symptoms are caused by CD, which hampers confirmation of the diagnosis. Among those symptoms are weight loss, bowel obstruction, abdominal pain, fever, and chronic or nocturnal diarrhea, although less frequently than other symptoms. These are all critical parameters for the initial diagnosis (25, 26).

IBD at any age is considered a risk factor for the onset of colon cancer due to the development of chronic inflammation that causes immune-mediated tissue destruction. The disease manifests itself in genetically susceptible individuals (i.e. mutations in IBD susceptibility loci including those of STAT3, TYK2, JAK2, CARD9 and IL10RA genes) (27), as a cause or consequence to an imbalance in commensal microbes, or if different environmental factors favor dysbiosis; poor hygiene (28), unbalanced diets (29), smoking, and stress (27). Several factors have been found to impair the functions of immune cells, including lymphocyte activation, autophagy, GC response, and chemotaxis (2, 30).

Specific and curative treatment for IBD is lacking. The focus is on supportive measures as well as the use of anti-inflammatory and immunosuppressive drugs (e.g., aminosalicylates, GCs, anti-TNF agents, such as infliximab, adalimumab, certolizumab pegol and CDP571) (31). The goals of therapy are to improve the quality of life, reduce the risk of disease-related complications, and avoid the need for surgery.

FIRST-GENERATION GCs

All GCs can be considered to be valid options when treating IBD. The most commonly used GCs are prednisone, methylprednisolone, and hydrocortisone (**Figure 2**). They can be used alone or in combination with mesalamine for the induction and maintenance of clinical remission in patients suffering from chronic IBD (32–34).

The primary purpose of GC use is to induce clinical remission. A controlled therapeutic regimen guarantees a reduction in the symptoms and side effects caused by these drugs. The most efficacious dose of prednisone is 1 mg/kg up to 40–60 mg/day, and a higher dose seems to not change therapy efficacy (35). The dose administered initially is 40–60 mg/day, but it must be reduced gradually to achieve therapy interruption

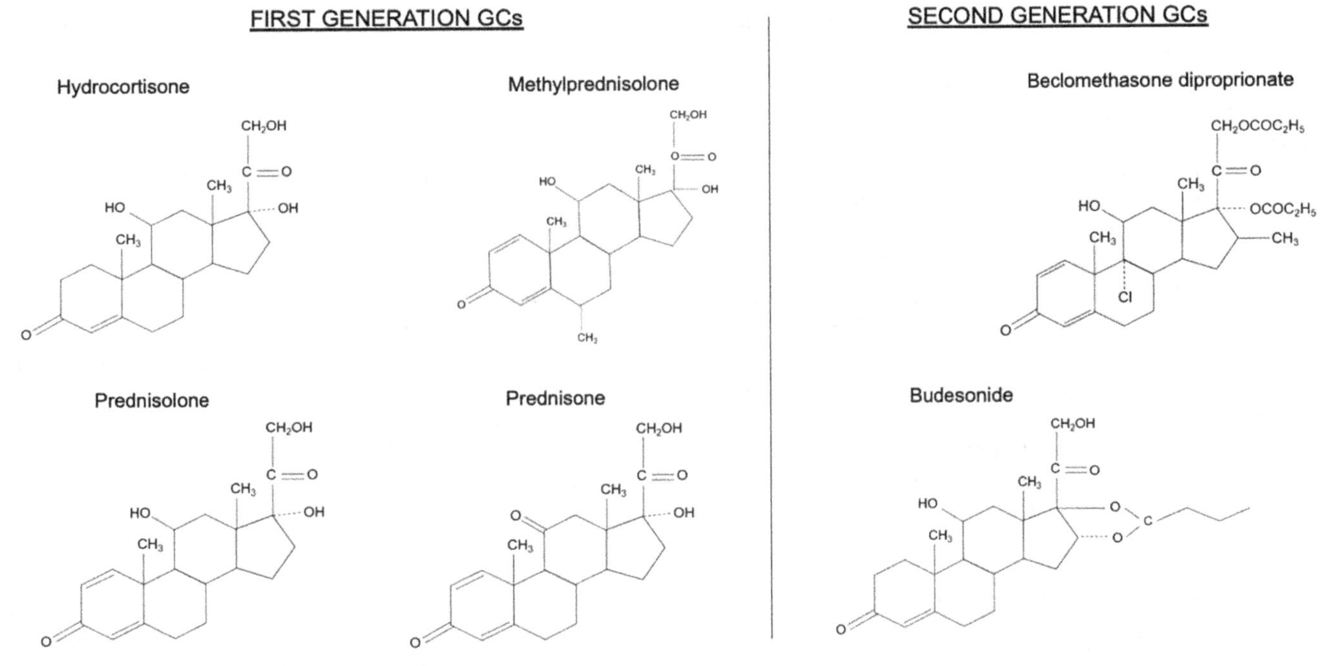

FIGURE 2 | Chemical structures of first and second generation glucocorticoids (GCs).

while maintaining control of IBD symptoms. At the same time it has been shown that alternate-day treatment helps to reduce and prevent the adverse effects on the central nervous system. Concomitant use with other drugs (e.g., azathioprine) also permits to avoid further use of GCs, while allowing maintenance therapy (36). It is important that prednisone can be considered lifesaving in severe diseases and this is especially true of chronic cases of UC after treatments from six weeks to three months. The effects are however temporary, as patients tends to miss out on the benefits after nine months of therapy (37).

It has been shown that intake of first-generation GCs, such as methylprednisolone (12–48 mg/day), if combined with other drugs, such as sulfasalazine (3 g/day), is important for symptom improvement. It was shown that these improvements occurred faster than if patients were treated with sulfasalazine alone (3).

Another factor in the choice of treatment (and consequently the dose) is the administration route because this is dependent upon the disease location. In people suffering from UC, drug administration can be topical if proctitis is present, or topical and systemic in the case of left-side colitis. In CD, disease severity is the main criterion for GC use because patients might not respond well to treatment and might need surgery if disease severity is high (38). To note, non-response to GCs is comparable between CD and UC.

Despite the efficacy of first-generation GCs, several serious side effects can be associated with their use, including osteoporosis, hyperglycemia, hypertension, mood disorders, gastric ulcer, and increased susceptibility to infections (3, 17). This characteristic limits their long-term use. Maintenance treatment with systemic GCs is not recommended.

SECOND-GENERATION GCs

Due to the limitations of prolonged therapy with first-generation GCs, compounds such as budesonide and BDP have been developed that maintain topical anti-inflammatory efficacy but minimize their bioavailability and, consequently, their systemic adverse effects (**Figure 2**) (3).

Budesonide undergoes hepatic inactivation before reaching the systemic circulation to diminish corticosteroid-related side effects. Several clinical trials have been conducted to establish the efficacy of oral budesonide. A randomized, double-blind controlled trial conducted in patients with mild, active CD demonstrated that budesonide, if administered at 9 mg/day for 2 months, was as efficacious as prednisone (which was used at 40 mg/day for the first 2 weeks) followed by 30 mg/day in the third month (39). Budesonide carried a lower prevalence of systemic adverse effects (33% of cases) than that of conventional GCs (55%). Budesonide use has not been reported to directly cause changes in the bone mineral density or adrenal insufficiency, however individual sensitivity may vary and therefore cause their onset. Consequently there is no direct correlation to the appearance of osteoporosis symptoms or decreased/inadequate cortisol production (40, 41). Multiple meta-analyses have demonstrated the efficacy of budesonide in inducing remission, and that a once-daily dose is just as efficacious as 3 mg taken thrice daily. In the context of more severe disease, budesonide is not as efficacious as prednisolone in achieving remission (42).

The second-generation GC BDP is a derivative of cortisone. It has topical effects and minimal systemic activity. It is administered as a prodrug and is partially metabolized in the lower gastrointestinal tract. If used at low doses, BDP has been shown to be free of many of the deleterious side effects associated with GCs absorbed systemically. The induction of remission in CD using BDP has not been investigated in double-blind randomized trials. The efficacy of BDP in patients with UC has been well established: eight double-blind randomized trials have been published (43). Oral BDP for UC has been approved in several countries. In one randomized controlled trial, oral BDP was administered as a daily dose of 5 mg for 4 weeks, then alternated weekly for 4 weeks. A similar efficacy to that observed with prednisolone was evident, and there was no difference in the prevalence of adverse events. However, as a second-generation GC with low systemic absorption, it is associated with fewer adverse events than that of first-generation GCs (44, 45).

NEW THERAPEUTIC GC-BASED APPROACHES IN CHRONIC IBD

Several studies have aimed to develop new delivery methods for existing drugs to improve the efficacy of therapeutic approaches by limiting the side effects associated with the use of specific drugs or resistance to therapy. Complexity of molecular pathways and networks regulating living organisms has become a central issue of molecular biology. Thus, "molecular stratification" is a new approach based on the needs of patients, their susceptibility to disease, and their gene variability. Studies are carried out on specific elements belonging to different molecular pathways. This can take the form of choosing biologically active molecules bound to cells such as erythrocytes, the targeting of selective GR agonists or the targeting of specific elements able to regulate the inflammatory reaction upon their activation. *GILZ* is a target linked to GC action, so it can be considered a new approach for the regulation of inflammatory diseases such as IBD or even as a molecular marker of inflammation (10, 24).

Drug-Delivery Strategies in IBD Therapy

Drug-delivery systems aim to improve the pharmacological activities of drugs. They play a key part in regulating solubility, drug aggregation, low bioavailability, poor biodistribution, and reducing side effects (46).

Red blood cells (RBCs) are the largest population of blood cells. Their main function is to carry oxygen to all body tissues. To use erythrocytes as carriers of biologically active substances, pores must be formed reversibly in their membrane, through which the drug can penetrate. To achieve this aim, the cell is stimulated with external influences, such as ultrasound. Drug molecules can also enter by endocytosis in the presence of certain chemical compounds, such as hydrocortisone. Active substances of different molecular weights can be delivered by incorporation in the cell or by binding to its surface (47). The average life of RBCs guarantees a therapeutic effect for 120 days, so biologically inactive compounds such as dexamethasone-21-phosphate are used (48). In recent years, drug selection and the relationship between specific drugs and RBCs have been adapted to reduce some of the limitations that their use could present. Prodrugs, such as corticosteroid prodrugs and nucleotide prodrugs, can improve the action of RBCs as carriers. If the molecule to be delivered is inactivated, erythrocytes can transform and release it in its active form (49).

A type of colonic-delivery technology called Multi-Matrix System (MMX®) has been developed to provide controlled release of budesonide throughout the entire colon. The most common adverse effects in studies using MMX were headache, nausea, and urinary-tract infection (50).

Therapy with systemically active GCs, including budesonide MMX, is associated with suppression of endogenous cortisol levels and HPA function. Oral budesonide MMX at 9 mg/day has been shown to be significantly more efficacious than placebo and can induce remission in mild-to-moderate UC, being as efficacious as 5-aminosalicylic acid (5-ASA, which is first-line therapy for mild-to-moderate active UC) (51). GC effects appear in a shorter time, while 5-ASA takes approximately 2 weeks and therefore it cannot be used in moderate disease as a sole therapeutic regimen (52).

Another strategy for drug delivery involves nanoparticles (NPs) which are organic, inorganic or polymeric particles that ranges between 1 to 100 nanometres in size. Among synthetic polymers used in pharmaceutical formulations there are poly-L-lactic acid, polyvinyl alcohol, poly(lactic-co-glycolic acid), and polyethylene glycol (53). NP efficacy is linked mainly to rapid and preferential intestinal uptake and decreased excretion of the drug following diarrhea (one of the main symptoms of IBD). Cellular internalization of NPs is characterized by paracellular transport or endocytosis into epithelial cells. It has been shown that NPs of diameter 200 nm prepared with cetyltrimethylammonium bromide and relatively neutral charge adhered to healthy colonic tissue in controls as well as inflamed colonic tissue in a colitis model using 2,4,6-trinitrobenzene sulfonic acid (TNBS). Simultaneously, polylactide–coglycolide FK506-NPs were shown to enhance drug penetration into inflamed tissue significantly in a TNBS-induced model and oxazolone-induced colitis model. Other parameters capable of influencing uptake (in addition to diameter) must be studied in detail. *In vivo* and *ex vivo* studies have shown that the surface charge of NPs can affect targeting in the colon. Cationic systems adhere to the mucosal surface due to the interaction between the positively charged nanocarrier and the negatively charged intestinal mucosa. Anionic systems adhere preferentially to targeted sites *via* electrostatic interaction with the higher concentration of positively charged proteins (53). Use of hydrophilic and uncharged NPs is also under development. The creation of NPs bound to the surface with poly(ethylene glycol) (PEG) seem to increase NP translocation through the mucus and to ensure a substantially increased half-life. Another type of nanoformulation used for GC delivery is polymeric micelles in which PEG is present to allow an extended circulation time and slower release of the compound (54). Zeng et al. showed that a resin microcapsule composed of 717 anion exchange resin and Eudragit S100 could target dexamethasone to the colon, improve the efficacy of UC therapy, and reduce the overall toxic side effects (55).

Selective Glucocorticoid Receptor Agonists (SEGRAs)

Identification and development of SEGRAs is of particular interest because their therapeutic potential is uncertain (56, 57). SEGRAs are also defined as "dissociated GCs" because they could allow anti-inflammatory activities and the avoidance of metabolic effects. SEGRAs allow the mediation of only repressive effects on various controlled target genes from the GR, and not those of gene activation, because they work by operating through one of two main pathways: transactivation or transrepression (58). The concept that the activating action is responsible for the metabolic (and therefore collateral) effects, whereas immunosuppressive mechanisms are dependent upon the repressive effects, is controversial. Some SEGRA compounds have been shown to have anti-inflammatory properties with reduced collateral effects, such as Compound A [2-((4-acetophenyl)-2-chloro-N-methyl) ethylammonium-chloride))], or ZK216348 N-(4-methyl-1-oxo-1H-2,3-benzoxazine-6-yl)-4-(2,3-dihydrobenzofuran-7-yl)-2-hydroxy-2-(trifluoromethyl)-4-methylpentanamide (59). Therefore, their efficacy *in vivo* for treatment of inflammatory diseases, such as colitis, asthma, and rheumatoid arthritis, is being evaluated (60, 61).

GILZ-Based Therapy

One possible therapeutic solution involves GILZ being induced rapidly by CGs. GILZ protein has been recognized as a downstream inducer of anti-inflammatory effects (**Figure 3**). GILZ is a protein of 135 amino acids. It is highly conserved in humans and mice, and its binding activity can interfere with MAPK/extracellular receptor kinase and protein kinase B pathways (62, 63). Its action is mediated by the binding of GRs to the GREs present in the proximal region of the GILZ transcriptional start site. At the molecular level, GILZ can interact with proteins such as NF-κB, thereby obstructing the transcription of proinflammatory mediators (64). GILZ is expressed in virtually all cells, including macrophages, granulocytes, dendritic cells and T lymphocytes, as well as other non-lymphoid tissues (10). The function of GILZ has been identified only partially and its role (like that of GCs) is being studied in several mouse models of inflammatory and autoimmune diseases. Attention has focused mostly on various transduction pathways that act on suppression of the immune system (65). Several studies have focused on the role of GILZ and analyzed its protective aspect in dinitrobenzene sulfonic acid (DNBS)-induced colitis. It has been shown that transgenic mice overexpressing GILZ had lower levels of colonic inflammation. This result was reliant on a decrease in the number of Th1 cells in the lamina-propria lymphocytes and increase in the number of Th2 cells induced by GILZ overexpression (24, 66). Also, treatment with a recombinant form of TAT-GILZ has been

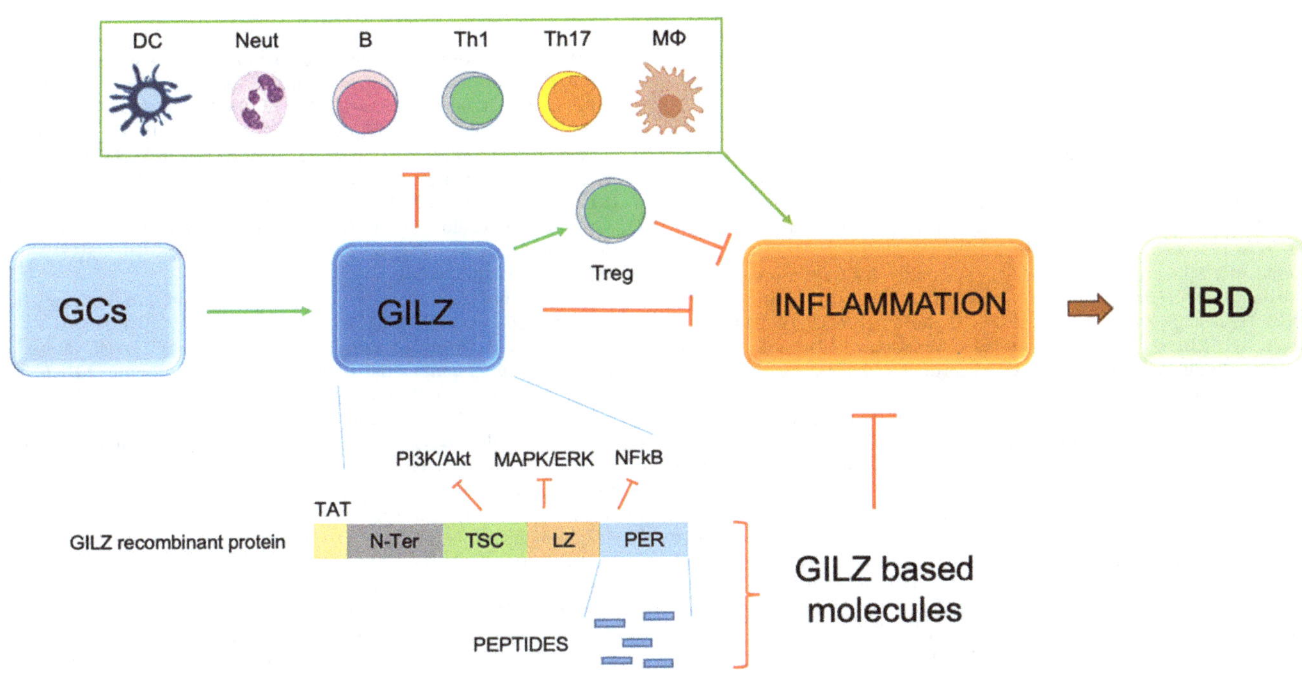

FIGURE 3 | Schematic representation of GILZ efficacy in inflammatory processes and IBD and anti-inflammatory activity of GILZ based molecules, such as peptides deriving from the Proline anf Glutamic acid rich (PER) region of the GILZ protein and TAT-GILZ full length protein. Green arrows indicate positive regulation; red lines indicate negative regulation. DC, dendritic cells; Neut, neutrophils; B, B cells; TH1, T helper Type-1 cells; Th17, T helper Type-17 cells; MΦ, monocytes/ macrophages; T regulatory cells.

studied in animals with IL-10 knockout. The presence of GILZ has been shown to lower the prevalence of spontaneous UC, thereby demonstrating a protective action of GILZ against severe inflammation (66). Moreover, we and other groups demonstrated the efficacy of GILZ based molecules (full recombinant GILZ protein or peptides) in different experimental models of inflammatory diseases. The main inflammatory target of GILZ is NF-kB. GILZ binds and inhibits p65/NF-kB subunit, thus exerting its anti-inflammatory activity (7, 64). The GILZ interaction with NF-kB is mediated by proline-rich (PXXP) domains present in proline and acid glutamic rich (PER) region of GILZ COOH-terminal portion. Consequently, the possibility to synthesize and use GILZ peptides, that include PXXP domains of the GILZ protein, could be an alternative to the administration of the entire recombinant GILZ protein with possible pharmacokinetic and pharmacodynamic advantages. Notably, no apparent toxic effects have been observed in mice upon *in vivo* administration (intraperitoneally or subcutaneously) of TAT-GILZ protein or GILZ-peptides in mice (66, 67, and Bruscoli, unpublished data). Thus, GILZ represents a new approach for IBD treatment, and to have an immunosuppressant effect comparable with that of GCs (24, 66, 68). GILZ has also has been associated with several inflammatory diseases other than IBD, such as rheumatoid arthritis and fibromyalgia (69, 70). An advantage of GILZ therapy could be that side effects have not been associated with administration of GILZ recombinant protein in cellular systems or in established *in vivo* models of IBD.

Therefore, novel drugs in inflammatory/autoimmune diseases (including IBD) can be developed based on the structure and molecular interactions of GILZ. Moreover, GILZ could be of interest for several inflammation-based degenerative diseases and possibly cancer.

AUTHOR CONTRIBUTIONS

SB and MF wrote the article. CR substantially contributed to the conception and design of the article and interpreting the relevant literature. GM revised it critically for important intellectual content. All authors contributed to the article and approved the submitted version.

FUNDING

This work was supported by the Crohn's & Colitis Foundation, award number 504854, USA and by the Italian Ministry of Education and Research, grant PRIN 2017-2017XZMBYX.

REFERENCES

Fiocchi C. Inflammatory Bowel Disease: Etiology and Pathogenesis. *Gastroenterology* (1998) 115:182–205. doi: 10.1016/S0016-5085(98)70381-6

Ananthakrishnan AN. Environmental Risk Factors for Inflammatory Bowel Diseases: A Review. *Dig Dis Sci* (2015) 60:290–8. doi: 10.1007/s10620-014-3350-9

Dubois-Camacho K, Ottum PA, Franco-Munoz D, de la Fuente M, Torres-Riquelme A, Diaz-Jimenez D, et al. Glucocorticosteroid Therapy in Inflammatory Bowel Diseases: From Clinical Practice to Molecular Biology. *World J Gastroenterol* (2017) 23:6628–38. doi: 10.3748/wjg.v23.i36.6628

Dunn AJ. Cytokine Activation of the HPA Axis. *Ann NY Acad Sci* (2000) 917:608–17. doi: 10.1111/j.1749-6632.2000.tb05426.x

Diamond MI, Miner JN, Yoshinaga SK, Yamamoto KRTranscription Factor Interactions: Selectors of Positive or Negative Regulation From a Single DNA Element. *Science* (1990) 249:1266–72. doi: 10.1126/science.2119054

Riccardi C, Bruscoli S, Migliorati. Molecular Mechanisms of Immunomodulatory Activity of Glucocorticoids. *Pharmacol Res* (2002) 45:361–8. doi: 10.1006/phrs.2002.0969

Ayroldi E, Migliorati G, Bruscoli S, Marchetti C, Zollo O, Cannarile L, et al Modulation of T-Cell Activation by the Glucocorticoid-Induced Leucine Zipper Factor *Via* Inhibition of Nuclear Factor Kappab. *Blood* (2001) 98:743–53. doi: 10.1182/blood.V98.3.743

Ayroldi E, Zollo O, Macchiarulo A, Di Marco B, Marchetti C, Riccardi C. Glucocorticoid-Induced Leucine Zipper Inhibits the Raf-Extracellular Signal- Regulated Kinase Pathway by Binding to Raf-1. *Mol Cell Biol* (2002) 22:7929- 41. doi: 10.1128/MCB.22.22.7929-7941.2002

Vago JP, Tavares LP, Garcia CC, Lima KM, Perucci LO, Vieira EL, et al. The Role and Effects of Glucocorticoid-Induced Leucine Zipper in the Context of Inflammation Resolution. *J Immunol* (2015) 194:4940–50. doi: 10.4049/jimmunol.1401722

Bereshchenko O, Migliorati G, Bruscoli S, Riccardi C. Glucocorticoid-Induced Leucine Zipper: A Novel Anti-Inflammatory Molecule. *Front Pharmacol* (2019) 10:308 doi: 10.3389/fphar.2019.00308

Quatrini L, Ugolini S. New Insights Into the Cell- and Tissue-Specificity of Glucocorticoid Actions. *Cell Mol Immunol* (2021) 18:269–78. doi: 10.1038/s41423-020-00526-2

Croxtall JD, Choudhury Q, Flower RJ. Glucocorticoids Act Within Minutes to Inhibit Recruitment of Signalling Factors to Activated EGF Receptors Through a Receptor-Dependent, Transcription-Independent Mechanism. *Br J Pharmacol* (2000) 130:289–98. doi: 10.1038/sj.bjp.0703272

Marchetti MC, Di Marco B, Cifone G, Migliorati G, Riccardi C. Dexamethasone-Induced Apoptosis of Thymocytes: Role of Glucocorticoid Receptor-Associated Src Kinase and Caspase-8 Activation. *Blood* (2003) 101:585–93 doi: 10.1182/blood-2002-06-1779

Ramamoorthy S, Cidlowski JA. Corticosteroids: Mechanisms of Action in Health and Disease. *Rheum Dis Clin North Am* (2016) 42:15–31. doi: 10.1016/ j.rdc.2015.08.002

Desmet SJ, De Bosscher K. Glucocorticoid Receptors: Finding the Middle Ground. *J Clin Invest* (2017) 127:1136–45. doi: 10.1172/JCI88886

Bereshchenko O, Bruscoli S, Riccardi C. Glucocorticoids, Sex Hormones, and Immunity. *Front Immunol* (2018) 9:1332. doi: 10.3389/fimmu.2018.01332

Cain DW, Cidlowski JA. Immune Regulation by Glucocorticoids. *Nat Rev Immunol* (2017) 17:233–47. doi: 10.1038/nri.2017.1

Ronchetti S, Migliorati G, Bruscoli S, Riccardi C. Defining the Role of Glucocorticoids in Inflammation. *Clin Sci (Lond)* (2018) 132:1529–43. doi: 10.1042/CS20171505

Mulder DJ, Noble AJ, Justinich CJ, Duffin JM. A Tale of Two Diseases: The History of Inflammatory Bowel Disease. *J Crohns Colitis* (2014) 8:341–8. doi: 10.1016/j.crohns.2013.09.009

Zhang YZ, Li YY. Inflammatory Bowel Disease: Pathogenesis. *World J Gastroenterol* (2014) 20:91–9. doi: 10.3748/wjg.v20.i1.91

Harbour SN, Maynard CL, Zindl CL, Schoeb TR, Weaver CT. Th17 Cells Give Rise to Th1 Cells That Are Required for the Pathogenesis of Colitis. *Proc Natl Acad Sci USA* (2015) 112:7061–6. doi: 10.1073/pnas.1415675112

Imam T, Park S, Kaplan MH, Olson MR. Effector T Helper Cell Subsets in Inflammatory Bowel Diseases. *Front Immunol* (2018) 9:1212. doi: 10.3389/fimmu.2018.01212

Shimomura Y, Mizoguchi E, Sugimoto K, Kibe R, Benno Y, Mizoguchi A, et al. Regulatory Role of B-1 B Cells in Chronic Colitis. *Int Immunol* (2008) 20:729–37. doi: 10.1093/intimm/dxn031

Bruscoli S, Sorcini D, Flamini S, Gagliardi A, Adamo F, Ronchetti S, et al. Glucocorticoid-Induced Leucine Zipper Inhibits Interferon-Gamma Production in B Cells and Suppresses Colitis in Mice. *Front Immunol* (2018) 9:1720. doi: 10.3389/fimmu.2018.01720

Wilkins T, Jarvis K, Patel J. Diagnosis and Management of Crohn's Disease. *Am Fam Physician* (2011) 84:1365–75.

Yeshi K, Ruscher R, Hunter L, Daly NL, Loukas A, Wangchuk P. Revisiting Inflammatory Bowel Disease: Pathology, Treatments, Challenges and Emerging Therapeutics Including Drug Leads From Natural Products. *J Clin Med* (2020) 9:2–10. doi: 10.3390/jcm9051273

Khor B, Gardet A, Xavier RJ. Genetics and Pathogenesis of Inflammatory Bowel Disease. *Nature* (2011) 474:307–17. doi: 10.1038/nature10209

Bach JF. The Hygiene Hypothesis in Autoimmunity: The Role of Pathogens and Commensals. *Nat Rev Immunol* (2018) 18:105–20. doi: 10.1038/nri.2017.111

David LA, Maurice CF, Carmody RN, Gootenberg DB, Button JE, Wolfe BE, et al. Diet Rapidly and Reproducibly Alters the Human Gut Microbiome. *Nature* (2014) 505:559–63. doi: 10.1038/nature12820

Jostins L, Ripke S, Weersma RK, Duerr RH, Mcgovern DP, Hui KY, et al. Host-Microbe Interactions Have Shaped the Genetic Architecture of Inflammatory Bowel Disease. *Nature* (2012) 491:119–24. doi: 10.1038/nature11582

Steeland S, Libert C, Vandenbroucke RE. A New Venue of TNF Targeting. *Int J Mol Sci* (2018) 19(5):1442. doi: 10.3390/ijms19051442

Lennard-Jones JE, Longmore AJ, Newell AC, Wilson CW, Jones FA. eq An Assessment of Prednisone, Salazopyrin, and Topical Hydrocortisone Hemisuccinate Used as Out-Patient Treatment for Ulcerative Colitis. *Gut* (1960) 1:217–22. doi: 10.1136/gut.1.3.217

Truelove SC, Watkinson G, Draper G. Comparison of Corticosteroid and Sulphasalazine Therapy in Ulcerative Colitis. *Br Med J* (1962) 2:1708–11. doi: 10.1136/bmj.2.5321.1708

Ham M, Moss AC. Mesalamine in the Treatment and Maintenance of Remission of Ulcerative Colitis. *Expert Rev Clin Pharmacol* (2012) 5:113–23. doi: 10.1586/ecp.12.2

Bello C, Goldstein F, Thornton JJ. Alternate-Day Prednisone Treatment and Treatment Maintenance in Crohn's Disease. *Am J Gastroenterol* (1991) 86:460–6.

Ewe K, Press AG, Singe CC, Stufler M, Ueberschaer B, Hommel G, et al. Azathioprine Combined With Prednisolone or Monotherapy With Prednisolone in Active Crohn's Disease. *Gastroenterology* (1993) 105:367–72. doi: 10.1016/0016-5085(93)90709-L

Truelove SC, Witts LJ. Cortisone in Ulcerative Colitis; Final Report on a Therapeutic Trial. *Br Med J* (1955) 4947:1041–8. doi: 10.1136/bmj.2.4947.1041

De Cassan C, Fiorino G, Danese S. Second-Generation Corticosteroids for the Treatment of Crohn's Disease and Ulcerative Colitis: More Effective and Less Side Effects? *Dig Dis* (2012) 30:368–75. doi: 10.1159/000338128

Bar-Meir S, Chowers Y, Lavy A, Abramovitch D, Sternberg A, Leichtmann G, et al. Budesonide Versus Prednisone in the Treatment of Active Crohn's Disease. *Israeli Budesonide Study Group Gastroenterol* (1998) 115:835–40. doi: 10.1016/S0016-5085(98)70254-9

Lofberg R, Danielsson A, Suhr O, Nilsson A, Schioler R, Nyberg A, et al. Oral Budesonide Versus Prednisolone in Patients With Active Extensive and Left- Sided Ulcerative Colitis. *Gastroenterology* (1996) 110:1713–8. doi: 10.1053/ gast.1996.v110.pm8964395

Schoon EJ, Bollani S, Mills PR, Israeli E, Felsenberg D, Ljunghall S, et al. Bone Mineral Density in Relation to Efficacy and Side Effects of Budesonide and Prednisolone in Crohn's Disease. *Clin Gastroenterol Hepatol* (2005) 3:113–21. doi: 10.1016/S1542-3565(04)00662-7

Rezaie A, Kuenzig ME, Benchimol EI, Griffiths AM, Otley AR, Steinhart AH, et al. Budesonide for Induction of Remission in Crohn's Disease. *Cochrane Database Syst Rev* (2015) 6:CD000296. doi: 10.1002/14651858.CD000296.pub4

Prantera C, Marconi S. Glucocorticosteroids in the Treatment of Inflammatory Bowel Disease and Approaches to Minimizing Systemic Activity. *Therap Adv Gastroenterol* (2013) 6:137–56. doi: 10.1177/1756283X12473675

Manguso F, Bennato R, Lombardi G, Riccio E, Costantino G, Fries W. Efficacy and Safety of Oral Beclomethasone Dipropionate in Ulcerative Colitis: A Systematic Review and Meta-Analysis. *PLoS One* (2016) 11:e0166455. doi: 10.1371/journal.pone.0166455

Lamb CA, Kennedy NA, Raine T, Hendy PA, Smith PJ, Limdi JK, et al. British Society of Gastroenterology Consensus Guidelines on the Management of Inflammatory Bowel Disease in Adults. *Gut* (2019) 68:s1–s106. doi: 10.1136/gutjnl-2019-318484

Li C, Wang J, Wang Y, Gao H, Wei G, Huang Y, et al. Recent Progress in Drug Delivery. *Acta Pharm Sin B* (2019) 9:1145–62. doi: 10.1016/j.apsb.2019.08.003

Koleva L, Bovt E, Ataullakhanov F, Sinauridze E. Erythrocytes as Carriers: From Drug Delivery to Biosensors. *Pharmaceutics* (2020) 12:1–3. doi: 10.3390/pharmaceutics12030276

Leuzzi V, Micheli R, D'agnano D, Molinaro A, Venturi T, Plebani A, et al. Positive Effect of Erythrocyte-Delivered Dexamethasone in Ataxia-Telangiectasia. *Neurol Neuroimmunol Neuroinflamm* (2015) 2:e98. doi: 10.1212/NXI.0000000000000098

Xu P, Wang R, Wang X, Ouyang J. Recent Advancements in Erythrocytes, Platelets, and Albumin as Delivery Systems. *Onco Targets Ther* (2016) 9:2873– 84. doi: 10.2147/OTT.S104691

Sandborn WJ, Travis S, Moro L, Jones R, Gautille T, Bagin R, et al. Once-Daily Budesonide MMX® Extended-Release Tablets Induce Remission in Patients With Mild to Moderate Ulcerative Colitis: Results From the CORE I Study. *Gastroenterology* (2012) 143:1218–26.e1-e2. doi: 10.1053/j.gastro.2012.08.003

Danese S, Siegel CA, Peyrin-Biroulet L. Review Article: Integrating budesonide-MMX Into Treatment Algorithms for Mild- to-Moderate Ulcerative Colitis. *Aliment Pharmacol Ther* (2014) 39:1095–103 doi: 10.1111/apt.12712

Katz S, Lichtenstein GR, Safdi MA. 5-Asa Dose-Response: Maximizing Efficacy and Adherence. *Gastroenterol Hepatol (NY)* (2010) 6(2 Suppl 3):1–16.

Hua S, Marks E, Schneider JJ, Keely S. Advances in Oral Nano-Delivery Systems for Colon Targeted Drug Delivery in Inflammatory Bowel Disease: Selective Targeting to Diseased Versus Healthy Tissue. *Nanomedicine* (2015) 11:1117–32. doi: 10.1016/j.nano.2015.02.018

Luhder F, Reichardt HM. Novel Drug Delivery Systems Tailored for Improved Administration of Glucocorticoids. *Int J Mol Sci* (2017) 18:3–5. doi: 10.3390/ijms18091836

Zeng A, Dong K, Wang M, Sun J, Dong Y, Wang K, et al. Investigation of the Colon-Targeting, Improvement on the Side-Effects and Therapy on the Experimental Colitis in Mouse of a Resin Microcapsule Loading Dexamethasone Sodium Phosphate. *Drug Deliv* (2016) 23:1992–2002. doi: 10.3109/10717544.2015.1046569

Heck S, Kullmann M, Gast A, Ponta H, Rahmsdorf HJ, Herrlich P, et al. A Distinct Modulating Domain in Glucocorticoid Receptor Monomers in the Repression of Activity of the Transcription Factor AP-1. *EMBO J* (1994) 13:4087–95. doi: 10.1002/j.1460-2075.1994.tb06726.x

Vandewalle J, Luypaert A, De Bosscher K, Libert C. Therapeutic Mechanisms of Glucocorticoids. *Trends Endocrinol Metab* (2018) 29:42–54. doi: 10.1016/j.tem.2017.10.010

Sundahl N, Bridelance J, Libert C, De Bosscher K, Beck IM. Selective Glucocorticoid Receptor Modulation: New Directions With Non-Steroidal Scaffolds. *Pharmacol Ther* (2015) 152:28–41. doi: 10.1016/j.pharmthera.2015.05.001

Reuter KC, Grunwitz CR, Kaminski BM, Steinhilber D, Radeke HH, Stein J. Selective Glucocorticoid Receptor Agonists for the Treatment of Inflammatory Bowel Disease: Studies in Mice With Acute Trinitrobenzene Sulfonic Acid Colitis. *J Pharmacol Exp Ther* (2012) 341(1):68–80. doi: 10.1124/jpet.111.183947

Coghlan MJ, Jacobson PB, Lane B, Nakane M, Lin CW, Elmore SW, et al. A Novel Antiinflammatory Maintains Glucocorticoid Efficacy With Reduced Side Effects. *Mol Endocrinol* (2003) 17:860–9. doi: 10.1210/me.2002-0355

Zhang Z, Zhang ZY, Schluesener HJ. Compound A, a Plant Origin Ligand of Glucocorticoid Receptors, Increases Regulatory T Cells and M2 Macrophages to Attenuate Experimental Autoimmune Neuritis With Reduced Side Effects. *J Immunol* (2009) 183:3081–91. doi: 10.4049/jimmunol.0901088

Ayroldi E, Zollo O, Bastianelli A, Marchetti C, Agostini M, Di Virgilio R, et al. GILZ Mediates the Antiproliferative Activity of Glucocorticoids by Negative Regulation of Ras Signaling. *J Clin Invest* (2007) 117:1605–15. doi: 10.1172/JCI30724

Venanzi A, Di Sante M, Bruscoli S, Biagioli M, Sorcini D, Cimino M, et al. Recombinant Long-Glucocorticoid-Induced Leucine Zipper (L-GILZ) Protein Restores the Control of Proliferation in Gilz KO Spermatogonia. *Eur J Pharm Sci* (2014) 63:22–8. doi: 10.1016/j.ejps.2014.06.013

Di Marco B, Massetti M, Bruscoli S, Macchiarulo A, Di Virgilio R, Velardi E, et al. Glucocorticoid-Induced Leucine Zipper (GILZ)/NF-Kappab Interaction: Role of GILZ Homo-Dimerization and C-terminal Domain. *Nucleic Acids Res* (2007) 35:517–28. doi: 10.1093/nar/gkl1080

Ronchetti S, Migliorati G, Riccardi C, GILZ A. GILZ as a Mediator of the Anti-Inflammatory Effects of Glucocorticoids. *Front Endocrinol (Lausanne)* (2015) 6:170. doi: 10.3389/fendo.2015.00170

Cannarile L, Cuzzocrea S, Santucci L, Agostini M, Mazzon E, Esposito E, et al. Glucocorticoid-Induced Leucine Zipper is Protective in Th1-mediated Models of Colitis. *Gastroenterology* (2009) 136:530–41. doi: 10.1053/j.gastro.2008.09.024

Srinivasan M, Janardhanam S. Novel p65 Binding Glucocorticoid-Induced Leucine Zipper Peptide Suppresses Experimental Autoimmune Encephalomyelitis. *J Biol Chem* (2011) 286:44799–810. doi: 10.1074/ jbc.M111.279257

Bereshchenko O, Coppo M, Bruscoli S, Biagioli M, Cimino M, Frammartino T, et al. GILZ Promotes Production of Peripherally Induced Treg Cells and Mediates the Crosstalk Between Glucocorticoids and TGF-beta Signaling. *Cell Rep* (2014) 7:464–75. doi: 10.1016/j.celrep.2014.03.004

Macedo JA, Hesse J, Turner JD, Meyer J, Hellhammer DH, Muller CP. Glucocorticoid Sensitivity in Fibromyalgia Patients: Decreased Expression of Corticosteroid Receptors and Glucocorticoid-Induced Leucine Zipper. *Psychoneuroendocrinology* (2008) 33:799–809. doi: 10.1016/j.psyneuen.2008.03.012

Eades LE, Thiagarajah AS, Harris J, Jones SA, Morand EF, Leech M. GILZ: A New Link Between the Hypothalamic Pituitary Adrenal Axis and Rheumatoid Arthritis? *Immunol Cell Biol* (2014) 92:747–51. doi: 10.1038/icb.2014.56

Permissions

All chapters in this book were first published by Frontiers; hereby published with permission under the Creative Commons Attribution License or equivalent. Every chapter published in this book has been scrutinized by our experts. Their significance has been extensively debated. The topics covered herein carry significant findings which will fuel the growth of the discipline. They may even be implemented as practical applications or may be referred to as a beginning point for another development.

The contributors of this book come from diverse backgrounds, making this book a truly international effort. This book will bring forth new frontiers with its revolutionizing research information and detailed analysis of the nascent developments around the world.

We would like to thank all the contributing authors for lending their expertise to make the book truly unique. They have played a crucial role in the development of this book. Without their invaluable contributions this book wouldn't have been possible. They have made vital efforts to compile up to date information on the varied aspects of this subject to make this book a valuable addition to the collection of many professionals and students.

This book was conceptualized with the vision of imparting up-to-date information and advanced data in this field. To ensure the same, a matchless editorial board was set up. Every individual on the board went through rigorous rounds of assessment to prove their worth. After which they invested a large part of their time researching and compiling the most relevant data for our readers.

The editorial board has been involved in producing this book since its inception. They have spent rigorous hours researching and exploring the diverse topics which have resulted in the successful publishing of this book. They have passed on their knowledge of decades through this book. To expedite this challenging task, the publisher supported the team at every step. A small team of assistant editors was also appointed to further simplify the editing procedure and attain best results for the readers.

Apart from the editorial board, the designing team has also invested a significant amount of their time in understanding the subject and creating the most relevant covers. They scrutinized every image to scout for the most suitable representation of the subject and create an appropriate cover for the book.

The publishing team has been an ardent support to the editorial, designing and production team. Their endless efforts to recruit the best for this project, has resulted in the accomplishment of this book. They are a veteran in the field of academics and their pool of knowledge is as vast as their experience in printing. Their expertise and guidance has proved useful at every step. Their uncompromising quality standards have made this book an exceptional effort. Their encouragement from time to time has been an inspiration for everyone.

The publisher and the editorial board hope that this book will prove to be a valuable piece of knowledge for researchers, students, practitioners and scholars across the globe.

List of Contributors

Tea Lanišnik Rižner
Institute of Biochemistry, Faculty of Medicine, University of Ljubljana, Ljubljana, Slovenia

Theresia Thalhammer
Department of Pathophysiology and Allergy Research, Centre for Pathophysiology, Infectiology and Immunology, Medical University of Vienna, Vienna, Austria

Csilla Özvegy-Laczka
Momentum Membrane Protein Research Group, Research Centre for Natural Sciences, Institute of Enzymology, Hungarian Academy of Sciences, Budapest, Hungary

Isabella Ellinger
Pathophysiology of the Placenta, Department of Pathophysiology and Allergy Research, Center for Pathophysiology, Infectiology and Immunology, Medical University of Vienna, Vienna, Austria

Waranya Chatuphonprasert
Pathophysiology of the Placenta, Department of Pathophysiology and Allergy Research, Center for Pathophysiology, Infectiology and Immunology, Medical University of Vienna, Vienna, Austria
Faculty of Medicine, Mahasarakham University, Maha Sarakham, Thailand

Kanokwan Jarukamjorn
Research Group for Pharmaceutical Activities of Natural Products Using Pharmaceutical Biotechnology (PANPB), Faculty of Pharmaceutical Sciences, Khon Kaen University, Khon Kaen, Thailand

Maša Sinreih, Tamara Kni ic, Maja Anko, Neli Hevir and Katja Vouk
Institute of Biochemistry, Faculty of Medicine, University of Ljubljana, Ljubljana, Slovenia

Aleš Jerin
Institute of Clinical Chemistry and Biochemistry, University Medical Centre, Ljubljana, Slovenia

Snježana Frković Grazio
Division of Obstetrics and Gynecology, Department of Pathology, University Medical Centre, Ljubljana, Slovenia

Martin Svoboda, Felicitas Mungenast, Theresia Thalhammer and Diana Mechtcheriakova
Department of Pathophysiology and Allergy Research, Center for Pathophysiology, Infectiology and Immunology, Medical University of Vienna, Vienna, Austria

Andreas Gleiss
Institute of Clinical Biometrics, Center for Medical Statistics, Informatics, and Intelligent Systems, Medical University of Vienna, Vienna, Austria

Ignace Vergote and Adriaan Vanderstichele
Division of Gynaecological Oncology, Department of Gynaecology and Obstetrics, Leuven Cancer Institute, University Hospital Leuven, Katholieke Universiteit Leuven, Leuven, Belgium

Jalid Sehouli and Elena Braicu
Department of Gynecology, Charité – Universitätsmedizin Berlin, Corporate Member of Freie Universität Berlin, Berlin Institute of Health, Humboldt-Universität zu Berlin, Berlin, Germany

Sven Mahner
Department of Gynecology, University Medical Center Hamburg-Eppendorf, Hamburg, Germany

Walter Jäger
Department of Clinical Pharmacy and Diagnostics, University of Vienna, Vienna, Austria

Dan Cacsire-Tong
Translational Gynecology Group, Department of Obstetrics and Gynaecology, Comprehensive Cancer Center, Medical University of Vienna, Vienna, Austria

Robert Zeillinger
Molecular Oncology Group, Department of Obstetrics and Gynaecology, Comprehensive Cancer Center, Medical University of Vienna, Vienna, Austria

Dietmar Pils
Institute of Clinical Biometrics, Center for Medical Statistics, Informatics, and Intelligent Systems, Medical University of Vienna, Vienna, Austria
Department of Surgery, Medical University of Vienna, Vienna, Austria

Markus Grube, Paul Hagen and Gabriele Jedlitschky
Department of Pharmacology, Center of Drug Absorption and Transport, University Medicine Greifswald, Greifswald, Germany

Alexander M. Scherbakov, Margarita A. Yastrebova and Olga E. Andreeva
Department of Experimental Tumor Biology, N.N. Blokhin National Medical Research Center of Oncology, Moscow, Russia

Alexander V. Komkov, Anna S. Komendantova, Valerii Z. Shirinian, Igor V. Zavarzin and Yulia A. Volkova
N.D. Zelinsky Institute of Organic Chemistry, Russian Academy of Sciences, Moscow, Russia

Alakananda Hajra
Department of Chemistry, Visva-Bharati University, Santiniketan, India

Gonda Konings, Linda Brentjens, Bert Delvoux, Marlies Bongers, Karlijn Cornel, Roy Kruitwagen, Sofia Xanthoulea and Andrea Romano
GROW-School for Oncology and Developmental Biology, Maastricht University, Maastricht, Netherlands, Department of Obstetrics and Gynaecology, Maastricht University Medical Centre, Maastricht, Netherlands

Tero Linnanen and Pasi Koskimies
Forendo Pharma Ltd., Turku, Finland

András Gyovai and Renáta Minorics
Department of Pharmacodynamics and Biopharmacy, University of Szeged, Szeged, Hungary

Anita Kiss, Erzsébet Mernyák and Gyula Schneider
Department of Organic Chemistry, University of Szeged, Szeged, Hungary

András Szekeres and Erika Kerekes
Department of Microbiology, University of Szeged, Szeged, Hungary

Imre Ocsovszki
Department of Biochemistry, University of Szeged, Szeged, Hungary

István Zupkó
Department of Pharmacodynamics and Biopharmacy, University of Szeged, Szeged, Hungary, Interdisciplinary Centre for Natural Products, University of Szeged, Szeged, Hungary

Emre Karakus, Daniel Zahner, Gary Grosser, Regina Leidolf and Joachim Geyer
Institute of Pharmacology and Toxicology, Faculty of Veterinary Medicine, Justus Liebig University Giessen, Giessen, Germany

Cemal Gundogdu
Department of Pathology, Private Practitioner of Medicine, Erzurum, Turkey

Alberto Sánchez-Guijo and Stefan A. Wudy
Steroid Research and Mass Spectrometry Unit, Pediatric Endocrinology and Diabetology, Center of Child and Adolescent Medicine, Justus Liebig University Giessen, Giessen, Germany

Stefan Poschner, Alexandra Maier-Salamon, Bettina Pachmann and Konstantin L. Sterlini
Division of Clinical Pharmacy and Diagnostics, Department of Pharmaceutical Chemistry, University of Vienna, Vienna, Austria

Martin Zehl
Department of Analytical Chemistry, Faculty of Chemistry, University of Vienna, Vienna, Austria

Judith Wackerlig and Daniel Dobusch
Division of Drug Design and Medicinal Chemistry, Department of Pharmaceutical Chemistry, University of Vienna, Vienna, Austria

Walter Jäger
Division of Clinical Pharmacy and Diagnostics, Department of Pharmaceutical Chemistry, University of Vienna, Vienna, Austria
Vienna Metabolomics Center (VIME), University of Vienna, Vienna, Austria

Lorna C. Gilligan, Ali Gondal, Vivien Tang, Maryam T. Hussain, Anastasia Arvaniti and Anne-Marie Hewitt
Institute of Metabolism and Systems Research, Centre for Endocrinology, Diabetes, and Metabolism, University of Birmingham, Birmingham, UK

Paul A. Foster
Institute of Metabolism and Systems Research, Centre for Endocrinology, Diabetes, and Metabolism, University of Birmingham, Birmingham, UK
Centre for Endocrinology, Diabetes, and Metabolism, Birmingham Health Partners, Birmingham, UK

Erika Bandini, Francesca Fanini, Ivan Vannini, Tania Rossi, Francesco Fabbri, Meropi Plousiou and Maria Maddalena Tumedei
Biosciences Laboratory, Istituto Scientifico Romagnolo per lo Studio e la Cura dei Tumori (IRST) IRCCS, Meldola, Italy

Francesco Limarzi and Roberta Maltoni
Istituto Scientifico Romagnolo per lo Studio e la Cura dei Tumori (IRST) IRCCS, Meldola, Italy

Silvana Hrelia
Department for Life Quality Studies, Alma Mater Studiorum - University of Bologna, Rimini, Italy

William C. S. Cho
Department of Clinical Oncology, Queen Elizabeth Hospital, Kowloon, Hong Kong

Muller Fabbri
Cancer Biology Program, University of Hawai'i Cancer Center, Hawaii, HI, United States

Stefano Bruscoli, Marta Febo, Carlo Riccardi and Graziella Migliorati
Section of Pharmacology, Department of Medicine and Surgery, University of Perugia, Perugia, Italy

Index

www.ingramcontent.com/pod-product-compliance
Lightning Source LLC
LaVergne TN
LVHW082217200926
848484LV00008B/2267